Promoting Patient Engagement and Participation for Effective Healthcare Reform

Guendalina Graffigna
Catholic University of the Sacred Heart of Milan, Italy

A volume in the Advances in Medical Diagnosis, Treatment, and Care (AMDTC) Book Series

Medical Information Science Reference
An Imprint of IGI Global

Published in the United States of America by
Medical Information Science Reference (an imprint of IGI Global)
701 E. Chocolate Avenue
Hershey PA, USA 17033
Tel: 717-533-8845
Fax: 717-533-8661
E-mail: cust@igi-global.com
Web site: http://www.igi-global.com

Library of Congress Cataloging-in-Publication Data

Names: Graffigna, Guendalina, 1979- editor.
Title: Promoting patient engagement and participation for effective healthcare reform / Guendalina Graffigna, editor.
Description: Hershey, PA : Medical Information Science Reference, [2016] | Includes bibliographical references and index.
Identifiers: LCCN 2016000391| ISBN 9781466699922 (hardcover) | ISBN 9781466699939 (ebook)
Subjects: LCSH: Patient participation. | Health promotion. | Health care reform.
Classification: LCC R727.42 .P76 2016 | DDC 362.1--dc23 LC record available at http://lccn.loc.gov/2016000391

This book is published in the IGI Global book series Advances in Medical Diagnosis, Treatment, and Care (AMDTC) (ISSN: Pending; eISSN: Pending)

British Cataloguing in Publication Data
A Cataloguing in Publication record for this book is available from the British Library.

All work contributed to this book is new, previously-unpublished material. The views expressed in this book are those of the authors, but not necessarily of the publisher.

For electronic access to this publication, please contact: eresources@igi-global.com.

Advances in Medical Diagnosis, Treatment, and Care (AMDTC) Book Series

ISSN: Pending
EISSN: Pending

Mission

Advancements in medicine have prolonged the life expectancy of individuals all over the world. Once life-threatening conditions have become significantly easier to treat and even cure in many cases. Continued research in the medical field will further improve the quality of life, longevity, and wellbeing of individuals.

The **Advances in Medical Diagnosis, Treatment, and Care (AMDTC)** book series seeks to highlight publications on innovative treatment methodologies, diagnosis tools and techniques, and best practices for patient care. Comprised of comprehensive resources aimed to assist professionals in the medical field apply the latest innovations in the identification and management of medical conditions as well as patient care and interaction, the books within the AMDTC series are relevant to the research and practical needs of medical practitioners, researchers, students, and hospital administrators.

Coverage

- Emergency Medicine
- Disease Management
- Chronic Conditions
- Critical Care
- Medical Procedures
- Experimental Medicine
- Patient Interaction
- Alternative Medicine
- Disease Prevention
- Cancer Treatment

IGI Global is currently accepting manuscripts for publication within this series. To submit a proposal for a volume in this series, please contact our Acquisition Editors at Acquisitions@igi-global.com or visit: http://www.igi-global.com/publish/.

The Advances in Medical Diagnosis, Treatment, and Care (AMDTC) Book Series (ISSN Pending) is published by IGI Global, 701 E. Chocolate Avenue, Hershey, PA 17033-1240, USA, www.igi-global.com. This series is composed of titles available for purchase individually; each title is edited to be contextually exclusive from any other title within the series. For pricing and ordering information please visit http://www.igi-global.com/book-series/advances-medical-diagnosis-treatment-care/129618. Postmaster: Send all address changes to above address.

Titles in this Series

For a list of additional titles in this series, please visit: www.igi-global.com

Effective Methods for Modern Healthcare Service Quality and Evaluation
Panagiotis Manolitzas (Technical University of Crete, Greece) Evangelos Grigoroudis (Technical University of Crete, Greece) Nikolaos Matsatsinis (Technical University of Crete, Greece) and Denis Yannacopoulos (Piraeus University of Applied Sciences, Greece)
Medical Information Science Reference • copyright 2016 • 315pp • H/C (ISBN: 9781466699618) • US $190.00 (our price)

Handbook of Research on Trends in the Diagnosis and Treatment of Chronic Conditions
Dimitrios I. Fotiadis (University of Ioannina, Greece)
Medical Information Science Reference • copyright 2016 • 659pp • H/C (ISBN: 9781466688285) • US $385.00 (our price)

Table of Contents

Detailed Table of Contents

Section 2
Individual, Relational, and Social Barriers and Facilitators of Patient Engagement

The primary purpose of this chapter is to determine factors that shape client dropout and adherence to Cardiac Disease Prevention and Rehabilitation Programs. The sample consists of 68 individuals, including those currently in the program (adherents) and those who have dropped out (dropouts). Findings show that clients undergoing rehabilitation are much likely to drop out when they are in the critical zone. This is a point where institutional factors, individual factors and environmentally-related factors are not favorable to clients. The risk of clients dropping out can be drastically reduced through the provision of an enabling environment comprising a set of factors that foster adherence such as financial sponsorship, institutional support, high intrinsic motivation, improved illness perception. In that context, there is the need for program administrators to closely monitor at-risk clients, especially those whose social, economic and psychological profiles predict non-adherence.

Non-adherence to health recommendations (e.g. medical prescriptions) presents potential costs for healthcare, which could be prevented or mitigated. This is often attributed to a person's rational choice, to not adhere. However, this may also be determined by individual and contextual factors implied in the recommendations communication process. In accordance, this chapter focuses specifically on barriers to and facilitators of adherence to recommendations and engagement with the healthcare process, particularly concerning the communication between health professionals and patients. For this, the authors present examples of engagement increment through different degrees of participation, from a one-way/directive towards a two-way/engaging communication process. This focuses specifically on a vulnerable population group with increasing healthcare needs: older adults. Future possibilities for two-way engaging communications are discussed, aimed at promoting increased adherence to health recommendations and people's self-regulation of their own health.

Research on the engagement of patients and their partners and the literature on couple relationships have remained surprisingly separated. In response to this gap, the first aim of the chapter is to show the advantages of an integration of these two lines of research in the context of promoting engagement in patients and their partners. Particular attention is devoted to couples' stress and coping literature and to those few studies that investigated the role played for patient engagement by characteristics of patients, partners, and their relationship. Couple-based research can inform engagement literature about facilitators and barriers to couples' coping with illness and about how to promote engagement in the context of the couple. Within this research, the concept of dyadic coping can be especially helpful in understanding how partners can effectively deal with the stress related to acute and chronic illness as well as the barriers to this process. A second aim of the chapter is to connect the suggestions from couple-based research with the field of engagement promotion.

Preterm infants need long-lasting hospitalization in the Neonatal Intensive Care Unit (NICU). On the one hand, the NICU stay constitutes an early adverse experience, due to highly stressful experiences. On the other hand, Developmental Care (DC) interventions, including caregiver engagement, can exert neuro-protective effects for preterm infants. Recent evidence in the field of behavioral epigenetics is revealing the biochemical pathways through which adverse and care experiences are embedded in early human development through epigenetic mechanisms. Nonetheless, the application of behavioral epigenetics to preterm birth and NICU stay is still at its beginning. In the present chapter, insights are provided for the application of behavioral epigenetics to the study of the biochemical underpinnings of NICU-related stress and care, with a specific focus on caregiver engagement. This contribute should be intended as a preliminary roadmap to guide future behavioral epigenetic research on the adverse and protective effects of early NICU care of preterm infants.

Despite the relevance of the topic, an exhaustive psychosocial reflection on the processes that may facilitate patients' protest is still missing. The chapter provides a theoretical and empirical overview of psychosocial pathways for patients' collective action. Five core factors are reviewed: perceived injustice, group efficacy, group identification, moral convictions and social embeddedness. Each of them provides a different explanation of collective action processes and is examined for its potential impact among patients. The chapter closes suggesting some core elements for a theoretical explanation of patients' collective action and its relationship with patient engagement. Practical and theoretical implications of patients' collective action are discussed to identify new directions for future research and interventions.

The concepts of patient-centered care and patient engagement are often used interchangeably in health policy debates. In fact, it is frequently – and implicitly – assumed that putting patients at the centre of care will more or less spontaneously lead to fully engaged patients. This chapter questions these assumptions. By focusing on the hospital's patient-centered reform in Italy, the chapter discusses the overlaps but also the discrepancies between the practices of putting patients at the centre and those of engaging patients. Discrepancies may appear at three levels: the new hospital model may challenge the establishment of a close alliance between patients and professionals, the new hospital spaces may not be perceived as a catalyst for improving patients' experiences, and the inter- and intra- professional struggles derived from the new configuration of hospital teams at an early stage may hinder patient care delivery. The chapter proposes some strategies for patient-centered hospitals to increase their capacity to engage patients and families in the management of their care plan.

The chapter investigates the dynamic of encounters between staff and patients in two case studies on hospital organisation, taking special account of the emotional and psychological aspects associated with practices in the use of organisational space. By drawing on two empirical cases set in different hospital contexts (the waiting rooms of two outpatients wards and an emergency unit), analysis is made of two examples of practices which represent express violations of the rules on the use of space by patients and their relatives. Violations that could be analysed as demand of engagement - by patients and relatives - in the process of care. In these empirical cases the governance defensive reaction strategies used by hospital staff in their interaction with waiting patients is shown in light of the rules that define the behaviour acceptable for patients and relatives. The study is based on a qualitative methodological approach using the techniques of observation and in-depth interviews with hospital staff, patients and relatives.

The concept of patient engagement offers a unique opportunity to inform our understanding of patients' ability to be active in managing their care. However, unless promoting the active role of patients is

Dramatic changes in the age structure of the population have led to a rise in the age of retirement. An ageing working population may be a problem for companies and for their health and safety services that must face the long-term management of active, chronically ill workers. For sustainability reasons the discipline of occupational medicine must be replaced by occupational health, which not only combats occupational diseases, but actively works to promote the health of older workers. More in general, occupational health has a strong interest in promoting engagement in professional activities. Shifting from a reactive to a proactive logic will take time and require a big effort on the part of employers, employees and health and safety staff in order to develop participatory ergonomics and best health promotion practices in the workplace.

Foreword

Promoting patients' participation and engagement for a more and more effective, efficient and sustainable healthcare offer.

This goal is crucial from various perspectives and it's also attracting the interest of several healthcare professionals and political-economical decision makers who are in charge in welfare systems. The interest of scientific research is growing as well, challenged by an issue, which is certainly socially relevant, but still needs roots both at the theoretical and empirical level.

The research program Horizon 2020, recently launched by the European Commission, is a good example – surely not the only one – of this trend: the section of this program dedicated to the societal challenges frames health as the main committing topic at the European level and claims for the activations of research guidelines oriented towards an integrated and sustainable and citizen-centered care and to the active participation of people in health promotion, prevention and care, even with the aid of new technologies.

With the contribute of a conspicuous number of experts from different scientific fields, the book deals with this task in a straightforward way, by achieving a double result: a) setting the current "state of the art"; b) suggesting future lines for research aimed at developing the topic both at the theoretical and pragmatic level.

I will let the Reader deepen the book's content. Here I would just suggest some considerations which may help in better linking its various contributes with each other, within a dynamic retrospective and prospective vision.

1. The research on Patients' Engagement and Participation in Health (PEPH) appears the outcome of a path started long time ago and reached today this theoretical and pragmatic elaboration. Its beginnings may be retrieved in the paradigmatic turn promoted by Engel at the end of the '70 with the proposal of a bio-psycho-social approach in healthcare, in substitution of the dominant medical model previously elaborated by Parsons. From this new approach and on the basis of the numerous drivers of change (i.e. cultural, organizational, political…) that were actual in occidental societies, in the 80' and 90' many considerations started to be made in order to innovate the healthcare vision from both a theoretical and a pragmatic point of view.
   On the one hand, the humanization movement in medicine developed the topic at the level of values (ethical and political) by refusing the simplified representation of patients as passive receivers of medical action and claiming for them a more active and participative role in the management of health (e.g. the elaboration of patients' rights cards, the informed consent practice, the evaluation and measurement of patients' satisfaction…).
   On the other hand, studies on the effectiveness of medical practices led to recognize the patient's role as a determinant of medicine's success. By furthering the analysis of the conditions for patients'

compliance and adherence to care, the patient-centered approach to medicine (able to acknowledge and value the patient's role) was asserted as the necessary condition to assure the effectiveness of the medical actions.

Finally, the encounter between a managerial culture – coming from the business field – and the welfare systems highlighted that the efficiency of such systems should be a priority issue. Answering uniquely in medical terms to the increasing and various needs of healthcare appears impossible; the activation of patients and of their social networks is a precious resource in order to maintain a balanced relationship between healthcare demand and offer and also in order to promote healthcare sustainability.

These three pathways can be easily considered as the historical roots of PEPH. Indeed, from the early 2000's, the PEPH perspective has progressively asserted itself as an approach that may offer an integrated and coherent answer to the needs of healthcare humanization, effectiveness in prevention/promotion/care, sustainability and efficiency of healthcare systems.

2. During the last two decades much has been done. Nonetheless, much still needs to be done. We may consider PEPH as a research agenda that is today testing its own ability to generate good research and good practices. Which conditions might better sustain the virtuous development of this research agenda? The necessity to overcome the partiality of previous approaches and to deal with the complexity and multiple facets of the phenomenon suggests two prior advices for future research on PEPH.

   First, a stronger link among different scientific disciplines involved in the study on PEPH (i.e. theoretical and empirical disciplines, life and human: philosophy, medicine, psychology, sociology, technological sciences, linguistics, economics, communication sciences, management and organization sciences …) is required. Certainly, this is not an easy goal to be achieved! In other words, a transdisciplinary perspective is warranted to embrace a "messy" comparative mode (i.e. not linear, hybrid, reflexive, heterogeneous…) based on the principle of "transformative contamination" (crossbreeding) among various scientific disciplines.

   Second, it is crucial to promote a more interactive dialogue among the various actors involved in the management of this topic. Both the field of scientific research and the "extra-scientific" fields (i.e. politics, business, public opinion) can fully contribute to orient the realization of PEPH in the social contexts. The "extra-scientific" fields are indeed not only destined to receive the operative outcomes of scientific research, but they also orient such research in terms of thematic priorities and development. From this perspective, it should be underlined that concepts such as *trans-sectoriality* and *co-authorship* are more and more adopted in the literature in order to highlight the deep and generative link between science and social worlds.

In sum, *trans-disciplinarity* and *trans-sectoriality* appear to be two crucial challenges which the research on PEPH is asked to face in order to avoid the risk of being a mere suggestive and fascinating (maybe mainstream and fashionable) topic, with a poor scientific and pragmatic impact. These two challenges have been clearly dealt with in the development of this volume and they are well represented by the thematic variety of the diverse contributes.

Procedamus igitur!

A. Claudio Bosio
Catholic University of the Sacred Heart of Milan, Italy

Preface

THE 21st CENTURY HEALTHCARE CHALLENGES

The ageing population, the rise of chronic conditions and the decrease of economic resources, directly or indirectly impact on healthcare systems.

Healthcare organizations, in the era of "chronicity," are particularly concerned with the long-term management of patients, especially the elderly ones. While the management of acute conditions is primarily restricted within the traditional hospital or clinic setting for short periods of time, chronic conditions need long-term and integrated approach to care, which implies an enhanced dialogue with the territory, both at the level of formal and unformal care (Graffigna, Barello & Triberti, 2015).

More and more social relationships and peer exchanges that happen in the lay community, indeed, play a crucial role in the healthcare process and may constitute a potential resource to improve the effectiveness and the efficiency of healthcare systems. Peers influence patients' knowledge about health and illness, contribute to shape shared practices of health management, and influence good or bad health conduct. Peers are also a source of pragmatic and emotional support for patients.

Furthermore, the last century Technological Revolution deeply impacted on healthcare systems and on the processes of delivering care. The advent of new technologies, in particular, enabled new processes of knowledge construction and exchange in the general democratization of information fluxes (Deluca & Enmark, 1999; Livingstone, 2004, Riva et al., 2012). This continuous development of technological and bio-medical solutions are not only increasing patients networks and improving doctor-patients communication: they are also alimenting the expectation for longer life expectancy and for a good quality of this renewed time of life (Diener et al., 1999).

Due to the evolution of socio-cultural health values and to the promise of new medical and technological discoveries, today people expect to be in good health and active for a longer period of time. Furthermore, people assess their quality of life not only in term of absence of disease and symptoms, but also in terms of good performance and ability to maintain their work activities for a longer period of time, a private satisfactory life, and active roles in their communities (Barello & Graffigna, 2015). In this light, patients expect that healthcare services not only are able to treat their disease in its symptomatic manifestations, but that they also guarantee the maintenance of a satisfactory private life and the possibility of being positively included in their community, despite the occurrence of a chronic condition (Haber, 2013).

Finally, today's patients are more aware of their rights as consumers and more literate about their health conditions and available treatment options. They require to be higher involved in the decision making about their care and are willing to deeply entangle all the possible treatment options, their advantages, and their risks (Coulter, 2011).

Healthcare systems, thus, today have to face increased healthcare needs and demand but in a scope of limited economic and human resources. In other terms, healthcare systems are today required "to do more with less" to successfully face their clients' needs and expectations and to be economically sustainable. This implies the urgency for a deep revision of healthcare systems' practices and organizational models in order to become better responsive to the present challenges highlighted above (Gorli et al, 2015). In the long run, the survival of the national health systems will depend on the extent to which this goal will be achieved (Baran, Kiani & Samuel, 2014).

PARTICIPATIVE MEDICINE AND PATIENT ENGAGEMENT: A POSSIBLE SOLUTION

Patient participation and engagement in healthcare management is today acknowledged by policy makers and healthcare experts as a valuable option to orient changes and actions of the healthcare systems. Several empirical studies have demonstrated the positive outcomes of a participatory care approach at the clinical, psychosocial, and economic levels (Osborn & Squires, 2012). The participatory medicine approach has given prominence to the patient role in the management of his/her health and have connoted this role with many different terminologies such as "patient participation", "patient activation", "patient empowerment", "patient involvement". It is notable that, in more recent years, both academic and grey literature have increasingly adopted the term "patient engagement" to indicate the active role of individuals in their healthcare (Barello, Graffigna & Vegni, 2012; Menichetti et al., 2015). The adoption of the term *engagement* in the healthcare field indicates a renewed partnership between the different actors and institutions (more often a patient and his/her healthcare provider) implied in the health and care management. Patient engagement is related to better quality of care and patient/health provider relationship, thus improving a patient's clinical indicators and compliance to recommended therapeutic regimens (Green & Hibbard, 2012). Making people aware of their health service options by supporting them in the decision-making process and engaging them in preventive health behaviors is vital to achieve successful health outcomes (Bellardita et al., 2012). Favoring a good psychological and emotional tenure will foster a self-image as active and may improve an internal locus of control over disease, by improving disease prevention and healthy behaviors (Cosgrove et al., 2013). Thus, patient engagement may not only contribute to the reduction of direct costs of the healthcare system, but it also can concur with the (re)orientation of economic resources in the management of healthcare systems to reduce waste of money (Hibbard et al., 2013).

PROMOTING PATIENTS PARTICIPATION AND ENGAGEMENT IN HEALTHCARE: RESEARCH AGENDA

However, many gaps still exist for the implementation of a truly participative medicine able to engage patients and their families in the care management, starting from the lack of a shared definition and of shared guidelines for medical practice. First, the meaning of "patient engagement" is not clear and a shared and a univocal and holistic explanations of patient engagement is still missed in the literature. Carman and colleagues (2013) define patient engagement as *a set of behaviors by patients, family members, and health professionals and a set of organizational policies and procedures that foster both the inclusion of patients and family members as active members of the health care team and collaborative partnerships with providers and provider organizations with the desired goals of patient and family engagement include improving the quality and safety of health care.* Other scholars define patient engagement in terms of level of "activation", by describing an engaged patient as *an active agent in the management of his/her own health* including developmental stages *of 1) believing the patient role is important, 2) having the confidence and knowledge necessary to take action, 3) actually taking action to maintain and improve one's health and 4) staying the course even under stress* (Hibbard et al, 2009). Furthermore, Gruman and colleagues' patient engagement behavioral framework (2010) defines patient engagement as a *set of behaviors including two overarching domains: (1) "managing health" behaviors, which is both the self-management of chronic disease and the adoption of healthy behaviors, and (2) "managing healthcare" behaviors, which can be both patient and "consumeristic" behaviors.* Finally Graffigna et al. (2014) offers a psycho-social perspective on patient engagement and define it as a *process-like and multi-dimensional experience, resulting from the conjoint cognitive (think), emotional (feel) and conative (act) enactment of individuals towards their health management. In this process patients go through four subsequent positions (blackout, arousal, adhesion and eudaimonic project).*

However, patients' and healthcare professionals' perspectives about the factors that may sustain or hinder patient engagement have not being sufficiently studied yet. Scientific research in this complex area is still at its beginning and the facilitators and barriers for patient engagement need to be further addressed for finding optimal ways of improving these aspects: currently, there are no clear recommendations on the interventions best effective or which may work best with the various patient populations. Future evidences are needed to orient future education and training of healthcare providers in order to make patient engagement not only an "holy grail" but a concrete guidance for practice.

THE AIMS AND THE STRUCTURE OF THIS BOOK

The broadness of the phenomenon of patient participation and engagement in healthcare is such that only a multi-disciplinary approach can investigate its manifold aspects. Furthermore, the high social expectations placed in additional scientific research in this field require that patient engagement scholars become able to establish linkage between the production of scientific knowledge and its application in the real context of healthcare practices. Favoring the encounter between science and its applications is an increasingly crucial task for healthcare academics and practitioners devoted to the establishment of a really participative medicine.

This book aims to be a first contribution in this direction, by offering some insights both towards the theoretical foundation of the patient engagement concept and for the planning of strategies aimed at sustaining it in healthcare settings.

In order to achieve these ambitious goals, the chapters hosted in the book are authored by healthcare scholars and professionals from around the World and belonging to different disciplines. This editorial project, indeed, was conceived as the occasion to promote a participative "bottom up" process in which different experts may contribute to the development of theory and practices of patient engagement from their different stand-points. The inevitable difficulty related to the effort of putting in dialogue so many different cultural instances and disciplinary domains is - in our opinion - "repaid" by the achievement of a multifaceted discussion of the several crucial aspects implied in the promotion of patient participation and engagement and of their implications for effective healthcare reform.

In order to facilitate the Reader, the book is structured in 3 thematic sections which organize the chapters on the basis of their main thematic focus.

The first section ("Theoretical perspectives") is devoted to epistemologically set the ground to the following discussions about patients participation and engagement and it proposes some paradigmatic, theoretical and ethical insights for modern healthcare reform.

In particular, Chapter 1, "Habilitation, Healthy Agency, and Patient-Participation" by Lawrence C. Becker offers a philosophical discussion of the ethical principles behind health, healing, agency and participation in healthcare. This chapter critically point at some "given for granted" assumptions of modern medicine and discusses the "light" and the "dark side" of current claims for patients' engagement and participation. This depth elucidation offers important theoretical and philosophical insights to open the discussion about patients participation and engagement.

Follows in this section Chapter 2, "The patient-centered medicine as the theoretical framework for patient engagement" by Lidia Borghi, Federica Galli, Elena Anna Maria Vegni, which offers an historical excursus about the main paradigmatic shifts that occurred in medical models in order to describe the theoretical roots of the current participative medicine and patient engagement movement. Moreover, the authors discuss theoretical and empirical implications of patient engagement for a patient centered medicine.

The second section of the book ("Individual, relational and social barriers and facilitators of patients participation and engagement") hosts some theoretical and empirical contributions about the factors that may sustain of hinder patients engagement and participation.

Chapter 3, "Individual, Institutional and Environmental Factors Promoting Patient Retention and Dropout" by Precious Arnan and Emmanuel Adugu, reports evidences from an empirical study devoted to determine factors that shape client dropout and adherence to prevention and rehabilitation in the area of cardiovascular diseases. On the basis of their research work, these authors suggest important implications for practice.

Chapter 4, "Barriers to and Facilitators of Older Adult's Adherence to Health Recommendations Towards an EngAging Two-way Health Communication" by Rui Gaspar, Samuel Domingos, António Diniz and Roberto Falanga, addresses the factors that may hinder or facilitate the adherence to health and care management of a particularly challenging patients population: older adults. The increasing of ageing and the high recurrence of chronical conditions in this target of the population is making particularly urgent the analysis of specific requirements and needs of engagement of these patients. The chapter, moving from a broad analysis of current literature in this field, offers an interesting systematization of barriers and facilitators related to older patients' adherence to health recommendations and set some concrete implications for practice.

Chapter 5, "A Relational Perspective on Patient Engagement: Suggestions from Couple-Based Research and Intervention" by Silvia Donato and Anna Bertoni, highlights the importance of taking care of the unformal caregivers of patients - and in particular of partners - along the participation and engagement process in healthcare. Chronic patients are often not alone during their care pathway. The role of patients' partners in the daily management of care or during encounters with the healthcare providers is extremely crucial: patients often relay on their partners to better adhere to health prescriptions, to decode medical communication, to successfully cope with the daily requirement of their healthcare. However often the debate about patient engagement has neglected the study of caregivers' needs and expectations of engagement. This chapter summarizes the main evidences of the literature on couple relationship and bridges them with the debate about patients engagement and participation in order to cast light on promising new lines of research and interventions.

Chapter 6, "The Light Side of Preterm Behavioral Epigenetics: An Epigenetic Perspective on Caregiver Engagement" by Livio Provenzi, Renato Borgatti and Rosario Montirosso, suggests the application of behavioral epigenetics to the study of the biochemical underpinnings of Neonatal Intensive Care Unit (NICU) related stress and care, with a specific focus on caregiver engagement. The authors suggest how interventions aimed to foster the engagement in healthcare of caregivers of preterm infants may have a beneficial clinical impact, also at the biochemical level. This contribute, by critically discussing recent literature in the field, offers a preliminary roadmap to guide future behavioral epigenetic research on the adverse and protective effects of early NICU care of preterm infants based on caregiver engagement.

Chapter 7, "Why do Patients Protest? Collective Action Processes in People with Chronic Illnesses: a Psychosocial Perspective" by Davide Mazzoni and Augusta Isabella Alberici, adopts a social psychology perspective to analyze the individual and interpersonal roots of patients' collective action and its relationship with patient engagement. The authors argument how patients' protests and critical actions may be considered as the other side of their active participation in healthcare. Practical and theoretical implications of patients' collective action are discussed to identify new directions for future research and interventions.

The last section of the book ("Reforming healthcare organizations and practices in the light of patients participation and engagement") adopts an organizational perspective in analyzing the implications or the potential levers for promoting patients participation and engagement in care management.

Chapter 8, "The patient centered organizational model in Italian hospitals: practical challenges for patient engagement" by Mara Gorli, Elisa G. Liberati, Laura Galuppo and Giuseppe Scaratti, questions the assumption that adopting a patient centered model of care in managing an hospital may directly lead to an improvement of patient engagement. By constructing on the analysis of real cases, the authors point at the contradictions, gaps, hindrances and resistances that may result in an healthcare organization when trying to reform their practices in the light of patient centered medicine and patient engagement.

Chapter 9, "No Entry. Prohibitions and violations in organizational spaces across the patient-staff interface in hospital" by Livia Bruscaglioni, points at the problematic negotiation of spaces in healthcare organizations and discusses how this aspect may be the scenario of interesting (but often counterproductive) power dynamics among different healthcare professions and between experts and patients in the daily management of healthcare. The author, based on real cases of research, discusses how these processes may hinder patients participation and engagement in healthcare.

Chapter 10, "The value of measuring patient engagement in healthcare: new frontiers for healthcare quality" by Guendalina Graffigna and Serena Barello, points at the importance of adopting performance indicators to assess the level of engagement of patients in their healthcare. The adoption of validated scale to measure patient engagement is argued by the authors as the first crucial step to transform patient engagement from a mere claim to a real guidance for practice. The chapter reviews the characteristics and psychometrics properties of the main validated tools existing in scientific literature to measure the levels of engagement of patients and their needs and expectations in order to better manage their care.

Chapter 11, "Accountability and public reporting. Publication of performance to improve quality" by Maria Tanzariello, Sabina Bucci, Walter Ricciardi and Antonio Giulio de Belvis, discusses how accountability, transparency, and public reporting are some key factors in promoting patients participation and engagement in healthcare. In particular, public reporting is one of the major tools in supporting patients' decisions making process, by providing structure, process and outcome measures. The authors performed a web-based analysis of the major initiatives of public reporting in order to highlight their main characteristics and properties and to detect actual gaps and directions for improvement in the aim of enhancing patients participation and engagement in healthcare.

Chapter 12, "Could patient engagement promote a health system free from malpractice litigation risk?" by Massimo Miglioretti, Francesca Mariani, Luca Vecchio, suggests how patient engagement in healthcare may be addressed as a possible method for reducing the risks of doctors being sued for medical malpractice. The authors test their hypothesis in two recent studies, and, on the bases of their results, they argument that future initiatives to promote patient engagement may offer a support in this direction.

Chapter 13, "Engagement in Health and Safety at the Workplace: a new Role for the Occupational Health Physician" by Nicola Magnavita, elucidates how ageing working population may be a problem for companies and for their health and safety services that must face the long-term management of active, chronically ill workers. On the basis of these premises, the author discusses how the discipline of occupational medicine must be replaced by occupational health, which not only combats occupational diseases, but actively works to promote the engagement of older workers in health prevention and care management. New directions for research and practices in this field are highlighted in the chapter.

REFERENCES

Baran, G. R., Kiani, M. F., & Samuel, S. P. (2014). *Healthcare and biomedical technology in the 21st century*. Springer. doi:10.1007/978-1-4614-8541-4

Barello, S., & Graffigna, G. (2014). Engaging patients to recover life projectuality: An Italian cross-disease framework. *Quality of Life Research: An International Journal of Quality of Life Aspects of Treatment, Care and Rehabilitation*, 1–10. PMID:25373927

Barello, S., Graffigna, G., & Vegni, E. (2012). Patient engagement as an emerging challenge for healthcare services: Mapping the literature. *Nursing Research and Practice*, *2012*, 1–7. doi:10.1155/2012/905934 PMID:23213497

Bellardita, L., Graffigna, G., Donegani, S., Villani, D., Villa, S., Tresoldi, V., & Valdagni, R. (2012). Patient's choice of observational strategy for early-stage prostate cancer. *Neuropsychological Trends*, *12*, 107–116.

Carman, K. L., Dardess, P., Maurer, M., Sofaer, S., Adams, K., Bechtel, C., & Sweeney, J. (2013). Patient and family engagement: A framework for understanding the elements and developing interventions and policies. *Health Affairs*, *32*(2), 223–231. doi:10.1377/hlthaff.2012.1133 PMID:23381514

Cosgrove, D. M., Fisher, M., Gabow, P., Gottlieb, G., Halvorson, G. C., James, B. C., & Toussaint, J. S. (2013). Ten strategies to lower costs, improve quality, and engage patients: The view from leading health system CEOs. *Health Affairs*, *32*(2), 321–327. doi:10.1377/hlthaff.2012.1074 PMID:23381525

Coulter, A. (2011). *Engaging patients in healthcare*. UK: McGraw-Hill Education.

Deluca, J. M., & Enmark, R. (1999). E-health: The changing model of healthcare. *Frontiers of Health Services Management*, *17*(1), 3–15. PMID:11184427

Diener, E., Suh, E. M., Lucas, R. E., & Smith, H. L. (1999). Subjective well-being: Three decades of progress. *Psychological Bulletin*, *125*(2), 276–302. doi:10.1037/0033-2909.125.2.276

Gorli, M., Galuppo, L., & Liberati, E. G. (2015). Hospital innovations in the light of patient engagement: Insights from the organizational field. In *Patient engagement: A consumer-centered model to innovate healthcare*. Walter de Gruyter GmbH & Co KG. doi:10.1515/9783110452440-011

Graffigna, G., Barello, S., Riva, G., & Bosio, A. C. (2014). Patient engagement: The key to redesign the exchange between the demand and supply for healthcare in the era of active ageing. *Studies in Health Technology and Informatics*, (203): 85–95. PMID:26630515

Graffigna, G., Barello, S., & Triberti, S. (Eds.). (2015). *Patient engagement: A consumer-centered model to innovate healthcare*. Walter de Gruyter GmbH & Co KG. doi:10.1515/9783110452440

Greene, J., & Hibbard, J. H. (2012). Why does patient activation matter? An examination of the relationships between patient activation and health-related outcomes. *Journal of General Internal Medicine*, *27*(5), 520–526. doi:10.1007/s11606-011-1931-2 PMID:22127797

Gruman, J., Rovner, M. H., French, M. E., Jeffress, D., Sofaer, S., Shaller, D., & Prager, D. J. (2010). From patient education to patient engagement: Implications for the field of patient education. *Patient Education and Counseling*, *78*(3), 350–356. doi:10.1016/j.pec.2010.02.002 PMID:20202780

Haber, D. (2013). *Health promotion and aging: Practical applications for health professionals*. Springer Publishing Company.

Hibbard, J. H., Greene, J., & Overton, V. (2013). Patients with lower activation associated with higher costs; delivery systems should know their patients' 'scores'. *Health Affairs*, *32*(2), 216–222. doi:10.1377/hlthaff.2012.1064 PMID:23381513

Hibbard, J. H., Greene, J., & Tusler, M. (2009). Improving the outcomes of disease management by tailoring care to the patient's level of activation. *The American Journal of Managed Care*, *15*(6), 353–360. PMID:19514801

Livingstone, S. (2004). Media literacy and the challenge of new information and communication technologies. *Communication Review*, *7*(1), 3–14. doi:10.1080/10714420490280152

Menichetti, J., Libreri, C., Lozza, E., & Graffigna, G. (2014). Giving patients a starring role in their own care: A bibliometric analysis of the on-going literature debate. *Health Expectations*, n/a. doi:10.1111/hex.12299 PMID:25369557

Osborn, R., & Squires, D. (2012). International perspectives on patient engagement: Results from the 2011 Commonwealth Fund Survey. *The Journal of Ambulatory Care Management*, *35*(2), 118–128. doi:10.1097/JAC.0b013e31824a579b PMID:22415285

Riva, G., Banos, R. M., Botella, C., Wiederhold, B. K., & Gaggioli, A. (2012). Positive technology: Using interactive technologies to promote positive functioning. *Cyberpsychology, Behavior, and Social Networking*, *15*(2), 69–77. doi:10.1089/cyber.2011.0139 PMID:22149077

Section 1
Theoretical Assumptions

Chapter 1
Habilitation, Healthy Agency, and Patient-Participation

Lawrence C. Becker
Hollins University, USA

ABSTRACT

This chapter argues, on ethical grounds, that wherever possible patient-participation must be kept consistent with the level of healthy rational agency that is, or might be, available to the patient. Merely compliant patient-participation is not enough. This is also true of patient-adaptation or adjustment. Mere adaptive compliance is not enough. Accepting patient-consent, cooperation, and compliance as an adequate indication of genuine agentic participation is often hard to avoid, but such acceptance is also often inconsistent with appropriate healthcare. These conclusions follow, as a matter of empirically informed practical ethics, from an analysis of the lifelong habilitative tasks that face every human being, and the role that the patient's healthy agency plays in the development, protection, or restoration of the patient's agency itself and the patient's basic good health generally.

INTRODUCTION

The Aims of This Chapter and Its Relation to the Book as a Whole

The purpose of this chapter is to argue for the practical and ethical importance, in all healthcare contexts, of a certain conception of individual human agency – called here "healthy" agency. This form of agency is too often neglected or underemphasized in philosophy, psychology, and healthcare contexts.

In philosophy, this happens when discussions of agency are confined to metaphysical or moral problems about agent causation, volition, and moral responsibility. See, for a recent book length example, *Understanding Human Agency* (Mayr, 2011). In psychology, it happens when agentic activity is thought of in terms of the individual's consciously self-centric pursuits, either together with or in opposition to more communal ones. See the recent anthology called *Agency and Joint Attention* (Metcalfe & Terrace, 2013).

As other chapters in the present volume will show, explicitly or implicitly, a distinction between active agents and passive patients is readily available in healthcare contexts. Moreover, in some healthcare

DOI: 10.4018/978-1-4666-9992-2.ch001

contexts a persistent effort is made to engage patients' active agentic powers in their own wellness and healthcare treatment programs. Nonetheless, situations abound in which the health of the patient's agency is neglected in healthcare research, policy, funding, and treatment decisions. Instead, it is relegated to matters of nonmedical training rather than medical treatment, and coaching rather than therapy.

This does not happen as much, of course, in places where healthy agency is by definition close to the center of treatment concerns – for example in "performance medicine" for soldiers, athletes, and other high-risk and high stress occupations, and in behavioral health contexts for people who are persistently self-destructive or compulsively antisocial. Even there, however, the relatively meager social resources allocated to the problems of agentic health may lead to its neglect in practice.

Overview of the Argument

This chapter will argue that there is an identifiable form of agency that is an essential aspect of basic good health for human beings. Thus for the same reasons healthcare professionals accept an ethical requirement to treat patients properly for broken bones, spinal cord injuries, diabetes, and life-threatening cancer they ought to accept that the proper treatment of a patient's unhealthy agency is an ethical requirement also. It then follows that just as it is unethical to set the patient's broken femur but leave his coincidently discovered kidney disease untreated, so too it is unethical to treat the femur and the kidneys but leave his coincidently discovered unhealthy agentic abilities untreated. Putting that into practice calls for some significant changes.

The argument to those conclusions will open with a set of BACKGROUND considerations. Because this chapter will be a piece of ground-level, practical, philosophical ethics – and not a report of research findings, policy analysis, or clinical practice – it will begin with some remarks about the nature of practical versus theoretical ethics, and the use practical ethics can make of the places where competing forms of ethical theory intersect, in practice, over a large area of common ground. Those remarks will include reminders about the way in which practical ethics must be well-informed by empirical work in history and the medical and behavioral sciences about that common ethical ground. This section will conclude with attention to the "circumstances of justice" – a schematic, common-ground account of special relevance for guiding normative arguments.

The main body of the argument is divided into two major parts. The first of these is the ARGUMENT FROM HABILITATION TO BASIC GOOD HEALTH, and it begins with a discussion of the lifelong human need for habilitation. This is followed by a discussion of the conceptions of basic good health and healthy agency – both in terms of standard treatments of the definition of health itself and in terms that come from focusing on habilitative necessities. Basic good health in habilitative terms is then defined as a large segment of a continuum of health states and conditions ranging from worst to best – a segment that includes both physical and psychological indices and both negative and positive dimensions. In a nutshell: in habilitative terms, basic good health is an age-appropriate, environment-specific combination of the absence of ill health and the presence of some important physical and psychological powers and strengths that are necessary for achieving and receiving habilitative necessities. Basic good health is quite distinct from ideal health, or even extremely robust health.

The second major part is the ARGUMENT FROM BASIC GOOD HEALTH TO AGENTIC PARTICIPATION. It begins with the premise that basically healthy agentic powers and strengths are a necessary component of basic good health. The significance of this for practical ethics is then described first in general terms, followed by a formal restatement of the argument that shows its logical validity and soundness. Strong conclusions about the ethics of patient-participation are drawn in and around this formal restatement of the argument.

Following the main body of argument are brief sections on SOLUTIONS AND RECOMMENDATIONS as well as FUTURE RESEARCH DIRECTIONS. Most of that material (as befits a philosophical essay) is woven throughout the main sections of the argument and its conclusion. The CONCLUSION is organized around the discussion of an ordinary example, easily multiplied, that reprises the purpose of the argument as a whole and emphasizes its ethical significance.

BACKGROUND

This section assembles some preliminaries to the arguments made in subsequent sections. Some readers may wish to go directly to the argument itself, and come back to this section later, if necessary.

Common Ground for Practical Ethics

The preliminaries will begin with some reasonable assumptions about two parcels of common ground: one from ethical theory and one from human history and the human sciences.

Convergence in Ethical Theory

Competing ethical theories appear to endorse the same ultimate goal for human beings. That goal is some form of happiness, joy, satisfaction, or tranquility achieved by living in accord with the principles of right conduct and virtue, and in the sort of physical and social environment necessary for such a life. However, the accounts of happiness, forms of a good life, and the list of social norms necessary for it differ dramatically in ethical theories. This is reflected in the priorities given to the items within the lists of the component goods, principles, and virtues found in various theories, and to the social norms regarded as necessary to produce and sustain those goods. For an overview of this variety, organized around the notion of a good life, see Becker (1992).

But whatever differences there may be between theories on these points, there is a surprising convergence among them on clusters of goods and social norms that are required for a good life. Lists of goods, for example, typically include pleasure, security, tranquility, health, knowledge, practical intelligence, successful goal-directed activity, and satisfying social activities – including those characterized by mutual affection and care. See Nussbaum (2000; 2007; 2011) for a list of ten of these drawn from an Aristotelian foundation for her capabilities approach to ethics. Lists of principles of right conduct typically include obligations of hospitality, reciprocity, impartiality and partiality, mutual concern, restrictions on purely self-interested activity, and some characterization of the boundaries of the moral community (that is, to whom the principles apply: whether to all sentient animals, all human beings, all human beings except enemies, all human beings except enemies and strangers, etc.). Lists of virtues typically include courage, moderation, justice, practical wisdom, wisdom about ends, benevolence, and what might be called the agentic powers of active, effective, goal-directed activity.

In that process, every ethical theory must indicate how various goods are logically related to right and wrong conduct, justice and injustice, virtue and vice. It will be a consequentialist theory (think of utilitarianism) if its account of rights, duties, and virtues are constructed in terms of good and bad consequences. It will be a deontological theory if its account of good or virtuous conduct is based on whether or not the conduct conforms to antecedent principles, such as duties or rules to which people are bound regardless of the direct consequences. It will be a virtue theory if its account of good or dutiful conduct is based on whether or not the conduct exhibits virtuous character.

It is remarkable that though the resulting ethical theories are quite different at an abstract level, their ultimate accounts of specific *types* of good and bad conduct, required and prohibited conduct, virtuous and vicious character traits, and ideals for a good life and a good society are quite similar in many respects. The theories converge on many particulars. Murder, rape, theft, fraud, lack of concern for others, a failure to cooperate with others for the common good, or to reciprocate for benefits received from others are prima facie wrong. Self-defense and pursuit of self-interest are good, if combined with a similar commitment to the welfare of others, and virtuous if stabilized in reliable dispositions. From time to time sharply divergent ethical theories are proposed, but historically have had little success in remaining plausible after careful scrutiny. Egoistic hedonism, for example, has a short life each time it raises its head. So do various versions of amoralism. Consider how little traction the amoralist Thrasymachus gets in his argument with Socrates (Plato, 2004, Bk I). Or consider how the views of the Hellenistic Cynics and Cyrenaics fared in the Hellenistic period (Long, 1986).

The similarity should not be overstated, of course. The details of the ancient conceptions of the virtues and justice, for example, especially when thickly described, sometimes seem quite alien to modern readers. This has been noted repeatedly, and sometimes at length (Crisp, 2013; McIntyre, 2007). And it is certainly true that the history of philosophically approved racism, misogyny, and slavery is not much different than the history of the socially – and scientifically – approved versions of those things. Moreover, historically, ethical theories have differed greatly in their accounts of distributive justice and the scope of the moral community (Fleischacker, 2004). Nonetheless, all the plausible contemporary ethical theories do converge on many important points. The same seems to be true for ethical theories in their own contemporary circumstances.

Convenient surveys of the extent of convergence and divergence in ethical theories can be found in various histories of ethics (Sidgwick, 1902; McIntyre, 2006; Becker & Becker, 2003), and in recent peer-reviewed handbooks and encyclopedias (Crisp, 2013; LaFollette, 2013; Becker & Becker, 2001).

Convergence in History and the Human Sciences

Historians and scientists who focus on human health and behavior have their own competing theories, oriented in part toward the same basic goals: describing, explaining, and predicting individual human well-being and its absence or opposite, and the existence and stability of the physical and social environments needed for individual well-being. Such theories generate lists of typical and important human goals, principled behavior, character traits, and social norms. There is considerable divergence in such lists, due to the divergence in emphasis among competing theories. Evolutionary biology and psychology, for example, may explain what looks like altruistic behavior in terms of what looks like egoistic behavior, while social psychology may focus on the features of human development and social interaction through which individual identity and personality arise.

Nonetheless, there is a good deal of convergence among these competing theories, just as there is among competing ethical theories. The lists of the things that need description, explanation, and prediction are similar from scientific theory to scientific theory – and in each such theory they divide into elements of positive, negative, or neutral functioning both for individuals and for social groups.

The contours of this similarity between ethical theory and the history and science of human behavior are summarized on the negative side in material on ill health, dysfunction, and collapse, both physical and psychological, individual and social (American Psychiatric Association [APA], 2013; Diamond, 2005). It is summarized on the positive side in handbooks on positive psychology (Peterson & Seligman, 2004; Snyder & Lopez, 2009) which include references to the work on helping behavior, reciprocity, and prosocial traits and behavior – as well as work in eudaimonistic psychology (Keyes, 2009; Keyes & Annas, 2009). The conclusions reflected in such sources that are relevant here are derived from empirical descriptions, explanations, and/or predictions of the emergence (or absence) of various human goals and social norms. And again, they divide those that are functionally stable, self-sustaining, efficient, and productive of health and happiness from those that are not.

Although these descriptive materials are not proposed as implying prescriptive or ethical norms directly, it is hard to avoid the impression that they are being proposed as relevant to accepting or rejecting such norms. Practical ethics is wise to consider this carefully, since it wants to be practical rather than utopian.

The Role of Empirical Evidence in Practical Ethics

The common ground just described opens the way for an obvious form of inquiry in practical ethics – one in which ethical theory is strongly guided by empirical realities. Moreover, it looks as though that guidance will be subject to change as long as descriptive, explanatory, and predictive knowledge of the empirical realities continues to develop. This means that ethical theory will have to adjust to such changes. And that changeableness sets up an obvious three-phase type of argument in practical ethics. As follows.

First, practical ethics is understood as offering tentative prescriptions for a good life for human individuals flourishing in a reasonably good society. Those prescriptions, for or against various goal-directed activities and character traits, are offered in the form of proposed requirements, prohibitions, favorable or unfavorable recommendations, or mere permissions. Such prescriptions, as usual, include the clause that "ought implies can" – meaning that they are not meant to prescribe conduct that is physically or psychologically impossible or self-defeating to achieve. Nor are they meant to prescribe conduct that would be self-defeating to attempt.

So, in the second phase, empirical evidence from history and the human sciences is brought to bear on a set of questions about the possibility of following, or attempting to follow, the tentative prescriptions of ethical theory. For example, is an absolute prohibition of lying reasonable? Or an absolute requirement of promise keeping? That is, could people conform to such prescriptions without self-defeating consequences? Have they ever done so in large numbers? Have they ever enforced such prescriptions by law? Under what circumstances? Could they conform to the level of impartiality and self-sacrifice that seems to be required in some versions of utilitarian theory?

Moreover, empirical evidence needs to be brought to bear on the social arrangements necessary for implementing various ethical prescriptions. How much, or how little, can safely be left to individuals operating under sanctionless social norms? How much can be left to the social norms sanctioned only by organized social pressure? How much requires at least the sanctions of private law? Or the sanctions of criminal law?

In the third phase, the prescriptions of practical ethics are revised as necessary in the light of empirical evidence. This needs to be done to make sure that its prescriptions do not become self-defeating – either through making a good life for individuals impossible or unlikely, or by compromising the chances for a stable, well-functioning society in which such good lives can develop and be sustained.

This three-phase process seems innocent enough, but is not thoroughly followed consistently either by philosophers or by historians and scientists. Philosophers are often impatient with the empirical material, relying on their sense of the common wisdom on the subject, or on a few celebrated studies. And ethical theorists often do not want to tie their theorizing to volatile empirical results. They prefer the stability of *a priori* proofs when they can get them. Historians and scientists are often similarly impatient with both practical ethics and ethical theory, but for different reasons. They sometimes don't see the point of it – thinking that the empirical necessities and possibilities alone are enough to determine appropriate policy and practice. For a broader picture of the history of practical ethics, see Jamieson (2013). For notable recent attempts to do practical ethics directly from a particular ethical theory see Singer (2011), who uses utilitarian theory, but also considers results from other theories; Daniels (1985, 2007), who favors Rawls' theory of justice; or Beauchamp and Childress (2012), who appeal to a plural set of fundamental principles.

The Circumstances of Ethical Theory

A useful way to resolve this reluctance to use the methods of empirically based practical ethics is to use only the empirical material that can plausibly be regarded as part of the pre-theoretical background – in this case, only those stable features of the human condition that raise fundamental questions of ethics. Why is it that philosophers got interested in the topic of justice in the first place, for example? What aspects of the human condition raise those questions? Why are they not just settled by people powerful enough to command others to do as they say? Plato (2004; 2002) outlines the answers to such questions in the first two books of his *Republic* (and in the dialogue *Euthyphro*) in ways that have been compelling ever since. Plato's account of these matters has been reworked repeatedly, beginning with Aristotle, but the main themes remain consistent.

David Hume gave them an especially pithy summary, and dubbed them the circumstances of justice (1978, III.ii.ii; 1993, I.iii). He said that justice was an artificial virtue, not arising inevitably from nature, but made necessary by four factors characteristic of human life in its typical physical and social environments. Those four factors are limited altruism, rough equality of power, rough equality of vulnerability, and the moderate scarcity of resources characteristic of human life in life-sustaining environments. In those circumstances, questions of justice always arise because there are conflicts that need to be resolved, cooperation problems that need to be solved, and coordination problems that require the general acceptance of decisions. In different circumstances, he thought, questions of justice would not arise. They would not arise in conditions of an overabundance of equally accessible resources, because in such circumstances there would be no occasion for conflict over resources. Everyone would have a surfeit. For similar reasons, questions of justice do not arise in conditions of perfect altruism, since any deficits would be shared equally. Interestingly, Hume thought that questions about justice do not have a chance to get started in the presence of *extreme* inequalities of power and vulnerability, or *extreme* scarcity of resources, either. Survival will be strongly motivated, but philosophical discussions about it or about justice will not be. Or so he thought.

Questions about what to include under the heading of "the circumstances of justice" continue. (Rawls, 1971, pp. 126-131) and various subsequent arguments for the inclusion of gender and the family (Okin, 1989), the inclusion of disability and dependency (Kittay, 1998), an emphasis on habilitation (Becker, 2012), and various accounts of the "currency" in which justice is to be counted for egalitarian purposes, most notably capabilities and luck (Sen, 2009; Nussbaum, 2011; Cohen, 1989; 2008; Segall, 2010).

These matters about the circumstances of justice are very useful questions for practical ethics, since they call for only the most basic and stable empirical information about human nature, conduct, and the human condition. And the answers to such questions have surprisingly powerful consequences for both ethical theory and practical ethics.

In the following argument, this chapter in effect proposes some amendments to two items in Hume's summary of the circumstances of justice. Specifically, it can be understood as proposing that facts about human habilitation, basic good health, and healthy agency must have a prominent role in our understanding of Hume's notions of rough equality of *power* and rough equality of *vulnerability*.

ARGUMENT FROM HABILITATION TO BASIC GOOD HEALTH

The aim in this section and the next is simply to develop an explicit appreciation of the role that habilitation, basic good health, and healthy agency should play in practical ethics about patient participation in healthcare contexts. In this, it will follow only the bare outlines of an account that might be offered for a theory of justice (Becker, 2012), heavily recast for present purposes.

Habilitated Powers and Vulnerabilities

Habilitation

The *Oxford English Dictionary* defines habilitation as "the action of enabling or endowing [a person or thing] with ability or fitness; capacitation; qualification." Here that meaning will sometimes be expressed as equipping an individual (including oneself) with functional abilities, usually relative to a specific range of physical or social environments which themselves may be the object of human habilitative or rehabilitative activities. Thus habilitation can be sorted into combinations of three things: the habilitation of others, self-habilitation, and the habilitation of physical and social environments. Human beings are typically involved in all three sorts for most of their lifetimes. The consequences of this for ethical theory and theories of justice generally are discussed at length in (Becker, 2012). Here, a few clarifying remarks will suffice.

- **Habilitation of Others:** Human infants are born lethally underdeveloped and dependent on others. If healthy, they are equipped to receive life-sustaining care from others, and a range of habilitative care that helps them gradually develop further abilities that make a good deal of independent activity possible. They cannot do this on their own, or in physical or social environments that are especially hostile to their healthy development. The same is true throughout childhood, adolescence, adulthood, and old age. Intermittent periods of more or less complete dependence occur. Even the strong have to sleep. And unless one is reduced to a completely isolated, solitary life there will be many occasions in which thoroughly interdependent activity is necessary – e.g., in cooperative or coordinated multigenerational social activity that requires a division of labor and expertise.

  Such interdependent activity is mutually habilitative in the sense that it equips people to flourish as specialists, acting independently in providing others as well as themselves with expertly made shoes, for example, while relying on others for a plentiful supply of grain or fish. The preservation of an interdependent social environment requires that it be organized so as to provide this sort of mixture of independence and interdependence.

- **Self-Habilitation:** Many of the abilities human beings need to survive and thrive are ones that cannot be successfully given to them by others, because their acquisition also requires the persistent and effective efforts of the individual acquiring them. Language acquisition is a good example. Dedicated habilitative efforts from primary caregivers help. But children can learn language in a social environment saturated with it even without such help from caregivers. They can do so because what helps most is the child's persistent efforts to participate in the use of language in the surrounding social environment – through imitation, trial and error learning, with constant feedback from others. Such learning is self-habilitation, which is necessary for the acquisition of many physical and intellectual abilities – as well as the moral virtues. On the point about the moral virtues, see the classic confrontation between Plato (2002, *Meno* at 87b-100) and Aristotle (2009, *Nicomachean Ethics*, Bk II beginning at 1103a-b). Plato has Socrates argue that virtue cannot be taught. The evidence is that there are no excellent teachers of it who are successful. Aristotle agrees that virtue cannot be taught, but makes the obvious point that virtue can nonetheless be *learned* – in fact has to be learned, as a habit or disposition, from practice. One becomes courageous by acting courageously, repeatedly and successfully, avoiding the excesses of foolhardiness and the deficiencies of cowardice.
- **Habilitation of the Physical and Social Environment:** Some physical and social environments are lethal for human beings. Others are hostile or inhospitable. Still others are minimally, moderately, or perhaps maximally hospitable. Human beings who are healthy, properly self-habilitative, and capable of both independent and interdependent living of various types often need to turn their attention to improving their environments – or to preserving them. This means devoting some of their cooperative and coordinative activity to the habilitation of their physical and social environments.

Habilitation of all these types is a lifelong necessity for human beings, and a large component in determining the extent of the equality or inequality in power and vulnerability involved in Hume's account of the circumstances of justice, and ethics generally. It therefore should figure prominently, at least implicitly, in all ethical theories. And it should have a prominent role in practical ethics.

The Health Continuum from Worst to Best

Health Defined in Functional Terms

The definition of health is contested on some points, philosophically and scientifically. For a summary of this – and the intensity of it – as it shows up in bioethics, see Humber and Almeder (1997). But for practical purposes, we can note that in the context of healthcare, health conditions are always defined in functional terms, whether they are on the medical side (physiological functioning) or the mental side (psychological functioning). Health has to do with how well or poorly individuals function, physiologically or psychologically, in the physical and social environments they inhabit.

Healthy Functioning Defined Negatively, Positively, or as a Combination of the Two

Some people focus on the negative side of things – pathology or dysfunction – and may be satisfied with a "negative" definition of health itself. That is, they may think of health itself as the *absence* of physiological or psychological dysfunction due to disease, deficit, disorder, impairment, injury, or distress. Other people, by contrast, are reluctant to define health in merely negative terms. Instead, they want a "combined" or "complete" definition of health which includes not only the *absence* of serious dysfunction but the *presence* of various positive degrees of physiological and psychological strength, stability, resistance, and resilience.

The presence of those positive things makes it possible to put various upward levels of good, better, and best health on the continuum of health in general – above the downward levels of good, bad, worse, and worst health represented in the familiar hospital nomenclature of increasingly grave conditions leading to death – e.g., good, fair, serious, critical, extremely critical. After all, a hospitalized patient in "good" condition (negatively defined) may not yet be in good enough health to be discharged. (In hospital nomenclature, the term good health is usually glossed as something like "vital signs are stable and within normal limits; indicators for recovery are excellent; patient is progressing well.") That is fully consistent with the patient's being quite weak and unable to do many of the activities of daily living. Hospitals will often discharge patients who are in "good" health (negatively defined) if it is thought that they can finish their recovery at home – or *ought* to be able to do so, in some undefined sense of ought.

So the negative definition of health does not easily capture the ordinary meaning of good health. Many times, attention to health positively defined – that is, to the levels of strength, stability, resistance, and resilience necessary for daily living – seems to be called for.

But advocates of the negative definition are suspicious of more expansive, positive definitions of good health, perhaps because it looks as though it will be hard to draw a boundary between those desirable states on the continuum that need to be medicalized in ways routinely covered by healthcare insurance (such as abscessed teeth) and those that usually do not (annoyingly yellowed teeth). Healthcare policy looks for a sharp distinction between treatment and training, and between therapy and coaching. Even some positive psychologists appear to be in this camp. For example, one of the first major handbooks in positive psychology has no indexed reference to health at all (Peterson & Seligman, 2004). The reference to health, however, is in the subtitle of Langer's more recent monograph on mindfulness (2009), based on her decades-long social psychological research (Langer, 1989).

For a philosophical defense of the negative definition of health, see Boorse (1975; 1976; 1977; 1997). For the controversy generally see the discussion of "complete" health used by the World Health Organization (Bok, 2008), and the discussion of the usefulness and limitations of a combined definition in Becker (2012, pp. 45-80).

Habilitative Necessities Require Both the Absence of Pathology and the Presence of Strength

It turns out that focusing on what is needed for habilitation can avoid entanglement in this controversy over negative versus positive definitions of health. In particular, it turns out that what is needed for present purposes is a conception of basic good health that includes some but not all of its positive dimension, above the mere absence of pathology. As follows.

Think about the type of good health that is necessary for habilitation throughout one's life – necessary for thriving, functionally, in a range of physical and social environments. Such habilitative necessities will include what is necessary for accomplishing the three habilitative tasks that fall on all human beings: receiving habilitation from others when necessary; self-habilitation when possible and necessary; and habilitating others, and one's physical and social environments, when possible and necessary.

It is clear that a significant amount of strength, resistance to ill health, resilience in recovering from it, agentic energy, initiative, and persistence in the face of difficulties will be needed at every stage along the way – from learning to walk and talk to suffering losses and coping with the difficulties of old age. These are traits with a positive, physiological and psychological dimension as well as the mere absence of pathology. In fact, the necessities of self-habilitation in particular require a substantial amount of active, effective agency in every healthy human adult – that is, consciously planned, situationally aware, goal-directed activity. So it is important to define basic good health in this context so as to include not only the absence of dysfunction (physical or psychological) but as the presence of the necessary amount of functional habilitative strength, given the range of reasonably hospitable environments.

A Nutshell Definition of Basic Good Health with Some Important Restrictions

In a nutshell, basic good health in habilitative terms is an age-appropriate and environment-specific combination of stable, functional, physical and psychological strengths that preserve the absence of ill health and include the presence of those powers and strengths that are necessary for recovering from ill health and resisting a relapse into it – in a range of accessible, hospitable, and ethically defensible physical and social environments. But note the qualifiers in that definition.

- **Age-Appropriateness:** The age-appropriateness restriction is important. Infants can be healthy or not even though they require receiving almost all their habilitation, at first, from others. What counts as basic good health for an infant will soon count as a form of unhealthiness if the child does not begin and then continue to develop in many self-habilitating ways. Thus the capacity for the development of active effective individual agency – for the purposes of self-habilitation – is a part of basic good health.
- **Range of Environments:** The environmental restriction is also important. Adults can be basically healthy even though they may be unable to achieve or sustain habilitative necessities in chaotic or extreme physical or social environments. Many reasonably healthy adults are unable to cope with the physical and psychological chaos of warfare, incarceration in solitary confinement for long periods, or living in the space station, the Antarctic, or the Amazon basin. And many superbly successful athletes in one sport are unable to succeed in another, or in the decathlon. Even basically good health is situational; it always comes with implicit environmental qualifications. (Basically healthy, but not for deep-sea diving.)
- **Environments Hospitable to Human Development:** And there is an important ethical restriction that is usually implicit in this functional definition. It assumes that the notion of basic good health will not apply to what happens in inhospitable or hostile social environments that sharply truncate functional habilitative development. Understanding basic good health in habilitative terms acknowledges, for example, that physiological and psychological traits in a person necessary to produce an abject, non-resisting acceptance of thoroughgoing and brutal enslavement cannot reasonably be called basically *good* psychological health. (Slaves may well be in basic good

health, as Epictetus was, but probably not if they are uninterested in freedom when it is offered. Epictetus took his, and flourished.)

Thus basic good health, as the concept will be used here, combines both the "negative" and "positive" definitions of health one finds in the literature, as well as its physical and social dimensions. The inclusion of positive health, both physical and psychological, is crucial, because it is almost always implicated in the individual's ability to receive or achieve the habilitative necessities for surviving and thriving in a given range of environments. See the accounts of positive mental health in Jahoda (1958) and Vaillant (2003), as well as the account of positive psychological strengths and virtues in Peterson and Seligman (2004), and Langer's work on mindfulness (1989, 2009).

Basic Good Health Includes Age-Appropriate Individual Human Agency

The typical track of human development, in basic good health, from newborn to adult includes the development of increasing agentic powers. Like every other physiological or psychological aspect of human development, agency can be healthy or unhealthy in the functional contribution it makes to the whole. So basic good health, including the development of the individual agency necessary for self-habilitation, is among the factors that define the practical necessities of the human condition. This has significant ethical consequences for healthcare policy and practice, particularly with respect to patient participation in healthcare contexts.

ARGUMENT FROM BASIC GOOD HEALTH TO AGENTIC PARTICIPATION

Healthy Agency

The Irrelevance of Metaphysical Freedom of the Will

For present purposes, there is no need to tarry at the question of whether human beings have genuine freedom of will at some exalted metaphysical level. Individual human beings are links in many causal chains of events. In some of those causal chains, a given human being will function only as an *object* – a living organism that occupies space, consumes resources, and may be a causal factor in the activities of other living organisms. So far, there is no agency involved in that human being's functioning.

In other causal chains, the same human being may function as a *subject* – a living organism who is *passively* aware of the surrounding world, or even of some particular causal chains within it, but makes no effort to act with respect to it, as opposed to responding to stimuli or requests. (Think of the paralyzed patient under awake sedation of a sort that disrupts the formation of new memories.) Again, as long as this subjectivity is completely passive, there is no agency involved in it.

Individual agency does arrive on the scene, however, if and when a given human individual functions as an *active* subject in one or more causal chains of events – one who not only has the ability to be passively aware, but who is also active with respect to trying to start, stop, or modify various causal chains. Such subjective activity is at the core of human agency, as the term is used both in ethical theory and in related behavioral sciences. Whether or not such agency, or agentic functioning, constitutes a form of autonomy or freedom, or is ever actually effective in starting, stopping, or modifying causal chains is not the issue here. The issue is rather that the existence of agentic functioning is a particularly interesting set of physiological and psychological abilities that most human individuals have.

Ethical theorists tend to describe and study those functional abilities in terms of the agent's conscious, cognitive, and conative abilities. For a recent example in ethical theory, see Korsgaard (2008), and for an example in practical ethics Becker (2003). Behavioral scientists tend to study the physiological and psychological determinants of those agentic abilities, and their age-appropriate development throughout the lifespan. For the relevant literature in developmental psychology see Zelazo (2013), the two massive volumes of which may be used to flesh out the details of what follows.

The Developmental Track of Healthy Human Agency

Healthy human agency is a part of basic good health, and it develops through the same age-appropriate stages. Agentic abilities may be absent, present, undeveloped, developed, dysfunctional, or reliably competent in any given individual, in every developmental stage, and be reliably competent or not in some specifiable range of environments. Thus,

Healthy agency is age-appropriate reliably competent physiological and psychological agentic functioning, with respect to habilitative necessities, in a given range of environments.

The account here will focus mainly on developmental matters from the perspective of practical ethics. So it will be useful to make some coarse-grained distinctions based on ordinary observations about the sequence of age-appropriate developments in the powers of human agency, and thus of varieties of healthy agency.

Impersonal agency is characteristic of healthy human infants from the beginning, prior to their acquiring the sort of self-awareness and awareness of circumstances characteristic of personhood. Impersonal agency involves only simple purposive behavior, elicited by situational memory and awareness of possibility together with aversive reactions to some things; repeated exploration of other things; seeking more of some of them, while avoiding others. This is distinguishable from reflexive responses to stimuli, though it may begin with such reflexes. The sucking involved in nursing is an example. It may begin with reflexive responses, but in favorable circumstances soon also becomes simple purposive behavior – given the appropriate habilitation provided by others and successfully received and repeated by the infant.

This then becomes a useful model for habilitation throughout the lifecycle. Its success typically depends on three things: favorable physical and social circumstances, help from others, and self-habilitative activity.

Personal agency of a simple sort arises in various forms during the first two years of life (or more) with the emergence of some elements of personality. The simplest forms of this involve early forms of self-awareness, memory, anticipation, sociality, gestural communication, and explicit, persistent, goal-directed activity that are possible *prior* to the acquisition of full-fledged language – though not before the acquisition of a vocal and non-vocal vocabulary. In healthy humans, this sort of agency is usually well-developed by the age of two.

Rational agency of increasing complexity develops from simple personal agency, ultimately becoming what philosophers label moral agency. Rational agency involves the acquisition of a full-fledged language in which agents can represent themselves to themselves as beings with a history, a present, and a possible future in describable physical and social environments. They also acquire what philosophers and some psychologists call "a theory of mind" that imputes to others something analogous to their own subjective experience. Rational agents are thus agents with autobiographical powers as well as descriptive ones that include others' self-conscious points of view. The full-fledged language required for this will typically make possible (given the appropriate habilitation) the emergence and development of increasingly complex forms of self-consciousness, attachment, aversion, desire, preference structure, memory, imagination, anticipation, dread, goal-setting, planning, deliberation, choice, and (more or less) effective goal-directed action.

Simple forms of rational agency are found in early childhood, but are often not fully comprehensible to the children themselves, and not consistently coherent or successful. This is healthy in an age-appropriate way, but gradually becomes age-inappropriate if it remains that simple. To put it in (ancient) philosophical terms, the rudimentary practical intelligence involved in simple rational agency will gradually become unhealthy if it does not develop into genuine practical wisdom (*phronesis*) in three senses, each of which is a major developmental milestone.

First, practical intelligence must be able to prioritize goals and organize goal-directed activity in a coherent and effective manner in short-term, parametric or non-strategic situations in which the responses of others do not need to be considered. (Playing solitaire is a nonstrategic enterprise.) To be coherent and effective even in nonstrategic situations, however, choices must track preferences ordered by the rules and goals of the enterprise, and such preferences must track the player's desires and aversions. In addition, to be consistently effective, choices must also track accurate deliberative decisions about the possibilities for successful conduct, and conduct itself must track those decisions – uncomplicated by paralyzing ambivalence, for example, suspended between equally attractive options.

This complicates simple rational agency in two important ways: one is by complicating the practical intelligence involved in it, but another is by complicating and strengthening the agentic powers which yield consistent, effective action in parametric situations. If a label is needed for this development, call it "parametric rational agency." Its presence is a healthy, developmental milestone.

Second, practical intelligence must be able to filter out unwise (dysfunctional) goals and courses of conduct in *strategic* social situations, so as to direct agency always toward wise or functional ones. In order to do that, rational agents need to be able to anticipate what others might do in response to their actions – things that might assist or defeat those actions. (Playing chess is a strategic enterprise.) And in order to anticipate what others might do, rational agents need to be able to read the intentions and motives of others. This involves rational agents in a more or less continuous effort to understand the subjective point of view of others in particular situations. All of this takes time, a great deal of agentic activity of a trial and error sort (some of it deliberately guided by others), as well as a good deal of agentic self-reflection on that activity.

To the extent that the agent is able to develop coherent and successful "strategic rational agency" in addition to the nonstrategic sort – and to make both sorts into a coherent, complex form of rational activity that is habitual, dispositional, and highly motivated – a second milestone has been reached. But note that reaching this level of rational agency is compatible with some dramatic forms of pathology. Psychopaths can have strategic rational agency.

Third, practical intelligence needs to become full-fledged practical wisdom in the context of the transformation of rational agency into "moral" agency. Since this transformation typically occurs gradually, over the whole course of the development of rational agency – and since it prevents some pathologies found in purely rational agency, including psychopathy – its development is of great importance to habilitation and to practical ethics. It is therefore best to characterize it separately. As follows.

Moral agency is a form of psychologically healthy agency characterized negatively by the absence of dysfunctional, self-destructive, antisocial, or asocial pathologies (e.g., in suicidal, psychopathic, or sociopathic personalities). It is characterized positively by the presence of reliably functional, self-respecting, prosocial strengths of positive health (e.g., in stable dispositions of enduring self-protective and self-promoting interest, but self-interest that is limited by an interest in the welfare of others; an interest in mutual love, friendship, affection, and benefit; and an interest in mutually advantageous forms of conflict resolution, cooperation, and coordination).

Nascent natural virtues. It is clear from the developmental literature reported in Zelazo (2013) that healthy human infants come equipped with the agentic powers to explore not only the possibilities of pain avoidance, pleasure seeking, and need reduction but also various sorts of reciprocal social interactions. Early versions of the prosocial motivations of moral agency are internalized (or not) as strongly motivated behavioral dispositions by infants and children if such behaviors are functional for them within their preferred social environments. The dispositions involved are acquired both through deliberate training from their caregivers (from toileting to paying attention to the expectations of others), and through active, agentic learning on the part of the children themselves – through observation, imitation, exploration, repetition, and eventual habituation.

Ethical theorists who pay attention to childhood development sometimes think of these prosocial traits as nascent "natural" goals, goods, duties, rights, and virtues. They are natural not only because they are part of healthy development in its earliest stages, but because when they persist in adult behavior in a powerful way they are central to the "health" of stable, well-functioning, multi-generational social environments generally. They are natural and healthy, then, not only for human individuals but for the environments in which they live.

A sense of causal accountability. There is an additional consequence of these natural dispositions that characterize moral agency. Rational agents, even at an early stage, are able to appreciate how they themselves might be causally accountable for the consequences of their conduct. This aspect of moral agency is a very useful development for the purposes of both social science and practical ethics. Moral agents understand the notion of moral accountability, and tend to respond predictably and sometimes usefully to habilitation aimed at reinforcing the strength of their natural dispositions to act toward good, right, or virtuous ends. This is so even though the concept of accountability raises, rather than resolves, the theoretical question of how such accountability can be compatible with determinism.

Practical ethics and social science can usefully distinguish the concept of moral responsibility (with its implications of moral praiseworthiness or blameworthiness) from a concept of accountability that is severed from such implications. The term 'moral responsibility' can then be reserved for theoretical discussions about freedom and determinism, and 'accountability' can be used merely for the practical problem of identifying plausible targets for human interventions in such causal chains in the future.

Specifically, in this case, the concept of accountability can be used to identify plausible targets for human habilitative efforts – habilitation designed to reinforce functional (healthy, good, virtuous) conduct and character, and to reduce or extinguish its opposite (dysfunctional, unhealthy, bad, vicious conduct and character).

The Centrality of Healthy Moral Agency, Theoretical, and Practical

Ethical theories always call for more than merely healthy moral agency as just described. Rather, each ethical theory promotes a theory-specific form of moral agency in which the ideal agent is reliably motivated to act for the theoretically correct reasons – and with the theoretically correct affective attitudes – as specified by the theory, rather than by the physiological and psychological requirements of health. Utilitarians want moral agents to act so as to maximize aggregate welfare, with attitudes that can be similarly justified. Kantians want moral agents to follow the moral law, with attitudes that are similarly law-respecting. Aristotelians want conduct that proceeds from virtuous character, and which is understood to be a reliable route (given some moderately good luck) to an objectively good life considered as a whole. Similar amendments to the notion of healthy agency are found in theological ethics. It is not that ethical theories want to recommend *un*healthy moral agency. It is rather that they want to recommend something beyond it (or perhaps to redefine the notion of health by adding something about the unhealthy consequences of sin).

But there are competing ethical theories. So theory-specific descriptions of moral agency will tend to scatter away from the common ground shared by all those theories, and shared as well with the biological and psychological sciences. Practical ethics, if it remains on the common ground, cannot follow. It will stay with a common-ground version of moral agency that is not infused with a specific ethical theory.

- **Practical Moral Agency:** Focusing on practical rather than theoretical moral agency amounts to focusing on a form of especially healthy rational agency. As noted above, unconstrained rational agency can be pathological for the agent and for the agent's social environment. Healthy moral agency (both theoretical and practical) can correct for those pathologies. The correction comes from two things already discussed. One is the development of nascent natural virtues that define persistent ends to be prioritized and coordinated by practical wisdom. The other is the appreciation of one's causal responsibility for one's conduct and character.

But practical moral agency, as discussed here, also calls attention to another source of pathology, and its correction. This is the powerful, often necessary role of self-habilitation throughout the lifespan. Even infant agency has a direct role in the further development of agentic powers themselves. Self-habilitation goes on to have a direct role throughout the agent's lifetime in the strength and scope of the agency so achieved and sustained – the age-appropriate *health* of the agency. Moreover, as the agent achieves more and more independence those age-appropriate agentic powers become more and more central to sustaining the agent's health generally – not only in avoiding ill health but in recovering from it. Medical advice and medical treatment are often futile if the agent doesn't seek them from the right people in a timely way, and then actively follow out the necessary preventative and rehabilitative measures. This is well understood in medicine, but one recent literature review (Thórarinsdóttir & Kristjánsson, 2014) suggests a lack of interest in trying to study, in a quantitative way, how frequently and how much patients' practical agency fails in this respect, and how such agentic dysfunction might be appropriately and effectively treated.

There is a second, and equally important role that self-habilitation plays in human health. Self-habilitative activity will often be directed toward making the physical and social environment hospitable to individual health throughout the population. Every well-functioning society needs the cooperative efforts of many healthy agents in order to sustain and develop that hospitability. That typically requires the development of healthy moral agency in a large portion of the society – agents with prosocial as well as self-interested dispositions, and the agentic energy needed to pursue them.

To the extent that sustaining or restoring healthy practical agency gets ignored in healthcare research, policy, and practice – leaving weakly-agentic patients on their own (see the case of Martha in the Conclusion) – unethical consequences can follow.

Agentic Patients in Healthcare

The argument to this point now yields a fairly direct and powerful consequence for the topic of patient-participation and adaptability. It is that every aspect of healthcare needs to make the age-appropriate health, development and strength of the patient's moral agency a prominent goal of the care. That means that every aspect of healthcare needs to address psychological health, and more specifically positive psychological health, and most specifically agentic health.

Not many attempts to study patient-participation in medical terms seem to take this up. See the literature review in Simmons, Wolever and Bechard (2014). Perhaps a formal statement of the ethical argument to the conclusions implicit in the foregoing reminders can help to motivate such study.

[Technical Note: The health sciences, both in practice and policy, effectively endorse a powerful list of relevant explanatory and predictive propositions of varying probabilities – some of which are implicit in the discussion and argument given above. In those propositions, made explicit below, the verb-phrase "*requires but is not guaranteed by*" is a reference to causal probabilities. It is sometimes shortened to "requires" or is replaced by the logical connective "only if," which is itself equivalent to the "if-then" material conditional of truth-functional logic written as $p \rightarrow q$. This sets up a hypothetical syllogism, which practical ethics can complete simply by endorsing an ethical duty in support of the first antecedent (A), in the list of explanatory and predictive propositions. As follows.]

Explanatory and Predictive Propositions

- **The Necessity of Habilitation:** (A) The survival, development, and age-appropriate basic good health of any human individual *requires but is not guaranteed by* (B) effective age-appropriate self-habilitative and cooperative activity from that given individual, and some others who are adults, in the context of a survivable, and at least intermittently hospitable physical and social environment. That is, A only if B.
- **The Necessity of Basic Good Health:** (B) *requires but is not guaranteed by* (C) age-appropriate basic good health in that given individual, and some others who are adults, including age-appropriate positive psychological health and healthy agency. That is, B only if C.
- **Basic Good Health in Adults Includes Healthy Rational and Moral Agency:** (C) *requires but is not guaranteed by* (D) the age-appropriate development and maintenance of the elements of physiological and psychological health that can become and sustain healthy, complex rational and moral agency. That is, C only if D.
- **The Habilitative Necessity of a Multigenerational Social Environment:** (D) *requires but is not guaranteed by* (E) effective, sustained habilitative activity, from some adult human beings with age-appropriate healthy rational and moral agency, for themselves, for some other human beings, and for the social environment, so as to create and sustain a multigenerational social environment that is survivable, and at least intermittently hospitable for basic good health in each generation. That is, D only if E.

- **The Habilitative Necessity of Coordinated Group Activity:** (E) *requires but is not guaranteed by* (F) effective, coordinated and cooperative group habilitative activity devoted to sustaining age-appropriate basic good health, including positive psychological health and healthy rational and moral agency of the human individuals within the care of the group. That is, E only if F.
- **The Habilitative Necessity of Healthy Rational and Moral Agency in Caregivers:** (F) *requires but is not guaranteed by* (G) age-appropriate healthy agency including complex forms of rational agency and practical moral agency in most individuals engaged in group habilitative activity devoted to caring for members of the group. That is, F only if G.

There are many other propositions, and arrangements of them, that can be extracted from the common ground used by practical ethics. The ones given above are the ones most relevant to the points about habilitation and agency. But from those alone we can derive compound propositions such as

only if (B & C & D & E & F & G)
only if (C &….)
only if (D &…) etc.

Translating this into Practical Ethics

One easy way of translating this into a normative argument in practical ethics is to put a normative premise above item "A" that recognizes the necessity of habilitation for human beings, and endorses an age-appropriate and role-appropriate ethical requirement on all human beings to secure, insofar as possible, the survival, development, and basic good health of other human individuals specified by a relevant group-defining distributive principle.

That would amount to asserting a normative duty on every *moral* agent to act effectively to achieve item (A), which then entails normative requirements to act effectively to achieve the things required by (A) – namely, in this case, (B & C & D & E & F & G).

Of course, requirements endorsed by practical ethics carry with them priority rankings and excusing conditions. One cannot be required, ethically, to do the impossible. Nor can one be required, coherently, to do things that are self-defeating – unless such sacrifice is necessary for a higher priority (for example, compromising one's health to carry out a competing duty to rescue).

And ethical theories differ dramatically about relevant group-defining distributive principles – from egalitarian universalism to libertarian isolationism. Common-ground practical ethics cannot by itself solve the distributive problem, except in pluralistic political systems or institutions *which must resolve distributive matters in terms of common ground principles*. Practical ethics there will endorse practical politics of a common-ground sort.

As a consequence, those excusing conditions and distributive matters, though in one sense left unresolved, nonetheless leave intact a powerful ethical requirement to put the health of the patient's rational and moral agency in an urgent, and prominent place in the discussion of patient-participation, and in treatment decisions. The application of this argument to making sure that patient-participation is, insofar as possible, agentic participation – and does not damage or interrupt the development of the patient's healthy agency – will be discussed again in the Conclusion section below.

SUGGESTIONS AND RECOMMENDATIONS

A few suggestions and recommendations may be extracted from the argument and listed here.

One is that there seems to be a need for increased scholarly and practical interest in the topic of healthy agency – both among philosophers and among people working in the scientific and healthcare contexts represented in this volume.

Another is that this appears to be particularly acute for understanding the developmental track of agentic powers throughout adulthood – and particularly for understanding its plasticity (or lack of it) throughout adulthood.

And a third is to encourage the coordination – in terms of health and healthcare – of several overlapping streams of research: the human capabilities approach to questions about the good life, health, and justice (as represented in the activities of the Human Development and Capabilities Association); the research on human happiness and well-being (as represented in both life satisfaction and eudaimonistic research in social science); and the fields of positive psychology and developmental psychology.

FUTURE RESEARCH DIRECTIONS

Philosophers should probably be wary of predicting or making suggestions for future research to anyone, including themselves. This is especially true when philosophers are speaking to scientists. (One thinks of the logical positivists of the 1930s telling physicists to forget about the neutrino.)

But there is one problem among those mentioned in the argument of this chapter that is clearly a candidate for future research. It is the "combined" conception of health, and particularly its definition of basic good health. It would be nice to have an operationalized, quantifiable health scale for basic good health – one that could not only be used in healthcare contexts, but also in political ones as well, as a part of an account of distributive justice with respect to health. There is an illustration of how such a health scale might look in Becker (2012, pp. 81-94). But it is clearly in need of further development by others.

CONCLUSION

The argument of this chapter is meant to be convincing for the purposes of common-ground practical ethics as it relates to health care policy, and similarly convincing for common-ground healthcare policy and practice. But an ordinary example (fictionalized from cases known to the author and easily multiplied) indicate the reverse – that there is significant resistance to the central conclusion of the argument in both healthcare policy and practice, and in the practical ethics supporting them. As follows.

The Example of Martha

In the United States, the cost of long-term professional care for quadriplegics is very high. It is particularly high if a quadriplegic is dependent on a ventilator – either completely or for sleep and rest each day. Sometimes such people cannot be cared for safely, or at all, at home. And in that case, sometimes they will be placed in a long-term care facility especially licensed for the care of ventilator dependent patients of all ages and conditions.

Suppose such a facility has 36 beds, in 12 rooms, three to a room. Suppose state licensure does not require anything beyond the custodial medical care necessary to keep the patients' physical and mental health stable – meaning, in practical terms, good enough not to require readmission to a hospital unless some new life-threatening condition arises. Suppose state regulations require that the facility be staffed at all times by at least one registered nurse, and a "sufficient number" of licensed nurses and certified nursing assistants. So such a facility can be fully licensed without providing any on-staff physical, occupational, or psychological therapy. No other amenities are legally required.

Now suppose that Martha, a 50-year-old woman, is transferred to this facility from a rehabilitation center. She is a relatively recent C-5 spinal cord injury patient, quadriplegic with a weak diaphragm and limited function in her hands, who is (noninvasive) ventilator-dependent for sleep and rest. She has become proficient with an expensive power wheelchair and computer that she learned to use in the rehabilitation unit of the hospital. This has helped ease her depression, but purchase of that equipment is still pending, so it did not come with her. Nor does she get many visits from friends or colleagues from work, because the facility is in a city over a hundred miles from where she had been living and working as the manager of a small café. She has no surviving immediate family members. They all died in the accident that injured her. She was fully informed of the financial necessity for the transfer, the nature of the facility, and the high quality of the nursing care she could expect there, but its lack of on-site physical and occupational therapy. She was apprehensive about the change, but discussed it cooperatively with the rehabilitation center's staff, and ultimately accepted it in the same cooperative spirit.

Martha now finds herself in a room with two other women who are on invasive ventilation 24/7. One of them is almost completely unresponsive. The other one has persistent control of the room's television set, which is always on throughout the day.

The nursing assistants are underpaid and overworked. Every time Martha mentions a power wheelchair and computer, the staff says they don't see how she will be able to use it except to get back and forth to the day room. They take her there in a wheeled reclining chair if she asks, but there is rarely anyone else in the day room who isn't occupied with family visitors. And several times Martha has been left there alone, reading, apparently forgotten for long periods. There is no Internet connection for patients, so she doesn't press for a computer. And the facility does not provide regular transportation to and from accessible locations in nearby towns.

Martha becomes increasingly passive and discouraged, while remaining courteous and cooperative. She remains a model patient, but increasingly becomes a patient who is not an active, effective agent at all.

The staff is meticulous about keeping her clean, hydrated, fed, free of bedsores, and comfortable – both physically and in terms of feeling safe and secure. Her nurses bring books and magazines for her to read, but she gradually loses interest in reading. Volunteers of various sorts make visits, especially around the holidays, but she gradually withdraws from all of them. Always politely, or by feigning sleep.

Now Consider the Following Proposition

If you are going to save a life without initially arguing about the cost, then always save the moral agent in it as an equally urgent priority, and don't argue about that cost either (Becker, 2000, modified). And then consider how far the reality for Martha is from what practical ethics and decent healthcare require.

Such Cases Can Be Multiplied

There is apparently considerable resistance to treating threatened, damaged, or weak agency in the context of healthcare, unless there is an explanation for it in physical or psychological health *negatively* defined (e.g., child neglect; alcoholism; depression). Yet it is clear that adult human beings who lose or lack some of their capacity for *self*-habilitation often continue to need habilitation from others to repair, sustain or improve their healthy agency. It does not look as though neglecting this could possibly be justified.

An Ethical Prescription

As matter of practical ethics it seems safe to say that habilitation for survival and basic good health – both at an individual level and the public health level – should be, uncontroversially, among the highest priorities recognized by healthcare practice and policy. More to the point here, insofar as practical ethics recognizes the necessity of habilitation for human life generally, it will recognize the centrality of habilitation for basic good health along both its negative and positive dimensions.

In recognizing this, healthcare practice and policy should also recognize the centrality – and priority – of healthy rational and moral agency. Moreover, the centrality of such agency should be at least an implicit feature of any general discussion of patient-participation.

REFERENCES

American Psychiatric Association. (2013). *Diagnostic and statistical manual of mental disorders* (5th ed.). Arlington, VA: American Psychiatric Publishing.

Aristotle. (2009). The Nicomachean ethics (trans. by L. Brown, ed. by W. D. Ross). Oxford: Oxford University Press.

Beauchamp, T. L., & Childress, J. F. (2012). *Principles of biomedical ethics* (7th ed.). New York: Oxford University Press.

Becker, L. C. (1992). Good Lives: Prolegomena. *Social Philosophy & Policy*, *9*(02), 5–37. doi:10.1017/S0265052500001382

Becker, L. C. (2000). The Good of Agency. In L. P. Francis & A. Silvers (Eds.), *Americans with disabilities: Exploring implications of the law for individuals and institutions* (pp. 54–63). New York: Routledge.

Becker, L. C. (2003). Human Health and Stoic Moral Norms. *The Journal of Medicine and Philosophy*, *28*(2), 221–238. doi:10.1076/jmep.28.2.221.14206 PMID:12943215

Becker, L. C. (2012). *Habilitation, health, and agency: A framework for basic justice*. New York: Oxford University Press. doi:10.1093/acprof:oso/9780199917549.001.0001

Becker, L. C., & Becker, C. B. (2001). *Encyclopedia of ethics* (2nd ed.). New York: Routledge.

Becker, L. C., & Becker, C. B. (2003). *A history of western ethics* (2nd ed.). New York: Routledge. doi:10.4324/9780203426937

Bok, S. (2008). Rethinking the WHO Definition of Health. In K. Heggenhougen & S. Quah (Eds.), *International encyclopedia of public health* (Vol. 6, pp. 590–597). San Diego, CA: Academic Press. doi:10.1016/B978-012373960-5.00550-5

Boorse, C. (1975). On the Distinction between Disease and Illness. *Philosophy & Public Affairs*, *5*(1), 49–68.

Boorse, C. (1976). What a Theory of Mental Health Should Be. *Journal for the Theory of Social Behaviour*, *6*(1), 61–84. doi:10.1111/j.1468-5914.1976.tb00359.x

Boorse, C. (1977). Health as a Theoretical Concept. *Philosophy of Science*, *44*(4), 542–573. doi:10.1086/288768

Boorse, C. (1997). A Rebuttal on Health. In J. Humber & R. Almeder (Eds.), *What is disease?* (pp. 1–134). Totowa, NJ: Humana Press. doi:10.1007/978-1-59259-451-1_1

Cohen, G. A. (1989). On the Currency of Egalitarian Justice. *Ethics*, *99*(4), 906–944. doi:10.1086/293126

Cohen, G. A. (2008). *Rescuing justice and equality*. Cambridge, MA: Harvard University Press. doi:10.4159/9780674029651

Crisp, R. (2013). *The Oxford handbook of the history of ethics*. Oxford: Oxford University Press. doi:10.1093/oxfordhb/9780199545971.001.0001

Daniels, N. (1985). *Just health care*. New York: Cambridge University Press. doi:10.1017/CBO9780511624971

Daniels, N. (2007). *Just health: Meeting health needs fairly*. New York: Cambridge University Press. doi:10.1017/CBO9780511809514

Diamond, J. (2005). *Collapse: How societies choose to fail or succeed*. New York: Viking.

Fleischacker, S. (2004). *A short history of distributive justice*. Cambridge, MA: Harvard University Press.

Humber, J., & Almeder, R. (1997). *What is disease?* Totowa, NJ: Humana Press. doi:10.1007/978-1-59259-451-1

Hume, D. (1978). *Treatise of human nature* (L. A. Selby-Bigge, Ed.). Oxford: Oxford University Press.

Hume, D. (1993). Enquiry concerning the principles of morals (2nd Ed., E. Steinberg). Indianapolis: Hackett Publishing Company.

Jahoda, M. (1958). *Current concepts of positive mental health*. New York: Basic Books. doi:10.1037/11258-000

Jamieson, D. (2013). Constructing Practical Ethics. In R. Crisp (Ed.), *The Oxford handbook of the history of ethics* (pp. 843–866). Oxford University Press.

Keyes, C. L. (2009). Toward a Science of Mental Health. In C. R. Snyder & S. J. Lopez (Eds.), *Oxford handbook of positive psychology* (2nd ed., pp. 89–96). New York: Oxford University Press.

Keyes, C. L., & Annas, J. (2009). Feeling Good and Functioning Well: Distinctive Concepts in Ancient Philosophy and Contemporary Science. *The Journal of Positive Psychology*, *4*(3), 197–201. doi:10.1080/17439760902844228

Kittay, E. (1998). *Love's labor: Essays on women, equality, and dependency*. New York: Routledge.

Korsgaard, C. M. (2008). *The constitution of agency: Essays on practical reason and moral psychology*. New York: Oxford University Press. doi:10.1093/acprof:oso/9780199552733.001.0001

Lafollette, H. (2013). *International encyclopedia of ethics*. Hoboken, NJ: Wiley-Blackwell.

Langer, E. J. (1989). *Mindfulness*. Boston: Perseus Books.

Langer, E. J. (2009). *Counterclockwise: Mindful health and the power of possibility*. New York: Ballantine Books.

Long, A. A. (1986). *Hellenistic Philosophy: Stoics, Epicureans, Sceptics* (2nd ed.). Berkeley: University of California Press.

Mayr, E. (2011). *Understanding human agency*. New York: Oxford University Press. doi:10.1093/acprof:oso/9780199606214.001.0001

McIntyre, A. (2006). *A short history of ethics* (2nd ed.). New York: Routledge.

McIntyre, A. (2007). *After virtue* (3rd ed.). South Bend, IN: Notre Dame Press.

Metcalfe, J., & Terrace, H. S. (2013). *Agency and joint attention*. New York: Oxford University Press. doi:10.1093/acprof:oso/9780199988341.001.0001

Nussbaum, M. C. (2000). *Women and human development: The capabilities approach*. New York: Cambridge University Press. doi:10.1017/CBO9780511841286

Nussbaum, M. C. (2007). *Frontiers of justice*. Cambridge, MA: The Belknap Press of Harvard University Press.

Nussbaum, M. C. (2011). *Creating capabilities: The human development approach*. Cambridge, MA: The Belknap Press of Harvard University Press. doi:10.4159/harvard.9780674061200

Okin, S. M. (1989). *Gender, justice, and the family*. New York: Basic Books.

Peterson, C., & Seligman, M. (2004). *Character strengths and virtues: A handbook and classification*. New York: Oxford University Press.

Plato. (2002). Five dialogues (trans. by J. M. Cooper, ed. by G. M. Grube). Indianapolis, IN: Hackett Publishing Company.

Plato, . (2004). *Republic* (C.D. Reeve, Trans.). Indianapolis, IN: Hackett Publishing Company.

Rawls, J. (1971). *A theory of justice*. Cambridge, MA: The Belknap Press of Harvard University Press.

Segall, S. (2010). *Health, luck, and justice*. Princeton, NJ: Princeton University Press.

Sen, A. (2009). *The idea of justice*. Cambridge, MA: The Belknap Press of Harvard University Press.

Sidgwick, H. (1902). *Outlines of the history of ethics* (4th ed.). London: Macmillan.

Simmons, L. A., Wolever, R. Q., Bechard, E. M., & Snyderman, R. (2014). Patient engagement as a risk factor in personalized health care: A systematic review of the literature on chronic disease. *Genome Medicine*, *6*(2), 1–21. doi:10.1186/gm533 PMID:24571651

Singer, P. (2011). *Practical Ethics* (3rd ed.). New York: Cambridge University Press. doi:10.1017/CBO9780511975950

Snyder, C. R., & Lopez, S. J. (2009). *Oxford handbook of positive psychology* (2nd ed.). New York: Oxford University Press.

Thórarinsdóttir, K., & Kristjánsson, K. (2014). Patients' perspectives on person-centred participation in healthcare: A framework analysis. *Nursing Ethics*, *21*(2), 129–147. doi:10.1177/0969733013490593 PMID:23812560

Vaillant, G. (2003). Mental health. *The American Journal of Psychiatry*, *160*(8), 1373–1384. doi:10.1176/appi.ajp.160.8.1373 PMID:12900295

Zelazo, P. D. (2013). *The oxford handbook of developmental psychology*. Oxford: Oxford University Press.

KEY TERMS AND DEFINITIONS

Agency, Agent, Agentic: The ability to function as an active, conscious subject in various causal chains of events by trying to start, stop, modify, or otherwise control such events.

Basic Good Health: Reliably competent physiological and psychological functioning in a given range of physical and social environments; the absence of ill health combined with the presence of the physical and psychological powers and strengths necessary for recovering from ill health, and resisting a relapse into it.

Empirical Ethics: Ethics informed by empirical work in history and the human sciences.

Ethics, Ethical Theory, Philosophical Ethics: A central field of philosophy devoted to examining questions about what moral agents ought to do and be, all things considered, and offering thoroughgoing reasoned justifications for fundamental ethical goals, duties, rights, virtues, and good lives; classically understood to include social and political philosophy, and thus theories of justice.

Habilitation: Equipping an individual, including oneself, or aspects of the physical and social environment, with functional abilities, capabilities, or capacities.

Health, Complete Health: The absence of physical and psychological ill health combined with the presence of the physical and psychological powers, strengths, and traits necessary for active, effective agency.

Healthy Agency: Reliably competent physiological and psychological *agentic* functioning in a given range of environments.

Moral Agency, Agent: A form of complex rational agency characterized by the presence of prosocial dispositions corresponding to ethical virtues, and an appreciation of agentic accountability for individual actions, including self-habilitation.

Normative Ethics: Substantive ethical theory; the part of ethics devoted to getting a philosophical account of good, right, and virtue that will yield general goals, principles, rules, and ideals for moral agents.

Practical Ethics: General guidance from philosophical ethics about what various *types* of moral agents ought to do and be in various *types* of cases; such guidance derived by reasoning from a given normative ethical theory or a combination of them, together with practical realities.

Practical Moral Agency: A form of agentic ability and activity that is not pursued within one specific ethical theory alone, but is instead pursued in terms of the normative elements such theories have in common, together with an appreciation of practical possibilities.

Rational Agency: A form of agentic ability and activity in which practical intelligence prioritizes goals, organizes goal-directed activity in a coherent and effective manner in both nonstrategic and strategic situations, and effectively translates goods, goals, preferences, and deliberative decisions into coherently planned action.

Chapter 2
The Patient-Centered Medicine as the Theoretical Framework for Patient Engagement

Borghi Lidia
University of Milan, Italy

Galli Federica
University of Milan, Italy

Vegni Elena Anna Maria
University of Milan, Italy

ABSTRACT

The present contribution will describe the origin, development and main characteristics of the patient-centered medicine; the literature on patient-centeredness, in particular in the field of chronic disorders, will be discussed and the importance of this approach underlined; arguments about the importance of patient-centered medicine as theoretical frame founding and supporting the concept of patient engagement will be highlighted, considering that only within this medical epistemology the patient's engagement can find a full and complete expression.

INTRODUCTION

Engagement is a relatively new concept, as far as the healthcare system is concerned. Its application is very interesting and useful in a variety of different health contexts, not only in regard to patient care, such as the management of chronic diseases, but also as a possible concept at an organizational level. The issue of "patient engagement" is often linked to other concepts as those of patient activation, patient participation, patient's adherence, and patient empowerment. The term is frequently used to convey different meanings and a unique definition is missing. The aim of this chapter is to introduce a theoretical discussion of the concept connecting it, in a pure conceptual view, to the framework of patient-centered medicine (PCM). In our view, a fruitful and actual patient engagement may be better realized within

DOI: 10.4018/978-1-4666-9992-2.ch002

the theoretical framework of the PCM. It is difficult to conceive the engagement of a patient without considering the existence of at least two actors playing in a healthcare context, in a communicative and relational exchange. The importance of engaging patient and the ways to reach this involvement could not be seen out of the doctor-patient relationship. To support this view, we will describe the origin of PCM, its conceptual evolution, and the related practice in order to better involve patients in the management of their illness conditions. Patients are increasingly facing with multiple chronic disorders (comorbidity) and more and more aware of their rights; moreover an increased lay health literacy favor a more conscious public of people not passive but actively requiring to the health care system. This (r) evolution in the domain of care concerned all the western healthcare organizations all over the recent years, generating new issues both at the level of doctor-patient relationship and at organizational level (public health systems). We will discuss PCM and patient engagement in this modified environment. But, because the relations between doctor and patient is a core issue in the theoretical framework of PCM, the patient engagement may be reached in a relational view only assuming the PCM as a conceptual setting of the medical practice.

BACKGROUND

Patient centered medicine is above all a revolution in medicine, a method that changes the way of practicing medicine, the way in which physicians communicate and relate with their patients during medical consultations and the role that these two actors play within the visit. It originated and spread from North America and northern Europe during the 1970s.

This way of relating to a patient has its roots on the theoretical thinking of two British psychoanalysts Michael Balint and his wife Edin, who coined the term "patient-centered medicine" in 1969. Balint (1969) wrote "there is another way of medical thinking which we call 'patient-centered medicine'. Here, in addition to trying to discover a localizable illness or illnesses, the doctor also has to examine the whole person in order to form what we call an 'overall diagnosis'. This should include everything the doctor knows and understands about his patient; the patient, in fact, has to be understood as a unique human-being. The illness which can be described in terms of a 'traditional diagnosis' is either an incident like a broken leg, or a part like accident proneness which makes better sense if understood in terms of the whole" (Balint, 1969).

Balint, as a psychoanalyst, described a form of psycho-therapeutic intervention that general practitioners could use for people who had disorders that were partially or wholly psychosomatic; but the revolution in her thoughts and words went beyond: a new way of understanding the complaints reported by the patients, not in terms of pathology, but in terms of the unique individuality of the patient was described (Balint, 1957). In this sense, the new concept contrasted with the "doctor-centered care", by allowing patients more control of the medical visit, and from "disease-centered care", by focusing not only on the disease but also on the patient who suffers (Bensing, 2000).

The development of this method should be viewed in light of a revolution in the model of medicine, an epistemological change shifting the science of medicine from a biological reductionist approach - the biomedical model - to a bio-psychosocial point of view. This shift was theorized by the American psychiatrist George L. Engel, who in 1977 posited a new epistemological paradigm expanding the biomedical model. The bio-psychosocial perspective (Engel, 1977, 1981) constitutes the theoretical frame of patient-centered medicine, presenting it as a broadening of the scope of medicine from organic disease, focused on diagnosis and treatment, to also encompass the patient's experience of disease. In the bio-psychosocial model (Engel, 1977, 1981), disorders are conceptualized as existing at a number of interacting, hierarchical levels (from biological to psychological and social levels). According to this point of view, every patient has a story that demonstrates the interactions among the biologic, psychological, and social components of his or her life.

Engel (1977) wrote that the bio-psychosocial model would "take into account the patient, the social context in which he lives, and the complementary system devised by society to deal with the disruptive effects of illness".

These changes in the medical epistemology have significant impacts on the clinical method with a shifting from disease-centered to patient-centered perspective.

The disease-centered method has been, so far, the dominant model in medical practice; as previously stated, it is based on the biomedical paradigm in which patients' reports of their medical conditions are read as the expression of disease processes and the clinical method focuses on identifying standard disease entities and numeric entities, and on this basis proposes an evidence based therapeutic treatment. This clinical method has several strengths according to McWhinney (1989, 1993): it is simple, clear, verifiable and allows not only formulation of diagnostic hypotheses but, as the disease is the effect of a cause that is biologically identifiable and given the constancy of the cause-effect relations, also allows clinicians to identify a prognosis. Nevertheless, in the past few years, it has been criticized for oversimplifying the problems of illness, assuming that disease is fully accounted for by deviations from the norm of measurable biological variables and not taking into account the patient's perspective.

Development of the concept of patient-centeredness is closely linked to these perceived limitations in the disease-centered method of practicing medicine. As we have discussed above, patient-centered medicine gives clinicians a more complex goal to achieve during the process of caring for the patient.

The complexity is the result of various factors. First, it considers the patient as a unique person with his/her own experience of the disease and with an active role in the care process; it integrates the traditional understanding of disease with each patient's point of view on his condition, moving from TO CURE the disease centered medicine TO CARE. As Kleinman (1989) stated, beyond the dimension of the "disease", intended as the doctor's understanding of the biomedical disorders, there is the "illness", that refers to the patient's subjective experience of feeling sick. Patient-centered medicine deals with the non-biological aspects of the disease: even personal, psychological and social aspects are recognized as current and important, so that the tasks of the consultation are focusing not only on disease but also on the "patient agenda", his/her personal illness experience, which may be broken down into four main factors (his/her feelings, his/her ideas about the illness, the impact of his/her problems on his life, his/her expectations about what should be done and his desires) (Moja & Vegni, 2000).

Secondly, the patient-centered method suggests that communication and relational skills and techniques are a core professional competence to be used by clinicians; for example, interviewing skills and communication techniques are proposed in order to achieve the comprehension of the patient's agenda, e.g. attentive listening, open questions, paraphrasing and asking for understanding.

Thirdly, it also takes into account the perspective of the physician with the own emotional experience.

These concepts outline that the main differences between the two clinical methods are played out in the context of the doctor-patient relationship, where the content and style of the relationship is defined as "an abstraction embodying the activities of two interacting systems (persons)" (Szasz & Hollender, 1956). The relationship between doctor and patient is no longer a means to make a diagnosis, but it becomes the aim of the medicine itself. The relationship is recognized as part of a process where the patient is the protagonist, the only true expert of his own health.

So it can be said that a clinical consultation that is patient-centered elicits and explores patients' expectations, feelings, and illness beliefs, and tries to activate the patient to take some control in the medical visit (Platt et al., 2001).

The patient-centered perspective promotes changes not only in the field of the clinical practice, but also, in the fields of education and research. In particular, new modes of teaching and learning, e.g., the use of role-playing and videotaping, are proposed as tools necessary for real understanding of the importance of doctor-patient communications and relationships. In the field of research, and in particular in the outcome of research, the evaluation of the results of health interventions in clinical practice, patient-centered medicine has been the basis of various studies quantifying the state of health, not only through clinical outcomes but also through measurements of outcomes reported by the patient - the so-called patient-reported outcomes. Ample literature has found associations between the patient-centered model of communication and patient satisfaction (Kinmonth, Woodcock, Griffin, Spiegal, & Campbell, 1998; Kinnersley, Stott, Peters, & Harvey, 1999; Rosenberg, Lussier, & Beaudoin, 1997; Williams, Weinman, & Dale, 1998; McMillan et al., 2013; Rathert, Wyrwich, & Boren, 2012), treatment adherence (Rosenberg et al., 1997; Safran et al., 1998; Street, Makoul, Arora, & Epstein, 2009), medical outcomes (Arora, 2003; Kaplan, Greenfield, & Ware, 1989; Maisiak, Austin, West, & Heck, 1996; Rao, Weinberger, & Kroenke, 2000; Rosenberg et al., 1997; Robinson, Callister, Berry, & Dearing, 2008; Ekman et al., 2012) and decreased rates of malpractice claims (Levinson, Roter, Mullooly, Dull, & Frankel, 1997). Furthermore, clinician failure to elicit and discuss patient expectations predicts dissatisfaction with the visit and the persistence of symptoms (Jackson, Kroenke, & Chamberlin, 1999; Kravitz, Callahan, Azari, Antonius, & Lewis, 1997).

A synthetic overview of this long and ongoing process may be that PCM grounds on the biopsychosocial context, and lies on the exploration of the so-called patient's agenda (the interplay of ideas and interpretations, expectations and desires, feelings and personal context the patient brings with him/her during the medical encounter) by the mean of specific communication techniques (Moja & Vegni, 2001). The achievement of such professional skills between doctor and patient is the outcome of structured educational/academic interventions. Academic curriculum or post-graduate education should be planned taking into consideration such a goal (Street & de Haes, 2013). Unfortunately, the Italian context is not representative of a widespread and common training on communication skills for health professionals (with some rare exception), while in English speaking countries this issue is widely addressed (e.g., Fortin, Dwamena, Frankel, & Smith, 2012; Stewart et al., 2003). Within this scenario, the contribution to the spread of patient-centered medicine has been led by the new challenges the healthcare system has to face and the new outcomes the medicine has to deal with.

CHRONICITY AND MULTIMORBIDITY: NEW CHALLENGES FOR MEDICINE

Besides cultural and epistemological changes, there are other important factors and contemporary forces that have bolstered the shift towards the origin of the patient-centered method within the wider bio-psychosocial paradigm transformation. The growing demands for quality and safety in health care have refocused attention on patient outcomes. Moreover, the shift stems from the attempt to cut health care costs and is expressed in particular in the field of general practice. For example, in the United States, serious concerns about the excessive price of medical care have resulted in consideration of whether shifting care from the subspecialist to the primary care physician could reduce costs (Bardes, 2012). Last but not least, and probably most interesting as far as this contribution is concerned, the increase in prevalence and incidence of chronic disease, as well as the increase of the aging population, played a crucial role in the need for a new medical model.

Chronic conditions are defined as illnesses that last longer than three months and are not self-limiting. Common examples of chronic conditions are diabetes, asthma, congestive heart failure, stroke, low back pain and arthritis. Most of these diseases have major physical, psychological, social and financial consequences and impact the lives of individuals and their families in many ways. From the societal perspective, chronic diseases are a major source of health care utilization (Vlieland, 2002). At a younger age, chronic conditions are increasing also as consequence of the development of specialized pediatric intensive care unit care (PICU). On one hand, PICU contributed to the improved survival rates for critically ill children, but on the other historical data suggest that pediatric critical care may have exchanged mortality for morbidity over the last several decades, with a prevalence of new morbidity that is 4.8%, twice the mortality rate (Pollack et al., 2014). In the most cases, the transition from childhood/adolescent care to adult care is guaranteed.

In all developed countries, chronic conditions are spreading as consequence of the increase of the aging population (Beaglehole et al., 2008; Wiederhold, Riva, & Graffigna, 2013). On adults, data from US report that nearly half of the adult population is affected from chronic conditions with one-fourth of all adults have multiple (2 or more) chronic conditions (Ward, 2013). In the US population, studies projecting the prevalence of chronic conditions in upcoming years estimate an increase of diabetes by more than 80 percent, of Parkinson's disease by 30 percent and Alzheimer is projected to increase by 40 percent. The National Cancer Institute projects that by 2020 there will 30 percent cancer survivors more than in 2010 (Dall et al., 2013).

A chronic medical condition is often comorbid with other medical and/or psychopathological disorder(s): it has been demonstrated that over 50% of depressed patients show multiple chronic medical conditions as well (Wells, Rogers, Burnam, Greenfield, & Ware Jr, 1991), with additional consequences for health care services and primary care providers for costs, treatment planning and outcome. Multi-morbidity has been defined as the "most common chronic condition", and its prevalence progressively increases with age, affecting more than 60% of people aged 65 or older (Barnett et al., 2013).

These conditions result in numerous adverse health outcomes, increased health care needs, and subsequently higher medical costs. These patients are more likely to be admitted to hospital, have poorer quality of life, and receive multiple drugs with consequent difficulties in adherence (Marengoni et al., 2011). In the past, strategies have focused on preventing and ameliorating a single disease at a time; however, the large percentage of people with two or more conditions, or multiple chronic conditions, has added a level of complexity to developing intervention strategies. Moreover, the presence of physical and mental multi-morbidity also significantly impacts the costs of health care, with estimates of increasing costs by at least 45% for each person with a chronic physical disease and a co-morbid mental health problem (Naylor et al., 2012).

Patients with multi-morbidity have the most complex health needs, but due to the traditional disease-oriented approach in healthcare, they risk facing highly fragmented care that may lead to partial, ineffective, and potentially inadequate interventions.

As illustrated above, health care systems around the world have been worldwide modeled around the epistemology of the disease model. This presumes a series of assumptions such as: organ or system-based pathology cause disease, symptoms are "caused" by the underlying disease, the treatment is focused on removing the underlying cause of pathology and it is identical for everyone. The patient is simply the holder of the disease, which is the same for everyone. The doctor is the only holder of the medical knowledge to be transmitted to the patient, in a hierarchical way. This approach to disease fails to detect differences in patients' needs, does not take into account patient expectations, beliefs, impact on function, quality of life and his/her relational and inner world. The traditional disease-oriented approach does not take into account the overall health status of patients with multi-morbidity, since it is focused on a single disease and neglecting fundamental aspects of health, like frailty and functional ability as well as cognitive and affective state.

It is immediately clear how chronic diseases are extremely complex and how they can be better understood within a bio-psychosocial perspective, and therefore, that the most suitable clinical method to approach chronic disease is the patient-centered method. In this complex context new approaches to improve care are needed, with the aim to diminish suffering of patients, improving their quality of life and satisfaction of the clinicians, and the concept of engagement seems to be particularly promising in this model.

DRAWING THE ROADMAP TOWARDS PATIENT ENGAGEMENT, PATIENT-CENTRED MEDICINE AND CHRONIC DISEASE

We know that the patient-centred approach is built on several premises such as the fact that patients often do not seek healthcare only because a symptom, that usually bring more than one concern to their clinicians, that empathic communication allows patients to experience the clinician's compassionate presence (Fortin et al., 2012). Setting up the clinical interview in a way attuned with the emotional and personal status of the patient is the *sine qua non* of the patient-centred approach, the fast track in the direction of patient engagement. This is exceedingly true in the case of chronic disorders (Eaton, Roberts, & Turner, 2015), when the patient is usually older and forced to cope with multiple disabling conditions.

The increase of chronic disease and multi-morbidity poses new questions and challenges to the traditional health system and doctor-patient relationship. Complexity of care in patients with multi-morbidity requires the involvement of a large number of healthcare providers and resources. Rethinking the doctor-patient relationship based on the traditional disease-centered model by shifting to a patient-centered model may be the common ground for promoting new methods for care management. The Picker Institute (Gerteis, Edgman-Levitan, Daley, & Delbanco, 1993) in partnership with patients and families, conducted a multiyear research project and identified eight characteristics of care as the most important indicators of quality and safety, from the patients' perspective: respect for the patient's values, preferences, and expressed needs; coordinated and integrated care; clear, high-quality information and education for the patient and family; physical comfort, including pain management; emotional support and alleviation of fear and anxiety; involvement of family members and friends, as appropriate; continuity, including through care-site transitions; and access to care. Care that achieves these goals is deemed to be patient-centered (Mead & Bower, 2000).

We consider the patient-centredness as "the" method to be used in each doctor-patient encounter, the essential tool in the hands of the health professionals towards a fruitful PE, mostly in the case of chronic disorders. De Haes (2006) brilliantly evidenced some different meanings and conceptual background of the PCM, outlining the importance of tailoring care according to patient's peculiarities. Communication in the medical encounter has several functions: building relationships, information gathering, information provision, making decisions, responding to emotions, managing uncertainty and last, but not least, enabling patient self-management (Moja & Vegni, 2000; Street & De Haes, 2013). We wonder if it might be useful to tailor PCM interventions bearing in mind some characteristics of the patients' adjustment to the illness course towards a better PE.

As we pointed out, there is no shared consensus on the definition of patient engagement, but the general consensus is that it is related to the importance of taking an active role in one's health, having knowledge, skills, and confidence to manage health/chronic conditions and performing health-promoting behaviors. The term "engagement" is also used in very different contexts as marketing and consumer behavior literature to describe the attitude of a consumer toward a brand, product, service, or even media event (Gambetti & Graffigna, 2010).The adoption of the term engagement in the healthcare field is recent and indicates a renewed partnership between patient and healthcare professional involved in the health and care management (Hibbard, Stockard, Mahoney, & Tusler, 2004; Coulter, 2012).

The difficulties in the definition of PE are related to the existence of several constructs having indefinite boundaries or handled interchangeably because not having (often) a clear-cut definition: shared decision making, patient participation, involvement, empowerment or activation, self-management, compliance or adherence are examples of constructs linked to PE, but not exhaustive of the meaning we confer to PE. We agree with Graffigna, Barello and Triberti (2015b) that PE is an umbrella concept encompassing all the previous definitions, without replacing them (Barello & Graffigna, 2015).

The role of patient engagement in chronic disease care is increasingly being cited as critical for improving health outcomes and reducing costs. A recent review of the literature on chronic diseases and patient engagement (Simmons, Wolever, Bechard, & Snyderman, 2014) supported the link between improved outcomes and patient engagement, demonstrating that relatively short interventions can increase and promote positive health outcomes. Moreover, specific behavioral targets and their tracking appear essential to assess the role of patient engagement over time to achieve positive health outcomes. In contrast, poor patient engagement is a risk factor for worse chronic disease outcomes. In this framework, early identification of individuals who are low in patient engagement coupled with tailored behavioral interventions to enhance participation may provide a reasonable and low cost target for personalized health care innovation (Simmons et al., 2014). In other words, the adjustment of a patient to changed health conditions is a long and complex psychological process where the personality, the age, the familial, social and cultural context of life of *that* patient play a critical role.

Graffigna et al. (2015b) described patient engagement as the final outcome of a long process encompassing emotional, cognitive, and behavioral reframing of the patient's health condition (PHE model), where the success of each phase depends on the success of the previous one. In the last phase of the model the patients successfully reframed the pathological condition, incorporating it into their life projects, where they are no longer overwhelmed by their health conditions. By our perspective, it is difficult to think that the engagement of the patient can be realised without passing through an empathic dyadic exchange realised in healthcare contexts, without a sound patient-doctor alliance, and overlooking the building of a trustworthy relationship. The patient-centred medicine may be seen as characterised by two main streams (Liberati et al., 2015): the first one is *dyadic* and pertains to the more traditional stream belonging to the approach having as main objective the exploration both of patient's objective disease and symptoms and their subjective illness experience (patient's agenda). The second one is *organiza-*

tional and is addressed to identify organizational and system-level facilitators of and barriers to PCC. Both could be an interesting and valuable frames within which to conceptualize the patient engagement. But, to address our main aim in this contribution, the conceptual grounding of patient engagement in the context of a patient-centredness medicine, we focus on the dyadic, relational view of PCM exploring its fundamental role to reach a fruitful and real engagement of the patient.

The Patient Health Engagement (PHM) model (Graffigna et al., 2015b) suggests that the patients steadily get over changes in their health condition through the so-called "patient journey". It means that the patient adjusts to a changed health condition through a process articulated in four steps characterised by specific emotional, behavioural and cognitive factors. The first one is the "Black out": the patient in this stage appears overwhelmed by the illness experience, blocked and with a passive attitude toward the healthcare system (e.g., it might be preferred a paternalistic approach by the physician). In the second step, the patient is in "Arousal": it means to be "hyper-attentive" to every signal in their body, but also to be better informed about their health condition, even though in a superficial manner and in a way that does not allow the self-management of their disease and treatment. The third step is the "Adhesion": the patient acquires a broader spectrum of behavioural skills to cope with their illness, starting to perceive the importance of their role. The final step is the "Eudaimonic project": the patients fully accept their condition, are no more overwhelmed by illness and are prone to become "partner" with the healthcare system in managing the changed health condition.

Health professionals should always bear in mind the existence of a process of psychological modification and adaptation to changed health conditions, and PE might be better realised if grounded on the different steps of this process on the basis of PCM framework, considering 1) The other (the patient) as a necessary subject of information regarding the personal and changing perspective about being ill; 2) The necessary relational and communication skills tailored on the basis of the patient journey; and 3) Taking into account the relevance of the physician's inner experience of being with a patient who will never recover. A possible challenge in the connection between the patient engagement journey and the patient centred medicine may be that of conceptualizing a specific way of interacting with the patient (goal to reach, communication skills to use, personal reaction of the doctor) during each stage of the journey as it has been done as far as the concept of process of patient education with his/her motivational levels and readiness to act (Prochaska & Di Clemente, 1982; Grüninger, 1995). In each critical point of the patient engagement during a chronic illness the principles of PCM could represent a guide for the physician's work with patients. Communication skills are the principal way in the direction of decoding and labelling the psychological state of *that* patient in *that* clinical situation. Communication skills may be taught, learnt and practised, and most of all may aid the identification of the stage the patient is experiencing and his/her agenda to tailor every exchange we have with the specific characteristics of *that* patient, always in the direction of PE. If the patient is allocated in the "black-out" stage any attempt towards active engagement may result ineffectual. In that stage, the patient seems to be overwhelmed by emotions: it is not the time for acting, planning, giving statistics. It is the time to dedicate a lot of effort to empathic reflection, stating partnership, legitimating and respectful support. We have to wait the awkward transition to the "Arousal" stage to broaden the repertoire of communicative skills and techniques: tactful questioning skills (we recommend in this stage open questions), facilitation and active listening, eliciting patients view of the problem, surveying the field may be very useful in this stage to accompany the patient to shift from passive to active role in the coping with illness. With the transition to "Adhesion" the patients are gradually more aware of the primary role to undertake in coping with illness: it may be especially helpful negotiating priorities, focusing and more directive comments. Once it has been reached the final stage of the "Eudaimonic project" probing, challenging, checking back and summarizing have to be used to strengthen the active role of the patients and their complete and informed engagement. The connection between PCM and PE seems to be a promising practical way to discover, giving achievable goals in the doctor-patient relations and interesting challenges for clinical and experimental research.

SOLUTIONS, RECOMMENDATIONS AND FUTURE DIRECTIONS

Facing the new challenges that are arising in health care, such as the spread of chronic disease, aging population, the need of reducing health care costs, and looking at the possible answers as the health resource optimization and the spread of good health practice, the concept of patient engagement may be a keystone.

Achieving effective patient engagement could reduce health care costs in the sense that patients would decrease the demand for check-ups or general practitioner consultations, or the phenomenon of doctor shopping because of being better able to manage their own disease and treatment and to implement good health practices.

In this context, the promotion of patient activation and satisfaction, treatment adherence, and medical outcomes are critical issues, in particular when dealing with chronically ill patients, and are concepts intimately related to patient engagement, that we consider an umbrella concept encompassing several meanings and objectives that may be reached through the aid of PCM.

Nevertheless, in the opinion of the authors, all of these concepts remain "orphan" without the conceptual framework of patient-centered medicine, that means *in primis* tailored care accordingly to the exploration of the patient's agenda by specific communication techniques. Only within a patient-centered method of care a fruitful engagement can be fully realized. Patient-centered medicine entails a shifting by the classical outcomes (e.g. adherence, patient satisfaction) to new ones, such as promoting an active role of the patients in their healthcare or evaluating patient engagement, to allow a real full share-decision making and to facilitate health literacy. Helping patients to be more active in medical consultations change centuries of physician-dominated dialogues to dialogues that engage patients as active participants. This change has become possible thanks to the epistemological, clinical and methodological revolution brought in by patient-centered medicine. In regards to the health system, the adoption of a patient-centered care entails a review of the educational system in healthcare to achieve a patient-centered working method. Patient-centered methods of care could be taught in the context of structured training programs.

Lines of research for the future should go in the direction of measuring patient engagement after the fulfillment of patient-centered interventions. It opens to several lines of research considering all the different constructs PE is made, the steps the patients experience in the adjustment process to chronic illness and the different instruments the PCM makes available to health professionals. To the best of our knowledge, no study has been conducted that correlates measurements of patient engagement, such as the Patient Activation Measure (PAM) (Hibbard et al., 2004) or the Patient Health Engagement (PHE) (that is the first instrument specifically aimed to measure engagement) (Graffigna, Barello, Bonanomi, & Lozza, 2015a), with classic measures of patient-centeredness, like the Roter Interaction Analysis System (RIAS) (Roter, 1991; Roter & Larson, 2002) or the Patient Centred Score Sheet (PCSS) (Henbest & Stewart, 1989). If patient engagement will found to be directly associated with measures of patient-centeredness, it could be supported the authors' hypothesis of considering PE as a new goal for PCM.

Another important field for future research, in a framework shifting from and individual to a familiar and societal context, is to consider what means to engage a third party in the care process and how this may be inserted in a patient-centered visit. In particular conditions, as the frail elderly, diseases that severely limit individual capacity and autonomy (e.g., dementia), and pediatric conditions, the role of the third party becomes more and more crucial: in these particular conditions engaging the caregivers in the patients' journey is a new challenge and try to achieve this goal within a patient-centered clinical consultation seems to be not enough: consultations should become also caregiver-centered and familiar-centered in a wider, social perspective.

CONCLUSION

If PE represents a new goal for the medicine, the PCM may be considered an epistemological framework towards this objective. The public healthcare system may benefit in terms of reduction of costs: engaged patients in a patient-centered perspective are more satisfied, more compliant, less prone to instigate legal action in case of medical error, more engaged in their social context, and so on. New lines of research entails the measurement of PE and PCM, and the promotion of good health practices in the framework of patient-centered consultations, assessing the impact on outcomes, both in clinical, patient-reported and social terms.

REFERENCES

Arora, N. K. (2003). Interacting with cancer patients: The significance of physicians' communication behavior. *Social Science & Medicine*, *57*(5), 791–806. doi:10.1016/S0277-9536(02)00449-5 PMID:12850107

Balint, E. (1969). The possibilities of patient-centred medicine. *The British Journal of General Practice*, *17*(82), 269–276. PMID:5770926

Balint, M. (1957). *The doctor, his patient and the illness*. London: Tavistock Publications.

Bardes, C. L. (2012). Defining "patient-centered medicine". *The New England Journal of Medicine*, *366*(9), 782–783. doi:10.1056/NEJMp1200070 PMID:22375968

Barello, S., & Graffigna, G. (2015). Patient engagement in healthcare: Pathways for effective medical decision making. *Neuropsychological Trends*, *17*(1), 53–65. doi:10.7358/neur-2015-017-bare

Barnett, K., Mercer, S. W., Norbury, M., Watt, G., Wyke, S., & Guthrie, B. (2012). Epidemiology of multimorbidity and implications for health care, research, and medical education: A cross-sectional study. *Lancet*, *380*(9836), 37–43. doi:10.1016/S0140-6736(12)60240-2 PMID:22579043

Beaglehole, R., Epping-Jordan, J., Patel, V., Chopra, M., Ebrahim, S., Kidd, M., & Haines, A. (2008). Improving the prevention and management of chronic disease in low-income and middle-income countries: A priority for primary health care. *Lancet*, *372*(9642), 940–949. doi:10.1016/S0140-6736(08)61404-X PMID:18790317

Bensing, J. (2000). Bridging the gap.: The separate worlds of evidence-based medicine and patient-centered medicine. *Patient Education and Counseling*, *39*(1), 17–25. doi:10.1016/S0738-3991(99)00087-7 PMID:11013544

Coulter, A. (2012). Patient engagement—what works? *The Journal of Ambulatory Care Management*, *35*(2), 80–89. doi:10.1097/JAC.0b013e318249e0fd PMID:22415281

Dall, T. M., Gallo, P. D., Chakrabarti, R., West, T., Semilla, A. P., & Storm, M. V. (2013). An aging population and growing disease burden will require a large and specialized health care workforce by 2025. *Health Affairs*, *32*(11), 2013–2020. doi:10.1377/hlthaff.2013.0714 PMID:24191094

De Haes, H. (2006). Dilemmas in patient centerdness and shared decision making: A case for vulnerability. *Patient Education and Counseling*, *62*(3), 291–298. doi:10.1016/j.pec.2006.06.012 PMID:16859860

Eaton, S., Roberts, S., & Turner, B. (2015). Delivering person centred care in long term conditions. *British Medical Journal*, *350*(feb10 14), 181. doi:10.1136/bmj.h181 PMID:25670186

Ekman, I., Wolf, A., Olsson, L. E., Taft, C., Dudas, K., Schaufelberger, M., & Swedberg, K. (2012). Effects of person-centred care in patients with chronic heart failure: The PCC-HF study. *European Heart Journal*, *33*(9), 1112–1119. doi:10.1093/eurheartj/ehr306 PMID:21926072

Engel, G. L. (1977). The need for a new medical model: A challenge for biomedicine. *Science*, *196*(4286), 129–136. doi:10.1126/science.847460 PMID:847460

Engel, G. L. (1981). The clinical application of the biopsychosocial model. *The Journal of Medicine and Philosophy*, *6*(2), 101–124. doi:10.1093/jmp/6.2.101 PMID:7264472

Fortin, A. H., Dwamena, F. C., Frankel, R. M., & Smith, R. C. (2012). *Smith's Patient Centered Interviewing: An Evidence-Based Method: An Evidence-Based Method*. McGraw Hill Professional.

Gambetti, R. C., & Graffigna, G. (2010). The concept of engagement: A systematic analysis of the ongoing marketing debate. *International Journal of Market Research*, *52*(6), 7. doi:10.2501/S147078531020166

Gerteis, M., Edgman-Levitan, S., Daley, J., & Delbanco, T. (1993). *Through the patient's eyes: Understanding and Promoting Patient-Centered Care Paperback*. San Francisco: Jossey-Bass.

Graffigna, G., Barello, S., Bonanomi, A., & Lozza, E. (2015a). Measuring patient engagement: Development and psychometric properties of the patient health engagement (PHE) scale. *Frontiers in Psychology*, 2015, 6. PMID:25870566

Graffigna, G., Barello, S., & Triberti, S. (2015b). *Patient engagement: a consumer-centered model to innovate healthcare*. Warsaw, Poland: DeGruyter Open. doi:10.1515/9783110452440

Grüninger, U. J. (1995). Patient education: An example of one-to-one communication. *Journal of Human Hypertension*, *9*(1), 15–25. PMID:7730996

Henbest, R. J., & Stewart, M. A. (1989). Patient-centredness in the consultation. 1: A method for measurement. *Family Practice*, *6*(4), 249–253. doi:10.1093/fampra/6.4.249 PMID:2632300

Hibbard, J. H., Stockard, J., Mahoney, E. R., & Tusler, M. (2004). Development of the Patient Activation Measure (PAM): Conceptualizing and measuring activation in patients and consumers. *Health Services Research, 39*(4p14 Part 1), 1005–1026. doi:10.1111/j.1475-6773.2004.00269.x PMID:15230939

Jackson, J. L., Kroenke, K., & Chamberlin, J. (1999). Effects of physician awareness of symptom-related expectations and mental disorders: A controlled trial. *Archives of Family Medicine, 8*(2), 135–142. doi:10.1001/archfami.8.2.135 PMID:10101984

Kaplan, S. H., Greenfield, S., & Ware, J. E. Jr. (1989). Assessing the effects of physician-patient interactions on the outcomes of chronic disease. *Medical Care, 27*(3 Suppl.), S110–S127. doi:10.1097/00005650-198903001-00010 PMID:2646486

Kinmonth, A. L., Woodcock, A., Griffin, S., Spiegal, N., & Campbell, M. J. (1998). Randomised controlled trial of patient centred care of diabetes in general practice: Impact on current wellbeing and future disease risk. *British Medical Journal, 317*(7167), 1202–1208. doi:10.1136/bmj.317.7167.1202 PMID:9794859

Kinnersley, P., Stott, N., Peters, T. J., & Harvey, I. (1999). The patient-centredness of consultations and outcome in primary care. *The British Journal of General Practice, 49*(446), 711–716. PMID:10756612

Kleinman, A. (1989). *The illness narratives: suffering, healing, and the human condition.* New York: Basic Books.

Kravitz, R. L., Callahan, E. J., Azari, R., Antonius, D., & Lewis, C. E. (1997). Assessing patients' expectations in ambulatory medical practice. *Journal of General Internal Medicine, 12*(1), 67–72. doi:10.1007/s11606-006-0010-6 PMID:9034949

Levinson, W., Roter, D. L., Mullooly, J. P., Dull, V. T., & Frankel, R. M. (1997). Physician-patient communication: The relationship with malpractice claims among primary care physicians and surgeons. *Journal of the American Medical Association, 277*(7), 553–559. doi:10.1001/jama.1997.03540310051034 PMID:9032162

Liberati, E. G., Gorli, M., Moja, L., Galuppo, L., Ripamonti, S., & Scaratti, G. (2015). Exploring the practice of patient centered care: The role of ethnography and reflexivity. *Social Science & Medicine, 133*, 45–52. doi:10.1016/j.socscimed.2015.03.050 PMID:25841094

Maisiak, R., Austin, J., West, S., & Heck, L. (1996). The effect of person-centered counseling on the psychological status of persons with systemic lupus erythematosus or rheumatoid arthritis. A randomized, controlled trial. *Arthritis and Rheumatism, 9*(1), 60–66. doi:10.1002/art.1790090111 PMID:8945114

Marengoni, A., Angleman, S., Melis, R., Mangialasche, F., Karp, A., Garmen, A., & Fratiglioni, L. et al. (2011). Aging with multimorbidity: A systematic review of the literature. *Ageing Research Reviews, 10*(4), 430–439. doi:10.1016/j.arr.2011.03.003 PMID:21402176

McMillan, S. S., Kendall, E., Sav, A., King, M. A., Whitty, J. A., Kelly, F., & Wheeler, A. J. (2013). Patient-centered approaches to health care: A systematic review of randomized controlled trials. *Medical Care Research and Review, 70*(6), 567–596. doi:10.1177/1077558713496318 PMID:23894060

McWhinney, I. (1989). The need for a transformed clinical method. In M. Stewart & D. Roter (Eds.), *Communicating with medical patients.* London: Sage.

McWhinney, I. (1993). Why we need a new clinical method. *Scandinavian Journal of Primary Health Care*, *11*(1), 3–7. doi:10.3109/02813439308994894 PMID:8484077

Mead, N., & Bower, P. (2000). Patient-centredness: A conceptual framework and review of the empirical literature. *Social Science & Medicine*, *51*(7), 1087–1110. doi:10.1016/S0277-9536(00)00098-8 PMID:11005395

Moja, E. A., & Vegni, E. (2000). *La visita medica centrata sul paziente*. Milano: Cortina Editore.

Naylor, C., Parsonage, M., McDaid, D., Knapp, M., Fossey, M., & Galea, A. (2012). *Long-term conditions and mental health: the cost of co-morbidities*. London: The King's Fund and Centre for Mental Health.

Platt, F. W., Gaspar, D. L., Coulehan, J. L., Fox, L., Adler, A. J., & Weston, W. W. et al.. (2001). "Tell me about yourself": The patient-centered interview. *Annals of Internal Medicine*, *134*(11), 1079–1085. doi:10.7326/0003-4819-134-11-200106050-00020 PMID:11388827

Pollack, M. M., Holubkov, R., Funai, T., Clark, A., Berger, J. T., Meert, K., & Jenkins, T. L. et al. (2014). Pediatric Intensive Care Outcomes: Development of New Morbidities During Pediatric Critical Care. *Pediatric Critical Care Medicine*, *15*(9), 821–827. doi:10.1097/PCC.0000000000000250 PMID:25226501

Prochaska, J. O., & Di Clemente, C. C. (1982). Transtheoretical therapy: Toward a more integrative model of change. *Psychotherapy (Chicago, Ill.)*, *19*(3), 276–288. doi:10.1037/h0088437

Rao, J. K., Weinberger, M., & Kroenke, K. (2000). Visit-specific expectations and patient-centered outcomes: A literature review. *Archives of Family Medicine*, *9*(10), 1148–1155. doi:10.1001/archfami.9.10.1148 PMID:11115222

Rathert, C., Wyrwich, M. D., & Boren, S. A. (2013). Patient-Centered Care and Outcomes A Systematic Review of the Literature. *Medical Care Research and Review*, *70*(4), 351–379. doi:10.1177/1077558712465774 PMID:23169897

Robinson, J. H., Callister, L. C., Berry, J. A., & Dearing, K. A. (2008). Patient-centered care and adherence: Definitions and applications to improve outcomes. *Journal of the American Academy of Nurse Practitioners*, *20*(12), 600–607. doi:10.1111/j.1745-7599.2008.00360.x PMID:19120591

Rosenberg, E. E., Lussier, M. T., & Beaudoin, C. (1997). Lessons for clinicians from physician-patient communication literature. *Archives of Family Medicine*, *6*(3), 279–283. doi:10.1001/archfami.6.3.279 PMID:9161356

Roter, D., & Larson, S. (2002). The Roter interaction analysis system (RIAS): Utility and flexibility for analysis of medical interactions. *Patient Education and Counseling*, *46*(4), 243–251. doi:10.1016/S0738-3991(02)00012-5 PMID:11932123

Roter, D. L. (1991). *Roter Interaction Analysis System: Coding Manual*. Baltimore, USA: Johns Hopkins University.

Safran, D. G., Taira, D. A., Rogers, W. H., Kosinski, M., Ware, J. E., & Tarlov, A. R. (1998). Linking primary care performance to outcomes of care. *The Journal of Family Practice*, *47*(3), 213–220. PMID:9752374

Simmons, L. A., Wolever, R. Q., Bechard, E. M., & Snyderman, R. (2014). Patient engagement as a risk factor in personalized health care: A systematic review of the literature on chronic disease. *Genome Medicine*, *6*(2), 16. doi:10.1186/gm533 PMID:24571651

Stewart, M., Brown, J. B., & Weston, W. W., NcWhinney, I. R., McWilliam, C.L., & Freeman, T.R. (2003). Patient-centered medicine-Transforming the clinical method. Bristol, UK: Radcliffe medical Press.

Street, R. L. Jr, & De Haes, H. (2013). Designing a curriculum for communication skills training from a theory and evidence-based perspective. *Patient Education and Counseling*, *93*(1), 27–33. doi:10.1016/j.pec.2013.06.012 PMID:23890580

Street, R. L. Jr, Makoul, G., Arora, N. K., & Epstein, R. M. (2009). How does communication heal? Pathways linking clinician–patient communication to health outcomes. *Patient Education and Counseling*, *74*(3), 295–301. doi:10.1016/j.pec.2008.11.015 PMID:19150199

Szasz, T. S., & Hollender, M. H. (1956). A contribution to the philosophy of medicine: The basic models of the doctor-patient relationship. *A.M.A. Archives of Internal Medicine*, *97*(5), 585–592. doi:10.1001/archinte.1956.00250230079008 PMID:13312700

Vlieland, V. T. P. (2002). Managing chronic disease: Evidence-based medicine or patient centred medicine? *Health Care Analysis*, *10*(3), 289–298. doi:10.1023/A:1022951808151 PMID:12769416

Ward, B. W. (2013). Prevalence of multiple chronic conditions among US adults: Estimates from the National Health Interview Survey, 2010. *Preventing Chronic Disease*, 2013, 10. PMID:23618545

Wells, K. B., Rogers, W., Burnam, A., Greenfield, S., & Ware, J. E. Jr. (1991). How the medical comorbidity of depressed patients differs across health care settings: Results from the Medical Outcomes Study. *The American Journal of Psychiatry*, *148*(12), 1688–1696. doi:10.1176/ajp.148.12.1688 PMID:1957931

Wiederhold, B. K., Riva, G., & Graffigna, G. (2013). Ensuring the best care for our increasing aging population: Health engagement and positive technology can help patients achieve a more active role in future healthcare. *Cyberpsychology, Behavior, and Social Networking*, *16*(6), 411–412. doi:10.1089/cyber.2013.1520 PMID:23751102

Williams, S., Weinman, J., & Dale, J. (1998). Doctor-patient communication and patient satisfaction: A review. *Family Practice*, *15*(5), 480–492. doi:10.1093/fampra/15.5.480 PMID:9848436

KEY TERMS AND DEFINITIONS

Bio-Psychosocial Model: The bio-psychosocial model is a general model stating that biological, psychological and social factors, all play a significant role in human functioning in the context of disease or illness. It posits that, health is best understood in terms of a combination of biological, psychological, and social factors rather than purely in biological terms.

Chronic Disease: The term chronic is usually applied when the course of the disease lasts for more than three months. A chronic condition is a persistent or otherwise long-lasting in its effects or a disease that comes with time.

Disease-Centered Medicine: Disease-centered method is based on the biomedical paradigm in which patients' reports of their medical conditions are read as the expression of disease processes and the clinical method focuses on identifying standard disease entities and on this basis proposes an evidence based therapeutic treatment.

Health Literacy: It is the ability to obtain, read, understand and use healthcare information to make appropriate health decisions and follow instructions for treatment.

Patient Agenda: It is a key concept of the patient-centered medicine. Patient's personal illness experience becomes a critical aspect of the care process in its four principal dimensions (feelings, ideas, the impact of problems on their lives, expectations).

Patient Reported Outcome: It is a measurement of health status directly reported by the patient.

Patient-Centered Medicine: The patient-centered medicine deals with the non-biological aspects of the disease: even the personal, psychological and social aspects are recognized as current and important, so that the tasks for the consultation are focusing not only on disease but also on patients' illness experience.

Section 2

Individual, Relational, and Social Barriers and Facilitators of Patient Engagement

Chapter 3
Individual, Institutional, and Environmental Factors Promoting Patient Retention and Dropout

Precious Arnan
University of West Indies, Barbados

Emmanuel Adugu
University of West Indies, Barbados

ABSTRACT

The primary purpose of this chapter is to determine factors that shape client dropout and adherence to Cardiac Disease Prevention and Rehabilitation Programs. The sample consists of 68 individuals, including those currently in the program (adherents) and those who have dropped out (dropouts). Findings show that clients undergoing rehabilitation are much likely to drop out when they are in the critical zone. This is a point where institutional factors, individual factors and environmentally-related factors are not favorable to clients. The risk of clients dropping out can be drastically reduced through the provision of an enabling environment comprising a set of factors that foster adherence such as financial sponsorship, institutional support, high intrinsic motivation, improved illness perception. In that context, there is the need for program administrators to closely monitor at-risk clients, especially those whose social, economic and psychological profiles predict non-adherence.

INTRODUCTION

The issue of client dropout from Cardiac Disease Prevention and Rehabilitation Programs (CDPRP) is a global problem. Client dropout from CDPRPs has generated concern at the institutional level, prompting the need to determine barriers to adherence as a means to both address the problem and improve institutional planning (Leon et al, 2005). It is in that context that determining barriers to client adherence and retention have been the concern of the Heart and Stroke Foundation of Barbados.

DOI: 10.4018/978-1-4666-9992-2.ch003

The following are the objectives of this chapter:

1. To investigate reasons that influence client adherence dropout from the program.
2. To determine the effectiveness of the program.
3. To assess if there are differences in adherents (current participants) and dropouts with respect to client satisfaction, intrinsic motivation, social support, institutional support, family support, illness perception and psychological distress.

BACKGROUND

Barbados is a densely populated island of 431 square kilometers with a population of 284,644 (World Bank, 2013). The Heart and Stroke Foundation of Barbados initiated the Cardiac Disease Prevention and Rehabilitation Program in 1994. It aims at rehabilitating clients through the use of medically monitored exercise, dietary advice, psychological counseling and education to enable participants (clients) become more informed and empowered to adopt a healthy lifestyle and ultimately sustain the benefits of rehabilitation over a lifetime (Heart and Stroke Foundation of Barbados). Unfortunately, client participation and adherence to the CDPRP have been declining over the years.

Despite the evidence of benefits, many patients fail to participate in or adhere to cardiac rehabilitation (Ades as cited in Leon et al., 2005). Adherence rate is operationally defined as 'the number of persons who remained active in a program at a given time compared with the total number of persons who began the program' (American Heart Association, 1994, p. 1605). According to the American Heart Association, adherence rate is highest in the first three months of exercise training programs, typically above 80%, down to 60% -71% in the sixth month, 45% -60% in twelfth month, 30%-50% after the second to fourth years. While factors linked to client drop-out are varied and somewhat interconnected, Aldosary and Garba (1999) stated that these factors could be grouped into two main categories namely (1) individual factors-those factors associated with individual traits and (2) institutional factors-those factors associated with the institutional environment.

Barriers to Participation and Adherence

There are barriers to client participation and adherence to health rehabilitation. Evidence from survey research indicates that there are several obstacles faced by patients who are eligible to participate in outpatient cardiac rehabilitation. In that context, Yohannes, Yalfani, Doherty, and Bundy (2007) studied a group of 189 patients who had been referred to a six-week outpatient cardiac rehabilitation program. The specific focus of their research was to identify the predictors of early drop-out from a cardiac rehabilitation program perceived to contribute to the drop-out problem, and assess the major differences between adherents and drop-outs. Yohannes and colleagues found significant differences between adherents and drop-outs, hence concluded that gender, younger age, Hospital Anxiety Depression Scale score, illness perception consequences, illness perception personal control and illness perception treatment control to be the major predictors of persisting or dropping-out. Similarly, Wittmer, Volpatti, Piazzalonga, and Hoffmann (2012) reported that low exercise capacity, high body mass index, smoking, diabetes, and widowhood were significant factors associated with early withdrawal. Daly et al. (2007) reported that factors associated with adherence included non-referral by physicians, associated illness, specific cardiac diagnoses, reimbursement, self-efficacy, perceived benefits of CR, distance and transportation, self-concept, self-motivation, family support, social support, self-esteem, and job. Whereas, factors associated with non-adherence included being elderly, female, having fewer years of formal education, CR perception benefits, having angina, and lower activity level during leisure time.

While views for improving retention are wide reaching, they are reflective of the fact that peoples' non-participation or adherence often draws on a number of contributing factors, rather than just one main issue. A relevant conceptual framework will offer insight into the dynamics of client adherence/ retention and dropout.

CONCEPTUAL FRAMEWORK

The purpose of the conceptual framework is to present a clear picture to help in understanding client dropout and adherence to the program and how it impacts program success.

Figure 1 is a diagram of the conceptual framework which depicts the factors associated with dropouts and adherence to treatment- individual factors, institutional and environmental related factors. The authors posit that clients do not act in isolation hence conceptualizing that there are certain factors contributing to and or inhibiting the development of long-term adherence to Cardiac Disease Prevention and Rehabilitation Programs. The core problem of low rates of adherence which subsequently inhibits the ability of the program to achieve its shorter, intermediate and long-term outcomes, comprise individual, institutional and environmental factors.

The complexes of dynamic individual factors which are obstacles to adherence include: low intrinsic motivation, psychological distress, illness perception beliefs and financial constraints. Institutional obstacles to adherence include lack of institutional support, service cost, and negative or low client satisfaction. Environmental factors that can also pose a challenge to adherence are lack of family and social support. The above obstacles to adherence may put clients at risk of dropping out of the program.

On the other hand, a number of positive set of factors can foster clients' adherence to the program. There are: high intrinsic motivation; improved illness perception beliefs; improved psychological functioning; financial sponsorship; positive institutional support; adequate equipments; gym environment conducive to do more exercises; positive family support; high level of customer satisfaction.

It is important to note that subjecting (exposing) clients at-risk of dropping out to the above positive factors fostering adherence may change their status from dropout to adherent. This change may ultimately lead to program success. In other words, obstacles to client motivation can be removed through the provision of an enabling environment of set factors that foster adherence such as high intrinsic motivation, improved illness perception, financial sponsorship, institutional support, etc. Using reverse logic, it means that where factors fostering adherence are absent, an environment may be created which predispose clients to the risk of dropping out.

MEASUREMENT OF VARIABLES

The main variables measured are as follows.

Figure 1. Conceptual framework

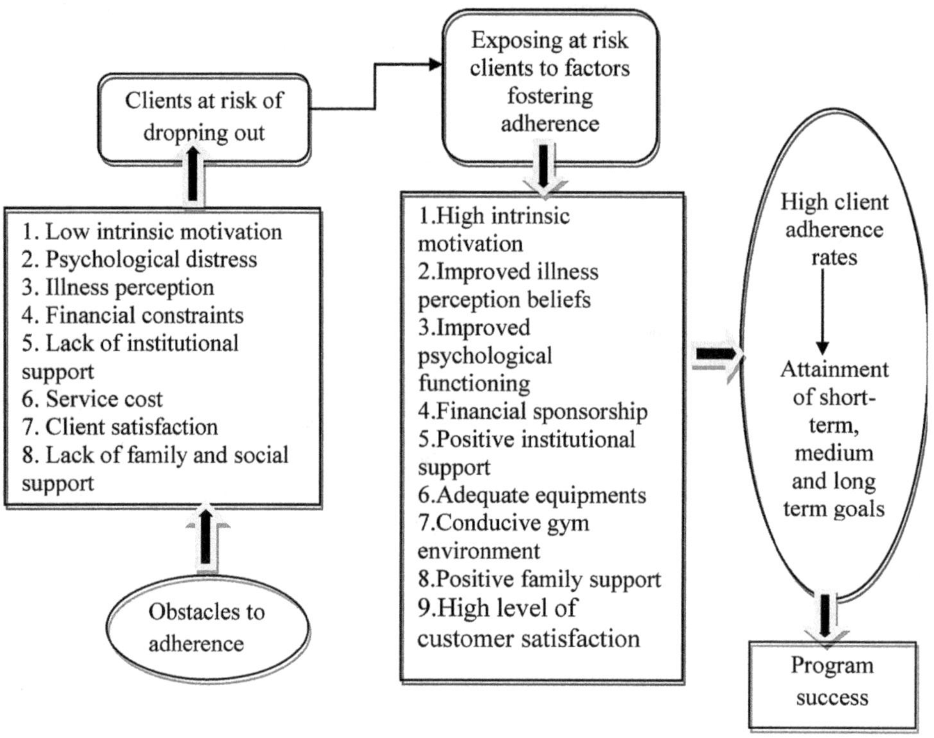

Institutional Support

The institutional support that is provided by a program tends to influence client retention (Wittmer et al, 2012). In that regard, respondents were asked to indicate their level of agreement regarding six questions measuring institutional support, with strongly disagree (1) to strongly agree (5). These were: I believe the CDPRP staff care about me; My personal difficulties are understood by the CDPRP staff; It is important to the CDPRP staff that my health improves; I look forward to interacting with the CDPRP staff during the week; The CDPRP staff create a gym environment conducive to do more exercises; I can always find a CDPRP staff to explain things to me about the program.

Client Satisfaction

It was measured by asking respondents the following questions: I believe my overall wellbeing has improved as a result of joining this program; if necessary, I will recommend this program to other friends and family; This program meets my expectations; I like this program. The response options ranged from strongly disagree (1) to strongly agree (5).

Intrinsic Motivation

Ades and Allen as cited in Leon et al. (2005) posited that intrinsic motivation influences adherence to cardiac rehabilitation. Intrinsic motivation was measured by asking respondents the following questions:

I decide my goals in life by myself; I challenge myself to exercise; I believe I have control over the way my life turns out; I am motivated because I believe this program (CDPRP) will make my health better; I do my best to improve my health; I make a lot of effort to live up to what my friends expect. The response options ranged from strongly disagree (1) to strongly agree (5).

Social Support

Wittmer et al. (2012) stated that social support that is provided by program staff also influences client retention. In order to investigate this, respondents were asked to rate on a scale of 1 to 5, with 1 coded as never, and 4 coded as always, social support system that they have during the period of rehabilitation. Specific questions asked were: There is someone in your life who you can count on to listen to you when you need to talk; There is someone available to give you good advice about a problem; There is someone available to you who shows you love and affection; You can count on someone to provide you with emotional support, such as talking over problems or helping you make difficult decisions.

Family Support

Marzolini, Brooks and Oh (2008) found out that clients were more likely to dropout from cardiac rehabilitation programs if they have no family support systems available. It is in that context that three sets of questions were developed to measure family support, with response options ranging from strongly disagree (1) to strongly agree (5). These were: I have family who encourage me to maintain a healthy lifestyle; my family encouraged me to join this program (CDPRP); it is important to most of my family members that I stay in this program (CDPRP).

Psychological Distress

Available literature shows that individuals' mood may affect whether they drop out of a program or stay in it (Yohannes et al., 2007). Following that, five sets of questions were developed and used to measure the mood/psychological distress of respondents. These were: I feel miserable and sad; I feel life is not worth living; I feel scared or frightened; I feel as if I have slowed down; worrying thoughts constantly go through my mind. The response options were not at all (1) to always (4).

Illness Perception

Similar to psychological distress, the literature has shown that illness people's perception may influence whether they stay in or drop out from health rehabilitation (Broadbent, Petrie, Main, & Weinman, 2006). In that regard, a battery of two questions was used, with response options ranging from 0 to 10: how much control do you feel you have over your illness?; and how well do you feel you understand your illness?

DATA

As indicated earlier, the primary foci of this evaluation research is to determine factors that shape client dropout and adherence to the program. Given the data needs, a mostly quantitative research technique was employed by involving the major stakeholders (adherents and dropouts) of the program. This approach was desirable for this study as the underlining evaluation research objectives were to determine the effectiveness of the program, to investigate factors that shape client dropout from the program and assess if there are differences in adherents and dropouts with respect to institutional support, client satisfaction, intrinsic motivation, social support, family support, psychological distress and illness perception.

The study population for this survey consisted of two groups. These are: those who are currently in the program (adherents) and those who had earlier enrolled in the program (CDPRP) and dropped out (dropouts). The total study population is 279.

Availability sampling procedure was used to select the samples from both dropout and adherents. Using this random procedure, a sample of 30 individuals who had dropped out of the program was selected. With respect to those participants currently in the program (adherents), availability sampling procedure was used to select the sample from a population of 142. Availability sample studies cases or units that are readily accessible (Weisberg, 2005; Zikmund, 2003). Using this sampling procedure is consistent with available information from the CDPRP which shows that most of those currently enrolled in the program and dropouts are at least 50 years old, retired or unemployed. They constitute a homogenous population. In that context, there is very little variation in the population which justifies the use of convenience sampling (Saunders, Lewis, & Thornhill, 2009). It must be emphasized that this research is correlational in nature, thus a sample size of about 30 participants is considered appropriate (Daniel, 2012).

Using a structured questionnaire, data was collected from adherents within a four-week span. Program staff approached all eligible participants and provided an explanation of the study. Interested persons were given a questionnaire upon verbal agreement to fill-out. Similarly, data was collected from dropouts within a four-week timeframe. The selected dropouts were first contacted by the researcher via telephone to ascertain their willingness to participate. Then they were later contacted at an agreed scheduled time. Administering the telephone questionnaire took approximately 15-25 minutes each to complete.

There were ethical considerations in the conduct of this research. The dignity and welfare of all respondents were ensured by protecting them from any harm, unnecessary risks, or mental and physical discomfort that might be inherent in the research procedure. The respondent's participation in the survey was not obligatory and they were informed that they had the right not answer any question, or withdraw from the study at any point. Additionally, they were assured that all information would be treated in a confidential manner and that no individual would be identifiable in the study findings to ensure confidentiality and anonymity.

EVIDENCE/FINDINGS

The research findings are presented with respect to individual, institutional and environmentally-related factors.

Individual Factors

Three main factors are discussed under this section. These are: intrinsic motivation, psychological distress and illness perception.

Table 1. Intrinsic motivation

	Adherents				Dropouts			
	Mean	Min	Max	SD	Mean	Min	Max	SD
I decide my goals in life by myself	4.3	2	5	.8	4.1	2	5	.74
I challenge myself to exercise	4.3	1	5	.96	3.8	2	5	.91
I believe I have control over the way my life turns out	4.2	1	5	1	3.9	2	5	.91
I am motivated because I believe this program (CDP & RP) will make my health better	4.7	3	5	.48	3.9	3	5	.55
I do my best to improve my health	4.6	4	5	.50	4.1	2	5	.66
I make a lot of effort to live up to what my friends expect	2.6	1	5	1.5	2.7	1	5	1.14
Intrinsic Motivation Scale (Cronbach's alpha reliability): Adherents=0.6 Dropouts=0.6	25	18	30	3.3	22.7	15	27	2.8

Intrinsic Motivation

A six item summated scale of intrinsic motivation (Cronbach's alpha reliability=0.6 for each group) was created. The above Cronbach's alpha reliability value means that the internal consistency of the intrinsic motivation scale is quite good. The results are presented in Table 1 below. An independent-sample t-test was conducted to compare intrinsic motivation scale scores for adherents and dropouts. There was a significant difference in scores for adherents (M=25, SD=3.36) and dropouts, M=22.7, SD=2.8; t (60) = 2.92, p=.005 (two tailed). This finding is consistent with Evenson and Fluery (2000) study which revealed that patients are more likely to drop out of outpatient Cardiac Disease Prevention and Rehabilitation due to lack of motivation. This finding is consistent with Ades and Allen as cited in Lean et al. (2005) which noted that a contributing factor to dropout is low client intrinsic motivation. In this regard, the services of a psychologist might help in motivating clients to have a more positive attitude to life in general and their health in particular.

Psychological Distress

Individuals' mood/psychological distress may affect whether they stay or drop out of a program. In that regard, a five item summated psychological distress scale (Cronbach's alpha reliability of 0.6 for adherents and 0.6 for dropouts) was created. This suggests that the internal consistency of the psychological distress scale is quite good. The scale ranged from 5 to 15 for adherents and 5 to 19 for dropouts. The results are shown in Table 2.

An independent-sample t-test was conducted to compare psychological distress scale scores for adherents and dropouts. There was no significant difference in scores for adherents (M=8.8, SD=2.6) and dropouts, M=10.3, SD=3.7; t (64) = -1.885, p=.073 (two tailed). However, a closer look at the mean psychological distress scores shows that dropouts had a higher score of 10.3 compared with 8.8 for adherents. This supports Yohannes et al. (2007) study which revealed that dropouts had higher psychological

Table 2. Psychological distress

	Adherents				Dropouts			
	Mean	Min	Max	SD	Mean	Min	Max	SD
I feel miserable and sad	1.9	1	3	.94	2.1	1	4	.91
I feel life is not worth living	2.1	1	4	.91	1.6	1	4	1.9
I feel scared or frightened	1.4	1	3	.71	1.7	1	4	.92
I feel as if I have slowed down	2.2	1	3	.76	2.7	1	4	.83
Worrying thoughts constantly go through my mind	2.18	1	4	.98	2.17	1	4	1.02
Psychological Distress Scale (Cronbach's alpha reliability): Adherents=0.6 Dropouts=0.6	8.8	5	15	2.6	10.3	5	19	3.7

distress scores than adherents. Hence psychological distress scores can be considered as predictors of early dropout from Cardiac Disease Prevention and Rehabilitation programs.

Illness Perception

The literature has shown that people's illness perception may influence whether they stay in or drop out from health rehabilitation (French, Cooper & Weinman, 2006). Two main questions were used to assess the illness perception of adherents and dropouts. In terms of control over the illness, adherents have a mean value of 6.03 compared with 7.4 for dropouts (on a 10-point scale). Similarly, for understanding of illness, adherents have a mean value of 8.14 compared with 9.17 for dropouts. When an independent t-test was conducted to compare adherents' understanding of illness; and feelings of control over illness, the tests were statistically significant. The mean scores for dropouts were higher than those for adherents. These suggest that dropouts feel they have much control over their lives; and also have better understanding of their health status compared with adherents.

Institutional Factors

Institutional factors deal with influences (issues) relating to the Cardiac Disease Prevention and Rehabilitation Program. These factors may foster clients' retention or dropout from the program. For analytical purposes, institutional factors are subdivided into client satisfaction and institutional support.

Institutional Support

The institutional support that is provided by a program tends to influence client retention. An institutional support scale (Cronbach's alpha reliability of 0.84 for adherents and 0.92 for dropouts) was created using a battery of six questions. This suggests that the scale has good internal consistency (Pallant, 2007). In general, the responses ranged from 13-29. Table 3 shows the distribution of the responses from both adherents and dropouts.

Table 3. Respondents' views on institutional support

	Adherents				Dropouts			
	Mean	**Min**	**Max**	**SD**	**Mean**	**Min**	**Max**	**SD**
I believe the CDP &RP staff care about me	4.6	4	5	.49	4.2	2	5	.73
My personal difficulties are understood by the CDP &RP staff	4.3	3	5	.68	3.9	2	5	.73
It is important to the CDP &RP staff that my health improves	4.6	3	5	.55	4.1	2	5	.52
I look forward to interacting with the CDP &RP staff during the week	4.6	3	5	.56	3.9	2	5	.64
The CDP &RP staff create a conducive gym environment for clients	4.5	4	5	.50	3.7	2	5	.67
I can always find a CDP &RP staff to explain things to me about the program	4.5	3	5	.60	3.7	2	5	.64
Institutional Support Scale (Cronbach's alpha reliability): Adherents=0.84 Dropouts=0.92	27.3	23	30	2.4	23.6	13	29	3.4

An independent-sample t-test was conducted to compare the institutional support scale scores for adherents and dropouts. There was a significant difference in scores for adherents (M=27.3, SD=2.4) and dropouts, M=23.6, SD=3.4; t (61) = 5.037, p=.000 (two tailed).

There is a significant difference in scores for adherents compared with dropouts. The magnitude of this difference in terms of eta squared statistic is large. This strongly suggests that unlike dropouts, adherents have a better perception of program support with respect to caring about them; creating conducive atmosphere, understanding of their personal difficulties, etc. This finding is consistent with Pack et al. (2013) and Zarani, Besharat, Sadeghian, and Sarami (2010) in their studies which concluded that providing institutional support improved patient adherence. Their findings showed a significant increase in attendance and completion of Cardiac Rehabilitation when purposeful encouragement and reinforcement strategies are employed.

Examining the reasons given by respondents for dropping out of the program, about half of them stated that they dropped out due to financial constraints or lack of sponsorship. Given the fact that about 50% of the respondents are retirees, it means that they may not have enough income to afford paying for the program services.

Apart from financial constraints leading to client dropouts, some clients dropped out because they felt they did not have enough assistance on equipment use; and others did so due to lack of sufficient monitoring during exercise; inflexible time schedules; and bad experience with program staff. Thus in general, client dropout is shaped by lack of sufficient sponsorship, staff attitudes to clients and equipment. These may become obstacles to client adherence and ultimately the effectiveness of the program.

It is worthy of note that when dropouts were asked about their willingness to rejoin the program, about 62% answered in the affirmative. This suggests that they may have been impacted by the program. For example, when asked about their improved overall wellbeing as a result of joining the program, the mean score (on a five-point scale) were 4.63 and 4.1 for adherents and dropouts respectively. This further suggests that the program has been quite effective even for dropouts too (though there is also a

Table 4. Client satisfaction

	Adherents				Dropouts			
	Mean	Min	Max	SD	Mean	Min	Max	SD
I believe my overall well-being has improved as a result of joining this program	4.6	3	5	.54	4.1	2	5	.68
If necessary, I will recommend this program to other friends and family	4.7	4	5	.46	4.2	2	5	.81
This program meets my expectations	4.5	3	5	.60	3.9	2	5	.66
I like this program	4.5	4	5	.50	4	2	5	.85
Client Satisfaction Scale (Cronbach's alpha reliability): Adherents=0.76 Dropouts=0.85	18.5	15	20	1.6	16.2	9	20	2.5

statistically significant difference between adherents and dropouts in terms of their improved overall wellbeing score). It is in that that regard that it may be understandable why a good number of them are willing to rejoin the program—if given the necessary support and resources.

Client Satisfaction

A four item summated scale (Cronbach's alpha reliability of 0.76 for adherents and 0.85 for dropouts) was created from a series of questions related to client satisfaction. This means that the internal consistency of the client satisfaction scale is good. The scale ranged from 15 to 20 for adherents and 9 to 20 for dropouts. The results are presented in Table 4 below.

An independent-sample t-test was conducted to compare client satisfaction scale scores for adherents and dropouts. There was a significant difference in scores for adherents (M=18.5, SD=1.6) and dropouts, M=16.2, SD=2.5; t (61) = 4.425, p=.000 (two tailed).

The research findings clearly show that the mean scores in all measures of client satisfaction are relatively higher for adherents compared with dropouts. This consistency in higher client satisfaction scores is ultimately reflected in the higher score for the summated scale measuring client satisfaction. Following Cohen (1988), this finding suggests that a high magnitude of the difference in client satisfaction is explained by the client's status (either adherent or dropout). Thus there is compelling evidence from the findings to show that adherents are more satisfied compared with dropouts. In essence, clients who adhere to the CDPRP are more satisfied compared with the dropouts. This is consistent with Wittmer et al. (2012) findings that highly satisfied participants had a low rate of dropout from Cardiac Disease Prevention and Rehabilitation Programs.

Given the above results in the context of respondents' views about strengths of the program, it can be inferred that in order to reduce clients' dropouts and increase adherence, the program has to improve upon the following: provide friendly and supportive environment; provide very good exercising machines; make clients feel they can ultimately achieve an improved overall wellbeing.

Environmentally-Related Factors

The factors that are discussed under this section are: family support, and social support. These factors may foster adherence to the program or facilitate dropout.

Family Support

Clients were more likely to dropout from CDPRP if they have no family support systems available. It is in that context that a three item summated scale (Cronbach's alpha reliability of 0.64 for adherents and 0.68 for dropouts) was created. These values suggest that the internal consistency of the family support scale is quite good. The results are shown in Table 5 below. An independent-sample t-test was conducted to compare family support scale scores for adherents and dropouts. There was a significant difference in scores for adherents (M=12.64, SD=1.95) and dropouts, M=10.97, SD=2.22; t (61) = 4.936, p=.002 (two tailed). In addition to that, the magnitude of the difference is large according to the eta squared statistic. This supports Marzolini et al. (2008) findings that family issues are linked to premature withdrawal from Cardiac Disease Prevention and Rehabilitation programs.

Social Support

As discussed in the methodology section, social support that is provided by program staff also influences client retention. In order to investigate this, a four item summated scale (Cronbach's alpha reliability of 0.87 for adherents and 0.86 for dropouts) was created as shown in Table 4. This suggests that the social support scale has good internal consistency. The scale ranged from 8 to 16. An independent-sample t-test was conducted to compare the social support scale scores for adherents and dropouts. There was a significant difference in scores for adherents (M=14.2, SD=2.4) and dropouts, M=11.5, SD=2 t (66) = 4.936, p=.000 (two tailed). Findings revealed that there is a statistically significant difference between the social support of adherents and dropouts. This difference according to the eta squared statistic is large. Adherents scored much higher in social support compared with dropouts. This is consistent with Chatham as cited in WHO (1993) finding that the social support provided to a patient is as important

Table 5. Family support

	Adherents				Dropouts			
	Mean	Min	Max	SD	Mean	Min	Max	SD
I have family who encourage me to maintain a healthy lifestyle	4.5	3	5	.56	4.1	2	5	.84
My family encouraged me to join this program (CDP & RP)	3.9	1	5	1.14	3.3	2	5	1.01
It is important to most of my family members that I stay in this program (CDP & RP).	4.2	2	5	.74	3.6	2	5	.96
Family Support Scale (Cronbach's alpha reliability): Adherents=0.64 Dropouts=0.68	12.6	7	15	1.95	10.97	6	15	2.2

as the intervention. This suggests that dropouts do not have the necessary social support to stay in the program.

LESSONS LEARNED: INTERACTION OF FACTORS AFFECTING PROGRAM EFFECTIVENESS

It can be inferred from the above discussion that three main factors affect the effectiveness of the Cardiac Disease Prevention and Rehabilitation Program. These are: institutional factors; individual factors; and environmentally-related factors. These factors can either be obstacles to adherence or foster adherence depending on the context. For example, institutional factors such as providing financial sponsorship, creating conducive atmosphere, being accessible to clients, etc. may foster adherence. On the other hand, lack of financial sponsorship, inaccessibility of staff to clients, etc. may become obstacles to client adherence, which may ultimately lead to dropout. Similarly, individual factors such as low intrinsic motivation, coupled with high psychological distress may act as obstacles to adherence. However, high intrinsic motivation coupled with low psychological distress may foster adherence. It follows logically that an environment that provides a good family and social support can foster adherence to the program. These interactions between the factors are depicted in Figure 2 below. For analytical purposes, the following typology was developed and used:

1a. Positive institutional factors = high institutional support plus high client satisfaction.
1b. Institutional support is considered negative when either institutional support or client satisfaction or both are negative.
2a. Positive individual factors = high intrinsic motivation plus high illness perception plus low psychological distress.
2b. Individual factors are considered negative when one at least one of the variables has a negative connotation. For example, high psychological distress or low illness perception or low intrinsic motivation.

Figure 2. Interactions of factors affecting program effectiveness

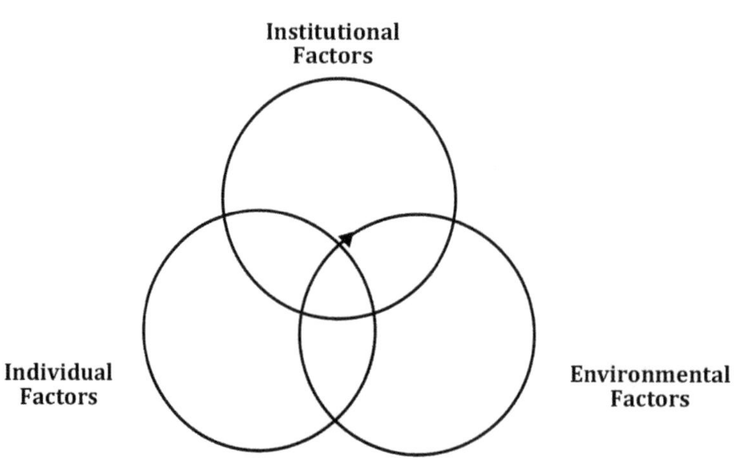

3a. Positive environmental factors = high family support plus high social support.
3b. Environmental factors are considered negative when either family support or social support or both are negative.

Based on the above typology, the following possible program outcomes (scenarios) are derived:

1. Positive institutional factors plus positive individual factors coupled with positive environmentally-related factors may lead to the most desirable program outcome. On the other hand, when all the afore-mentioned factors are negative, a critical point is reached. At the critical point, obstacles to adherence are at their highest levels and client dropout is guaranteed.
2. Positive institutional factors plus positive environmental factors coupled with negative individual factors may lead to weakened client adherence and hence dropout.
3. Positive institutional factors plus positive individual factors coupled with negative environmentally-related factors may facilitate client dropout.
4. Positive environmentally-related factors plus positive individual factors coupled with negative institutional factors may not foster program adherence.

CONCLUSION

In view of the findings, it can be concluded that a number of factors put clients of the Cardiac Disease Prevention and Rehabilitation Program (CDPRP) at risk of dropping out. These are: low intrinsic motivation, low illness perception, low client satisfaction, lack of institutional support, lack of family and social support, high psychological distress, and financial constraints/lack of sponsorship. On the other hand, certain factors may foster client adherence/retention. These are: high intrinsic motivation, high level of consumer satisfaction, positive institutional support, positive family support, improved illness perception, improved psychological functioning, financial sponsorship, adequate equipments, and conducive gym environment.

In general, the CDPRP has good client evaluations with respect to institutional support and client satisfaction. However, the fact that there is a significant difference between adherents and dropouts it implies that the program must improve its institutional support mechanisms and also strive better to improve the satisfaction levels of all clients in general, and dropouts in particular. Similar to client satisfaction and institutional support, in general, there is a consistent, significant and high magnitude difference between adherents and dropouts in terms of intrinsic motivation, social and family support, illness perception, and psychological distress. Thus the program facilitators must initiate measures to close these gaps between adherents and dropouts to improve the effectiveness of the program. Davies et al. (2010) alluded that adherence can marginally be improved with some interventions.

RECOMMENDATIONS

These research findings have practical implications for the Cardiac Disease Prevention and Rehabilitation Program. Clients undergoing rehabilitation are guaranteed to drop out when they are in the critical zone. The critical zone is a point where institutional factors, individual factors and environmentally-related factors are not favorable to clients. On the other hand, if all the above factors are favorable, client adherence is ensured. At any point in a client's journey of rehabilitation, when any of the aforementioned factors become unfavorable, client retention is weakened. Consequently, the following are recommended:

1. There is the need to closely monitor at-risk clients, especially those whose socio-economic, social and psychological profiles predict non-adherence.
2. Longer follow-up period with former clients (dropouts) need to be reinforced to convey a positive and supportive message from the Cardiac Disease Prevention and Rehabilitation Program. Regular telephone calls, emails, mail-in newsletters, etc. can serve as a good way of keeping former clients up to date with new and exciting improvements to the program. In addition to that, communication channels with current clients (adherents) should be maintained through meetings to keep them up to date thus fostering a culture of belonging.
3. Program administrators should continuously evaluate the institutional policies, practices and social environment of the program in order to cater for the evolving needs of their clients. In such evaluations, the concerns of the clients need to be reviewed carefully and incorporated into institutional planning, policies, and practices.

ACKNOWLEDGMENT

We would like to express our gratitude to the staff of Heart and Stroke Foundation of Barbados for facilitating the collection of data for this evaluation research. This book chapter would not have been possible without their support.

REFERENCES

Aldosary, A. S., & Garba, S. B. (1999). An analysis of factors contributing to college student dropout in a medium sized technical university: The case of the King Fahd University of Petroleum and Minerals Dhahran, Saudi Arabia. *Higher Education Policy*, *12*(4), 313–328. doi:10.1016/S0952-8733(99)00021-5

American Heart Association. (1994). Cardiac rehabilitation programs: A statement for healthcare professionals from the American Heart Association. *Circulation*, *90*(3), 1602–1610http://circ.ahajournals.org/content/90/3/1602.full.pdf+html?ijkey=c95f4e77ee2deea285d9361fb53c32d71957c126&keytype2=tf_ipsecsha. doi:10.1161/01.CIR.90.3.1602 PMID:8087975

Broadbent, E., Petrie, K. J., Main, J., & Weinman, J. (2006). The brief illness perception questionnaire. *Journal of Psychosomatic Research*, *60*(6), 631–637. doi:10.1016/j.jpsychores.2005.10.020 PMID:16731240

Cohen, J. W. (1988). *Statistical power analysis for the behavioral sciences* (2nd ed.). Hillsdale, NJ: Lawrence Erlbaum Associates.

Daly, J., Sindone, A. P., Thompson, D. R., Hancock, K., Chang, E., & Davidson, P. (2007). Barriers to participation in and adherence to cardiac rehabilitation programs: A critical literature review. *Progress in Cardiovascular Nursing*, *17*(1), 8–17. doi:10.1111/j.0889-7204.2002.00614.x PMID:11872976

Daniel, J. (2012). *Sampling essentials: Practical guidelines for making sampling choices*. Thousand Oaks, CA: Sage Publications Inc.

Davies, P., Taylor, F., Beswick, A., Wise, F., Moxham, T., Rees, K., & Ebrahim, S. (2010). Promoting patient uptake and adherence in cardiac rehabilitation. *Cochrane Database of Systematic Reviews*. doi:10.1002/14651858.CD007131.pub2 PMID:20614453

Evenson, K. R., & Fleury, J. (2000). Barriers to outpatient cardiac rehabilitation participation and *adherence. Journal of Cardiopulmonary Rehabilitation*, *20*(4), 241–246. doi:10.1097/00008483-200007000-00005 PMID:10955265

French, D. P., Cooper, A., & Weinman, J. (2006, December). Illness perceptions predict attendance at cardiac rehabilitation following acute myocardial infarction: A systematic review with meta-analysis. *Journal of Psychosomatic Research*, *61*(6), 757–767. doi:10.1016/j.jpsychores.2006.07.029 PMID:17141663

Heart and Stroke Foundation of Barbados. (n. d.). *Cardiac disease prevention and rehabilitation programme*. Retrieved from http://www.hsfbarbados.org/GymCDPR.aspx

Leon, A. S., Franklin, B. A., Costa, F., Balady, G. J., Berra, K. A., & Stewart, K. J. et al.. (2005). Cardiac rehabilitation and secondary prevention of coronary heart disease. *Circulation*, *111*(3), 369–376. doi:10.1161/01.CIR.0000151788.08740.5C PMID:15668354

Marzolini, S., Brooks, D., & Oh, I. P. (2008, December). Sex differences in completion of a 12-month cardiac rehabilitation programme: An analysis of 5922 women and men. *European Journal of Cardiovascular Prevention and Rehabilitation*, *15*(6), 698–703. doi:10.1097/HJR.0b013e32830c1ce3 PMID:18981927

Pack, Q. R., Johnson, L. L., Barr, L. M., Daniels, S. R., Wolter, A. D., Squires, R. W., & Thomas, R. J. et al. (2013). Improving cardiac rehabilitation attendance and completion through quality improvement activities and a motivational program. *Journal of Cardiopulmonary Rehabilitation and Prevention*, *33*(3), 153–159. doi:10.1097/HCR.0b013e31828db386 PMID:23595006

Pallant, J. (2007). *SPSS survival manual: A step by step guide to data analysis using SPSS for windows* (3rd ed.). Berkshire, England: Open University Press.

Saunders, M., Lewis, P., & Thornhill, A. (2009). *Research methods for business students* (5th ed.). Essex, England: Pearson Education Limited.

Weisberg, H. F. (2005). *The total survey error approach: A guide to the new science of survey research*. Chicago, IL: The University of Chicago Press. doi:10.7208/chicago/9780226891293.001.0001

Wittmer, M., Volpatti, M., Piazzalonga, S., & Hoffmann, A. (2012, October). Expectation, satisfaction, and predictors of dropout in cardiac rehabilitation. *European Journal of Preventive Cardiology*, *19*(5), 1082–1088. doi:10.1177/1741826711418163 PMID:21788251

World Bank. (n. d.). *World databank*. Retrieved from http://data.worldbank.org/indicator/SP.POP.TOTL

World Health Organization. (1993). *Needs and actions priorities in cardiac rehabilitation and secondary prevention in patients with CHD*. Retrieved from http://whqlibdoc.who.int/euro/-1993/EUR_ICP_CVD_125.pdf

Yohannes, A. M., Yalfani, A., Doherty, P., & Bundy, C. (2007, March). Predictors of drop-out from an outpatient cardiac rehabilitation programme. *Journal of Clinical Rehabilitation*, *21*(3), 222–229. doi:10.1177/0269215506070771 PMID:17329279

Zarani, F., Besharat, A. M., Sadeghian, S., & Sarami, G. (2010, September). The effectiveness of the Information-Motivation-Behavioral skills model in promoting adherence in CABG patients. *Journal of Health Psychology*, *15*(6), 828–837. doi:10.1177/1359105309357092 PMID:20453057

Zikmund, W. G. (2003). *Business research methods* (7th ed.). Mason, OH: South-Western.

KEY TERMS AND DEFINITIONS

Adherence Rate: The number of persons who remained as active participants in a program compared with the total number of persons who started the program.

Barriers: An influence that reduces the chances of participation in cardiac rehabilitation program.

Cardiac Rehabilitation: A medically supervised program aimed at improving the overall wellbeing of its participants/clients thereby reducing morbidity and mortality.

Clients: Persons whose needs are to be satisfied or whose behavior or circumstance the agency aims to change.

Critical Zone: This is a point where institutional factors, individual factors and environmentally-related factors are not favorable to clients.

Illness Perception: Subjective beliefs, attitudes, or ideas about health and illness.

Institutional Support: Influences relating to the program which may facilitate/foster clients' retention or dropout from the program.

Rehabilitation: The restoration to a former capacity through training or therapy.

APPENDIX

Table 6. Summary of T-tests and Eta Squared

Indicator	T-test	Eta Squared	
		Value	Interpretation
Client satisfaction scale	Significant	0.24 (24%)	Large effect. Magnitude of the difference between means of adherents and dropouts in relation to client satisfaction scale is large. Statistically, 24% of the variance in client satisfaction is explained by respondents' status (adherent/dropout).
Institutional support scale	Significant	0.29 (29%)	Large effect. Magnitude of the difference between means of adherents and dropouts regarding institutional support scale is large. Implies that 29% of the variance in institutional support is explained by respondents' status (adherent/dropout).
Improved overall wellbeing	Significant	0.15 (15%)	Large effect. Magnitude of the difference between means of adherents and dropouts with respect to improved overall wellbeing is large. This means that 15% of the variance in improved overall wellbeing is explained by respondents' status (adherent/dropout).
Understanding nutritional guidelines	Significant	0.12 (12%)	Moderate effect. Magnitude of the difference between means of adherents and dropouts with respect to understanding of nutritional guidelines is moderate. Implies 12% of the variance in understanding nutritional guidelines is explained by the status of respondents (adherent/dropout).
Intrinsic motivation scale	Significant	0.12 (12%)	Moderate effect. Magnitude of the difference between means of adherents and dropouts in relation to intrinsic motivation is moderate. Thus 12% of the variance in intrinsic motivation is explained by the respondents' status (adherent/dropout).
Control over illness	Significant	0.06 (6%)	Moderate effect. Magnitude of the difference between means of adherents and dropouts with respect to control over illness is moderate. Thus 6% of the variance in control over illness is explained by the respondents' status (adherent/dropout).
Family support scale	Significant	0.14 (14%)	Large effect. Magnitude of the difference between means of adherents and dropouts in relation to family support is large. Implies 14% of the variance in family support is explained by respondents' status (adherent/dropout).
Social support scale	Significant	0.27 (27%)	Large effect. Magnitude of the difference between means of adherents and dropouts with respect to social support is large. Thus 27% of the variance in social support is explained by the respondents' status (adherent/dropout).

Chapter 4
Barriers to and Facilitators of Older Adult's Adherence to Health Recommendations:
Towards an Engaging Two-way Health Communication

Rui Gaspar
William James Center for Research, ISPA- Instituto Universitário, Portugal

Samuel Domingos
William James Center for Research, ISPA- Instituto Universitário, Portugal

António M. Diniz
Universidade de Évora, Portugal

Roberto Falanga
Instituto de Ciências Sociais, Universidade de Lisboa, Portugal

ABSTRACT

Non-adherence to health recommendations (e.g. medical prescriptions) presents potential costs for healthcare, which could be prevented or mitigated. This is often attributed to a person's rational choice, to not adhere. However, this may also be determined by individual and contextual factors implied in the recommendations communication process. In accordance, this chapter focuses specifically on barriers to and facilitators of adherence to recommendations and engagement with the healthcare process, particularly concerning the communication between health professionals and patients. For this, the authors present examples of engagement increment through different degrees of participation, from a one-way/directive towards a two-way/engaging communication process. This focuses specifically on a vulnerable population group with increasing healthcare needs: older adults. Future possibilities for two-way engaging communications are discussed, aimed at promoting increased adherence to health recommendations and people's self-regulation of their own health.

DOI: 10.4018/978-1-4666-9992-2.ch004

INTRODUCTION

"Patients are adherent when they do what their health professionals recommend" (DiMatteo, 2004; p. 200). When patients do not do what health professionals recommend, i.e. they are non-adherent, this may increment healthcare costs, by wasting human and material resources. In accordance, lack of engagement with the healthcare process in general and specifically lack of adherence to recommendations as communicated by health professionals, has been an important setback for health promotion effectiveness, in various healthcare systems across the world (see DiMatteo, 2004). To provide a contribution in this regard, this chapter aims to provide an overview of barriers to recommendations adherence and facilitators of people's increased participation and engagement with their own health care process.

This chapter specifically focus on the older adult's population. There are some reasons that justify this focus. Over the past decades we have witnessed an increase in life expectancy, resulting in a greater prevalence of chronic diseases, with negative impact on the health systems (Bauer, Briss, Goodman, & Bowman, 2014; Sabate, 2003).It is estimated that most of the elderly have two or more diseases (van den Akker, Buntinx, Metsemakers, Roos, & Knottnerus, 1998; Ward & Schiller, 2013), and comorbidity often implies polypharmacy and subsequent undesirable drug-drug, drug-body, and/or drug-disease interactions (Arnold, 2008). This is frequently implemented through complex administration regimens that require daily habit changes implying effortful actions and strong adherence to what the health professionals recommend (Hajjar, Cafiero, & Hanlon, 2007). In agreement, a recent qualitative review focusing on randomized controlled trials interventions for chronic diseases, found that current methods of improving medication adherence are mostly complex and not very effective (Nieuwlaat et al., 2014; see also Haynes, Ackloo, Sahota, McDonald, & Yao, 2008). This is worrisome due to the fact that has been shown that the elderly have more difficulty in following recommendations than younger people, given that they ask for less clarification and tend to be less active regarding care for their own health, being therefore more susceptible to physical, psychological and social consequences from non-adherence (Branin, 2001). This has negative consequences as non-adherence to long-term therapy in chronic diseases achieves an average of 50% in developed countries (less in developing countries), increasing health costs and decrementing positive health outcomes. To tackle this, patient-tailored interventions should include not only the assessment of patient-related non-adherence factors but also contextual factors, namely those linked to the health professionals (Sabate, 2003) and the health recommendations communication process.

However, the consideration of these contextual factors is not the focus of many patient-tailored interventions, which potentially reduces their effectiveness. In fact, the reasons for non-adherence are often attributed to a rational choice from the individual and due to their individual characteristics and not as much to their surrounding context. This is in agreement with research that found a set of individual characteristics that may explain non-adherence (DiMatteo, 2004). However, equally important are factors related to the communication process itself and how engaged the actors of this process (e.g. patient, doctor.) are in it. When these are considered, they focus mainly on the relationship between the patient and the health professional and/or on the communication content (e.g. how information is framed). However, this tells us little about how motivated the person is to engage with the process and adhere to what is recommended.

It should be noted that upon communication of health information it is expected that people initiate a process of *deliberation* - a thoughtful, careful and lengthy consideration of the information (Davies, 2009) - and then implement the necessary actions to adhere to recommendations. However, providing information alone without people feeling engaged with the communication process and expecting the recommendation to translate into behaviours, may not achieve the desired results. The patient's engagement could be evidenced though affirmations such as "I have a question!" "May I comment on that?" or similar expressions, when faced with recommendations. However, these are less heard than it would be desirable, in healthcare settings. Not expressing their information needs and not manifesting elaboration on the health information received, may suggest lack of manifest deliberation on this information and engagement with the healthcare process. This may not necessarily evidence that the person chose to rationally distance her/himself from the process but rather that the process may not be sufficiently engaging. It is our contention that increased engagement can be achieved through strategies that may mitigate barriers and promote facilitators of people's engagement with the communication process and adherence to recommendations. Rather than having a one-way communication process in which recommendations are transmitted to the person and expected to be followed, a two-way engaging process centred not only on the person but also on the communication process, could be put forward.

With this goal in mind, this chapter first identifies examples of macro and micro level factors that may explain people's lack of adherence to recommendations. Moreover, reasons for lack of engagement with the healthcare process itself that may translate into people's lack of adherence to recommendations are identified. This will be followed by various examples through which this engagement can be increased, based both on person-centred and communication-centred perspectives. Lastly, we will discuss future possibilities and avenues for research and practice, towards the promotion of an engaging two-way health communication. In order to do this, we will focus specifically on a worldwide growing vulnerable population group with increasing needs with regard to healthcare: older adults.

BARRIERS TO OLDER ADULT'S ADHERENCE TO RECOMMENDATIONS

Over the past few decades, the European institutions have encouraged new forms of social participation in various domains, to implement shared consensus towards problem solving and create stronger support for public actions. New mechanisms and methods aimed at enhancing citizenship have entailed a large variety of activities across different scales and levels of analysis and intervention. This has been manifested worldwide in the construction of new connections and interactions between governmental institutions, non-governmental organizations and citizens. Despite this new "way of doing things" that has been emerging, in the healthcare domain there is still much to do, especially concerning older adult's healthcare. Specifically, there are still a number of barriers that inhibit people's intention to adhere and implement those intentions into behaviours.

One level in which these barriers can be found is the macro level, concerning for example socio-cultural, organizational and socio-political factors. At this level, the theoretical and methodological approaches to the study of older adult's participation and engagement, has become increasingly more complex, in order to face the rapidly changing world and social actors shifting roles. Socio-demographic transformations are making older age a very sensitive socio-political issue and challenges to healthcare systems are manifested worldwide. Significant changes concerning economic resource distribution, social exclusion, the strains posed on the welfare state and the necessary measures to mitigate it, all reflect structural changes at the macro-level. These in turn, have implied profound transformations in the last century, in how senior citizens are perceived worldwide. As one of the most dramatic results, older people often feel non-competent to influence the political debate, and show low levels of collective action – e.g. through petition, protests, occupations, etc. – in different fields, including the healthcare system.

Theories concerning social and economic disengagement have sought to explain the main factors for older adults' distancing from community life. Ironically, they have also often contributed to reinforce an image of elderly passivity in the hands of policymakers. Public policies regarding retirement have particularly contributed to build an image of dependence on State's economic resources and public healthcare services (Cumming & Henry, 1961). Another related negative perception is that the elderly have reduced abilities, needs and capacities in various dimensions of their personal and social life, also contributing to this perceived dependency. These are some of the perceived characteristics associated with an elderly stereotype, implying their view as a homogenous group sharing these negative characteristics. This view has been counteracted in the last few decades, given the senior users new demands concerning various personal and social services, new senior citizen-centred approaches in public services, and increasing demands for professional expertise in health and other domains. This has compelled scholars to shift towards new approaches to ageing (Walker, 2006). Increasing awareness has been reached on conditions that lead to dependence in later life, which may be produced and reproduced by economic mechanisms and social policies. In addition, senior citizens do represent a controversial target by being everything but a homogeneous social group and scholars have growingly testified how old age is highly diverse within the associated population group. As a result, needs and capacities to participate and engage in social and political life should take into account such diversity. This should allow counteracting the perceived passivity and lack of capacities to socially engage and be more participatory, as these may work as barriers by ironically contributing to induce dependency.

To counteract the influence of the negative elderly stereotype, new perspectives on ageing have gained room in the scientific debate in the last few years. The focus on sources and resources for "active ageing" has been critically underpinning the socio-political constraints that often reinforce ageist attitudes and measures (Timonen, 2008). Fight against ageist attitudes should mean actually removing structural, social and psychological barriers in order to improve accessibility to all senior citizens, which can then decide whether or not to engage and participate. Inclusion rather than exclusion of senior citizens by removing barriers that may prevent them from making choices with regard to their own healthcare represents an issue of great relevance when acknowledging demographic trends, and risks of marginalization run through the design of ineffective public services.

Senior citizens' involvement is seen increasingly as a priority against atomized consumerism trends, potentially corroborating neoliberal needs of low-paid labour force as well as of minimization of the state in health and social care services. While so, a critical approach to "active ageing" has also made explicit the risk for further discrimination when narrating "simple" stories of autonomous senior citizens expecting to be involved (Biggs, 2001; Beresford & Branfield, 2006). In these terms, the affirmation that senior citizens empowerment can be improved through voicing their claims and directly involving them in public services, can have also counter-effects. In this regard, Gilleard and Higgs (1998) pinpoint the risk of shifting the responsibility for health from the corporate representation of the people's needs to the individual's responsibility to preserve his or her own health. The authors argue that the market language is forced into citizen's discourse to "sustain a "hyper-reality" of user involvement and empowerment" (p. 246). The authors also state that older people represent one of the most impoverished groups of healthcare users, with inequalities stemming from socio-demographic, socio-economic, geographical and other factors, which may limit their engagement and participation efforts. Moreover, lack of resources to effectively engage and participate may be a limitation, including for example lack of symmetric information and skilled/competent personal assistants (Glendenning, 2008).

Apart from this macro level barriers to the participation of older adults and their engagement in the healthcare process in general, which may translate into lack of adherence to health recommendations, other important barriers exist in more concrete contexts. These concern the communication context and associated situational factors in which recommendations are shared, from the micro level dyadic patient-health professional interaction to the macro level of communication sharing by health organizations (and other stakeholders) to citizens. From these stakeholders, experts and laypeople in general point of view, reasons for non-adherence are often attributed to a rational choice to not adhere. These are often attributed to individual factors (their goals, needs, personality, etc.), namely personal goals that determine an individual to preserve her/his quality of life (DiMatteo, 2004; Schüz, Wolff, Warner, Ziegelmann, & Wurm, 2014). Differently, macro level and situational factors that interact with these and other individual factors are less frequently seen as reasons for non-adherence. For example, the type of therapeutic regimen prescribed to a patient and the perceived available social and individual resources to adhere to the recommendation have been considered important factors. Accordingly, the probability of adherence may decrease due to barriers such as high demanding regimens (e.g. medicine intake rather than lifestyle changes) and low levels of resources (e.g. education; income) (DiMatteo, 2004).

In addition to these factors, the dyadic relationship between the person and the health professional manifested in a micro level setting, between doctors and their patients, and at a macro level between health organizations and citizens, is considered equally important. These include factors for example related to the relationship itself; the health professional characteristics (Kjeldmand, Holmstrom, & Rosenqvist, 2006) and her/his capacities to convey the information and its meaning (Davis, 1968; Davis & von der Lippe, 1968); the information content (DiMatteo, Reiter &, Gambone, 1994).

Less frequently considered, are factors related to the communication process itself. In fact, it is insufficient to consider only the communicator's role (the health professional), the receiver's role (the patient) and the recommendations content (information provided), in promoting adherence to recommendations. The actual process, through which recommendations are communicated and disseminated, may also be determinant. Hence, in addition to a patient centred perspective (for a review, see Mead & Bower, 2000), a communication-centred perspective needs also be acknowledged, in order to increase the effectiveness in promoting adherence (see Mead & Bower, 2002). With regard to this, it should be noted that the interaction between individual characteristics and the way the information is perceived, may even prevent people from hearing/reading the information about the recommendation. In other words, before deciding to adhere or not, they may not even access the content of the information regarding the recommendation, because they may actively avoid it before hearing/reading it. Accordingly, it has been demonstrated that some people show a tendency to avoid information that is communicated by health practitioners (Brashers, Goldsmith, & Hsieh, 2002). For example, as shown by Gaspar et al. (2015), if an information on risk-benefits (e.g. maximum daily amount of red meat consumption) somewhat contradicts the previous information individual's had, their existing attitudes (e.g. towards red meat) and/or beliefs towards the issue (e.g. red meats consumption provides pleasure), they may avoid information that is communicated to them and not seek further information. This can occur for example, if people have positive attitudes towards a certain product (e.g. food product or food component; medicine) or perform certain behaviours, and receive information that it has risks to them.

Apart from individual factors, the communication environment itself may also contribute to people avoiding information. They may perceive health information as overly complex and feel lacking the capacity to deliberate on it, thus reducing their engagement with the information and the associated communication process (Rutsaert et al., 2015). This may occur because they feel that there is: 1) an information overload - too much information available in the "communication environment" surrounding them – thus deeming this information as inconsistent, confusing and hard to comprehend (van Kleef et al., 2006); 2) the communication context has increasingly become more complex and uncertain (Miles & Frewer, 2003; Renn, 2008); 3) there is too much conflicting information from different sources (e.g. Regan et al., 2014). This complex communication context may lead consumers to become more dependent on authorities and less engaged with socially relevant issues (Shepherd & Kay, 2012) and, ironically, more information avoidant (Gaspar, Carvalho, Luís, & Lima, 2014).

Therefore, it is essential to implement communication strategies that on one side, promote better understanding, reduce perceived complexity and are tailored to the individual's information needs, therefore facilitating deliberation. On another side, they should be more motivating and engaging, therefore reducing individual's avoidance. From these, we will focus on the second aspect, by presenting examples of strategies aimed at promoting older adult's engagement with the communication process. Ultimately, this can increase the probability of people deliberating on the information communicated by health professionals and use this information as guides to adjust their behaviour to the recommendations.

FACILITATORS OF OLDER ADULT'S ADHERENCE TO RECOMMENDATIONS

Forms of Participation and Engagement

Counteracting the increasing complexity of societies, participatory mechanisms have been promoted in policymaking for more effective and responsive public services (Fischer, 2003). The inclusion of social actors in a field that traditionally has barely provided spaces for public deliberation, has transformed the socio-political scenario in the last few decades. As pointed out by Arnstein (1969) in his milestone contribution regarding citizen participation, the redistribution of information, resources and influence on decision-making should be understood at the heart of these new processes. The author's analysis was framed within a specific context of struggles carried by low-income citizens and community organizations in the United States in the 1960s. The author operationalized the insights concerning participation through the articulation of a 'ladder' that posits eight rungs of progressive citizens' empowerment through different participatory methods, that provide a good analogy to analyse the subject of this chapter. At the bottom of the ladder we find the so-called 1) *manipulator methods*, followed in an increasing level of participation by 2) *like-therapy participation,* 3) *information,* 4) *consultation,* 5) *placation,* 6) *partnership,* 7) *delegated power,* and finally, 8) *citizen control*. Through means of this ladder, the author sought to capture the diverse degrees of power that citizens can either be given or self-attribute in public decisions. As manipulator and like-therapy methods are inserted at the very bottom of the ladder, the author advises against considering them as forms of genuine participation. Subsequently sets Information as key to empowerment, though not sufficient for the purpose of citizen participation and empowerment. Arguably, Arnstein describes the following approaches, from consultative to citizen-centred, in terms of increasing control over decision and, therefore, empowerment. Developed explanations of each "ladder" will be presented next.

From this contribution, numerous authors have since debated the opportunity to rely on this ladder, to advance it or contest its theoretical and methodological application. Pretty (1995) for example, improved the ladder by distinguishing: manipulative and passive participation whenever the decisions have already been taken; consultation, representing material incentives making people participate by contributing with resources; functional participation, whenever the aim is efficiency and cost reduction, after the main decisions have been made by external agents; interactive, when local groups take control over decisions; and self-mobilization of people controlling the resources and taking the initiative independently of external organizations. Fung (2006) also criticizes Arnstein's ladder (1969) and argues that different contexts demand different typologies of participation which cannot be defined as bad or good in a "normative" sense. They should be rather seen as a complex combination of different scopes, extents of authority, and modes of communication and decision. Differently, consistent with Arnstein's proposals, redistributing powers, gathering new agents for shared projects, reconsidering the borders between public and private, regenerating trust towards political institutions, are some of the complex issues emerging through participatory processes in the last few years (Sintomer, 2007). Participation can be designed in very different ways and this has opened to a lively debate in social and political sciences. The power exerted within the participatory initiatives may take different forms depending on dynamics among participants as well as on the relation between participants and institutions (Nie & Verba, 1975; Gaventa, 2006; Falanga, 2013, 2014).

Although being a classical approach to citizens' participation developed decades ago, we think that Arnstein's (1969) "ladder of citizen participation" provides a clear analogy to propose different ways through which older people can participate and be engaged in the area of health recommendations communication and promotion of patient's adherence to health programs. In our view, this area may be overly dominated by a one-way informative approach and thus, various forms of participation can be followed, moving forward towards a two-way communication. Some of these examples will be given next. From these, we will specifically focus on the last five levels of Arnstein's "ladder" (1969) from Consultation to Citizen Control. We will not consider the first three levels - (1) Manipulation, (2) Therapy and (3) Informing – as the first two are considered to be "substitutes" for genuine participation, and the third as representing only one-way directive communications. Differently, Consultation and Placation allow the distribution of a relative – yet low – degree of power. On one side, consultative approaches are concerned with collecting people's voice, opinions and feedback to devise possible changes. When citizens hear and are heard, the process of interaction between health professionals and patients is likely to enhance models for two way communication. On the other side, placation implies a more pro-active role for all the agents, in shedding power from established owners to recipients. However, in both cases no assurance is given on the impact of patients' views over final decisions. It should be noted then that, although Consultation and Placation provide approaches with the potential for increased citizen participation and engagement, they reflect a degree of tokenism in which an illusion of power for those "have-nots", is created. Hence, they may often be more of a barrier than a facilitator to citizen participation and engagement, as they provide this "illusion" and may prevent higher levels in the "ladder" of being achieved. Differently, from Partnership to Delegated Power and Citizen Control, we find increasing levels of participation and shared decisional power, where people can negotiate and make changes in the process and ultimately self-manage their health behaviour in a way that allows them to effectively adhere to recommendations.

It should be noted however, that we draw on Arnstein's "ladder" (1969) only as a way to provide structure to the chapter, with regard to the presentation of adherence facilitators and also because it is a much known analogy to citizen participation, which allows making arguments clearer by drawing on familiar examples. More recent approaches (e.g. Collins & Ison, 2006) have criticized Arnstein's "ladder" (1969), seeing it not as much as a participation approach but more as a social learning process towards true participation. Hence, next we present examples of facilitative strategies that may allow achieving increased participation/engagement, based on Arnstein's proposal as a familiar approach in this regard.

Consultation

In a broad sense, consultation implies the invitation made to citizens for sharing their opinions (Arnstein, 1969). This can take various forms, from more formal or informal interviews to more scientifically validated forms, including for example experimental and non-experimental studies on people's adherence to health recommendations. For example, through this, patients can be "consulted" to determine the facilitators and barriers to this adherence. We will next present some examples of studies held exactly with this goal in mind.

Considering the example of medical prescriptions and regimes, in accordance to Osterberg and Blaschke (2005), health professionals have been contributing to poor adherence to medication. This is due to failing to explain the drugs benefits and side effects, not taking into account the lifestyle of patients, the cost of drugs, prescription of complex administration regimens, and establishment of weak therapeutic relationships. All these function as barriers to adherence that should be taken into account if consultation is to be implemented. Given these findings, it should also be noted that communicating of information about medication prescription to elderly patients, should be carefully undertaken. Accordingly, assessments should be implemented with the goal of collecting information and feedback about the most prevalent factors in non-adherence. This should take into account not only the patients but also their surrounding contexts and its various elements (e.g. health professionals; communication content and framing) (Krueger, Berger, & Felkey, 2005; Vermeire, Hearnshaw, Van Royen, & Denekens, 2001).

In order to overcome the problem of patient's poor medication adherence (MA), various studies have been put forward, that we consider fitting the category of Consultation. In most studies, the MA factors were separately analysed. Nevertheless, through the experimental research model (Lamiell, 1995) it is possible to simultaneously study factors and processes that influence MA, namely the factors' relative weight and also between-factors interactions. The therapeutic relationship itself has an impact on MA as it generates less or greater trust in health professionals. Particularly the trust that patients have in health professionals was conceptualized by Hall, Camacho, Dugan and Balkrishnan (2002) in association with five factors: loyalty, competence, honesty, confidentiality, and global confidence (the "soul" of confidence, combining elements of some or all of the previous factors). Trust is generated in the reciprocal relations of the consultation process. Unfortunately, many health professionals are not formally trained to detect whether patients are adhering to medication and do not know how best to intervene when patients seemingly do not adhere to medication (Marcum, Sevick, & Handler, 2013). Also the non-compliance to prescription regimens may generate frustration in health professionals, leading to paternalistic attitudes (Wens, Vermeire, Van Royen, Sabbe, & Denekens, 2005). On the other hand, the health professionals' perception of drug adherence can influence prescription standards and lead to failure in the therapy intensity (el-Kebbi, Ziemer, Gallina, Dunbar, & Phillips, 1999; Roberts & Volberding, 1999; Huizinga, Bleich, Beach, Clark, & Cooper, 2010). For example, in the pre-prescription phase, HIV/AIDS's health professionals may make decisions based on their beliefs about the patient's likelihood of adhering to therapy, exploring their current psychosocial situations (Roberts & Volberding, 1999). In post-prescription phases, they may often suspect the emergence of non-adherence, even when patients admit to comply with therapy. Then, if professionals have difficulties in dealing with this perceived distrust in patients, this may induce a lack of exploration of reasons for non-adherence: this bias is an important barrier to in-depth adherence communication (Barfod, Hecht, Rubow, & Gerstoft, 2006).

The drug administration regimen complexity (RC) has also been found to determine adherence: the more complex the more likely it will not be followed, since simpler administration regimens tend to have higher adherence (Matsui, 2013; Russell, Conn, & Jantarakupt, 2006). The RC is related to the number of prescribed medications and it has a negative impact on MA, particularly in elderly patients, who on average receive more prescriptions than other age groups. This is an important issue because the elderly tend to be more vulnerable to cognitive deficits and seem to be less capable in decision-making processes based on information that requires in-depth analysis (Finucane & Lees, 2005; see also Diniz & Amado, 2014). Cooper et al. (2005) showed that the cognitive decline by itself does not decrease adherence but together with a resistance to care, may decrease adherence. The authors add that this association is typical in people with poor insight into their dementia, implying that health professionals can improve MA tailoring interventions to the dementia degree. Another relevant finding regards financial factors, namely the existence of low financial resources which have a negative impact on MA (Safran et al., 2005). In general, it is not mandatory for health professionals to ask patients how they pay for medication. For example, in the study of Ried (2010) the cost of medication (CM) played an important role on adherence in patients who have low adherence rates, but not in patients who normally adhere to medication, suggesting that despite financial difficulties, patients are influenced by their health beliefs. Thus, the relationship that patients establish with health professionals is important as it can influence the perception of valuation of medication prescription. Finally, the severity of clinical condition (SCC) is also important factor. When a clinical condition that poses a risk to life is communicated, it generates an aversive feeling, usually of great intensity, which raises feelings of dread. However, despite this, dread may also act as an emotional persuasion factor invoking risk mitigation measures (Sjöberg, 2002). For example, a person who considers her/his illness to be serious but controllable through medication will have a more adaptive response to the threat that the disease may represent (Schüz et al., 2011).

These MA determinants were mainly studied, separately, within quantitative, correlational and clinical experimental research models (Lamiell, 1995). These have included direct measures of adherence such as pill intake and medical tests; direct forms of feedback collection (e.g. through verbal reports collected from interviews or focus groups); and indirect measures of adherence and its determinants (e.g. risk perception) such as patient self-reports, patient spouse reports, medical reports and questionnaires. These are often mentioned in the literature as some of the most commonly used techniques to assess MA (Krueger et al., 2005; Osterberg & Blaschke, 2005; Vermeire et al., 2001). However, experimental research model use (Lamiell, 1995) can be advantageous to simultaneously study factors and processes that influence MA. An example of this is provided in a study developed by Santos (2014) with elders without depression and cognitive impairment, in a non-clinical context. Factors such as SCC (severity of clinical condition: normal, serious, life threatening), CM (cost of medication: 75€, 150€, 225€, matching a 15% proportion of 500€, 1000€, and 1500€ monthly income, respectively), RC (regimen complexity: complex and simple), and TC (trust in clinicians, operationalized as clinician experience: experienced vs. highly experienced), were analysed through a randomized sequence of 18 scenarios presented on a computer. Each scenario conveyed the same cover story depicting an ordinary medical consultation, wherein a fictitious elder patient had to decide whether to adhere to a new drug prescription for a heart condition, as suggested by a doctor. The participants reported how much they thought the fictitious patient was willing to adhere, on a Visual Analogical Scale ranging from "not at all adhering" to "totally adhering".

Results showed in both RC but not in both the TC, that SCC and CM had a main effect on adherence, and that their interaction effect added up until a "serious" level of SCC was achieved. The latter represented a ceiling effect of SCC precluding a further impact of CM even at its highest level (225€ among the patients' current expenses). This interaction means that CM strongly determined the adherence but in a situation of risk in which life is of concern, it progressively took less importance. Irrespectively of the CM, it appeared that the elderly (and people in general) possess affective rationality (Slovic, Finucane, Peters, & MacGregor, 2002; Slovic, Peters, Finucane, & MacGregor, 2005) implying that when facing a hazardous situation, the financial aspect becomes less important. Moreover, despite financial difficulties, patients may be influenced by their health beliefs (Piette, Bears, Rosland, & McHorney, 2011; Ried, 2010), which makes possible to decrease the therapy failure, even when there is high cost for drugs. Another finding was that participants previously clinically diagnosed with heart condition showed more willingness to adhere when confronted with trials combining prescribed complex regimen with highly experienced clinician, than trials simply with an experienced clinician.

The studies examples and the methodology underlying them, have theoretical and practical potential for designing communication protocols with the goal of enhancing MA among the elderly. Using a discourse similar to Santos (2014, pp. 52-53), health professionals can discuss the cost of drugs with patients, knowing that similar importance judgments are made for both "serious" and "life threatening" conditions of SCC. The implications of the affective process on risk communication, drawing on how the different levels of medical condition severity are presented to the elderly, may also help outlining strategies to increase adherence. However, information manipulation concerning the levels of disease severity is ethically unacceptable, even though it might be a benefit: its effect can only occur upon a full demonstration of appropriate information transparency (without excessive technicalities, and pointing out real consequences). At the same time, it should be associated with the value of decision-making autonomy of the patient, a dimension needing to be accounted for in MA.

Placation

Although important, consultation is not enough by itself to motivate elderly people to achieve higher levels of involvement and participation in health promotion programs. Through Placation, a form of consultation may also be implemented, although in this case people begin to have some degree of influence (Arnstein, 1969) over the healthcare process and specifically over the communication process. Although placation is not a true two-way communication between health professionals and people, it may be step towards its implementation. The reason for it not being a true two-way communication is related to the "power balance" given that the power to decide and adjust the communication process still lies with the communication managers (decision makers) and health professionals. Nevertheless, it can allow for example designing of communication adapted/tailored to people's everyday "language" and increase the effectiveness of healthcare communication in real time and as it develops. This may allow empowering both the health professionals and communication recipients (i.e. patients and general population). The feedback resulting from this interaction can be further used to provide input for communication managers and health professionals with valuable insights, allowing them to adjust future communication strategies and better manage their communicational resources.

The role played by both the health professionals and the communication recipients is very important, as they influence not only the way that communicational processes are shaped but also the building blocks towards a stronger involvement and participation. This can be achieved through the trust building and creation of a functional two-way practitioner-recipient channel, set to achieve relational and communicational goals. To start building this trust, it is important that health professionals are ready and able to listen and value the reactions and inputs/feedback shared by the recipients, upon receiving information. Hence, this process should be seen more as a form of social learning or co-constructed learning process that allows a convergence of goals, expectations, understandings and behaviours (Collins & Ison, 2006). This may allow the progression of all people involved towards higher levels of participation and mutual learning.

Examples of this communication-centred perspective are found in the literature, representing a form of placation. For example, a simple way for people to provide feedback is through the expression of comments, opinions, and questions. However, people are not used to do this nor are the health professionals used to promote this "habit", when some sort of information or other stimuli is presented. It is therefore more frequent to find placation in the form of feedback acquired through people expressing their views/ opinions on a certain subject(s) and not as much from feedback acquired through questions, opinions, and comments produced by people in real time. Accessing the later may allow tailoring communications to people's actual and perceived information needs, rather than to the information the health professionals perceive that people need. There are examples in the literature concerning tailored interventions that aim for this, such as for example the Adherence Therapy (Daley, Deane, Gray, Hill, & Myint, 2015). Although there are examples, these are more often found in the scientific literature rather than in practice.

To better understand the importance of listening to and valuing the feedback shared by people when confronted with information, we must look into the concept of Deliberation. Deliberation should be seen as a discursive knowledge construction and sense-making process, that is the basis for an informed decision-making with regard to health (namely risks and benefits). By promoting deliberation upon receiving information, people may compare the "new" received information with pre-existing information. This can allow for an "internal debate" with herself/himself and his/her own thoughts and weighing up information and (risk-benefit) trade-offs. By doing this, the creation and integration of new knowledge, new understandings, new decision and acting strategies may be achieved (Rutsaert et al., 2014; Barnett et al., 2008; De Cindo, Macintosh, & Peraboni, 2010). Under this assumption, comments, opinions and questions emerge as "deliberative markers", which can for example allow a qualitative analysis of this knowledge construction process (Marcu et al., 2014; Rutsaert et al., 2014). In order to foster participation and involvement, health professionals could see these deliberative markers as feedback, valuing it as a way of understanding people's deliberative processes (their "way of thinking") rather than discarding it as a sign of lack of information. It should be noted however, that deliberation is an inherently heterogeneous process that may differ between different people with different life experiences, knowledge, sociocultural and educational backgrounds. In addition, this type of feedback may also allow understanding the themes and strategies used by people to construct meaning, allowing health professionals to adapt their language and explanatory examples given, to the person's worldviews and cultural and educational backgrounds. This can be done for example by providing meaningful and familiar examples that can help people to understand information. This is important because when people use prior existing information to scrutinize new information, they tend to use the most readily accessible information and analogies to other pieces of information that are familiar to them and somewhat perceived as similar to what they know (see e.g. Morgan, Fischhoff, Bostrom, & Altman, 2002; Peters, Hess, Västfjäll, & Auman, 2007). This procedure may promote an initial form of participation and involvement, by eliciting comments and questions and ultimately, allowing the co-construction of the communication process. For example, in an exploratory study that addressed the deliberative processes upon confronting the participants with a health recommendation with regard to red meat consumption (Domingos, 2014) we found that very few participants used the numerical information conveyed by health authorities. Instead, deliberation was based on information on their own past behaviours and behaviours of others (e.g. family members and neighbours), used for social comparison.

Lastly these aspects should also be seen from the point of view of new forms of expression that are available nowadays. The emergence of the internet changed the way people engage with information, which combined with the increasing use of communication and information technologies in healthcare settings, implies that more and more people rely on health information conveyed by electronic communication tools. Particularly, the potential of social media to improve healthcare, health communication and health information sharing should not be underestimated (Chretien & Kind, 2013) for all people, including the elderly. Online information seeking habits and social media comments, opinions and questions should also be taken into consideration, and can be further used to understand and tailor communication to people's needs. It is important that health organizations, health program managers and health professionals follow this trend, by providing safe digital environments. In these, people may seek accurate information to address their health concerns, produce their own user-generated content, exchange their comments, opinions and questions with expert professionals and others, therefore satisfying their needs while building trust. Hence, social media data can be analysed and used to provide another form of placation, helping to move forward towards higher levels of participation.

Partnership and Delegated Power

While consultation and placation are valuable sources of information for adapting communications and health programs to older adults, the power that older people have is still low. This is because there is no assurance that feedback will actually be implemented into healthcare changes and in the communication of recommendations. In this regard, it should be noted that the concept of participation is visibly intertwined with different fields of older adults' daily life. When focusing on the effective integration of senior citizens into social and familiar networks, as well as into community life, we should better consider the impact over individual and collective standards of quality of life (Lavasseur, Richardc, Gauvinf, & Raymondi, 2010). Health and social care systems have often promoted new mechanisms for the involvement of senior users. The rise of more sophisticated and diverse consumerism, new demands from service users and carers, new questions concerning professionals and experts towards involvement-oriented practices, make participation of senior citizens a matter of high and global significance (Scourfield & Burch, 2010).

Opportunities for activity imply looking at the social, economic and political structures that either facilitate or constrain senior citizens' involvement in public life activities. Activity can also refer to physical abilities and continuity in labour force, as well as social, economic, cultural activities and participation in civic affairs (World Health Organization [WHO], 2002; European Commission [EC], 2012). In this regard, the International Classification of Functioning, Disability and Health (ICF), as provided guidelines for assessment, placing emphasis on the involvement of people in need of technical and/or human help to accomplish daily activities in life situations (WHO, 2001). Based on this, participation should be analysed with validated measures and focus on the degree to which a person fulfils roles, has relationships, and displays community presence as well as other actions that can be witnessed by an observer. In this regard, activity if seen (as a mere execution of tasks) is overtaken by participation (meant as functioning beyond impairment and performance, i.e. control of one's own life), even if the person may not actually do something themselves (Dijkers, Yavuzer, Ergin, Weitzenkamp, & Whiteneck, 2002).

Older people's access to organizations, institutions and agencies that have a role in their lives, in a way that may allow them to "have a say", is a primary challenge (Carter & Beresford, 2000). Looking at the different forms of older adults' participation through the lens of Arnstein's (1969) ladder, it is evident how the higher rungs – the delegated power and citizen's control – are not the most common experiences worldwide. In most cases, participation is mediated by organizations that provide the possibility to exercise their democratic rights through representatives that promote their material and immaterial interests. These organizations are mainly voluntary agencies, community groups and political parties, which have been emerging in the last few decades, attributed the role of wide range of functions on behalf of older people. Such functions mainly concern advocating, acting as pressure or lobbyist group, facilitating the interaction among other senior citizens' organizations, providing services to senior citizens, etc. Service user organizations generally reflect the right of service users to speak and act on their own behalf but have developed in different ways and with different strategies. Often these operate either independently or in partnership-based arrangements with State and social service systems (Beresford & Branfield, 2006).

Organized or non-organized forms of senior citizens' involvement can both encourage new forms of planning ahead for the elderly's own health and wellbeing. Cook and Klein (2005) argue that involving the public in services moves towards developing partnership with patients in the planning of services. Evans and Vallely (2007) state that the "Opportunities for service users to be involved in decisions about care delivery and service development on an ongoing basis are increasingly seen as central to a sense of well-being." (p. 15). The active involvement of senior citizens was considered an asset which potentially increases the chances of success of service planning and care management process. The Program "Better Government for Older People", run in United Kingdom at the end of the 1990s, has argued in favour of the need to go beyond mere consultations through a capillary implementation of new initiatives at the local level in Europe (Vegeris et al., 2007). On the one hand, the experiences carried out in UK reflect that health and social care issues predominate in the Local Authorities' thinking about older people's participation. In other words, the business and the context of major interaction are directed towards senior users of such services. More traditional models of consultation and information sharing were favoured by the Local Authorities, though in numerous cases the new forms of interaction led to the implementation of "wider and deeper" forms of engagement (Farrington, Bebbington, Wellard, & Lewis, 1993). All in all, the most innovative forms of engagement and positive effects on seniors' involvement typically contained elements of informality against business-like settings. This outcome confirmed that care services' users can be more effectively involved by opening to their role as "decision-makers" concerning their own health. In this regard, Barnes and Bennet (1998) assumed users' will to be involved not only in final decisions but also in "framing" the problems, as the basis to undertake participatory researches and citizen-led programs evaluations. Hayden and Boaz (2000) argued that the Program "Better Government for Older People" has ensured that healthcare services reflect the needs of older people and raised the awareness concerning the positive contribution of their participation. Nevertheless to actively engage older people in new democratic processes, some type of formal organization is nevertheless required.

With regard to the direct control exerted by senior citizens in self-regulatory forms of organization, one of the authors of this chapter is currently involved in a European Commission-funded Project aimed at identifying participatory practices in policymaking[1]. A small part of the evidence collected through this Project sheds a light on direct involvement of older adults in public services. Among them some interesting practices are being carried out in healthcare systems. The case of the Andalusia region in Spain, is a clear example of how senior citizens and users could take part in their well-being. There are more than 3,500 social centres regulated by the Regional Ministry, which work on issues relate with child care, drug addiction, disabilities, immigration and elderly people. Services are provided in coordination with local authorities and in collaboration with local NGOs. Almost two thousands centres are devoted also to senior citizens and The Regional Government of Andalusia issued the Decree 72/2012 which transformed the "Day Centres" for older people into "Active Participation Centres". These Centres promote a new form of healthcare service delivery by including senior users in the General Assembly board and elect their representatives within the Management and Participation Board of the Centres. It means that beyond promoting care, services and social activities, these Centres provide the tools to make senior citizens' voice heard, in decision-making. The Centres deal with a wide range of activities, including cultural and leisure, as well as ICT training, and advice on juridical matters and other services for low income seniors. Activities and workshops are decided together with the Regional authority and all services are discussed in the General Assembly and decided by the Management and Participation Board together with the Direction of the Centres.

Mere forms of consultation may not be effective if the results are ignored or even used to legitimate a pre-set agenda. Both UK and Andalusia cases make a point on senior citizens' role in decisional processes that directly affect them. The "Better Government for Older People" program in the UK owned a large variety of approaches that resulted into very different outcomes. The need to go further in providing decisional power to older users has been clearly pinpointed as one of the results by the people involved in the local experiences (Vegeris et al., 2007). At the same time, the ongoing case of Andalusia demonstrates that is possible to include older people's "voice" in the management of health and care services. While so, it also demonstrates that the socio-political context wherein these experiences take place plays a crucial role. In the last two decades, Andalusia has been one of the most "active" regions in Europe, with regard to the implementation of participatory mechanisms in policymaking.

Barriers and Facilitators across Different Levels of Participation and Engagement

Given the different "ladders" that may be crossed to achieve more effective and "true" forms of elderly participation/engagement, we now synthesize the barriers mentioned before, by considering their detrimental role in this progression. These are shown in the table 1 below.

It should be noted that our goal in this regard was not to be exhaustive in finding all possible barriers but rather to present a wide diversity of reasons for non-adherence, at macro and micro levels of analysis.

TOWARDS THE PROMOTION OF AN ENGAGING TWO-WAY HEALTH COMMUNICATION

In the examples given above, various forms of older adult's participation in the healthcare process we presented. These went from different levels from consultation – including direct and indirect information and feedback gathering – to "partnership" and "delegated power" in which older people may have a shared decisional power, can negotiate and make changes in the healthcare and communication process. All of these were presented as strategies through which participation in the healthcare process may be increased, implying a reduction of barriers to and increment of facilitators of older people's adherence to health recommendations. From all of these, however, the last step (8) of Arnstein's ladder (1969) – *Citizen Control* – is still unaccounted for. The power implied in it would allow people to have an active role in their care, for example by self-managing their behaviours, cognitions and emotions, to more effectively adhere to health recommendations.

There are various examples in the literature (e.g. concerning physical activity programs; diet and nutritional programs; etc.) showing that the most effective health programs involve a last stage in which

Table 1. Barriers to older adult's adherence to health recommendations across levels of participation/ engagement

Level of analysis	Barriers	Level of participation in which there is a detrimental effect
Macro	• Ageist attitudes and behaviours; negative stereotypes associated with a perceived homogeneity of the elderly population group, concerning various aspects of the elderly personal and social life with consequences on engagement and participation (e.g. passiveness, reduced capacities and interests) • Inequalities stemming from socio-demographic, socio-economic, geographical and other factors • Asymmetries of information concerning laws, procedures, and health policies • Communication context as determined by health organizations and other experts/stakeholders (e.g. lack of information sharing; ineffective communication framing and content)	• Consultation • Placation • Partnership & delegated power • Citizen control
	• Lack of resources to effectively engage and participate (e.g. information; professional support) • Over-emphasizing "active ageing" and elderly's autonomy, attributing the responsibility for preserving health to the individuals, rather than to the health care professionals and organizations	• Placation • Partnership & delegated power • Citizen control
Micro	• Communication environment and processes involved in the dyadic patient-health professional interaction (e.g. negative perceived relationship; ineffective communication process and setting) • Characteristics of the health professional/communicator (lack of capacities to convey information, to engage patients, etc.)	
	• High demanding regimens (e.g. medicine intake rather than lifestyle changes) • Low levels of social and individual resources (e.g. education; income) to adhere to recommendations – objectively available and perceived as available by the elderly • Characteristics of the elderly patient that conflict with collaborative methods (e.g. cognitive impairment; information avoidance; lack of interest/motivation in the communication process) • Characteristics of the communication context (health information perceived as overly complex and/or surpassing the capacity to deliberate on it)	• Partnership & delegated power • Citizen control

the development of self-regulation competencies is a priority (see Godinho, Alvarez, & Lima, 2013). Naturally, for this to occur, the necessary conditions need to be set, in a preceding stage. A study by Schüz, Wurm, Warner, Wolff and Schwarzer (2013), for example, showed that emphasising health as a subjective motive in older adults is necessary for intentions to be translated into healthy behaviours, via planning. This planning is one of the key features that may allow older adults to implement their intentions into actions and adhere to recommendations, as it may allow finding strategies to cope with barriers and reinforce the facilitators.

The importance of planning in self-management for health behaviours to take place is demonstrated through the Health Action Process Approach (see Schwarzer, 1992, 2008). This approach considers two main phases that need to be implemented, for healthy behaviour to occur - motivational phase and volitional phase – each determined by different factors: The motivational phase emphasizes the importance of (action) self-efficacy, outcome expectancies, and risk perception; the volitional phase emphasizes the importance of both action planning and coping planning, and of self-efficacy maintenance/recovery, for a person to change from an "intender" to an "actor". Planning demands the person to both plan their own behaviour(s) and plan the change in the necessary conditions for it to take place, including overcoming barriers to its implementation and devising (individual and contextual) facilitators for it. Additionally, the person needs to be capable of recovering from failures (e.g. forgetting to take medicine) and having optimistic (self-efficacy) beliefs that they can cope with these barriers (e.g. memory impairments) and recover from failures. All this demands self-regulation strategies, dependant on affective, cognitive and behavioural dimensions. Based on this approach, we consider that the motivational phase is the focus of the various forms of older people's participation referred before – consultation, placation, partnership and delegated power - as these clearly aim to increase older people's engagement with the healthcare process, i.e. increase their motivation and involvement with the various aspects of it (e.g. patient-health professional relationship; degree of shared decisional power; for a similar perspective, see Cox & Klinger, 2004, with regard to Systematic Motivational Counselling - SMC). However, in our view, the volitional phase can only be reached if the control over the process is placed upon the person. This can only be achieved if a form of Citizen Control (as presented by Arnstein, 1969) is promoted, in which people can self-manage their healthcare process.

A few recent health programs have been trying to reach these goals. One example is the Health and Welfare Information Portal (ZWIP) developed by Robben et al. (2012a) and Robben et al. (2012b) to be an intervention for older people with frailty, based on an online health community (OHC). This aimed at facilitating multidisciplinary communication between health professionals and information exchange in the care of older people. Moreover, it aimed to facilitate self-management and shared decision making between older people and their informal caregivers. This included for example the stimulation of engagement and two-way communication between the patients and a team of health professionals. Moreover, it was supported by strategies for increasing motivation that were tailored to older adults. This was focused on improving self-efficacy and beliefs in the elder's ability to complete the tasks requested and fulfil the pre-determined goals, thus allowing the necessary conditions for self-management to take place. A more recent example in this regard is the SMART-PD program presented by Lakshminarayana et al. (2014), aimed towards the self-management of Parkinson's disease. This program is based on technological assistance from smartphone and internet platforms, including a set of adherence promotion tools. Although still under evaluation, this program may be an effective tool to achieve "citizen control" of their own health, assisted by new technologies. Other examples, have also presented Online Health Seeking (OHS) – "the process by which people find, share and consume online health and wellness information" (Bonner & Mynatt, 2014, p. 1) – as a new trend for interventions focused on adherence and related aspects, based on Patient-Centered Care (PCC) approaches. Various examples (see Bonner & Mynatt, 2014) have shown that PCC may result in positive effects such as improving patient provider relationships and patient's satisfaction with the healthcare process.

It should be noted nevertheless that this type of programs is under development and modification, and still face several barriers (see Makai et al., 2014). First of all, people low digital literacy and low of internet use inhibit the use of OHC. Second, there are various factors that serve as barriers to self-management, even when people are motivated and engaged in the program. Accordingly, Robben et al. (2012a) identified various factors found in the literature, such as: people's attitude toward self-management; emotions (e.g. fear of losing independence); their perceived self-efficacy for self-management; their perceived knowledge (e.g. about the disease, symptoms, and treatments); personal skills and limitations (e.g. cognitive deficits); perceived social norms and social support (e.g. advocacy); financial constraints; and the high complexity of the health care system; the health professionals not providing adequate information for self-management; the health professionals not being genuinely interested in the older person; and lastly the health professionals not encouraging questions. In addition, from the health professional's point of view, various barriers were also identified, such as: their attitude toward patient self-management; their knowledge and skills for self-management support; and others aspects of the health care system[2]. Despite facing several barriers, the types of programs presented emerge as an interesting future path, towards self-regulation as a basis for citizen's control of their own healthcare.

CONCLUSION

From the various aspects referred in the previous sections, it is clear that there is still much work to do in finding strategies that on one side, increase older people's motivation, participation and engagement with the healthcare process and, on another side, provide the necessary conditions for self-regulation, with support/monitoring from formal and informal care providers. Nevertheless, it may be a matter of time, as the various existent programs are being improved and new ones being developed. Longitudinal evaluations of some of these programs (Makai et al., 2014) show that despite the existence of various barriers to their success, there are positive outcomes for the people involved in these (such as e.g. in their activities of daily living). Hence, as long as the necessary conditions are in place (e.g. increase in digital literacy and internet usage, regarding the ZWIP program), older people's motivation and self-management of their own healthcare process may be incremented through more effective two-way communications and self-regulation strategies promotion. Ultimately, this will allow reducing barriers and reinforcing facilitators, towards an increased adherence to health recommendations.

ACKNOWLEDGMENT

William James Center for Research, ISPA- Instituto Universitário is supported by the FCT Grant No. UID/PSI/04810/2013

REFERENCES

Arnold, M. (2008). Polypharmacy and older adults: A role for psychology and psychologists. *Professional Psychology, Research and Practice*, *39*(3), 283–289. doi:10.1037/0735-7028.39.3.283

Arnstein, S. (1969). A ladder of citizen participation. *Journal of the American Institute of Planners*, *26*(4), 216–233. doi:10.1080/01944366908977225

Barfod, T. S., Hecht, F. M., Rubow, C., & Gerstoft, J. (2006). Physicians' communication with patients about adherence to HIV medication in San Francisco and Copenhagen: A qualitative study using grounded theory. *BMC Health Services Research*, *6*(1), 154. doi:10.1186/1472-6963-6-154 PMID:17144910

Barnes, M., & Bennet, G. (1998). Frail bodies, courageous voices: Older people influencing community care. *Health & Social Care in the Community*, *6*(2), 102–111. doi:10.1046/j.1365-2524.1998.00105.x PMID:11560582

Barnett, J., Fife-Schaw, C., Shepherd, R., Timotijevic, L., Fletcher, J., & Fletcher, D. (2008). *Online deliberative engagement: A pilot study. A report for the Wellcome Trust*. Surrey, U.K.: University of Surrey/Brook Lyndhurst/White October.

Bauer, U. E., Briss, P. A., Goodman, R. A., & Bowman, B. A. (2014). Prevention of chronic disease in the 21st century: Elimination of the leading preventable causes of premature death and disability in the USA. *Lancet*, *384*(9937), 45–52. doi:10.1016/S0140-6736(14)60648-6 PMID:24996589

Beresford, P., & Branfield, F. (2006). Developing inclusive partnerships: User-defined outcomes, networking and knowledge – a case study. *Health & Social Care in the Community*, *14*(5), 436–444. doi:10.1111/j.1365-2524.2006.00654.x PMID:16918836

Biggs, S. (2001). Toward critical narrativity: Stories of aging in contemporary social policy. *Journal of Aging Studies*, *15*(4), 303–316. doi:10.1016/S0890-4065(01)00025-1

Bonner, M., & Mynatt, E. D. (2014). Gauging the patient-centered potential of online health seeking. *Proceedings of the 8th International Conference on Pervasive Computing Technologies for Healthcare PervasiveHealth '14*. Retrieved from https://research.cc.gatech.edu/ecl/sites/edu.ecl/files/PH-paper-v5-cameraReady.pdf

Branin, J. J. (2001). The role of memory strategies in medication adherence among the elderly. *Home Health Care Services Quarterly*, *20*(2), 1–16. doi:10.1300/J027v20n02_01 PMID:11987652

Brashers, D. E., Goldsmith, D. J., & Hsieh, E. (2002). Information seeking and avoiding in health contexts. *Human Communication Research*, *28*(2), 258–271. doi:10.1111/j.1468-2958.2002.tb00807.x

Carter, T., & Beresford, P. (2000). *Age and change: Models of involvement for older people*. New York, NY: Joseph Rowntree Foundation.

Chretien, K., & Kind, T. (2013). Social media as a tool in medicine. *Circulation*, *127*, 1351–1443. doi:10.1161/CIRCULATIONAHA.112.128017

Collins, K., & Ison, R. (2006). Dare we jump off Arnstein's ladder? Social learning as a new policy paradigm. *Proceedings of the PATH Conference*, Scotland. Retrieved from http://www.macaulay.ac.uk/PATHconference/outputs/PATH_abstract_3.1.2.pdf

Cook, G., & Klein, B. (2005). Involvement of older people in care, service and policy planning. *International Journal of Older People Nursing in association with Journal of Clinical Nursing, 14*(S1), 43-47.

Cooper, C., Carpenter, I., Katona, C., Schroll, M., Wagner, C., Fialova, D., & Livingstone, G. (2005). The AdHOC study of older adults' adherence to medication in 11 countries. *The American Journal of Geriatric Psychiatry*, *13*(12), 1067–1076. doi:10.1097/00019442-200512000-00006 PMID:16319299

Cox, M., & Klinger, E. (2004). Systematic motivational counseling: The motivational structure questionnaire in action. In W. M. Cox & E. Klinger (Eds.), *Handbook of motivational counselling: Concepts, approaches, and assessment* (pp. 3–28). Chichester: John Willey & Sons.

Cumming, E., & Henry, W. E. (1961). *Growing old: The process of disengagement*. New York, NY: Basic Books.

Daley, D., Deane, K., Gray, R., Hill, R., & Myint, P. (2015). Qualitative evaluation of adherence therapy in Parkinson's disease: A multidirectional model. *Patient Preference and Adherence*, *9*, 989–998. doi:10.2147/PPA.S80158 PMID:26203231

Davies, T. (2009). The blossoming field of online deliberation. In *Online deliberation: Design, research, and practice* (pp. 1-19).

Davis, M. S. (1968). Variations in patients' compliance with doctors' advice: An empirical analysis of patterns of communication. *American Journal of Public Health, 58*(2), 274–288. doi:10.2105/AJPH.58.2.274 PMID:5688773

Davis, M. S., & von der Lippe, R. P. (1968). Discharge from Hospital Against Medical Advice: A Study of Reciprocity in the Doctor-Patient Relationship. *Social Science & Medicine, 1*, 336–342.

De Cindio, F., Macintosh, A., & Peraboni, C. (2010). From e-Participation to Online Deliberation. *Proceedings of the Fourth International Conference on Online Deliberation OD2010*, Leeds, UK.

Dijkers, M. P., Yavuzer, G., Ergin, S., Weitzenkamp, D., & Whiteneck, G. G. (2002). A tale of two countries: Environmental impacts on social participation after spinal cord injury. *Spinal Cord, 40*(7), 351–362. doi:10.1038/sj.sc.3101310 PMID:12080463

DiMatteo, M. R. (2004). Variations in patients' adherence to medical recommendations: A quantitative review of 50 years of research. *Medical Care, 42*(3), 200–209. doi:10.1097/01.mlr.0000114908.90348.f9 PMID:15076819

DiMatteo, M. R., Reiter, R. C., & Gambone, J. C. (1994). Enhancing medication adherence through communication and informed collaborative choice. *Health Communication, 6*(4), 253–265. doi:10.1207/s15327027hc0604_2

Diniz, A. M., & Amado, N. (2014). Procedures for successful data collection through psychological tests in the elderly. *Psychology/Psicologia. Reflexão e Crítica, 27*(3), 491–497. doi:10.1590/1678-7153.201427309

Domingos, S. (2014). *Alimentação com conta, peso e medida: Um estudo exploratório da representação mental e da quantificação subjetiva do consumo de carne vermelha, numa amostra de idosos.* [Estimating, weighing and measuring food consumption: An exploratory study of the mental representation and subjective quantification of meat consumption, in an elderly sample] [Master thesis]. University of Évora, Évora, Portugal.

el-Kebbi, I. M., Ziemer, D. C., Gallina, D. L., Dunbar, V., & Phillips, L. S. (1999). Diabetes in urban African-Americans. XV: Identification of barriers to provider adherence to management protocols. *Diabetes Care, 22*(10), 1617–1620. doi:10.2337/diacare.22.10.1617 PMID:10526724

European Commission. (2012). The 2012 Ageing Report: Economic and budgetary projections for the EU27 Member States (2010-2060), European Economy 2/2012.

Evans, S., & Vallely, S. (2007). *Social well-being in extra care housing*. New York, NY: Joseph Rowntree Foundation.

Falanga, R. (2013). Participation and Public Sector: A Democratic Challenge. *Universitas Humanas, 10*, 11–20.

Falanga, R. (2014). Changes need change. A psychosociological perspective on participation and social inclusion. *Rivista di Psicologia Clinica, 2*, 24–38.

Farrington, J., Bebbington, A., Wellard, K., & Lewis, D. J. (1993). *Reluctant Partners: Non-governmental Organisations, the State and Sustainable Agricultural Development*. London: Routledge.

Finucane, M. L., & Lees, N. B. (2005). Decision-making competence of older adults: Models and methods. Retrieved from http://citeseerx.ist.psu.edu/viewdoc/download?doi=10.1.1.116.7585&rep=rep1&type=pdf

Fischer, F. (2003). *Reframing Public Policy. Discursive Politics and Deliberative Practices*. New York, NY: Oxford University Press. doi:10.1093/019924264X.001.0001

Fung, A. (2006). Varieties of Participation in Complex Governance. *Public Administration Review*, *66*(s1), 66–75. doi:10.1111/j.1540-6210.2006.00667.x

Gaspar, R., Carvalho, J., Luís, S., & Lima, M. L. (2014). Food risk communication: Empirical studies and practical resources. *Transcultural*, *4*, 25–37.

Gaspar, R., Luís, S., Seibt, B., Lima, M. L., Marcu, A., Rutsaert, P., & Barnett, J. et al. (2015). Consumers' avoidance of information on red meat risks: Information exposure effects on attitudes and perceived knowledge. *Journal of Risk Research*, 1–17. doi:10.1080/13669877.2014.1003318

Gaventa, J. (2006). Finding the spaces for change: A power analysis. *Ids Bulletin-Institute of Development Studies*, *37*(6), 23–33. doi:10.1111/j.1759-5436.2006.tb00320.x

Gilleard, C., & Higgs, P. (1998). Old people as users and consumers of healthcare: A third age rhetoric for a fourth age reality? *Ageing and Society*, *18*(2), 233–248. doi:10.1017/S0144686X98006904

Glendinning, C. (2008). Increasing Choice and Control for Older and Disabled People: A Critical review of New Developments in England. *Social Policy and Administration*, *42*(5), 451–469. doi:10.1111/j.1467-9515.2008.00617.x

Godinho, C., Alvarez, M. J., & Lima, M. L. (2013). Formative research on HAPA model determinants for fruit and vegetable intake: Target beliefs for audiences at different stages of change. *Health Education Research*, *28*(6), 1014–1028. doi:10.1093/her/cyt076 PMID:23856178

Hajjar, E. R., Cafiero, A. C., & Hanlon, J. T. (2007). Polypharmacy in elderly patients. *The American Journal of Geriatric Pharmacotherapy*, *5*(4), 345–351. doi:10.1016/j.amjopharm.2007.12.002 PMID:18179993

Hall, M. A., Camacho, F., Dugan, E., & Balkrishnan, R. (2002). Trust in the medical profession: Conceptual and measurement issues. *Health Services Research*, *37*(5), 1419–1439. doi:10.1111/1475-6773.01070 PMID:12479504

Hayden, C., & Boaz, A. (2000) *Making a Difference: Better Government for Older People Programme Evaluation Report*. The University of Warwick, Local Government Centre.

Haynes, R. B., Ackloo, E., Sahota, N., McDonald, H. P., & Yao, X. (2008). Interventions for enhancing medication adherence. *Cochrane Database of Systematic Reviews*. doi:10.1002/14651858.CD000011.pub3 PMID:18425859

Huizinga, M. M., Bleich, S. N., Beach, M. C., Clark, J. M., & Cooper, L. A. (2010). Disparity in physician perception of patients' adherence to medications by obesity status. *Obesity (Silver Spring, Md.)*, *18*(10), 1932–1937. doi:10.1038/oby.2010.35 PMID:20186132

Kjeldmand, D., Holmstrom, I., & Rosenqvist, U. (2006). How patient-centered am I? A new method to measure physicians' patient-centredness. *Patient Education and Counseling*, *62*, 31–37. doi:10.1016/j.pec.2005.05.017 PMID:16024208

Klinger, E., & Cox, M. (2004). Motivation and the Theory of Current Concerns. In W. M. Cox & E. Klinger (Eds.), *Handbook of motivational counselling: Concepts, approaches, and assessment* (pp. 3–28). Chichester: John Willey & Sons.

Krueger, K. P., Berger, B. A., & Felkey, B. (2005). Medication adherence and persistence: A comprehensive review. *Advances in Therapy*, *22*(4), 313–356. doi:10.1007/BF02850081 PMID:16418141

Lakshminarayana, R., Wang, D., Burn, D., Chaudhuri, K. R., Cummins, G., Galtrey, C., & Williams, A. et al.SMART-PD Investigators. (2014). Smartphone- and internet-assisted self-management and adherence tools to manage Parkinson's disease (SMART-PD): Study protocol for a randomised controlled trial. *Trials*, *15*(1), 374. doi:10.1186/1745-6215-15-374 PMID:25257518

Lamiell, J. T. (1995). Rethinking the role of quantitative methods in psychology. In J. A. Smith, R. Harré, & L. Van Langenhove (Eds.), *Rethinking methods in psychology* (pp. 143–162). London: Sage. doi:10.4135/9781446221792.n10

Levasseur, M., Richard, L., Gauvin, L., & Raymond, É. (2010). Inventory and analysis of definitions of social participation found in the aging literature: Proposed taxonomy of social activities. *Social Science & Medicine*, *71*(12), 2141–2149. doi:10.1016/j.socscimed.2010.09.041 PMID:21044812

Makai, P., Perry, M., Robben, S. H., Schers, H. J., Heinen, M. M., Olde Rikkert, M. G., & Melis, R. R. (2014). Evaluation of an eHealth intervention in chronic care for frail older people: Why adherence is the first target. *Journal of Medical Internet Research*, *16*(6), e156. doi:10.2196/jmir.3057 PMID:24966146

Marcu, A., Gaspar, R., Rutsaert, P., Seibt, B., Fletcher, D., Verbeke, W., & Barnett, J. (2014). Analogies, metaphors, and wondering about the future: Lay sense-making around synthetic meat. *Public Understanding of Science (Bristol, England)*, *24*(5), 547–562. doi:10.1177/0963662514521106 PMID:24553438

Marcum, Z. A., Sevick, M. A., & Handler, S. M. (2013). Medication non-adherence: A diagnosable and treatable medical condition. *Journal of the American Medical Association*, *309*, 2105–2106. doi:10.1001/jama.2013.4638 PMID:23695479

Matsui, D. (2013). Medication adherence issues on patients: Focus on cost. *Clinical Audit*, *5*, 33–42. doi:10.2147/CA.S30125

Mead, N., & Bower, P. (2000). Patient-centredness: A conceptual framework and review of the empirical literature. *Social Science & Medicine*, *51*(7), 1087–1110. doi:10.1016/S0277-9536(00)00098-8 PMID:11005395

Mead, N., & Bower, P. (2002). Patient-centred consultations and outcomes in primary care: A review of the literature. *Patient Education and Counseling*, *48*(1), 51–61. doi:10.1016/S0738-3991(02)00099-X PMID:12220750

Miles, S., & Frewer, L. J. (2003). Public perception of scientific uncertainty in relation to food hazards. *Journal of Risk Research*, *6*(3), 267–283. doi:10.1080/1366987032000088883

Morgan, M. G., Fischhoff, B., Bostrom, A., & Altman, C. J. (2002). *Risk communication*. Boston, MA, USA: Cambridge University Press.

Nie, N., & Verba, S. (1975). Political participation. In F. I. Greenstein & N. W. Polsby (Eds.), *Handbook of political science* (pp. 1–74). Reading, MA: Addison-Wesley.

Nieuwlaat, R., Wilczynski, N., Navarro, T., Hobson, N., Jeffery, R., & Keepanasseril, A. et al.. (2014). Interventions for enhancing medication adherence. *Cochrane Database of Systematic Reviews*. doi:10.1002/14651858.CD000011.pub4 PMID:25412402

Osterberg, L., & Blaschke, T. (2005). Adherence to medication. *The New England Journal of Medicine*, *353*(5), 487–497. doi:10.1056/NEJMra050100 PMID:16079372

Peters, E., Hess, T. H., Västfjäll, D., & Auman, C. (2007). Implications for the role of affective and deliberative processes in older adults' decision making. *Perspectives on Psychological Science*, *2*(1), 1–23. doi:10.1111/j.1745-6916.2007.00025.x PMID:26151915

Piette, J. D., Beard, A., Rosland, A. M., & McHorney, C. A. (2011). Beliefs that influence cost-related medication non-adherence among the "haves" and "have nots" with chronic disease. *Patient Preference and Adherence*, *5*, 389–396. doi:10.2147/PPA.S23111 PMID:21949602

Pretty, J. N. (1995). Participatory learning for sustainable agriculture. *World Development*, *23*(8), 1247–1263. doi:10.1016/0305-750X(95)00046-F

Regan, Á., McConnon, Á., Kuttschreuter, M., Rutsaert, P., Shan, L., Pieniak, Z., & Wall, P. et al. (2014). The impact of communicating conflicting risk and benefit messages: An experimental study on red meat information. *Food Quality and Preference*, *38*, 107–114. doi:10.1016/j.foodqual.2014.05.019

Renn, O. (2008). *Risk governance: coping with uncertainty in a complex world*. Earthscan.

Ried, L. D. (2010). Cost sharing and adherence, medication burden and adherence, and beta receptor selectivity. *Journal of the American Pharmacists Association*, *50*(3), 440. doi:10.1331/JAPhA.2010.10521 PMID:20452925

Robben, S. H., Huisjes, M., van Achterberg, T., Zuidema, S. U., Olde Rikkert, M. G., Schers, H. J., … & Zowel N.N. Study Group. (2012a). Filling the gaps in a fragmented health care system: Development of the Health and Welfare Information Portal (ZWIP). *JMIR Research Protocols, 1,* e10. doi:10.2196/resprot.1945

Robben, S. H., Perry, M., Huisjes, M., van Nieuwenhuijzen, L., Schers, H. J., van Weel, C., & Melis, R. J. F. et al. (2012b). Implementation of an innovative web-based conference table for community-dwelling frail older people, their informal caregivers and professionals: A process evaluation. *BMC Health Services Research*, *12*(1), 251. doi:10.1186/1472-6963-12-251 PMID:22894654

Roberts, K. J., & Volberding, P. (1999). Adherence communication: A qualitative analysis of physician-patient dialogue. *AIDS (London, England)*, *13*(13), 1771–1778. doi:10.1097/00002030-199909100-00022 PMID:10509580

Russell, C. L., Conn, V. S., & Jantarakupt, P. (2006). Older adult medication compliance: Integrated review of randomized controlled trials. *American Journal of Health Behavior*, *6*(6), 636–650. doi:10.5993/AJHB.30.6.10 PMID:17096621

Rutsaert, P., Barnett, J., Gaspar, R., Marcu, A., Pieniak, Z., Seibt, B., & Verbeke, W. et al. (2015). Beyond information seeking: Consumers' online deliberation about the risks and benefits of red meat. *Food Quality and Preference*, *39*, 191–201. doi:10.1016/j.foodqual.2014.07.011

Sabate, E. (2003). Adherence to long-term therapies: Evidence for action. Geneva: World Health Organization; Retrieved from http://www.who.int/chronic_conditions/en/adherence_report.pdf

Safran, D. G., Neuman, P., Schoen, C., Kitchman, M. S., Wilson, I. B., Cooper, B., et al. (2005). *Prescription drug coverage and seniors: Findings from a 2003 national survey*. Retrieved from http://content.healthaffairs.org/content/early/2005/04/19/hlthaff.w5.152

Santos, V. (2014). *Determinantes da resposta de adesão ao medicamento em idosos: Uma abordagem experimental* [Determinants of response to drug adherence in the elderly: An experimental approach] [Master thesis]. University of Évora, Évora, Portugal.

Schüz, B., Marx, C., Wurm, S., Warner, L. M., Ziegelmann, J. P., Schwarzer, R., & Tesch-Römer, C. (2011). Medication beliefs predict medication adherence in older adults with multiple illnesses. *Journal of Psychosomatic Research*, *70*(2), 179–187. doi:10.1016/j.jpsychores.2010.07.014 PMID:21262421

Schüz, B., Wolff, J. K., Warner, L. M., Ziegelmann, J. P., & Wurm, S. (2014). Multiple illness perceptions in older adults: Effects on physical functioning and medication adherence. *Psychology & Health*, *29*(4), 442–457. doi:10.1080/08870446.2013.863884 PMID:24224651

Schüz, B., Wurm, S., Warner, L. M., Wolff, J. K., & Schwarzer, R. (2013). Health motives and health behaviour self-regulation in older adults. *Journal of Behavioral Medicine*, *37*(3), 491–500. doi:10.1007/s10865-013-9504-y PMID:23512197

Schwarzer, R. (1992). Self-efficacy in the adoption and maintenance of health behaviours: Theoretical approaches and a new model. In R. Schwarzer (Ed.), *Self-efficacy: Thought control of action* (pp. 217–242). Washington, DC: Hemisphere.

Schwarzer, R. (2008). Modeling health behaviour change: How to predict and modify the adoption and maintenance of health behaviours. *Applied Psychology*, *57*, 1–29. doi:10.1111/j.1464-0597.2007.00325.x

Scourfield, P., & Burch, S. (2010). Ethical Considerations when involving older people in public service participation processes. *Ethics and Social Welfare*, *4*(3), 236–253. doi:10.1080/17496535.2010.516120

Shepherd, S., & Kay, A. C. (2012). On the perpetuation of ignorance: System dependence, system justification, and the motivated avoidance of sociopolitical information. *Journal of Personality and Social Psychology*, *102*(2), 264–280. doi:10.1037/a0026272 PMID:22059846

Sintomer, Y. (2007). *Le pouvoir au people: Jurys citoyens, tirage au sort et démocratie partecipative*. Paris: La Découverte.

Sjöberg, L. (2002). Factors in risk perception. *Risk Analysis*, *20*(1), 1–12. doi:10.1111/0272-4332.00001 PMID:12017352

Slovic, P., Finucane, M., Peters, E., & MacGregor, D. G. (2002). The affective heuristic. In T. Gilovich, D. Griffin, & D. Kahneman (Eds.), *Heuristics and biases: The psychology of intuitive judgment* (pp. 397–420). New York, NY: Cambridge University Press. doi:10.1017/CBO9780511808098.025

Slovic, P., Peters, E., Finucane, M., & MacGregor, D. G. (2005). Affect, risk and decision making. *Health Psychology*, *24*(4Suppl. 4), S35–S40. doi:10.1037/0278-6133.24.4.S35 PMID:16045417

Timonen, V. (2008). *Ageing societies: A comparative introduction*. London: McGraw Hill Open University Press.

van den Akker, M., Buntinx, F., Metsemakers, J. M., Roos, S., & Knottnerus, A. (1998). Multimorbidity in general practice: Prevalence, incidence, and determinants of co-occurring chronic and recurrent diseases. *Journal of Clinical Epidemiology*, *51*(5), 367–375. doi:10.1016/S0895-4356(97)00306-5 PMID:9619963

Van Kleef, E., Frewer, L. J., Chryssochoidis, G. M., Houghton, J. R., Korzen-Bohr, S., Krystallis, T., & Rowe, G. et al. (2006). Perceptions of food risk management among key stakeholders: Results from a cross-European study. *Appetite*, *47*(1), 46–63. doi:10.1016/j.appet.2006.02.002 PMID:16584811

Vegeris, S., Barnes, H., Campbell-Barr, V., Mackinnon, K., Taylor, R., Martin, D., & Harris, J. (2007). *Beyond the tick box: Older citizen engagement in UK local government*. London: Policy Studies Institute PSI and Better Government OPAG.

Vermeire, E., Hearnshaw, H., Van Royen, P., & Denekens, J. (2001). Patient adherence to treatment: Three decades of research. A comprehensive review. *Journal of Clinical Pharmacy and Therapeutics*, *26*(5), 331–342. doi:10.1046/j.1365-2710.2001.00363.x PMID:11679023

Walker, A. (2006). Aging and politics: An international perspective. In R. H. Binstock & L. K. George (Eds.), *Handbook of aging and the social sciences* (6th ed., pp. 339–359). San Diego, CA: Academic Press. doi:10.1016/B978-012088388-2/50022-5

Ward, B. W., & Schiller, J. S. (2013). Prevalence of multiple chronic conditions among US adults: Estimates from the national health interview survey, 2010. *Preventing Chronic Disease*, *10*, 1–15. doi:10.5888/pcd10.120203 PMID:23618545

Wens, J., Vermeire, E., Van Royen, P., Sabbe, B., & Denekens, J. (2005). GPs' perspectives of type 2 diabetes patients' adherence to treatment: A qualitative analysis of barriers and solutions. *BMC Family Practice*, *6*(1), 20. doi:10.1186/1471-2296-6-20 PMID:15890071

World Health Organization. (2001). *International Classification of Functioning, Disability and Health*. Geneva: WHO. Retrieved from http://psychiatr.ru/download/1313?view=1&name=ICF_18.pdf

World Health Organization. (2002). *Active ageing: A policy framework*. Retrieved from http://apps.who.int/iris/bitstream/10665/67215/1/WHO_NMH_NPH_02.8.pdf

KEY TERMS AND DEFINITIONS

Adherence: Intentional disposition to implement actions as prescribed in a recommendation(s) communicated by health professionals (e.g. taking medication) and/or organizations (e.g. recommended amount of nutrients intake).

Barriers: factors that may inhibit individual's intentions to adhere and reduce the probability of implementing these intentions into behaviours (actual adherence).

Facilitators: factors that may reinforce individual's intentions to adhere and increment the probability of implementing these intentions into behaviours (actual adherence).

Deliberation: Dispositional tendency to actively and consciously approach one-self (behaviourally, cognitively and/or emotionally) from information that is deemed personally relevant.

Engagement: Active involvement and participation in the different aspects of the healthcare process in general and health recommendations communication process in particular. This can have various manifestations, such as interest in information, information seeking behaviours, positive interactions with the health professionals and others.

Information Avoidance: Dispositional tendency to actively and consciously distance one-self (behaviourally, cognitively and/or emotionally) from information that may pose a threat to ones perceptions, beliefs and evaluations toward one or more issues.

Motivation: "The internal states of the organism that lead to the instigation, persistence, energy, and direction of behaviour towards a goal" (Klinger & Cox, 2004; p. 3).

Participation: Set of principles and practices aimed at complementing representative democracy, yet different from forms of direct democracy, such as petitions and referendums. This includes a wide range of experiences setting new spaces of legitimized deliberation between political institutions and civil society beyond the traditional adversary model of political debate.

ENDNOTES

1. More information on the Seventh Framework Programme funded Project MOPACT – Mobilising the Potential of Active Ageing in Europe is retrievable on: www.mopact.group.shef.ac.uk
2. For the full list of studies references, please see Robben et al. (2012a).

Chapter 5
A Relational Perspective on Patient Engagement:
Suggestions from Couple-Based Research and Intervention

Silvia Donato
Università Cattolica del Sacro Cuore, Milan, Italy

Anna Bertoni
Università Cattolica del Sacro Cuore, Milan, Italy

ABSTRACT

Research on the engagement of patients and their partners and the literature on couple relationships have remained surprisingly separated. In response to this gap, the first aim of the chapter is to show the advantages of an integration of these two lines of research in the context of promoting engagement in patients and their partners. Particular attention is devoted to couples' stress and coping literature and to those few studies that investigated the role played for patient engagement by characteristics of patients, partners, and their relationship. Couple-based research can inform engagement literature about facilitators and barriers to couples' coping with illness and about how to promote engagement in the context of the couple. Within this research, the concept of dyadic coping can be especially helpful in understanding how partners can effectively deal with the stress related to acute and chronic illness as well as the barriers to this process. A second aim of the chapter is to connect the suggestions from couple-based research with the field of engagement promotion.

INTRODUCTION

Today's increasing demand of care challenges healthcare systems to pool all available resources in the care environment. To face such a challenge health care systems need to effectively rely not only on professionals, but also on the patient himself/herself and on the patients' informal networks (e.g., the partner, relatives, and friends). Home-based self-care is considered in fact essential for the success of the

DOI: 10.4018/978-1-4666-9992-2.ch005

treatment and to avoid re-hospitalization (Agren, Evangelista, Davidson, & Stromberg, 2013). Patient engagement in disease management, that is regarded as the conjoint cognitive, emotional, and behavioral enactment of patients towards their disease management (Graffigna, Barello, & Riva, 2013), is therefore a pivotal element for making patients co-producers of their health and enhancing their care experience as well as gaining improved health outcomes and lower healthcare costs (Barello, Graffigna, & Vegni, 2012; Carman et al., 2013; Graffigna et al., 2013).

Patients, however, considerably vary in their ability and will to actively engage in the treatment, with patients' self-care being less-than-adequate in many cases (e.g., Jaarsma & Stromberg, 2014). Thus, pooling those resources that can enhance the patient self-care and support his/her engagement in the treatment is essential (Riegel, Lee, & Dickson, 2011). According to the interdependent self-perspective (Kayser, Watson, & Andrade, 2007) these resources are primarily relational, as *human beings are essentially connected to each other and that this connection among individual must be maintained in order for the self to be complete. In other words, the person is fully human only in relation to others* (p. 416). Along with this perspective, the patient is a person-in-relationships and the patient's close relationships are necessarily involved in the disease. Within patients' close relationships, especially the couple relationship plays a central role for partners' well-being and the care process and can be an important factor influencing the patient engagement with the treatment in both positive and negative ways (Bertoni, Donato, Graffigna, Barello, & Parise, 2015).

Research on the engagement of patients and their partners and the literature on couple relationships, however, have remained surprisingly separated. In response to this gap, the first aim of the present chapter is to show the advantages of an integration of these two lines of research in the context of promoting engagement in patients and their partners. The role of the caregivers, and of the partner in particular, has been for a long time considered within an individual perspective and mostly analyzed in terms of the caregiver's burden. Only recently, a call for a dyadic perspective has been made within the health literature (Vellone et al., 2014). At this regard, particular attention will be devoted to couples' stress and coping literature and to those few studies that -only recently- started to investigate the role played for patient engagement by characteristics of patients, partners, and their relationship. In general, findings from couples' stress and coping literature underscore that patients and partners disease and health management cannot be understood only at the individual level, but require a dyadic and couple perspective in order to reveal the complexities of such a process and to effectively promote patients' and partners' engagement in it.

A second aim of the chapters is to draw implications from couples' coping research for the promotion of patients' and partners' engagement. Awareness of the dyadic and relational features of each partners' cognition, emotions, and behaviors is in fact essential for partners' to cope effectively with the challenges of the care process along its development. Moreover, those skills and cognitions that are necessary for patients' and partners' participation in the care process need to be understood and trained also at the dyadic level and not only at the individual level.

Before starting, some caveats need to be considered. First, we will focus our discussion on patients in couples as for a substantial proportion of patients the spouse or partner is generally among the primary caregivers, together with adult children (Li & Loke, 2014). Moreover, partner support cannot be easily substituted by other sources (Coyne & DeLongis, 1986). It is arguable, however, that some of the present suggestions could apply to patient-caregiver dyads more generally. Second, our discussion presents studies that in most cases refer to a specific disease and not to a range of illnesses. In particular, cardiac illness and cancer have received the lion's share of attention in the lines of research considered. The present conclusions, nonetheless, will apply to a broad array of chronic diseases.

CHRONIC ILLNESS AND CARE: THE ROLE OF THE COUPLE RELATIONSHIP

In chronic illness patients often experience a gradual decline in functional capacity, symptom burden, impaired mental acuity and poor quality of life, and these aspects are accompanied by an increase in caregiving responsibilities. Many studies have demonstrated that caregivers are burdened and their stress has been associated with poor physical health (e.g., Grant, Glandon, Elliot, Giger, & Weaver, 2004). Caregivers contributing to patients' self-care experience exhaustion that impairs their physical quality of life (Vellone et al., 2014). In patients in couples, the spouse or partner is generally among the primary caregivers, together with the adult children (Li & Loke, 2014). When the caregiver is the spouse or partner, in addition to the emotional and physical burden he/she is subject to, the couple itself experience difficulties related to the disease and caregiving, especially in terms of communication problems (Vellone et al., 2014). Although illness and recovery make many complex demands on patients and their partners, the couple relationship can play a central role for sustaining partners' well-being, as it is been documented both in healthy partners (e.g., Bertoni & Bodenmann, 2010; Bertoni, Parise, & Iafrate, 2012; Donato et al., 2015; Pagani et al., 2015) and in partners facing health issues (e.g., Bertoni et al.,2015; Vilchinsky, Dekel, Leibowitz, Rages, & Khaskia, 2011). Research has shown that happily married patients have a longer life expectancy than non-married ones (e.g., King & Reis, 2012; Rohrbaugh, Shoham, & Coyne, 2006). The positive effect of having a stable and satisfying couple relationship on patients' survival when affected by a chronic illness seems due to the fact that several relationship processes, such as closeness, emotional support, communication, reciprocity, and mutual responsiveness between partners were identified as important factors associated with improved health outcomes (Sebern & Woda, 2012; Kayser et al., 2007). Reciprocity, in particular, that is giving and accepting of physical and emotional help with appreciation, is an important component of family care relationships (Sebern, 2005). Reinhardt (2001) found that an inability to reciprocate in family care predicted patient depression. Conversely, opportunities to reciprocate contribute to positive family outcomes and psychological well-being (Liang, Krause, & Bennett, 2001). Partners' mutual responsiveness, that is the combination of a focus on the relationship, an authentic attitude of partners, and an empathic responding to the other, was found to facilitate partners' coping with the illness as a couple (Kayser et al., 2007).

In addition to sustaining partners' well-being more generally, being in a couple relationship can also help to adopt a healthier life style and reduce modifiable risk factors (e.g., smoking; cholesterol levels; etc.) specifically related to the patients' disease management. A satisfying couple relationship, moreover, increases the likelihood that patients adhere to their treatment and participate to a complete program of rehabilitation (Rankin-Esquer, Deeter, & Barr Taylor, 2000). The partner's own engagement in the care process, moreover, is vital to achieve long-term positive health outcomes for patients (e.g., Carpenter et al., 2015). The couple relationship, however, may not always be a resource for the recovery (Fiske, Coyne, & Smith, 1991; Rankin-Esquer et al., 2000). The partner's tendency to substitute to the patient in dealing with his/her illness and to over-protect him/her undermines patients' psychological and physical well-being (Joekes, Van Elderen, & Schreurs, 2007; Stroebe et al., 2013), mostly because it conveys the message that the partner underestimates the patient's capabilities.

As evidence grows regarding the impact of illness on couples and families and the role of the relational context for patients' well-being and for the care process, a need for the health literature to expand its scope from the individual experience to of the one of both the patient and their caregivers (e.g., Lyons et al., 2014) as well as to implement couple-based care interventions (e.g., Scott & Kayser, 2009) has been recently acknowledged. Very few recent studies used a dyadic perspective to understand what happens in a couple affected by illness (see for a review Revenson & DeLongis, 2011; Regan et al., 2015) and even less assessed the interplay between couple processes and patient self-care and engagement (Buck et al., 2015; Lee et al., 2015; Lyons et al., 2014; Vellone et al., 2014). Lee and colleagues (2015) as well as Buck and colleagues (2015) highlight how self-care can affect both patients' and caregivers' quality of life. They also emphasize the need to consider the perspectives of both members of the couple as patient-reported and partner-reported variables may have unique contributions to the outcomes. Finally, they stress the fact that relational processes may be associated to both better and poorer outcomes of the care process, and that patients and caregivers should be considered as a unit. These few existing studies, however, do not target what relational factors may facilitate or hinder patients' and partners' collaborative self-care and engagement. What seems particularly lacking is a clear theoretical framework regarding couple-based processes that could complement theoretical models of patient engagement (Graffigna, Barello, Riva, & Bosio, 2014) as well as intervention to promote patient engagement, when applied to patients in couples.

Illness Appraisal and Management as Dyadic Processes

Couple-based research can inform the engagement literature about facilitators and barriers to couples' adjustment to illness and to the care process and, therefore, about how to promote engagement in the context of the couple relationship. At this regard, the line of couple-based research that can be particularly informative for the promotion of patient engagement is the one devoted to the study of couples' stress and coping processes. One partner's illness is a great challenge for both patients and their partners and can be considered among one of the major stressors couples may face in their life cycle (e.g., Randall & Bodenmann, 2009).

A diagnosis of illness, in fact, engenders numerous stressors and compelling tasks for couples, some of which emanate directly from the care process (e.g., making treatment decisions, managing medications and care activities; caregiving an ill or disabled partner; etc.) while others stem from the need to restructure family roles and responsibilities as well as people's daily lives (e.g., restructuring daily schedule to accommodate the treatment regimen; negotiating new allocation of chores to adjust to a severely disabled partner; restricting or adjusting the couple's social life; etc.). Illness of one partner in a couple relationship cannot be considered in a solely individualistic manner, in which patients and partners experience the illness separately and deal with it in isolation, but has to be understood as an interpersonal, dyadic experience that concerns both partners simultaneously, a genuine "we-desease" (e.g., Acitelli & Badr, 2005; Kayser et al., 2007). Illness-related stress, moreover, can add to general life stressors and daily hassles and such a pile-up of stress can erode patients' and partners' resources to deal with the care process (see Randall & Bodenmann, 2009). Couples dealing with illness are not only exposed to the challenges of the disease, but also to all the requirements of daily life. Knowledge on how couples deal with stress in both domains (illness and daily life) is particularly important as couples' coping is needed for both demands.

Patient engagement, as the conjoint cognitive, emotional, and behavioral enactment of patients towards their disease management (Graffigna et al., 2013), most probably co-varies with the quality of patients' and partners' efforts to cope with the disease and with their daily life routine. Patient engagement is, in fact, a dynamic, evolutive process patients go through while adjusting to their disease (Barello et al., 2012) and the relational context in which patients are embedded is an important factor potentially influencing such a process. Recent models of patient engagement have revealed the dynamic nature of it, highlighting 4 phases patients go through during the engagement process (Blackout, Arousal, Adhesion, Eudaimonic project; Graffigna et al., 2014). It is noteworthy that in each of these phases the partner, and specifically his/her way to cope together with the patient, can play a fundamental role by facilitating or -on the contrary- undermining the patient's transition from one phase to the other as well as his/her ability to finally reach a positive, active approach to health management. Along this evolutionary process, patients will need their partners to adopt different attitudes and coping behaviors. Moreover, the partner himself/herself will play different roles while coping with the patient's disease (Barello, Savarese, & Graffigna, 2015; Barello, Graffigna, Savarese, Donato, & Bertoni, 2014).

The following paragraphs, therefore, will examine couples' stress and coping processes both in the context of daily life and in the context of illness in order to derive potential implications for a couple-based, relational approach to the study and promotion of patient engagement.

Beyond the Individual Approach to Couples' Adjustment to Illness

The focus on the couple relationship in the study of the adjustment to illness is relatively new in the stress and coping literature. The first impetus towards the inclusion of this focus was given in the 1990s by a number of conceptual frameworks that started from expanding the seminal work by Lazarus and colleagues (Lazarus & Folkman, 1984). Their Transactional Model of Stress and Coping emphasizes the role of appraisals in the stress experience, on the one hand, and the role of personal resources and situational determinants for the coping process on the other. Within this model, supportive relationships are considered the primary resources an individual can pool to assist his/her coping efforts in a number of ways (e.g., providing information and feedback, instrumental assistance, emotional support, etc.). The role of the social context for the individual's coping, however, was limited to the exchange of social support (e.g., Manne, 1998) and to the effects of chronic illness on the spouse (see review by Manne & Badr, 2008; Manne & Zautra, 1990). Expanding this framework and considering the couple as the unit of analysis required the stress and coping literature to move beyond its individual frame of reference to embrace a proper dyadic and relational perspective (cfr. Iafrate & Donato, 2012; Donato, 2014). The concept of dyadic coping, in fact, recognizes mutuality and interdependence in partners' coping responses to illness, considering that the couple responds to stress as an interpersonal unit. This movement highlighted within the stress and coping literature parallels the recent, similar movement observed within the field of the health literature more generally and in the field of patient engagement more specifically (e.g., Lee et al., 2015). Within the stress and coping research in couples, two sets of findings have contributed to this movement: a) the cross-over effects emerged in partners' stress and coping, and b) the influence of the other's responses on partners' coping.

Cross-Over Effects in Couples

A consistent finding that suggests the importance of the interpersonal context of stress and coping with illness refers to the effects of individuals' stress on their intimates, and particularly on their partners, in both couples facing illness (e.g., Hagedoorn, Sanderman, Bolks, Tuinstra, & Coyne, 2008) as well as in couples facing other stressors (e.g., Bolger, DeLongis, Kessler, & Wethington, 1989; Repetti, 1989; Thompson & Bolger, 1999). When dealing with a chronic stress, *family members labor not only with their own distress, but also with the distress of their loved ones* (O'Brien & DeLongis, 1997, p. 161). For example, in a recent meta-analysis of role and gender effects on distress among couples coping with cancer, Hagedoorn and colleagues (2008) found a significant association between patient and partner's distress within couples, suggesting that the two partners may react as an "emotional system" (p. 19) rather than as individuals when facing a stressful event. Research has shown, in fact, that in couple relationships emotions are transmitted from one partner to another (e.g., Schoebi, 2008). Chung, Moser, Lennie and Rayers (2009) also showed that depressive symptoms exhibited actor effects of both patients and spouses and partner effects were evident on patients' quality of life. Patients and spouses with higher depressive symptoms had poorer quality of life. Patients whose partners had higher depressive symptoms were more likely to indicate their own quality of life was poorer. Anxiety had similar actor and partner effects on quality of life and depressive symptoms.

Cross-over effects refer also to the fact that the individual's way of managing his/her stress impacts the others' psychological functioning. In couples coping with infertility, wives using a support-seeking strategy in managing their stress (i.e., looking for the support of others) had husbands that were less psychologically distressed (Stanton, 1991). Moreover, wives using more self-controlling coping strategies (i.e., controlling one's reactions to the stressful situation) had husbands that reported higher levels of distress (Stanton, Tennen, Affleck, & Mendola, 1992). Overall these studies suggest that one partner's stress and coping responses have an impact that goes beyond the individual's own well-being and can erode or – on the contrary – activate important resources for disease management and partners' engagement within the couple relationship system.

Influences of the Other's Responses

Another research finding that has contributed to the growing attention on the social context in illness adjustment is represented by the influence that the other's responses exert on the individual's coping efforts (e.g., Griffin, Friend, Kaell, & Bennett, 2001; Manne & Zautra, 1989; Marin, Holtzman, DeLongis, & Robinson, 2007). In a study on couples coping with one partner's rheumatoid arthritis patients whose partners got angry and irritated at their expressions of pain were more likely to use maladaptive coping strategies, such as venting of negative emotions, and behavioral disengagement (Griffin et al., 2001). On the contrary, positive support was found to influence rheumatoid arthritis patients' pain severity indirectly, both through the promotion of specific coping strategies (e.g., positive reappraisal) and through affecting the effectiveness of such strategies. Moreover, partner support attenuated the impact of maladaptive responses to pain, such as catastrophizing (Holtzman & DeLongis, 2007). Not only illness, individual symptoms, and relational aspects are clearly related, but patients' and partners' perspectives were differently associated to their outcomes: for example, in the acute phase of illness, for both patients and partners, one's greater marital satisfaction was associated with one's lower levels of depression. In the chronic phase, instead, different patterns of associations were found: partner-reported marital satisfaction was associated with their own and the patients' decreased depression symptoms, whereas higher levels of patient-reported marital satisfaction were associated with elevated levels of depression both for themselves and for their partners (Dekel et al., 2014). In general, these studies show that the partner plays a critical role in influencing what strategies the individual eventually adopts to deal with illness and with the care process, the motivation to use such strategies, the effort made, and the effectiveness of them. These findings also warn researchers to assess both patients' and partners' perspectives in the disease management process.

A NEW RELATIONAL FRAMEWORK

To the aim of expanding traditional stress and coping concepts, novel notions and models, such as the ones of communal coping and dyadic coping, begun to emerge. These models do not simply re-conceptualize partners' individual coping strategies within their interpersonal context, but also target those partners' coping efforts that could not be considered as mere individual responses, but rather as truly relational processes. Lyons and colleagues (Lyons, Mickelson, Sullivan, & Coyne, 1998; Mickelson, Lyons, Sullivan, & Coyne, 2001) defined *communal coping* as involving a) a "social appraisal" of the stressor, that is the understanding of a stressor as a problem of the whole group and not only of a single member of it, and b) the cooperative actions of the group members in order to cope with it. Somehow similar to communal coping, but referring specifically to the couple relationship, *dyadic coping* is broadly defined as *the interplay between the stress signals of one partner and the coping reactions of the other, a genuine act of shared coping* (Revenson, Kayser, & Bodenmann, 2005, p. 4). In the past decades different, yet overlapping, conceptualizations of dyadic coping have been elaborated (cfr. Donato, 2014).

Theoretical Perspectives on Dyadic Coping

Within the various approaches to dyadic coping that can be identified in the stress and coping literature (see Bodenmann, 2005; Revenson, 2003; Revenson, Abraido-Lanza, Majerovitz, & Jordan, 2005), especially in the context of illness (Revenson & DeLongis, 2011), dyadic coping has been defined as: a) the mutual influence between each partner's individual coping, b) the fit or congruence between partners' coping, c) each partner's coping efforts focused on the other partner's well-being and on the maintenance of the relationship, and d) collaborative problem solving efforts made by both partners; e) a dyadic process in which both partners deal with stress as a couple; f) coping efforts aimed at building and sustaining the couple's intimacy.

Mutual Influence Models

The mutual influence approach focuses on the effects of each partner's coping efforts with regard to the other person's coping and adjustment (Barnoy, Bar-tal, & Zisser, 2006; Berghuis & Stanton, 2002; Levin, Sher, & Theodos, 1997; Wijngaards-de Meij et al., 2008). In couples coping with breast cancer, patients' reports of mutual constructive communication were associated to the partner psychological distress 9 months later, while patient-reported demand-withdraw communication and mutual avoidance were negatively associated to it (Manne et al., 2006). Similarly, relationship maintenance behaviors were associated with both patients' and partners' psychological and relational well-being, concurrently as well as over the next 6 months (Badr, Acitelli, & Carmack Taylor, 2008; Badr & Carmack Taylor, 2008).

These models highlight the importance of mutual influences and of reciprocal processes in the context of disease management in couples and of the involvement of both partners in research and intervention in this context.

Coping Congruence

Revenson and her colleagues (Revenson et al., 2005) argued that *the goal of couples' coping is to maximize the congruence or fit between the partners' coping styles in order to cope most effectively as a couple* (p. 141). According to Revenson (1994, 2003) congruence can involve either symmetry or complementarity of coping styles as long as partners' efforts work in concert to reach a desired goal: Symmetrical coping styles may help partners to reach their goals because they are coordinated and mutually reinforcing, whereas complementary coping styles may be useful because they broaden partners' options and their coping repertoire. On the contrary, incongruent strategies are the ones that work in direct opposition, canceling each other out or undermining the other's coping efforts. Studies on congruence have not always yield consistent results, probably because the effects of congruence vary as a function of the type of coping considered. Barnoy and colleagues (Barnoy et al., 2006), for example, found that in seeking medical information, for female cancer patients it was important to be congruent with their husbands on monitoring (i.e., high information seeking), while for male patients it was better to be congruent with their partners on blunting (i.e., low information seeking).

Another line of research on partners' congruence examined the fit between partners' perceptions. In particular, several studies examined the role for partners' satisfaction of partners' perceived similarity (i.e., how each partner perceived himself/herself to be similar to the other in coping) and accuracy (i.e., the congruence between one partner's coping responses and the other partner's perceptions of such responses) (Iafrate, Bertoni, Donato, & Finkenauer, 2012; Donato et al., 2015) as well as actual similarity (i.e., how partners reported similar coping styles; Iafrate, Bertoni, Barni, & Donato, 2009; Iafrate, Bertoni, Margola, Cigoli, & Acitelli, 2012). These studies highlighted that partners' relationship satisfaction is boosted by perceiving themselves similar to the partner in coping (Iafrate et al., 2012), even more than by actually being similar (Iafrate et al., 2009). Moreover, accurately understanding the other's coping responses was also important for partners' satisfaction (Donato et al., 2015), but these effects were found to be moderated by relationship duration (Iafrate et al., 2012). These models suggest that, in the promotion of patient engagement, the effects of congruence in the patients' and partners' cognitions and behaviors may vary in different types of couples and over the course of treatment.

Relationship-Focused Coping

This perspective conceptualizes dyadic coping as a third possible function of coping in addition to the two basic functions identified in classic models of individual coping (Endler & Parker, 1990; Lazarus & Folkman, 1984): when facing a stressful encounter, in addition to the goal of solving their own problem (problem-focused coping) or managing their own distress (emotion-focused coping), partners also aim to regulate and preserve their relationship (relationship-focused coping). As maintaining close relationships in the face of stress protects individuals from the negative impact of stressful circumstances (e.g., Badr, Acitelli, & Carmack Taylor, 2007), relationship maintenance is an important goal of partners dealing with illness-related stress. Relationship-focused coping refers to the coping efforts aiming to sustain the relationship during stressful events and involves a challenging balance between the well-being of the self, the other, and the relationship. Coyne and colleagues (Coyne, Ellard, & Smith, 1990; Coyne & Smith, 1991) identified three forms of relationship-focused coping: a) *active engagement* (involving the other in discussing the problem, asking how the partner feels, engaging in constructive problem-solving), b) *protective buffering* (protecting the other and the relationship by hiding concerns and worries and by giving in to the partner), and c) *overprotection*, which refers to one partner underestimating the other's ability to cope.

Active engagement was found to be associated with the well-being of patients (e.g., Buunk, Berkhuysen, Sanderman, Nieuwland, & Rancor, 1996), of partners (e.g., Ybeman, Kuijer, Buunk, DeJong, & Sanderman, 2001), and of the relationship (e.g., Hagedoorn et al., 2000; Hagedoorn et al., 2011). Overprotection and protective buffering, instead, have often been associated with negative individual and relational outcomes. Another specific mode of relationship-focused coping is considered *empathic coping* (DeLongis & O'Brien, 1990), which refers to the attempts to understand the other's feelings and emotions in the stressful situation and respond sensitively to them. The concept of relationship-focused coping highlights that, within the context of the couple relationship, the question is not only how individuals manage their stress and solve their problems in the care process, but also how they manage to do so while preserving their relationship and attending to the other's well-being as well. In the promotion of patients' and partners' engagement in the treatment these sometime competing needs should be taken into account.

Collaborative Coping

Within the Socio-Contextual Model of Coping (Berg, Meegan, & Deviney, 1998), collaborative coping is defined as *the active engagement of spouses in pooling resources and in joint problem-solving and coping* (Berg et al., 2008, p. 506). Collaborative strategies are the ones in which partners are both involved and share equal responsibility in actions and decision-making (Meegan & Berg, 2002) and are considered in contrast to *uninvolved* strategies (individual coping strategies in which partners act on their own), *supportive* strategies (instrumental or emotional supportive responses of the partner), and *control* strategies (over-involvement of partner by dominating and telling the other what to do). Collaborative coping aims at activating partners 'shared resources and promoting relationship satisfaction. Berg and colleagues (2008) found that in men with prostate cancer and their wives, the use of collaborative coping was associated with more same-day positive affect for both patients and partners and less same-day negative affect for wives only. Patients' and partners' perceptions of the effectiveness of collaborative coping mediated these effects, thereby suggesting that the intention to engage in behaviors that benefit the relationship, and the perception that such behaviors are actually effective, may be as important as enacting the behaviors themselves.

Systemic-Transactional Model

Bodenmann (1997, 2000) applied a dyadic approach to extend Lazarus and Folkman's (1984) classic model in all its three components of stress, appraisal, and coping. According to Bodenmann, in fact, in the context of the couple relationship, both common challenges or threats to their relationship (such as the ones that the illness might present) and 'cross-over' or transfer effects of stress from one partner to the other (Bodenmann, 2000, 2005) can be considered as "dyadic" rather than "individual" stress that both partners in a couple experience. Bodenmann's model was first developed in the context of couples' coping with daily hassles (minor stressors) and only later it was extended to critical life events such as illness.

The dyadic coping process is regarded as a circular sequence in which partner A's communication of stress is perceived, decoded and evaluated by partner B, who then responds with his/her coping reactions, that are in turn perceived, decoded and evaluated by partner A in a circular process. Dyadic coping is intended to restore or maintain both partners' individual well-being (not only the one of the stressed partner), by reducing the partners' levels of stress, and to promote couple functioning, by strengthening partners' sense of we-ness and reciprocal trust (Bodenmann, 2005; Cutrona, 1996). Partners, however, can engage in positive as well as negative forms of dyadic coping (e.g., Donato et al., 2009; Gagliardi et al., 2013). In particular, positive dyadic coping may include one partner showing understanding and being supportive (i.e., supportive dyadic coping), or both partners engaging in a problem-solving discussion (i.e., common dyadic coping). Negative responses include hostile, ambivalent, or superficial behaviors such as open disinterest, sarcasm, or minimizing the seriousness of the partner's stress.

Positive dyadic coping, especially common dyadic coping, was found to foster or protect relationship satisfaction in both community couples (Bertoni et al., 2007; Donato, Canzi, Parise, & Ferrari, 2014; Gasbarrini et al., *in press*; see for reviews: Donato, 2014; Iafrate & Donato, 2012) and in couples coping with chronic illness (Badr, Carmack Taylor, Kashy, Cristofanilli, & Revenson, 2010; Kayser et al., 2007). Dyadic coping introduces a new level in the study and promotion of an effective disease management and engagement with the treatment in which not only individual, but also shared appraisals and actions should be considered.

Relationship Intimacy Model

A recent review of research on couples coping with cancer (Regan et al., 2015) added another theoretical model to the ones already mentioned: the Relationship Intimacy Model (Manne et al., 2004; Manne & Badr, 2008).This model of couples' coping with cancer is based on Reis and Shaver's Interpersonal Process Model of Intimacy (Reis & Shaver, 1988). The authors identified several intimacy-enhancing behaviors (mutual constructive communication, reciprocal self-disclosure, partner responsiveness, and relationship engagement) as well as some intimacy-compromising behaviors (reluctance to discuss issues/feelings, criticism, and demand-withdraw communication) that partners may adopt in response to stress (Manne et al., 2004; Manne & Badr, 2008). Manne and colleagues (Manne, Badr, Zaider, Nelson, & Kissane, 2010) found that when patients coping with prostate cancer and their partners reported greater use of mutual constructive communication they also reported less psychological distress and greater levels of relationship intimacy. Moreover, perceptions of spousal disclosures and support were found to be associated with less distress, and greater (cancer-specific and relationship) intimacy (Manne et al., 2004; Belcher et al., 2011; Manne & Badr, 2010). On the contrary, patient-demand and partner-withdraw communication was associated with increased psychological distress (Manne & Badr, 2010). Even patients and partners' past negative communication was found to predict current levels of distress, mediated by current relationship intimacy (Manne, Badr, & Kashy, 2012).

This model suggests how intimacy, that is the degree of reciprocal recognition and validation between partners, is a crucial aspect in the process of disease management that can be enhanced in interventions devoted to the promotion of engagement in couples.

Couples' Coping with Illness: Implications for Patients' and Partners' Engagement

Broadly considered, all models of dyadic coping emphasize patients' and partners' shared, dyadic appraisal and shared, dyadic action in disease management. They suggest how the conceptualization of engagement in the treatment may be also expanded to acknowledge not only whether the individual (patient or partner) is engaged in his/her treatment and healthcare, but also whether the dyadic system is engaged in the care process. Accordingly, we propose that patients' and partners' engagement could be considered along a two-dimensional framework, in which one dimension refers to the type of appraisal (the degree to which health management is appraised as "my/your" *vs.* "our" problem) and the second to the type of action (the degree to which health management strategies involve both partners or only the individual).

According to the proposed model (see Figure 1), the degree of involvement in healthcare appraisals and actions can define three areas of patient-partner healthcare patterns that go from individual forms to progressively more relational and dyadic forms of engagement with treatment. The individual area refers to those situations in which partners consider their own and their partners' healthcare as individual matters that should be dealt with through individual actions. The interactive area, instead, refers to those patterns in which partners influence each other in dealing with their health, while the dyadic area refers to partners presenting joint engagement, characterized by a joint understanding and common actions.

In addition, the above dyadic coping models also suggest that those forms of engagement that go beyond the individual can be conceptualized in different ways: a) partners' behaviors and relational processes that can support or hinder the other's engagement, b) the mutual influence between patients' and partners' engagement, c) the congruence or incongruence between patients' and partners' engagement, and d) common, joint actions of engagement (e.g., shared decision making on treatment issues; shared discussions on emotional reaction to the care process, shared problem solving). Finally, dyadic coping models also highlight how shared actions of engagement may be both adaptive and maladaptive. In the

Figure 1. Model of individual, interactive and dyadic engagement

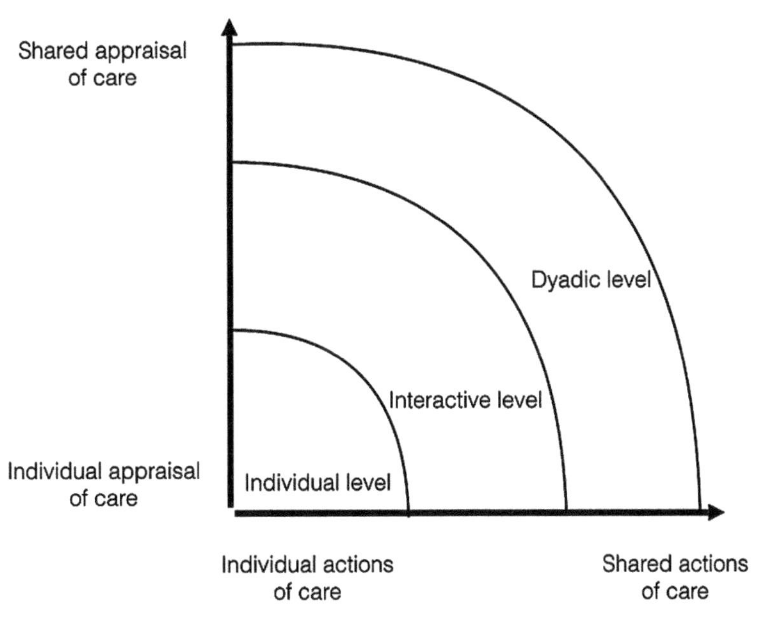

following paragraphs we will present some preliminary findings of a research study aimed at integrating couple-based research and the study of patient engagement. In particular, these findings pertain to the first of the above ways to consider patient engagement within a relational approach, that is the study of partners' behaviors and relational processes that can support or hinder the other's engagement.

Integrating Couple-Based Research and Patient Engagement: An example

Although partner support has been found to facilitate healthier behaviors such as exercise, eating better food, and not smoking, as well as greater adherence to medical regimens (Uchino, 2006), very few studies have assessed the associations of partner behaviors and relational processes with patient engagement. Indeed, a recent study focused explicitly on the integration between couple-based research and the study of patient engagement showing how partners and couple relationship factors are key in both facilitating and undermining patients' engagement in their treatment (Bertoni et al., 2015).

The study by Bertoni and colleagues (2015) aimed at exploring patients' (and partners') individual and relational functioning after an acute cardiac event as well the individual and relational factors associated with the patient engagement. Findings showed that, as compared to single patients, patients in a couple have a more optimistic perception of their illness and they are more engaged in their treatment. Moreover, findings highlighted that patients and partners showed similar levels of distress and that several relational variables (especially partner-reported ones) were correlated to the patient's engagement. In particular, the patient's perception of working actively at his/her relationship by putting forward also some self-sacrificing behaviors for the good of the other was positively associated with his/her engagement in the treatment. In addition, the partner's perception to support the patient's engagement and not to substitute to him/her facilitated the engagement process. Unexpectedly, patients whose partners endorsed in more negative dyadic coping responses were also more engaged in their disease management. It is possible that in this acute phase of the illness, in which patients are particularly dependent and disoriented, partners exhibiting less sympathy for the patient and less indulgence may provoke his/her own active involvement in his/her treatment. Indeed, other research has shown that negative partners' responses, such as demanding and withdrawing behaviors in conflict interactions, can be beneficial for the relationship in certain circumstances (e.g., Donato, Parise, Pagani, Bertoni, & Iafrate, 2014). Studies specifically focused on dyadic coping, however, have also shown the detrimental effects of negative dyadic coping over time (e.g., Donato & Parise, 2012), especially in light of the fact that partners tend to reciprocate negative dyadic coping responses (Donato, Iafrate, Bradbury, & Scabini, 2012). Further studies should explore whether in the longer run this benefits may backfire, in case the partner may continue to cope negatively with the other's illness-related stressors.

The study also showed that the couple may not always be a resource for the recovery. Not only partners were found to feel even worse than patients and not to be in the best conditions to help, but also the partner's tendency to substitute to the patient in dealing with their illness and to over-protect him/her undermined patient engagement. Moreover, having a depressed partner hindered the patient's engagement in the treatment. Unexpectedly, even the partner's relationship satisfaction correlated negatively with the patient's engagement. It may be that, being the acute event so close in time, high couple satisfaction may express a defensive movement (e.g., denial) which may be also translated into a difficulty of taking an active role in the treatment. Despite their preliminary nature, these findings have implications for the promotion of patient engagement as they highlight how the partner is an important actor to consider in the scene of the illness, both as an important resource to involve and as a potential burden, when not adequately included in the treatment process and instructed about his/her role. In the following section it will be highlighted how the findings reported above, together with the ones from the literature on stress and coping in couples, can inform couple-based interventions to promote patients' and partners' engagement.

PROMOTING PATIENT ENGAGEMENT: SUGGESTIONS FROM A RELATIONAL PERSPECTIVE

The research findings reported above offer some preliminary insights for interventions aiming at promoting the patient's and partner's engagement. The integrated, relational perspective proposed here to the understanding of illness is also useful when designing interventions with patients in couples. Within this perspective, in fact, disease management requires not only the patient himself/herself, but also his/her family members (and particularly the partner, when present) to play an active role. To support this role, interventions should not focus on the patient alone. Many studies suggested the importance to include the family caregivers in education and disease management interventions: *In the field of cardiac illness, up to half of heart failure patients are readmitted to hospitals within 6 months of discharge. Many read mission are linked to inadequate self-care or family support. To improve care, practitioners may need to intervene with both the patient and family caregiver* (Sebern & Woda, 2012, p. 289).Similarly to the shift from an individual to a dyadic focus proposed in research, it is fundamental that the interventions as well consider *the caregiver-patient dyad as a unit* (Li & Loke, 2014, p. 731). Indeed, Scott and Kayser (2009) highlighted that couple-based interventions produce greater effects sizes than interventions focused on patients only and several studies claimed that couple-based interventions improve the quality of life in patients and their partners as a dyad (Agren et al., 2013; Li & Loke, 2014).

The findings highlight that also the well-being of the partner and of the relationships is at stake when one member of a couple is ill and that partners dealing with illness are concerned with the well-being of the other and of the relationship at least as much as they are with their own. In addition to illness-related topics, therefore, couple-based interventions should aim at sustaining partners' relationship satisfaction and functioning more broadly. Considering that marital distress is associated with slower recovery trajectories and poorer outcomes (Yang & Schuler, 2009), it is important that marital satisfaction is regarded either as a moderator of couple-based interventions or as an outcome of these interventions. Interventions specifically targeting the enhancement of the couple's relationship satisfaction are relatively scarce and have mainly been conducted with breast and prostate cancer populations (McMahon, Gremore, Cella, & Sher, 2014). Among the few existing examples, Kayser, Feldman, Borstelmann and Daniels's (2010) Partners in Coping Program (PICP) that is a program aiming at integrating illness-related tasks into the couple's daily routine and at enhancing the couple's communication and supportive exchanges; the Partners empowered program (McMahon et al., 2014), that is a communication-focused couple-based intervention for patients and partners developed in the psycho-oncology area; the Shared Care Dyadic Intervention (SCDI; Sebern & Woda, 2012), based on the Shared Care Theory (Sebern,1996), that is aimed to improve dyadic communication, decision making, reciprocity, care planning, and family support.

To conclude, the main suggestions to inspire an integrative, relational intervention aimed to improve the patient's and partner's engagement skills and the couple's dyadic management of the illness can be summarized as follows:

A Clear Theoretical Framework

First, a clear theoretical framework is needed on how the couple and family deal with critical circumstances such as illness. Given that the patient is a person-in-relationship, patient engagement models could be usefully complemented by theoretical models on how couples and families adjust to normative and non-normative critical events (e.g., the Relational Symbolic Model by Cigoli & Scabini, 2006) as well as by dyadic coping models revealing how partners deal with illness as a dyad (e.g., the Systemic Transactional Model of dyadic coping by Bodenmann, 1997, 2000). Both the Relational Symbolic Model and the Systemic Transactional Model have been usefully applied to inform preventive interventions with community couples (Bodenmann & Bertoni, 2004; Bertoni, Donato, Morgano, Iafrate & Rosnati, in press).

The Couple as the Target

Second, the intervention should be addressed to both patients and their partners. As suggested by Li and Loke (2014) it is important that couple-based interventions focus on the couple as the unit of intervention and therefore work not only on the patient's skill training, or on supporting the caregiver's self-care, but also on sustaining couples' relationship processes, such as dyadic coping and couple engagement. Research suggested that the best interventions to improve self-care in heart failure targeted resources of both partners (Molloy, Johnston, & Witham, 2005; Reis & Collins, 2000) and stronger effect sizes were reported for those interventions that targeted both partners' relationship processes than for those targeting only the patients (Martire, Lusting, Schulz, Miller, & Helgeson, 2004).

Different Levels of Intervention

Within an integrated, relational perspective, to promote patient engagement the interventions should aim to sustain those processes that facilitate patients' and partners' engagement and to reduce those that undermine it. Such processes pertain to three different, but co-existent levels that can be integrated into the promotion of patient engagement (see Figure 1).

I. Individual level: This level, pertaining to the patient and partner as individuals, comprises intervention strategies aiming to prevent disengagement and to promote the individual's coping with the illness as well as the patient's and partner's engagement with their own healthcare, the individuals' well-being, and their self-care.

II. Interactive level: This level, referring to the connection between the patient's and partner's behaviors and relational processes, refers to intervention strategies aiming to prevent over-protectiveness and to promote partners' support to patient engagement, partners' open communication in order to share their needs and resources, and partners' relationship satisfaction.

III. Dyadic/relational level: This level, concerning the couple's joint appraisals and actions, involves intervention strategies devoted to prevent disengaged avoidance (Kayser et al., 2007) or incongruent strategies of coping (Revenson, 1994, 2003) and to promote mutual responsiveness (Kayser et al., 2007), symmetrical or complementary coping strategies (Revenson, 1994; 2003), and dyadic coping (Badr et al., 2010) to improve how couples use behavioral and cognitive strategies to manage stress, react to each other's responses, and appraise the illness-related stress.

CONCLUSION

In the present chapter it was proposed that a greater integration of the engagement literature with the couple relationship research and intervention may be a key to enhancing the efficacy of interventions aimed at promoting engagement among patients and their partners. Recognizing the importance of the patients' relational environment, and of a dyadic approach to the care process, will help healthcare systems to make a shift from a patient-centered model of intervention to a family-centered one and will make interventions more effective in promoting engagement and participation in healthcare.

REFERENCES

Acitelli, L. K., & Bard, H. (2005). My illness or our illness? Attending to the relationship when one partner is ill. In T. A. Revenson, K. Kayser, & G. Bodenmann (Eds.), *Emerging perspectives on couples' coping with stress* (pp. 121–136). Washington, DC: American Psychological Association. doi:10.1037/11031-006

Agren, S., Evangelista, L. S., Davidson, T., & Stromberg, A. (2013). Cost-effectiveness of a nurse-led education and psychosocial programme for patients with chronic heart failure and their partners. *Journal of Clinical Nursing*, *22*(15-16), 2347–2353. doi:10.1111/j.1365-2702.2012.04246.x PMID:23829407

Badr, H., Acitelli, L. K., & Carmack Taylor, C. L. (2007). Does couple identity mediate the stress experienced by caregiving spouses. *Psychology & Health*, *22*(2), 211–229. doi:10.1080/14768320600843077

Badr, H., Acitelli, L. K., & Carmack Taylor, C. L. (2008). Does talking about their relationship affect couples' marital and psychological adjustment to lung cancer? *Journal of Cancer Survivorship: Research and Practice*, *2*(1), 53–64. doi:10.1007/s11764-008-0044-3 PMID:18648987

Badr, H., & Carmack Taylor, C. L. (2008). Effects of relationship maintenance on psychological distress and dyadic adjustment among couples coping with lung cancer. *Health Psychology*, *27*(5), 616–627. doi:10.1037/0278-6133.27.5.616 PMID:18823188

Badr, H., Carmack Taylor, C. L., Kashy, D. A., Cristofanilli, M., & Revenson, T. A. (2010). Dyadic coping in metastatic breast cancer. *Health Psychology*, *29*(2), 169–180. doi:10.1037/a0018165 PMID:20230090

Barello, S., Graffigna, G., Savarese, M., Donato, S., & Bertoni, A. (2014). Patient engagement in chronic disease management: The pivotal role of partners. *Paper presented at the EACH - International conference on communication in healthcare*, Amsterdam, NL.

Barello, S., Graffigna, G., & Vegni, E. (2012). Patient engagement as an emerging challenge for healthcare services: Mapping the literature. *Nursing Research and Practice*, *1*, 1–7. doi:10.1155/2012/905934 PMID:23213497

Barello, S., Savarese, M., & Graffigna, G. (2015). The role of caregivers in the elderly healthcare journey: insights for sustaining elderly patient engagement. In G. Graffigna, S. Barello, & S. Triberti (Eds.), *Patient engagement: A consumer-centered model to innovate healthcare* (pp. 108–119). Warsaw: De Gruyter Open. doi:10.1515/9783110452440-010

Barnoy, S., Bar-tal, Y., & Zisser, B. (2006). Correspondence in informational coping styles: How important is it for cancer patients and their spouses? *Personality and Individual Differences*, *41*(1), 105–115. doi:10.1016/j.paid.2005.12.013

Belcher, A. J., Laurenceau, J. P., Graber, E. C., Cohen, L. H., Dash, K. B., & Siegel, S. D. (2011). Daily support in couples coping with early stage breast cancer: Maintaining intimacy during adversity. *Health Psychology*, *30*(6), 665–673. doi:10.1037/a0024705 PMID:21823795

Berg, C. A., Meegan, S. P., & Deviney, F. P. (1998). A social contextual model of coping with everyday problems across the life span. *International Journal of Behavioral Development*, *22*, 239–261. doi:10.1080/016502598384360

Berg, C. A., Wiebe, D. J., Butner, J., Bloor, L., Bradstreet, C., Upchurch, R., & Patton, G. et al. (2008). Collaborative coping and daily mood in couples dealing with prostate cancer. *Psychology and Aging*, *23*(3), 505–516. doi:10.1037/a0012687 PMID:18808241

Berghuis, J. P., & Stanton, A. L. (2002). Adjustment to a dyadic stressor: A longitudinal study of coping and depressive symptoms in infertile couples over an insemination attempt. *Journal of Consulting and Clinical Psychology*, *70*(2), 433–438. doi:10.1037/0022-006X.70.2.433 PMID:11952202

Bertoni, A., Barni, D., Bodenmann, G., Charvoz, L., Gagliardi, S., Iafrate, R., & Rosnati, R. (2007). Comunicazione dello stress, coping diadico e benessere della coppia: Uno studio cross-sectional e cross-nazionale. *Età Evolutiva*, *86*, 58–66.

Bertoni, A., & Bodenmann, G. (2010). Satisfied and dissatisfied couples: Positive and negative dimensions, conflict styles, and relationships with family of origin. *European Psychologist*, *15*(3), 175–184. doi:10.1027/1016-9040/a000015

Bertoni, A., Donato, S., Graffigna, G., Barello, S., & Parise, M. (2015). Engaged patients, engaged partnerships: Singles and partners dealing with an acute cardiac event. *Psychology Health and Medicine*, *20*(5), 505–517. doi:10.1080/13548506.2014.969746 PMID:25506636

Bertoni, A., Donato, S., Morgano, A., Iafrate, R., & Rosnati, R. (in press). A Qualitative Evaluation of a Preventive Intervention for Parents: The Groups for Family Enrichment_Parent Version (GFE_P). *Themed Issue of Journal of Prevention & Intervention in the Community*.

Bertoni, A., Parise, M., & Iafrate, R. (2012). Beyond Satisfaction: Generativity as a New Outcome of Couple Functioning. In P. E. Esposito & C. I. Lombardi (Eds.), *Marriage: Psychological Implications, Social Expectations, and Role of Sexuality* (pp. 115–131). New York, US: Nova Science Publishers.

Bodenmann, G. (1997). Dyadic coping - a systemic-transactional view of stress and coping among couples: Theory and empirical findings. *European Review of Applied Psychology*, *47*, 137–140.

Bodenmann, G. (2000). *Stress und Coping bei Paaren*. Göttingen: Hogrefe.

Bodenmann, G. (2005). Dyadic coping and its significance for marital functioning. In T. Revenson, K. Kayser, & G. Bodenmann (Eds.), *Couples coping with stress: Emerging perspectives on dyadic coping* (pp. 33–50). Washington: American Psychological Association. doi:10.1037/11031-002

Bodenmann, G., & Bertoni, A. (2004). *Promuovere le competenze della coppia. II Couple Coping Enhancement Training*. Roma: Carocci.

Bolger, N., DeLongis, A., Kessler, R. C., & Wethington, E. (1989). The contagion of stress across multiple roles. *Journal of Marriage and the Family*, *51*(1), 175–183. doi:10.2307/352378

Buck, H. G., Harkness, K., Wion, R., Carroll, S. L., Cosman, T., Kaasalainen, S., & Arthur, H. M. et al. (2015). Caregivers'contributions to heart failure self-care: A systematic review. *European Journal of Cardiovascular Nursing*, *14*(1), 79–89. doi:10.1177/1474515113518434 PMID:24399843

Buunk, B. P., Berkhuysen, M. A., Sanderman, R., Nieuwland, W., & Ranchon, A. V. (1996). The role of partner in heart disease: Active engagement, protective buffering, and overprotection. *Gedrag en Gezondheid*, *24*, 304–313.

Carman, K. L., Dardess, P., Maurer, M., Sofaer, S., Adams, K., Bechtel, C., & Sweeney, J. (2013). Patient and family engagement: A framework for understanding the elements and developing interventions and policies. *Health Affairs*, *32*(2), 223–231. doi:10.1377/hlthaff.2012.1133 PMID:23381514

Carpenter, D. M., Elstad, E. A., Sage, A. J., Geryk, L. L., DeVellis, R. F., & Blalock, S. J. (2015). The relationship between partner information-seeking, information-sharing, and patient medication adherence. *Patient Education and Counseling*, *98*(1), 120–124. doi:10.1016/j.pec.2014.10.001 PMID:25455797

Chung, M. L., Moser, D. K., Lennie, T. A., & Rayers, M. K. (2009). The effect of depressive symptoms and anxiety on quality of life in patients with heart failure and their spouses: Testing dyadic using Actor-Partner Interdependence Model. *Journal of Psychosomatic Research*, *67*(1), 29–35. doi:10.1016/j.jpsychores.2009.01.009 PMID:19539816

Cigoli, V., & Scabini, E. (2006). *Family identity: Ties, symbols, and transitions*. New York: Lawrence Erlbaum Associates Publishers.

Coyne, J. C., & DeLongis, A. (1986). Going beyond social support: The role of social relationships in adaptation. *Journal of Consulting and Clinical Psychology*, *54*(4), 454–460. doi:10.1037/0022-006X.54.4.454 PMID:3745597

Coyne, J. C., Ellard, J. H., & Smith, D. A. (1990). Unsupportive relationships, interdependence, and unhelpful exchanges. In I. G. Sarason, B. R. Sarason, & G. Pierce (Eds.), *Social support: An interactional view* (pp. 129–149). New York: Wiley.

Coyne, J. C., & Smith, D. A. F. (1991). Couples coping with a myocardial infarction: A contextual perspective on wives' distress. *Journal of Personality and Social Psychology*, *61*(3), 404–412. doi:10.1037/0022-3514.61.3.404 PMID:1941511

Cutrona, C. E. (1996). *Social support in couples: Marriage as a resource in times of stress*. Thousand Oaks: Sage. doi:10.4135/9781483327563

Dekel, R., Vilchinsky, N., Liberman, G., Leibowitz, M., Khaskia, A., & Mosseri, M. (2014). Marital satisfaction and depression among couples following men's acute coronary syndrome: Testing dyadic dynamics in a longitudinal design. *British Journal of Health Psychology*, *19*(2), 347–362. doi:10.1111/bjhp.12042 PMID:23552169

DeLongis, A., & O'Brien, T. (1990). An interpersonal framework for stress and coping: An application to the families of alzheimer's patients. In M. A. P. Stephens, J. H. Crowther, S. E. Hobfoll, & D. L. Tennenbaum (Eds.), *Stress and coping in later-life families* (pp. 221–240). New York: Hemisphere Publishing Corporation.

Donato, S. (2014). Il coping diadico, ovvero far fronte allo stress insieme: Una rassegna della letteratura. *Giornale Italiano di Psicologia, 36*, 471–499. doi:10.1421/78499

Donato, S., Canzi, E., Parise, M., & Ferrari, L. (2014). Partnership Questionnaire: Factorial structure, gender invariance, and concurrent validity. *TPM - Testing, Psychometrics. Methodology in Applied Psychology, 21*, 161–180. doi:10.4473/TPM21.2.4

Donato, S., Iafrate, R., Barni, D., Bertoni, A., Bodenmann, G., & Gagliardi, S. (2009). Measuring dyadic coping: The factorial structure of Bodenmann's "Dyadic Coping Questionnaire" in an Italian sample. *TPM - Testing, Psychometrics. Methodology in Applied Psychology, 16*, 25–47.

Donato, S., Iafrate, R., Bradbury, T. N., & Scabini, E. (2012). Acquiring dyadic coping: Partners and parents as models. *Personal Relationships, 19*(2), 386–400. doi:10.1111/j.1475-6811.2011.01368.x

Donato, S., & Parise, M. (2012). The role of enacted and perceived dyadic coping for young couples' satisfaction. In B. Molinelli & V. Grimaldo (Eds.), *Handbook of the Psychology of Coping: New research* (pp. 261–278). Hauppauge, NY: Nova Science Publisher.

Donato, S., Parise, M., Iafrate, R., Bertoni, A., Finkenauer, C., & Bodenmann, G. (2015). Dyadic coping responses and partners' perceptions for relationship satisfaction: An actor-partner longitudinal analysis. *Journal of Social and Personal Relationships, 32*, 580–600. doi:10.1177/0265407514541071

Donato, S., Parise, M., Pagani, A. F., Bertoni, A., & Iafrate, R. (2014). Demand-withdraw, couple satisfaction and relationship duration. *Procedia: Social and Behavioral Sciences, 140*, 200–206. doi:10.1016/j.sbspro.2014.04.410

Endler, N. S., & Parker, J. D. A. (1990). Multidimensional assessment of coping: A critical evaluation. *Journal of Personality and Social Psychology, 58*(5), 844–854. doi:10.1037/0022-3514.58.5.844 PMID:2348372

Fiske, V., Coyne, J. C., & Smith, D. A. (1991). Couples coping with myocardial infarction: An empirical reconsideration of the role of overprotectiveness. *Journal of Family Psychology, 5*(1), 4–20. doi:10.1037/0893-3200.5.1.4

Gagliardi, S., Bodenmann, G., Heinrichs, N., Bertoni, A., Iafrate, R., & Donato, S. (2013). Unterschiede in der Partnerschaftsqualität und imdyadischen Coping beiverschiedenenbindungsbezogenenPaartypen [Differences in relationship quality and dyadic coping for attachment-related couple types]. *Psychotherapie, Psychosomatik, Medizinische Psychologie, 63*, 185–192. doi:10.1055/s-0032-1333291

Gasbarrini, M. F., Snyder, D. K., Iafrate, R., Bertoni, A., Donato, S., & Margola, D. (in press). Investigating the Relation Between Shared Stressors and Marital Satisfaction: The Moderating Effects of Dyadic Coping and Communication. *Special Section of Family Science*. doi:10.1080/19424620.2015.1082044

Graffigna, G., Barello, S., & Riva, G. (2013). Technologies for patient engagement. *Health Affairs, 32*(6), 1172. doi:10.1377/hlthaff.2013.0279 PMID:23733998

Graffigna, G., Barello, S., Riva, G., & Bosio, A. C. (2014). Patient engagement: The key to redesign the exchange between the demand and supply for healthcare in the era of active ageing. *Active Ageing and Healthy Living, 203*, 85–95. doi:10.3233/978-1-61499-425-1-85 PMID:26630515

Grant, J. S., Glandon, G. L., Elliot, T. R., Giger, J. N., & Weaver, M. (2004). Caregiving problems and feelings experienced by family caregivers of stroke survivors the first month after discharge. *International Journal of Rehabilitation Research. Internationale Zeitschrift fur Rehabilitationsforschung. Revue Internationale de Recherches de Readaptation, 27*(2), 105–111. doi:10.1097/01.mrr.0000127639.47494.e3 PMID:15167107

Griffin, K. W., Friend, R., Kaell, A. T., & Bennet, R. S. (2001). Distress and disease status among patients with rheumatoid arthritis: Roles of coping styles and perceived responses from support providers. *Annals of Behavioral Medicine, 23*(2), 133–138. doi:10.1207/S15324796ABM2302_8 PMID:11394555

Hagedoorn, M., Dagan, M., Puterman, E., Hoff, C., Meijerink, W. J., Delongis, A., & Sanderman, R. (2011). Relationship satisfaction in couples confronted with colorectal cancer: The interplay of past and current spousal support. *Journal of Behavioral Medicine, 34*(4), 288–297. doi:10.1007/s10865-010-9311-7 PMID:21222025

Hagedoorn, M., Kuijer, R. G., Buunk, B. P., DeJong, G. M., Wobbes, T., & Sanderman, R. (2000). Marital satisfaction in patients with cancer: Does support from intimate partners benefit those who need it most? *Health Psychology, 19*(3), 274–282. doi:10.1037/0278-6133.19.3.274 PMID:10868772

Hagedoorn, M., Sanderman, R., Bolks, H., Tuinstra, J., & Coyne, J. C. (2008). Distress in couples coping with cancer: A meta-analysis and critical review of role and gender effects. *Psychological Bulletin, 134*(1), 1–30. doi:10.1037/0033-2909.134.1.1 PMID:18193993

Holtzman, S., & DeLongis, A. (2007). One day at time: The impact of daily spouse support on pain, negative affect and catastrophizing among individuals with rheumatoid arthritis. *Pain, 131*, 1633–1655. doi:10.1016/j.pain.2007.04.005

Iafrate, R., Bertoni, A., Barni, D., & Donato, S. (2009). Congruenza percettiva nella coppia e stili di coping diadico. *Psicologia Sociale, 1*, 95–114.

Iafrate, R., Bertoni, A., Donato, S., & Finkenauer, C. (2012). Perceived similarity and understanding in dyadic coping among young and mature couples. *Personal Relationships, 19*(3), 401–419. doi:10.1111/j.1475-6811.2011.01369.x

Iafrate, R., Bertoni, A., Margola, D., Cigoli, V., & Acitelli, L. K. (2012). The link between perceptual congruence and couple relationship satisfaction in dyadic coping. *European Psychologist, 17*(1), 73–82. doi:10.1027/1016-9040/a000069

Iafrate, R., & Donato, S. (2012). Coping in a relational context: The case of dyadic coping. In B. Molinelli & V. Grimaldo (Eds.), *Handbook of the Psychology of Coping: New research* (pp. 111–132). Hauppauge, NY: Nova Science Publisher.

Jaarsma, T., & Stromberg, A. (2014). Heart failure clinics are still useful (more than ever?). *The Canadian Journal of Cardiology*, *30*(3), 272–275. doi:10.1016/j.cjca.2013.09.022 PMID:24468418

Joekes, K., Van Elderen, T., & Schreurs, K. (2007). Self-efficacy and overprotection are related to quality of life, psychological well-being and self-management in cardiac patients. *Journal of Health Psychology*, *12*(1), 4–16. doi:10.1177/1359105306069096 PMID:17158836

Kayser, K., Feldman, B. N., Borstelmann, N. A., & Daniels, A. A. (2010). Effects of a randomized couple-based intervention on quality of life of breast cancer patients and their partners. *Social Work Research*, *34*(1), 20–32. doi:10.1093/swr/34.1.20

Kayser, K., Watson, L. E., & Andrade, J. T. (2007). Cancer as a "we-disease": Examining the process of coping from a relational perspective. *Families, Systems & Health*, *25*(4), 404–418. doi:10.1037/1091-7527.25.4.404

King, K. B., & Reis, H. T. (2012). Marriage and long-term survival coronary artery bypass grafting. *Health Psychology*, *31*(1), 55–62. doi:10.1037/a0025061 PMID:21859213

Lazarus, R. S., & Folkman, S. (1984). *Stress, appraisal, and coping*. New York: Springer Publishing Company.

Lee, C. S., Vellone, E., Lyons, K. S., Cocchieri, A., Bidwell, J. T., & D'Agostino, F. et al. (2015). Pattern and predictors of patient and caregiver engagement in heart failure care: A multi-level dyadic study. *International Journal of Nursing Studies*, *52*(2), 588–597. doi:10.1016/j.ijnurstu.2014.11.005 PMID:25468283

Levin, J. B., Sher, T. G., & Theodos, V. (1997). The effect of intracouple coping concordance on psychological and marital distress in infertility patients. *Journal of Clinical Psychology in Medical Settings*, *4*(4), 361–372. doi:10.1023/A:1026249317635

Li, Q., & Loke, A. Y. (2014). A systematic review of spousal couple-based intervention studies for couples coping with cancer: Direction for the development of interventions. *Psycho-Oncology*, *23*(7), 731–739. doi:10.1002/pon.3535 PMID:24723336

Liang, J., Krause, N. M., & Bennett, J. M. (2001). Social exchange and well-being: Is giving better than receiving? *Psychology and Aging*, *16*(3), 511–523. doi:10.1037/0882-7974.16.3.511 PMID:11554527

Lyons, K. S., Bennett, J. A., Nail, L. M., Fromme, E. K., Dieckmann, N., & Sayer, A. G. (2014). The role of patient pain and physical function on depressive symptoms in couples with lung cancer: A longitudinal dyadic analysis. *Journal of Family Psychology*, *28*(5), 692–700. doi:10.1037/fam0000017 PMID:25090253

Lyons, R., Mickelson, K. D., Sullivan, M. J. L., & Coyne, J. C. (1998). Coping as a communal process. *Journal of Social and Personal Relationships*, *15*(5), 579–605. doi:10.1177/0265407598155001

Pagani, A. F., Donato, S., Parise, M., Iafrate, R., Bertoni, A., & Schoebi, D. (2015). When Good Things Happen: The Effects of Implicit and Explicit Capitalization Attempts on Intimate Partners' Well-being. *Family Science*, *6*, 119–128. doi:10.1080/19424620.2015.1082013

Manne, S., & Badr, H. (2010). Intimacy processes and psychological distress among couples coping with head and neck or lung cancers. *Psycho-Oncology*, *19*(9), 941–954. doi:10.1002/pon.1645 PMID:19885852

Manne, S., Badr, H., Zaider, T., Nelson, C., & Kissane, D. (2010). Cancer-related communication, relationship intimacy, and psychological distress among couples coping with localized prostate cancer. *Journal of Cancer Survivorship: Research and Practice*, *4*(1), 74–85. doi:10.1007/s11764-009-0109-y PMID:19967408

Manne, S. L. (1998). Cancer in the marital context: A review of the literature. *Cancer Investigation*, *16*(3), 188–202. doi:10.3109/07357909809050036 PMID:9541634

Manne, S. L., & Badr, H. (2008). Intimacy and relationship processes in couples' psychosocial adaptation to cancer. *Cancer*, *112*(S11), 2541–2555. doi:10.1002/cncr.23450 PMID:18428202

Manne, S. L., Badr, H., & Kashy, D. A. (2012). A longitudinal analysis of intimacy processes and psychological distress among couples coping with head and neck or lung cancers. *Journal of Behavioral Medicine*, *35*(3), 334–346. doi:10.1007/s10865-011-9349-1 PMID:21556790

Manne, S. L., Ostroff, J., Rini, C., Fox, K., Goldstein, L., & Grana, G. (2004). The interpersonal process model of intimacy: The role of self-disclosure, partner disclosure, and partner responsiveness in interactions between breast cancer patients and their partners. *Journal of Family Psychology*, *18*(4), 589–599. doi:10.1037/0893-3200.18.4.589 PMID:15598164

Manne, S. L., Ostroff, J. S., Norton, T. R., Fox, K., Goldstein, L., & Grana, G. (2006). Cancer-related relationship communication in couples coping with early stage breast cancer. *Psycho-Oncology*, *15*(3), 234–247. doi:10.1002/pon.941 PMID:15926198

Manne, S. L., & Zautra, A. J. (1989). Spouse criticism and support: Their association with coping and psychological adjustment among women with rheumatoid arthritis. *Journal of Personality and Social Psychology*, *56*(4), 608–617. doi:10.1037/0022-3514.56.4.608 PMID:2709309

Manne, S. L., & Zautra, A. J. (1990). Couples coping with chronic illness: Women with rheumatoid arthritis and their healthy husband. *Journal of Behavioral Medicine*, *13*(4), 327–342. doi:10.1007/BF00844882 PMID:2246781

Marin, T., Holtzman, S., DeLongis, A., & Robinson, L. (2007). Coping and the response of others. *Journal of Social and Personal Relationships*, *24*(6), 951–969. doi:10.1177/0265407507084192

Martire, L. M., Lustig, A. P., Schulz, R., Miller, G. E., & Helgeson, V. S. (2004). Is it beneficial to involve a family member? A meta-analysis of psychosocial interventions for chronic illness. *Health Psychology*, *23*(6), 599–611. doi:10.1037/0278-6133.23.6.599 PMID:15546228

McMahon, M. E., Gremore, T. M., Cella, D., & Sher, T. G. (2014). Partners empowered: A couple-based intervention for newly diagnosed cancer. *Psycho-Oncology*, *23*(7), 832–834. doi:10.1002/pon.3490 PMID:24497302

Meegan, S. P., & Berg, C. A. (2002). Contexts, functions, forms, and processes of collaborative everyday problem solving in older adulthood. *International Journal of Behavioral Development*, *26*(1), 6–15. doi:10.1080/01650250143000283

Meij, L., W., , Stroebe, M., Schut, H., Stroebe, W., van den Bout, J., & Dijkstra, I. et al. (2008). Parents grieving the loss of their child: Interdependence in coping. *The British Journal of Clinical Psychology, 47*(1), 31–42. doi:10.1348/014466507X216152 PMID:17588295

Mickelson, K. D., Lyons, R. F., Sullivan, M. J. L., & Coyne, J. C. (2001). Yours, mine, ours: The relational context of communal coping. In B. R. Sarason & S. Duck (Eds.), *Personal relationships: Implications for clinical and community psychology* (pp. 181–200). New York: Wiley.

Molloy, G. J., Johnston, D. W., & Witham, M. D. (2005). Family caregiving and congestive heart failure. Review and analysis. *European Journal of Heart Failure, 7*, 592-603. doi:10.10167j.ejheart.2004.07.008

Northhouse, L. L., Katapodi, M. C., Song, L., Zhang, L., & Mood, D. W. (2010). Interventions with family caregivers of cancer patients meta-analysis of randomized trials. *CA: a Cancer Journal for Clinicians, 60*, 317–339. doi:10.3322/caac.20081 PMID:20709946

O'Brien, T. B., & DeLongis, A. (1997). Coping with chronic stress: An interpersonal perspective. In B. H. Gottlieb (Ed.), *Coping with chronic stress* (pp. 161–190). New York: Plenum Press. doi:10.1007/978-1-4757-9862-3_6

Randall, A. K., & Bodenmann, G. (2009). The role of stress on close relationships and marital satisfaction. *Clinical Psychology Review, 29*(2), 105–115. doi:10.1016/j.cpr.2008.10.004 PMID:19167139

Rankin-Esquer, L. A., Deeter, A. K., & Barr Taylor, C. (2000). Coronary heart disease and couples. In K. B. Schmaling & T. Goldman Sher (Eds.), *The psychology of couples and illness: Theory, research and practice* (pp. 43–70). Washington: American Psychological Association. doi:10.1037/10360-002

Regan, T. M., Lambert, S. D., Kelly, B., Falconier, M., Kissane, D., & Levesque, J. V. (2015). Couples coping with cancer: Exploration of theoretical frameworks from dyadic studies. *Psycho-Oncology, 24*(12), 1605–1617. doi:10.1002/pon.3854 PMID:26059915

Reinhardt, J. (2001). Effects of positive and negative support received and provided on adaptation to chronic visual impairment. *Applied Developmental Science, 5*(2), 76–85. doi:10.1207/S1532480XADS0502_3

Reis, H. T., & Collins, N. (2000). Measuring relationship properties and interactions relevant to social support. In S. Cohen, L. G. Underwood, & B. J. Gottlieb (Eds.), *Social support measurement and intervention* (pp. 136–192). New York: Oxford University Press. doi:10.1093/med:psych/9780195126709.003.0005

Reis, H. T., & Shaver, P. (1988). Intimacy as an interpersonal process. In S. Duck (Ed.), *Handbook of personal relationships* (pp. 367–389). Chichester, England: Wiley.

Repetti, R. L. (1989). Effects of daily workload on subsequent behavior during marital interaction: The roles of social withdrawal and spouse support. *Journal of Personality and Social Psychology, 57*(4), 651–659. doi:10.1037/0022-3514.57.4.651 PMID:2795436

Revenson, T. A. (1994). Social support and marital coping with chronic illness. *Annals of Behavioral Medicine, 16*, 122–130.

Revenson, T. A. (2003). Scenes from a marriage: Examining support, coping, and gender within the context of chronic illness. In J. Suls & K. Wallston (Eds.), *Social psychological foundation of health and illness* (pp. 530–559). Oxford: Blackwell Publishers. doi:10.1002/9780470753552.ch19

Revenson, T. A., Abraido-Lanza, A. F., Majerovitz, S. D., & Jordan, C. (2005). Couples coping with chronic illness: What's gender got to do with it? In T. A. Revenson, K. Kayser, & G. Bodenmann (Eds.), *Couples coping with stress: Emerging perspectives on dyadic coping* (pp. 121–136). Washington, DC: American Psychological Association. doi:10.1037/11031-007

Revenson, T. A., & DeLongis, A. (2011). Couples coping with chronic illness. In S. Folkman (Ed.), *The Oxford Handbook of Stress, Health, and Coping* (pp. 101–123). New York: Oxford University Press.

Revenson, T. A., Kayser, K., & Bodenmann, G. (2005). *Couples coping with stress: Emerging perspectives on dyadic coping*. Washington, DC: American Psychological Association. doi:10.1037/11031-000

Riegel, B., Lee, C. S., & Dickson, V. V. (2011). Self-care in patients with chronic heart failure. *Nature Reviews. Cardiology*, *8*(11), 644–654. doi:10.1038/nrcardio.2011.95 PMID:21769111

Rohrbaugh, M. J., Shoham, V., & Coyne, J. C. (2006). Effect of marital quality on eight-year survival of patients with heart failure. *The American Journal of Cardiology*, *98*(8), 1069–1072. doi:10.1016/j.amjcard.2006.05.034 PMID:17027573

Schoebi, D. (2008). The coregulation of daily affect in marital relationships. *Journal of Family Psychology*, *22*(4), 595–604. doi:10.1037/0893-3200.22.3.595 PMID:18729673

Scott, J. L., & Kayser, K. (2009). A review of couple-based interventions for enhancing women's sexual adjustment and body image after cancer. *Cancer Journal (Sudbury, Mass.)*, *15*(1), 48–56. doi:10.1097/PPO.0b013e31819585df PMID:19197174

Sebern, M. D. (1996). Explication of the construct of shared care and the prevention of pressure ulcers in home health care. *Research in Nursing & Health*, *19*(3), 183–192. doi:10.1002/(SICI)1098-240X(199606)19:3<183::AID-NUR2>3.0.CO;2-G PMID:8628907

Sebern, M. D. (2005). Psychometric evaluation of the Shared Care Instrument in a sample of home health care family dyads. *Journal of Nursing Measurement*, *13*(3), 175–191. doi:10.1891/jnum.13.3.175 PMID:16605041

Sebern, M. D., & Woda, A. (2012). Shared care dyadic intervention: Outcome patterns for heart failure care partners. *Western Journal of Nursing Research*, *34*(3), 289–316. doi:10.1177/0193945911399088 PMID:21383082

Stanton, A. L. (1991). Cognitive appraisals, coping processes, and adjustment to infertility. In A. L. Stanton & C. Dunkel-Schetter (Eds.), *Infertility: Perspectives from stress and coping research* (pp. 87–108). New York: Plenum Press. doi:10.1007/978-1-4899-0753-0_5

Stanton, A. L., Tennen, H., Affleck, G., & Mendola, R. (1992). Coping and adjustment to infertility. *Journal of Social and Clinical Psychology*, *11*(1), 1–13. doi:10.1521/jscp.1992.11.1.1

Stroebe, M., Finkenauer, C., Wijngaards-de Meij, L., Schut, H., Van den Bout, J., & Stroebe, W. (2013). Partner-oriented self-regulation among bereaved parents: The cost of holding in grief for the partner sake. *Psychological Science*, *24*(4), 1–8. doi:10.1177/0956797612457383 PMID:23406609

Thompson, A., & Bolger, N. (1999). Emotional transmission in couples under stress. *Journal of Marriage and the Family*, *61*(1), 38–48. doi:10.2307/353881

Uchino, B. N. (2006). Social support and health: A review of physiological processes potentially underlying links to disease outcomes. *Journal of Behavioral Medicine*, *29*(4), 377–387. doi:10.1007/s10865-006-9056-5 PMID:16758315

Vellone, E., Chung, M. L., Cocchieri, A., Rocco, G., Alvaro, R., & Riegel, B. (2014). Effects of self-care on quality of life in adults with heart failure and their spousal caregivers: Testing dyadic dynamics using the actor-partner interdependence model. *Journal of Family Nursing*, *20*(1), 120–141. doi:10.1177/1074840713510205 PMID:24189325

Vilchinsky, N., Dekel, R., Leibowitz, M., Reges, O., Khaskia, A., & Mosseri, M. (2011). Dynamics of support perceptions among couples with cardiac illness: The effect on recovery outcomes. *Health Psychology*, *30*(4), 411–419. doi:10.1037/a0023453 PMID:21480711

Yang, H., & Schuler, T. A. (2009). Marital quality and survivorship: Slowed recovery for breast cancer patients in distressed relationships. *Cancer*, *115*(1), 217–228. doi:10.1002/cncr.23964 PMID:18951520

Ybema, J. F., Kuijer, R. G., Buunk, B. P., DeJong, G. M., & Saderman, R. (2001). Depression and perceptions of inequity among couples facing cancer. *Personality and Social Psychology Bulletin*, *27*(1), 3–13. doi:10.1177/0146167201271001

KEY TERMS AND DEFINITIONS

Collaborative Coping: The active engagement of spouses in pooling resources and in joint problem-solving and coping.

Communal Coping: The understanding of a stressor as a problem of the whole group and not only of a single member of it (social appraisal) and the cooperative actions of the group members in order to cope with it.

Coping Congruence: Symmetry or complementarity of coping styles as long as partners' efforts work in concert to reach a desired goal.

Couple Relationship Processes: Dyadic processes as closeness, emotional support, communication, reciprocity, and mutual responsiveness.

Dyadic Coping: The interplay between the stress signals of one partner and the coping reactions of the other, a genuine act of shared coping.

Interdependent Self-Perspective: Theoretical point of view who considers the human beings as essentially connected to each other. Along with this perspective, the patient is a person-in-relationships and the patient's close relationships are necessarily involved in the disease.

Reciprocity: Giving and accepting of physical and emotional help with appreciation, is an important component of family care relationships.

Relationship-Focused Coping: The coping efforts aiming to sustain the relationship during stressful events.

Chapter 6
The Light Side of Preterm Behavioral Epigenetics:
An Epigenetic Perspective on Caregiver Engagement

Livio Provenzi
0-3 Center for the at-Risk Infant, Scientific Institute IRCCS Eugenio Medea, Bosisio Parini, LC, Italy

Renato Borgatti
0-3 Center for the at-Risk Infant, Scientific Institute IRCCS Eugenio Medea, Bosisio Parini, LC, Italy

Rosario Montirosso
0-3 Center for the at-Risk Infant, Scientific Institute IRCCS Eugenio Medea, Bosisio Parini, LC, Italy

ABSTRACT

Preterm infants need long-lasting hospitalization in the Neonatal Intensive Care Unit (NICU). On the one hand, the NICU stay constitutes an early adverse experience, due to highly stressful experiences. On the other hand, Developmental Care (DC) interventions, including caregiver engagement, can exert neuro-protective effects for preterm infants. Recent evidence in the field of behavioral epigenetics is revealing the biochemical pathways through which adverse and care experiences are embedded in early human development through epigenetic mechanisms. Nonetheless, the application of behavioral epigenetics to preterm birth and NICU stay is still at its beginning. In the present chapter, insights are provided for the application of behavioral epigenetics to the study of the biochemical underpinnings of NICU-related stress and care, with a specific focus on caregiver engagement. This contribute should be intended as a preliminary roadmap to guide future behavioral epigenetic research on the adverse and protective effects of early NICU care of preterm infants.

DOI: 10.4018/978-1-4666-9992-2.ch006

INTRODUCTION

Preterm birth is a major concern for healthcare services, ranging from about 5% to 18% worldwide (Field et al., 2009). Preterm birth is associated with a heightened risk for long-term detrimental consequences for development, including sensorial, behavioral, neurological, and emotional disorders (Stoll et al., 2010). Notably, even in absence of severe illness condition, preterm infants are especially fragile and they require long-term hospitalization and specialized multi-disciplinary interventions in a medical environment (i.e., Neonatal Intensive Care Unit, NICU), which clearly is not a surrogate of the maternal womb.

Specific features of NICU environment are sources of multiple stress for preterm infants, including painful stimuli, disruption of sleep, excessive noise and light levels, frequent handling associated with medical or nursing procedures, maternal separation and disrupted parenting (Peng et al., 2009). Effects of early exposure to NICU-related stress may be at least partially alleviated by caregiver engagement interventions. Despite there is considerable variations in caregiver engagement among different NICUs, Samra and colleagues (Samra et al., 2015) recently proposed a comprehensive definition. Caregiver engagement should be considered as a complex, dynamic, goal-oriented, and guided multifaceted process through which parents participate in the care of their infant to influence the outcome within a specific period and context (Samra et al., 2015). As such, caregiver engagement is a process aimed at enhancing parent parents' situational awareness (understanding of health care communication, awareness of cues in the environment, realistic perception of their infant's condition and cues), ability to problem solve, set goals, make appropriate care decisions, and acquire skills and knowledge to support their infant health needs. The caregiver engagement process in the NICU appears to be aimed at least at two main directions: engaging parents as partners of NICU staff and engaging parents in interacting with their own newborn and infant (Provenzi, Barello, & Graffigna, 2016a).

Caregiver engagement interventions encompass different Developmental Care (DC) practices (Westrup, 2007). DC includes a broad category of interventions designed to minimize the effects of NICU stress exposure encompassing control of external stimuli (vestibular, auditory, visual, tactile), kangaroo care and parental involvement (e.g., breastfeeding, policies of NICUs toward parental visiting, promoting infant-parent bonding), developmental activities of daily living (i.e., nesting, swaddling, prone position) and infant pain management (Symington & Pinelli, 2006). During last decades, parents have been increasingly engaged by NICU staff through a set of family-centered actions (Provenzi et al., 2016a). Caregiver presence in NICU has been shown to be beneficial for both the infants and their parents (Montirosso et al., 2012a). Specific ways of engaging parents in the NICU, such as skin-to-skin contact and kangaroo care, are able to exert positive long-lasting neuro-protective effects for the neuro-behavioral and psycho-biological development of preterm infants (Altimier, Kenner, & Damus, 2015). Hence, caregiver engagement in the NICU holds the potential to be a low-cost and high-quality intervention to provide positive influence on health outcomes of preterm infants (Samra et al., 2015).

Although several mechanisms may potentially link neonatal stress exposure with altered neurodevelopment, emerging evidence suggest that epigenetic changes are likely implied in the precocious programming of biological and physiological stress regulation systems in preterm infants (Montirosso & Provenzi, 2015). More specifically, behavioral epigenetic research (see below) is the study of environmental-driven modifications of the genotype resulting in long-lasting alterations of neuro-behavioral phenotype (Lester et al., 2011). In animals and humans, behavioral epigenetics is starting to provide insights about such biochemical mechanisms involved in the embedding of stressful and caring experiences in the developing biology of young individuals, programming the risk of health and disease later in life (Griffiths &

Hunter, 2014). Recently, behavioral epigenetics has started to be applied to the study of preterm infants' development (Kantake, Yoshitake, Ishikawa, Araki, & Shimizu, 2014; Provenzi et al., 2015), despite the study of epigenetic modifications associated with prematurity and NICU stay is still at its beginning and future research is needed (Provenzi & Montirosso, 2015).

The main objective of the present chapter is to provide an innovative framework for the study of the epigenetic mechanisms associated with DC practices of caregiver engagement for preterm infants hospitalized in the NICU. Preliminarily, the NICU environment will be discussed as both a source of stressful experiences for the preterm infants and their parents, as well as a place in which the caregiver engagement might act as a neuro-protective care strategy for infants' long-term development. Second, recent contributes within the field of behavioral epigenetics will be briefly reviewed, in order to offer an innovative point of view on the pathways through which early stressful and caregiving experiences might get under the skin, contributing to the long-lasting programming of health and disease. Finally, the application of behavioral epigenetics to prematurity will be discussed, providing emerging research on the epigenetic effects of NICU-related stress exposure and offering insights about the relevance of applying behavioral epigenetic to caregiver engagement practices in NICU.

One last annotation. Throughout the chapter, a metaphor on "dark" and "light" sides of NICU stay – and related epigenetic research – will be adopted to refer, on the one hand, to the NICU-related stressful/adverse experiences lived by preterm infants and their parents and, on the other hand, to the NICU-related caregiving support interventions thought to exert beneficial effects for infants and their family. This metaphor was chosen in order to underline there are two main research pathways through which epigenetics might be applied to the study of preterm birth and early hospitalization: one to improve our knowledge of premature babies' experience of the NICU and one to inform better neonatal healthcare practices. Nonetheless, we would like to warn the readers that this distinction only holds a didactical value. In the everyday life, neonatal healthcare professionals know that the dark and the light sides of NICU stay are deeply interwoven. Moreover, it is not always easy to distinguish how the dark and the light sides of NICU stay act independently or jointly on infants' long-term socio-emotional development.

BACKGROUND

The Dark Side of the NICU. Prematurity as an Early Adverse Experience

Preterm infants are born too soon, surrounded by an unfamiliar NICU environment, to which they are not prepared and without the comforting and protective support of the maternal uterus (Altimier et al., 2015). During this early period of development, the infant brain is extremely sensitive to environmental stimulations. As such, even in absence of medical complications, the NICU is a source of enormous distress for preterm infants, mainly due to three main aspects: sensorial adverse stimulations, invasive and painful procedures, forced maternal separation.

First, infants are exposed to physical and sensorial stimulations characterized by levels of intensity and length of exposure that are arduous to be tolerated (Brown, 2009; Ozawa, Sasaki, & Kanda, 2010). The NICU is characterized by high-intensity light – often exceeding the limit of 600 lux (Lee, Malakooti, & Lotas, 2005) – and noise – exceeding the average recommended standard of 45 decibels (Altuncu et al., 2009). As such, NICU lighting conditions and high-intensity noise have been shown to contribute to physiological instability of preterm infants, causing long-term detrimental consequences for visual and auditory development (Graven, 2004).

Moreover, clinical procedures – such as intubations, venipunctures, arterial insertions, surgery – are needed to improve the health status of preterm infants, but still they constitute invasive and painful stimulations for the immature preterm infant. Notably, due to their immature neuro-developmental state, preterm infants have a lower threshold and high sensitization to external perturbations, so that even routinely handling (e.g., diaper change) might be responded to with heightened physiologic response. Among NICU invasive procedures, skin-breaking procedures have been largely studied as a source of pain for preterm infants (Grunau, 2013). Skin-breaking interventions have been associated with several detrimental consequences for brief- and long-term development (Grunau et al., 2009), encompassing structural and functional alterations of brain development, which might persist through childhood (Smith et al., 2011). Furthermore, the level of NICU-related pain exposure is associated with neurodevelopment, including motor and cognitive development (Zwicker et al., 2013) as well as emotional problems during later childhood (Ranger, Synnes, Vinall, & Grunau, 2014).

These long-lasting developmental alterations appear to be at least partially mediated by an altered functioning of the main system of stress response, namely the hypothalamic-pituitary-adrenal (HPA) axis. The HPA axis acts as an energy mobilizer during stressful conditions through the activation of an hormonal cascade producing cortisol (Tsigos & Chrousos, 2002) and it is rapidly growing during the first months of life (Jansen, Beijers, Riksen-Walraven, & de Weerth, 2010). The HPA axis has two important implications for the development of adaptive stress response. First, the HPA axis grants the capacity to face stressful events (i.e., stress reactivity) through cortisol production. Second, the HPA axis is regulated via feedback mechanisms consisting in the binding of the cortisol to glucocorticoid receptors (GR) located in several brain regions, including hippocampus (Tsigos & Chrousos, 2002). This feedback regulation is essential for the stress regulation to be terminated when the stressful event is over (i.e., stress recovery). In other words, feedback mechanisms prevent the potential neuro-toxic effects of chronic brain exposure to stress-related high concentrations of cortisol. Several studies have documented that cumulative exposure to skin-breaking pain during the NICU stay might associate with altered resting cortisol levels (Brummelte et al., 2011), increased stress reactivity (Grunau et al., 2005) and altered HPA regulation (Haley, Weinberg, & Grunau, 2006) in preterm infants and children, independently from clinical confounders.

Finally, the preterm newborn is suddenly separated from the mother after birth. This forced separation is critical for both infants and their mothers, since it disrupts the biological and emotional caregiving bonding which was developing during the gestation (Latva, Lehtonen, Salmelin, & Tamminen, 2004). Animal studies documented that early life maternal separation might affect the development of the central nervous system (Bock, Rether, Gröger, Xie, & Braun, 2014) and of the HPA axis (Welberg & Seckl, 2001) in the offspring. In humans, the alteration of the caregiving environment due to forced maternal separation in the NICU alters the possibility of physical contact between the mother and her preterm newborn resulting in altered HPA reactivity to pain stimulations (Mörelius, Nelson, & Gustafsson, 2007).

From this point of view, mothers and fathers of preterm infants might be considered as premature parents, facing the unexpected preterm delivery and suddenly facing a long-lasting journey in the hospital (Provenzi & Santoro, 2015). On the one hand, mothers of preterm infants are exposed to the sight of their own infants connected with tubes and machineries, as well as the experience of the death of other infants, which are reported as critical sources of emotional disturbance from these parents. On the other hand, previous research has showed that these parents might suffer greatly from the unexpected separation from their own newborn (Montirosso, Provenzi, Calciolari, Borgatti, & NEO-ACQUA Study Group, 2012b), bearing a long-lasting and ambivalent emotional burden even after NICU discharge (Miles, Holditch-Davis, Schwartz, & Scher, 2007). Prolonged physical separations between the mother and her preterm infant is known to contribute to heightened maternal states of stress, anxiety, and depression (Montirosso et al., 2014). Moreover, during the NICU stay, these parents see their own infant handled by nurses, but usually they are prevented to touch the infant during the first period of the hospitalization, which might further contribute to alter the normal transition to parenthood (Provenzi & Santoro, 2015).

The Light Side of the NICU. Caregiver Engagement as Neuro-Protective DC Practice

As mentioned, DC practices include a broad category of interventions designed to minimize the effects of NICU stress exposure (Als et al., 2004). However, for the aims of the present chapter, we will focus on DC practices involving caregiver engagement as a mean to enhance NICU quality of care and to promote infants' outcomes and parental well-being. Based on recent literature (Altimier et al., 2015), caregiver engagement interventions in the NICU might be considered as multi-sensorial neuroprotective practices encompassing staff partnering with families, nutrition optimizing, facilitation of infants' positioning and handling, sleep and skin safeguard, and pain-related stress minimization.

A critical point is that the utilization of DC practices is not yet uniformly applied in NICUs (Ashbaugh, Leick-Rude, & Kilbride, 1999; Greisen et al., 2009). Interestingly, in a large multi-center investigation among 25 Italian NICUs, it has been documented that preterm infants from units with high quality of DC exhibited a better neuro-behavioral profile at the discharge (Montirosso et al., 2012a). The differences in the level of DC quality among different units is surprising in the light of recent evidence on the role of caregiver engagement. While infrequent maternal visits are a risk factor for later psychological development in preterm infants (Latva, Lehtonen, Salmelin, & Tamminen, 2007), a recent investigation has reported that the adoption of single-family room care was associated with improved neurobehavioral and medical outcomes in preterm infants (Lester et al., 2014). Specifically, a large group of very preterm infants was admitted to an open-bay NICU, whereas a counterpart group was admitted in a single-room facility. At the discharge, these latter infants had greater rate of weight gain, required a minor amount of medical procedures, reached full enteral feeding earlier, reported better attention and neurobehavioral indexes compared to infants cared for in the open-bay NICU. Taken together, these findings suggest that caregiver engagement is a critical and essential feature of NICU healthcare journey.

The main adopted caregiver engagement practices include facilitated visiting of parents in the NICU (Latva et al., 2007), skin-to-skin holding and kangaroo care (Feldman, Eidelman, Sirota, & Weller, 2002), and inclusion in pain management (Pillai Ridell et al., 2011). Skin-to-skin holding through kangaroo care consists in a prompt for precocious physical and emotional closeness, allowing the infant being prone and positioned upright on maternal chest. The preterm infant is kept diapered, but unclothed, and the contact of a kangaroo mother is simulated. Kangaroo care has shown to exert beneficial effects for the infants, including the promotion of physiologic stability (Cong, Ludington-Hoe, & Walsh, 2011), sleep organization (Calciolari & Montirosso, 2011), brain maturation (Scher et al., 2009), behavioral and emotional development (Keren, Feldman, Eidelman, Sirota, & Lester, 2003). Brain-imaging research has documented that kangaroo care improves cerebral blood flow in preterm infants during NICU stay (Korraa, El Nagger, Mohamed, & Helmy, 2014) and promotes the maturation of the infant brain (Scher et al., 2009). At the physiological level, preterm infants exposed to continuous skin-to-skin contact after birth have lower salivary cortisol reactivity to physical stimulation at one month (Mörelius, Örtenstrand, Theodorsson, & Frostell, 2015). At long-term, the adoption of caregiver engagement through DC intervention was found to be associated with minor psychomotor delay at 2 years of age, compared to the outcomes of infants provided with conventional care (Kiechl-Kohlendorfer et al., 2015).

As mentioned, caregiver engagement exerts beneficial effects for parents, too. DC practices are useful to reduce infants' painful experience, since they mitigate the stress and depressive symptomatology of the preterm mothers. Moreover, interventions addressed to promote parents' understanding of their infant's behavior were effective in reducing stress-role alteration in preterm mothers (Matricardi, Agostino, Fedeli, & Montirosso, 2013). Engaging parents in early physical contact and providing support to breastfeeding has been described by NICU mothers as the "step toward normality", fostering the parenthood transition and facilitating the establishment of an intimate bonding (Flacking, Ewald, Nyqvist, & Starrin, 2006). Furthermore, NICU mothers have reported that starting kangaroo care as soon as possible was critical in helping them to feel connected to their infants and developing a sense of self-efficacy and confidence in their own caregiving role. Importantly, despite they might more likely report fears of causing harm to the infant by manipulating and holding him, even fathers might ask to be facilitated in the early physical contact with their infant in order to sustain them in the transition to fatherhood (Provenzi & Santoro, 2015).

As such, despite the preterm birth appears to set a risk for the developing of an intimate bonding between the new mother and her newborn, DC practices involving caregiver engagement in NICU might exert beneficial effects for the developmental trajectory of preterm infants. The biological, neurological, behavioral and relational benefits provided by the active engagement of parents might contrast the detrimental effects of NICU-related stressors (Bader, 2015). From this point of view, NICU caregiver engagement emerges as a way to keep up with neuro-protective interventions for the brief- and long-term programming of preterm infants' health and wellbeing. Nonetheless, we still do not know the biological pathways through which these neuro-protective effects are provided. In the following sections, preliminary responses to this issue will be provided through recent advances in the field of behavioral epigenetics.

EPIGENETICS: HOW DO EARLY ADVERSE AND PROTECTIVE EXPERIENCES GET UNDER THE SKIN?

What is Epigenetics?

Behavioral epigenetics is a rapidly growing and innovative area of research, which is changing our view of the nature-nurture interrelations (Hyman, 2009). Epigenetics (from the ancient Greek epi, meaning above the genome) refers primarily to the fact that our genome is not a fixed structure. Whereas genetics has historically regarded genome changes as structural alterations (e.g., polymorphisms and mutations), epigenetic changes do not alter the structure of the DNA sequence. Specifically, epigenetics refers to processes capable of altering the accessibility of a coding portion of a given gene to the molecular transcriptional agents, resulting in the alteration of gene expression (Champagne & Curley, 2009). Changes at the level of genes expression result in altered availability of proteins that are necessary for the adequate development of young individuals (Meaney & Szyf, 2005). Authors use the term behavioral epigenetics to refer to the study of processes through which organisms modulate the fixed genome, altering protein production and resulting in different phenotypes. In other words, what is fascinating in behavioral epi-

Figure 1. DNA methylation process at the promoter region of an encoding gene. A: the transcriptional factor (T) is bound to the CpG-rich site within the promoter region of the gene. The transcriptional factor activates the process of gene expression. B: a methyl group (M) is bound to the CpG rich site within the promoter region of the gene. The methyl group inhibits transcriptional activity, resulting in gene silencing

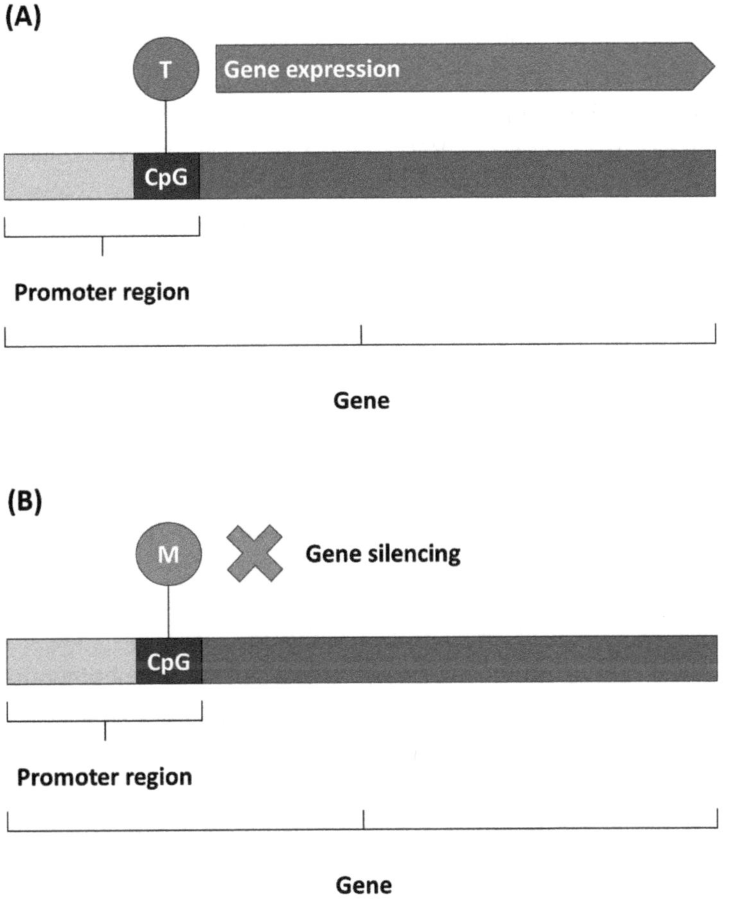

genetics is the fact that the genome dynamically interacts with environmental stimulations "learning" from experience (Hyman, 2009).

The epigenetic processes encompass DNA methylation, histone modification and small non-coding RNA molecules. Nonetheless, DNA methylation is the most investigated epigenetic mechanism in humans (Hyman, 2009). DNA methylation consists in the binding of a methyl group to a cytosine rich site (i.e., Cytosine-phosphate-Guanine, CpG dinucleotides) within a coding part of a given gene. This process results in the inhibition of the transcriptional activity of the gene, which is also known as "gene silencing" (see Figure 1).

DNA Methylation and Neuroplasticity

DNA methylation is a context-dependent process, which remains at least partially stable across the life span, contributing to the shaping of individual's phenotype and later-in-life health and disease. Moreover,

DNA methylation is greatly susceptible to environmental cues, both in the form of adverse (Griffiths & Hunter, 2014) and caregiving (Weaver et al., 2004) stimulations. Thus it is not surprising that the role of epigenetics during the early post-natal period of life is of great concern, above all during the first months of life which are considered a sensitive period for the development of the central nervous system and neuroendocrine systems of stress regulation (i.e., *neuroplasticity*) (Fagiolini, Jensen, & Champagne, 2009).

Two biological systems are of main concern about sensitive periods of brain neuroplasticity: the HPA axis and the serotoninergic system. On the one hand, the HPA axis is the key biological system for stress reactivity and regulation. During stressful events, the HPA axis initiate an hormonal cascade reaction involving hypothalamic release of CRH, pituitary synthesis of ATCH, and which finally ends in the release of corticosteroid (cortisol in human). Several mechanisms have evolved to control HPA axis activation and integrate the stress response. Specifically, if stressful conditions are prolonged in time, feedback mechanisms are needed to regulate cortisol secretion and to maintain homeostasis. Glucocorticoids binding to glucocorticoid receptors (GRs) in the hippocampus results in a negative feedback to the HPA axis. Consequently, under conditions of stress, sustained activation of the HPA axis is attenuated by negative feedback actions of circulating glucocorticoids. The hippocampus has a high density of GRs, which are a key factor the modulation of the stress response: while a high density of hippocampal GRs is associated with low stress reactivity, a low GRs density is associated with high stress reactivity. A critical point is that individuals exposed to stress during early development have reduced expression of GRs in the hippocampus. Indeed, a lower hippocampal density of GRs has been associated with stress dysregulation later in life (Witzmann, Turner, Meriaux, Meijer, & Muller, 2012) and a chronic and reiterated exposure to abnormally high levels of cortisol might be toxic for the developing brain, leading to higher risk of disease in adult life (Karatsoreos & McEwen, 2013).

On the other hand, the serotoninergic system is critical for the development of the HPA axis and contributes to the modulation of its functioning (Andrews & Matthews, 2004). Serotonin is a neurotransmitter widely distributed in the central nervous system. Serotonin is released in response to stressful events and the serotoninergic system is regulated thanks to the action of serotonin transporter proteins (5-HTT). The 5-HTT removes the serotonin from the synaptic cleft and relocate it in the pre-synaptic buttons, resulting in the serotonin turnover (Mueller, Brocke, Fries, Lesch, & Kirschbaum, 2010). Therefore, any variation of serotonin transporter may lead to dysregulation of the serotonin system and might contribute to altered HPA stress reactivity and emotional disorders. Importantly, the GRs expression is also mediated by activation of serotoninergic system. In animal model, serotonin regulates hippocampal GRs expression and increased serotonin levels in response to tactile stimulation, such as handling or maternal licking/grooming, increases the expression of transcription factors that regulate activation of the GRs (Laplante, Diorio, & Meaney, 2002). In humans, an alteration of the serotonin turnover has been linked to affective disorders (Schinka, Busch, & Robichaux-Keene, 2004).

The Dark Side of Epigenetics. DNA Methylation and Early Adverse Experiences

The first evidence of DNA methylation changes in relation to adverse environmental conditions emerged during the late nineties (Champagne & Curley, 2009). The classical experiments by Meaney and colleagues (Francis, Diorio, Liu, & Meaney, 1999) examined the effects of variations in the caregiving environment on GRs density in the offspring. Rat pups with mothers providing low quality of caregiving – e.g., less engaged in receptive nursing and in linking/grooming the offspring – were found to have lower levels of GRs in the hippocampus and elevated stress reactivity during adulthood. These effects were due to epigenetic processes, namely DNA methylation and decrease histone acetylation, at the level of the gene encoding for cortisol receptors in the rat hippocampus (Weaver et al., 2004). Similar findings were documented through maternal separation in rodents. Male offspring exposed to early maternal separation exhibited behavioral inhibition in maze exploration, mediated by DNA hyper-methylation of the gene encoding for the corticotropin-releasing hormone, which is key regulator of the stress response (Kember et al., 2012). Moreover, in mice, maternal separation was found to be associated with epigenetic alteration of the expression of the gene encoding for serotonin transporter, namely the SLC6A4 (Own, Iqbal, & Patel, 2013). Epigenetic alterations of the SLC6A4 lead to an altered re-uptake of serotonin in the brain, resulting in detrimental effects for emotional well-being and risk of affective disorders later in life in animals and in humans (Lesch, 2011).

Human studies documented similar epigenetic alterations in young individuals exposed to stressful adverse experiences during the prenatal and the postnatal life (Griffiths & Hunter, 2014). Importantly, both the HPA axis functioning and serotoninergic system have shown to be susceptible to epigenetic regulation. Prenatal exposure to maternal depression during the third trimester of pregnancy has been associated in full-term newborns with the methylation status of a specific CpG site of the *NR3C1* gene, which encodes for the hippocampal GRs (Oberlander et al., 2008). Interestingly, in the same study, the altered methylation of *NR3C1* gene was predictive of increased salivary cortisol response to a standardize laboratory stressful procedure at 3-month-age. More recently, exposure to parental stress during infancy and childhood was found to associate with global methylation in adolescents (Essex et al., 2013). As for postnatal adverse exposure, the genome-wide methylation status of 5-to-14-aged children with a previous history of parental abuse or neglect has been compared with that of a counterpart of children without exposure to family violence (Vijayendran, Beach, Plume, Brody, & Philibert, 2012). Maltreated and neglected children showed lower methylation for CpG sites that were highly methylated in control group, and higher methylation for CpG sites that were low-methylated in control group. In another study, adults with a post-traumatic stress disorders following exposure to early traumatic experiences were compared to adults without post-traumatic stress disorders, but without previous adverse experiences in childhood (Mehta et al., 2013). Individuals with a history of abuse showed non-overlapping areas of genome-wide methylation, when compared to individuals with similar history of abuse, but without anxiety disorder. On the other hand, the methylation status of the *SLC6A4* gene, which encodes for the 5-HTT (i.e., serotonin transporter), is affected by maternal depression during pregnancy (Devlin, Brain, Austin, & Oberlander, 2010) and by post-natal adversities (Wang et al., 2012).

The Light Side of Epigenetics: Reversible DNA Methylation

Animal studies have shown that, despite being stable across the life span, DNA methylation is susceptible to further environmental conditions and it might be further affected by positive experiences and environmental manipulations. Interestingly, when rats born from mothers characterized by low quality of caregiving are cross-fostered (i.e., adopted) by mothers characterized by high quality of care they show levels of methylation of the *NR3C1* gene which are similar to those of rats born and raised by high-quality of care mothers (Meaney & Szyf, 2005). Similarly, positive experiences for rats, such as being sensitively touched during the early post-natal period, has been shown to decreased the production of corticosteroid (the analogous of human stress-hormone cortisol) during the first day of life (Jutapakdeegul, Casalotti, Govitrapong, & Kotchabhakdi, 2003). Moreover, this change was associated with an increased expression of the gene encoding for the hippocampal GRs.

In humans, the epigenetic study of the effects of caring experiences, rather than stressful ones, is sparse. Nonetheless, recent research is suggesting that it might be possible to inquire for an epigenetic underpinning of positive experiences in human beings (Roberts et al., 2014). These authors have measured the level of methylation of the *SLC6A4* gene encoding for serotonin transporter in 116 children with anxiety disorder, before and after a cognitive-behavioral psychotherapy intervention. As before mentioned that *SLC6A4* is highly associated with the risk of developing emotional disorders, such as anxiety and depression (Lesch, 2011). Roberts and colleagues (2014) highlighted differential changes (increase or decrease) of *SLC6A4* methylation in children reporting improvements after a psychotherapeutic treatment, confronted with peers showing no improvement. Taken together, animal and human studies suggest that DNA methylation of specific genes correlated to the stress regulation might be affected by positive post-natal changes in the caring environment and through specific interventions.

PRETERM BEHAVIORAL EPIGENETICS

A Groundbreaking and Promising Research Field

In the light of evidence reported above, one might wonder how altered patterns of DNA methylation are involved in preterm infants' development. As they are born too soon, preterm infants are much more vulnerable to environmental insults, but also they might have great potential benefits if exposed to appropriate support, so that both NICU-related stress and DC practices involving caregiver engagement might exert relevant influence on their phenotype (Maddalena, 2013). Preterm Behavioral Epigenetics (PBE; Montirosso & Provenzi, 2015) is an innovative field applying behavioral epigenetic research to the study of prematurity and the effects of NICU stay, both through adverse experiences and DC caregiver engagement practices (see Figure 2). To date, the newborn research area of PBE has mainly focused on

Figure 2. A prospective model to inform the application of behavioral epigenetics to the field of preterm birth and NICU stay, including both the "dark" and the "light" side of preterm behavioral epigenetics

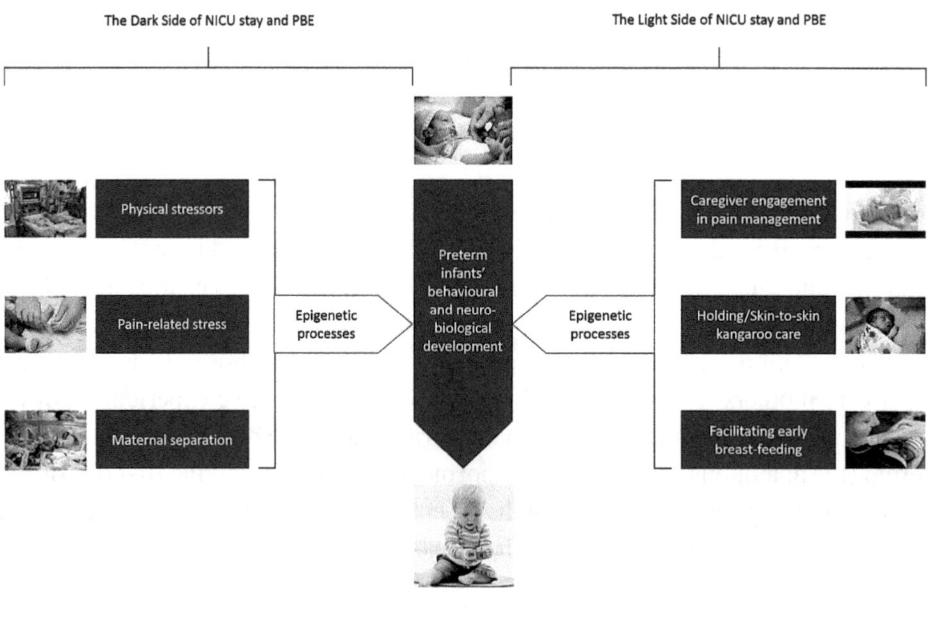

the "dark side" of the NICU environment, highlighting methylation correlates of NICU-related stressors (Chau et al., 2014; Provenzi et al., 2015). Nonetheless, it is also intriguing to hypothesize that epigenetic studies would increase our knowledge of the biological correlates of beneficial effects of DC practices and caregiver engagement in the NICU (Provenzi & Barello, 2015).

In the present section, the emerging available literature on the "dark side" of PBE is reviewed first, highlighting the epigenetic changes associated with NICU-related stress exposure in infants and children born preterm. Furthermore, the potential benefits of the application of PBE to the study of the neuroprotective effects of caregiver engagement in NICU will be discussed, providing insights for specific issues to be addressed through future investigations in the "light side" of PBE.

THE DARK SIDE OF PBE: UPCOMING RESEARCH FINDINGS

Recently, the methylation status of the *NR3C1* was measured in preterm and full-term newborns at birth and four days after birth (Kantake et al., 2014). The study showed that the methylation level of several CpG sites of the *NR3C1* gene increased from day 0 to day 4 in preterm infants, whereas it remained stable in full-term counterpart. Regression analyses revealed that the methylation rates at day 4 were predicted by gestational age, Apgar score, being small for gestational age, and NICU admission. Moreover, the heightened methylation rates were predictive of later complication during the neonatal period, such as chronic lung disease or cardiovascular instability.

To date, two studies have investigated the role of a specific NICU-related adverse condition, i.e., the exposure to painful skin-breaking procedures, in affecting the methylation status of the *SLC6A4* gene. When compared to full-term infants and to the preterm infants exposed to low levels of pain, preterm infants exposed to high levels of painful skin-breaking interventions during the NICU stay had higher DNA methylation at two specific CpG sites of the 5-HTT gene (Provenzi et al., 2015). Consistently, pain-related increase in DNA methylation of *SLC6A4* was found in 7-year-old preterm children (Chau et al., 2014). Importantly, the altered methylation profile of several CpG sites of the *SLC6A4* gene was also associated with behavior problems evaluated through self-report at 7-year-age (Chau et al., 2014). In another study, the methylation level of 20 CpG sites of the stress-related gene *SLC6A4* was measured in preterm infants at birth and at NICU discharge, and in full-term infants at birth (Montirosso et al., 2016). The study revealed no difference at birth in the methylation status of the *SLC6A4*. Notwithstanding, at NICU discharge, the methylation level of two specific CpG sites (CpG5 and CpG7) was higher in preterm infants compared to full-term and preterm infants' at birth. Furthermore, the methylation of CpG5 at discharge was found to be predictive of preterm infants' altered temperament at 3-month-age.

Taken together, these findings suggest that the early exposure to an unfamiliar environment characterized by high-intensive stressful stimulations might be considered as a risk factor for stable epigenetic alterations of specific genes associated with stress regulation. On the one side, altered methylation of the *NR3C1* might lead to a sub-optimal availability of hippocampal GRs, which further leads to a dysregulation of the HPA axis and to difficulties in stress regulation later in life (Laplante et al., 2002). On the other side, a reduced synthesis of 5-HTT by the *SLC6A4* might leaded to a deficiency in serotoninergic turnover (i.e., reduced 5-HT levels), which in turn may increase a susceptibility for lifetime risk for emotional disorders, reflecting a "serotonergic vulnerability" (Philibert et al., 2008).

THE LIGHT SIDE OF PBE: FUTURE RESEARCH DIRECTIONS

The application of PBE to the study of the biological underpinnings of caregiver engagement might provide NICU specialists with renewed insights about the pathways of neuro-protective effects of DC. Epigenetic changes may offer an array of targets that can be used for prevention and for treatment interventions. Three potential areas of investigation are provided to inform and guide the application of PBE research to the study of the epigenetic correlates of caregiver engagement in the NICU: measuring the neuro-protective effects of caregiver engagement; developing epigenetic markers for NICU quality of DC; monitoring short- and long-term outcomes of caregiver engagement.

These areas encompass different aspects of early intervention and prevention for the prematurely born infant (Altimier et al., 2015) and they are thought to unveil the light side of PBE, bringing new insights to developmental and psychobiology researchers as well as NICU clinicians (Samra et al., 2012).

Measuring the Neuro-Protective Effects of Caregiver Engagement

As mentioned before, caregiver engagement has been thought as a neuro-protective DC intervention for preterm infants being hospitalized in the NICU. Specific modalities of caregiver engagement, e.g., holding, kangaroo care, parental involvement in pain management have shown to exert long-term beneficial effects for preterm infants' development. The light side of PBE might be regarded as conveying a biologically grounded evidence-based proxy for better neonatal practices for the prematurely born infant. Animal studies have underlined that early stress-dependent methylation might be reversed through high-quality care interventions (Meaney & Szyf, 2005). These findings raise the intriguing possibility that NICU quality of care practices might be effective in reducing exposure of preterm infants to stress via epigenetic protective mechanisms

From this point of view, three objectives appear to be of interest. First, the epigenetic correlates of the different activities and practices of caregiver engagement should be investigated. As shown by Montirosso and colleagues (2012a), different features of DC associate with diverse behavioral outcomes for the preterm infant. As such, one might expect that not all the modalities of caregiver engagement exert similar, if any, epigenetic effect on the developing biology of prematurely born infants. Second, the PBE research should investigate which genes are better candidates for bearing the epigenetic marker of caregiver engagement. Epigenetic changes at different stress-related genes result in alterations of diverse physiologic systems of stress response. Early life changes in the HPA axis functioning or the serotoninergic system have different implications for socio-emotional development and for health conditions later in life. Finally, the most important point for NICU nurses and physicians regards the possibility that the epigenetic correlates of specific caregiver engagement strategies targets in a reversal way the same genes affected by NICU-related stressors.

Developing Epigenetic Markers for NICU Quality of DC Practices

The presence of wide variations in the types and amounts of caregiver engagement strategies might result in very different outcomes of preterm infants with similar characteristics at birth. For this reason, during recent years NICU research has moved toward identifying the effects of NICU quality of DC in a broader sense, identifying core features and their specific consequences on the neuro-behavioral development of infants. From this point of view, the application of epigenetic research to the light side of

NICU might provide innovative and objective markers to assess the quality of care provided in different facilities within and between diverse countries. For example, tools developed to inquire the presence and the amount of different features of DC, e.g., caregiver engagement, pain management, clustering of nursing activities etc., might be integrated by an investigation of the genome-wide or gene-specific methylation status at birth and at NICU discharge, in different populations of preterm infants.

Monitoring Short- and Long-Term Outcomes of Caregiver Engagement

Notably, stability of methylation is not given for granted and there is still need of longitudinal studies, especially in humans. Future studies are warranted to address the epigenetic correlates of neuro-protective DC practices at different time points across preterm infants, children and adults development.

On the one side, short-term outcomes would be relevant to understand the immediate impact of caregiver engagement interventions on the developmental biology of preterm infants. This would be of great importance to improve our knowledge of the more suitable time window to promote physical contact, massage, and skin-to-skin holding in a biologically sustainable and effective way for the infant.

On the other side, long-term neuro-protective effects of NICU DC practices need to be addressed with longitudinal studies. This research will be of great value to build a grounded and time-scaled meter of the biological and neuro-protective effects of caregiver engagement interventions in a life-span healthcare perspective. For example, coming to know if HPA axis or serotonergic system improvements associated with early DC interventions are stable or not during the lifetime of a preterm individual, has important implications for the programming of adult health and well-being from the beginning of life.

CONCLUSION

Focusing on Caregiver Engagement: The "Epigen-Ethic" Way of PBE

During the recent years, epigenetics is starting to reveal how early adversities are embedded into development and contribute to the programming of long-lasting health and disease. Nonetheless, animal studies suggest that epigenetics should also be applied to the "light side" of early life events (Meaney & Szyf, 2005). In humans, the application of epigenetics to the study of preterm birth and early NICU stay is still at its beginning (Montirosso & Provenzi, 2015). Upcoming research findings are revealing the methylation correlates of the "dark side" of NICU, such as the exposure to painful skin-breaking procedures, and their short- and long-term consequences for infants and children development. Nonetheless, to date there is a lack of studies investigating the epigenetic vestiges of caregiver engagement, which constitutes the light side of NICU stay and has been found to convey neuro-protective effects for the long-lasting development of preterm infants.

Applying behavioral epigenetic research to the field of prematurity and NICU stay would be a primer to take into our mind that human developmental trajectories are more complex than specific biological or environmental mechanisms and processes. In fact, even when efforts are made to improve caregiving with DC interventions, the incidence of poor neuro-behavioral outcomes cannot be ruled out. This might be at least partially related to the complex interactions among biological and environmental risks and caregiving factors, as well as to the timing and type of early interventions. An ambitious PBE program should encompass a double-track attention to both the NICU-related stressors and the neuro-protective effects of caregiver engagement. Integrating the dark and the light side of PBE research is warranted to deliver evidence-based findings, which might be useful for clinicians, keeping up with better outcomes conveyed by caregiver engagement and holding the promise of providing innovative insights and markers for better health-care practices in the NICU for preterm infants and their families.

Thus, although PBE research is fascinating and intriguing, careful should be taken when translating research findings into practice (Provenzi & Montirosso, 2015). Behavioral epigenetics holds the risk of a new form of reductionism grounded in a unilateral and deterministic interpretation of human epigenetic studies. On the one side, behavioral epigenetics underline the importance of caregiving environment for the developing biology of young individuals. Nonetheless, careless assumptions of epigenetic findings could result in blaming parents for their caregiving behavior, leaving out the importance of other factors, such a genetically settled risk and other environmental conditions (Richardson et al., 2014). From this point of view, PBE research focused on the multiple sources of care provided by DC practices might be considered as a way to stimulate a complex perspective on early caregiving environment, acknowledging that multiple sources of risk and protection surround human infants, especially at-risk preterm infants.

REFERENCES

Als, H., Duffy, F. H., McAnulty, G. B., Rivkin, M. J., Vajapeyam, S., Mulkern, R. V., & Eichenwald, E. C. et al. (2004). Early Experience Alters Brain Function and Structure. *Pediatrics*, *113*(4), 846–857. doi:10.1542/peds.113.4.846 PMID:15060237

Altimier, L., Kenner, C., & Damus, K. (2015). The Wee Care Neuroprotective NICU Program (Wee Care): The Effect of a Comprehensive Developmental Care Training Program on Seven Neuroprotective Core Measures for Family-Centered Developmental Care of Premature Neonates. *Newborn and Infant Nursing Reviews; NAINR*, *15*(1), 6–16. doi:10.1053/j.nainr.2015.01.006

Altuncu, E., Akman, I., Kulekci, S., Akdas, F., Bilgen, H., & Ozek, E. (2009). Noise levels in neonatal intensive care unit and use of sound absorbing panel in the isolette. *International Journal of Pediatric Otorhinolaryngology*, *73*(7), 951–953. doi:10.1016/j.ijporl.2009.03.013 PMID:19406484

Andrews, M. H., & Matthews, S. G. (2004). Programming of the hypothalamo-pituitary-adrenal axis: Serotonergic involvement. *Stress (Amsterdam, Netherlands)*, *7*(1), 15–27. doi:10.1080/10253890310001650277 PMID:15204029

Ashbaugh, J. B., Leick-Rude, M. K., & Kilbride, H. W. (1999). Developmental care teams in the neonatal intensive care unit: Survey on current status. *Journal of Perinatology*, *19*(1), 48–52. doi:10.1038/sj.jp.7200101 PMID:10685202

Bader, L. (2015). Brain-oriented care in the NICU: A case study. *Neonatal Network*, *33*(5), 263–267. doi:10.1891/0730-0832.33.5.263 PMID:25161134

Bock, J., Rether, K., Gröger, N., Xie, L., & Braun, K. (2014). Perinatal programming of emotional brain circuits: An integrative view from systems to molecules. *Frontiers in Neuroscience*, *8*(8), 1–16. PMID:24550772

Brown, G. (2009). NICU noise and the preterm infant. *Neonatal Network*, *28*(3), 165–173. doi:10.1891/0730-0832.28.3.165 PMID:19451078

Brummelte, S., Grunau, R. E., Zaidman-Zait, A., Weinberg, J., Nordstokke, D., & Cepeda, I. L. (2011). Cortisol levels in relation to maternal interaction and child internalizing behavior in preterm and full-term children at 18 months corrected age. *Developmental Psychobiology*, *53*(2), 184–195. doi:10.1002/dev.20511 PMID:21298633

Calciolari, G., & Montirosso, R. (2011). The sleep protection in the preterm infants. *The Journal of Maternal-Fetal & Neonatal Medicine*, *24*(Suppl. 1), 12–14. doi:10.3109/14767058.2011.607563 PMID:21942583

Champagne, F. A., & Curley, J. P. (2009). Epigenetic mechanisms mediating the long-term effects of maternal care on development. *Neuroscience and Biobehavioral Reviews*, *33*(4), 593–600. doi:10.1016/j.neubiorev.2007.10.009 PMID:18430469

Chau, C. M. Y., Ranger, M., Sulistyoningrum, D., Devlin, A. M., Oberlander, T. F., & Grunau, R. E. (2014). Neonatal pain and COMT Val158Met genotype in relation to serotonin transporter (SLC6A4) promoter methylation in very preterm children at school age. *Frontiers in Behavioral Neuroscience*, *8*, 1–12. doi:10.3389/fnbeh.2014.00409 PMID:25520635

Cong, X., Ludington-Hoe, S. M., & Walsh, S. (2011). Randomized crossover trial of kangaroo care to reduce biobehavioral pain responses in preterm infants: A pilot study. *Biological Research for Nursing*, *13*(2), 204–216. doi:10.1177/1099800410385839 PMID:21196428

Devlin, A. M., Brain, U., Austin, J., & Oberlander, T. F. (2010). Prenatal exposure to maternal depressed mood and the MTHFR C677T variant affect SLC6A4 methylation in infants at birth. *PLoS ONE*, *5*(8), e12201. doi:10.1371/journal.pone.0012201 PMID:20808944

Essex, M. J., Boyce, W. T., Hertzman, C., Lam, L. L., Armstrong, J. M., Neumann, S. M., & Kobor, M. S. (2013). Epigenetic vestiges of early developmental adversity: Childhood stress exposure and DNA methylation in adolescence. *Child Development*, *84*(1), 58–75. doi:10.1111/j.1467-8624.2011.01641.x PMID:21883162

Fagiolini, M., Jensen, C. L., & Champagne, F. A. (2009). Epigenetic influences on brain development and plasticity. *Current Opinion in Neurobiology*, *19*(2), 207–212. doi:10.1016/j.conb.2009.05.009 PMID:19545993

Feldman, R., Eidelman, A. I., Sirota, L., & Weller, A. (2002). Comparison of skin-to-skin (kangaroo) and traditional care: Parenting outcomes and preterm infant development. *Pediatrics*, *110*(1), 16–26. doi:10.1542/peds.110.1.16 PMID:12093942

Field, D., Draper, E. S., Fenton, A., Papiernik, E., Zeitlin, J., Blondel, B., & Van Reempts, P. et al. (2009). Rates of very preterm birth in Europe and neonatal mortality rates. *Archives of Disease in Childhood. Fetal and Neonatal Edition*, *94*(4), F253–F256. doi:10.1136/adc.2008.150433 PMID:19066186

Flacking, R., Ewald, U., Nyqvist, K. H., & Starrin, B. (2006). Trustful bonds: A key to "becoming a mother" and to reciprocal breastfeeding. Stories of mothers of very preterm infants at a neonatal unit. *Social Science & Medicine*, *62*(1), 70–80http://www.scopus.com/inward/record.url?eid=2-s2.0-28444467433&partnerID=40&md5=3132a5f7c93c56a187af23f82e6cc43c. doi:10.1016/j.socscimed.2005.05.026 PMID:15992983

Francis, D., Diorio, J., Liu, D., & Meaney, M. J. (1999). Nongenomic transmission across generations of maternal behavior and stress responses in the rat. *Science*, *286*(5442), 1155–1158. doi:10.1126/science.286.5442.1155 PMID:10550053

Graven, S. N. (2004). Early neurosensory visual development of the fetus and newborn. *Clinics in Perinatology*, *31*(2), 199–216. doi:10.1016/j.clp.2004.04.010 PMID:15289028

Greisen, G., Mirante, N., Haumont, D., Pierrat, V., Pallás-Alonso, C. R., & Warren, I. et al. (2009). Parents, siblings and grandparents in the Neonatal Intensive Care Unit A survey of policies in eight European countries. *Acta Paediatrica*: *International Journal of Pediatrics*, *98*(11), 1744–1750.

Griffiths, B. B., & Hunter, R. G. (2014). Neuroepigenetics of stress. *Neuroscience*, *275*, 420–435. doi:10.1016/j.neuroscience.2014.06.041 PMID:24976514

Grunau, R. E. (2013). Neonatal pain in very preterm infants: Long-term effects on brain, neurodevelopment and pain reactivity. *Rambam Maimonides Medical Journal*, *4*(4), e0025. PMID:24228168

Grunau, R. E., Holsti, L., Haley, D. W., Oberlander, T., Weinberg, J., Solimano, A., & Yu, W. et al. (2005). Neonatal procedural pain exposure predicts lower cortisol and behavioral reactivity in preterm infants in the NICU. *Pain*, *113*(3), 293–300. doi:10.1016/j.pain.2004.10.020 PMID:15661436

Grunau, R. E., Whitfield, M. F., Petrie-Thomas, J., Synnes, A. R., Cepeda, I. L., Keidar, A., & Johannesen, D. et al. (2009). Neonatal pain, parenting stress and interaction, in relation to cognitive and motor development at 8 and 18 months in preterm infants. *Pain*, *143*(1-2), 138–146. doi:10.1016/j.pain.2009.02.014 PMID:19307058

Haley, D. W., Weinberg, J., & Grunau, R. E. (2006). Cortisol, contingency learning, and memory in preterm and full-term infants. *Psychoneuroendocrinology*, *31*(1), 108–117. doi:10.1016/j.psyneuen.2005.06.007 PMID:16122876

Hyman, S. E. (2009). How adversity gets under the skin. *Nature Neuroscience*, *12*(3), 241–243. doi:10.1038/nn0309-241 PMID:19238182

Jansen, J., Beijers, R., Riksen-Walraven, M., & de Weerth, C. (2010). Cortisol reactivity in young infants. *Psychoneuroendocrinology*, *35*(3), 329–338. doi:10.1016/j.psyneuen.2009.07.008 PMID:19651476

Jutapakdeegul, N., Casalotti, S. O., Govitrapong, P., & Kotchabhakdi, N. (2003). Postnatal touch stimulation acutely alters corticosterone levels and glucocorticoid receptor gene expression in the neonatal rat. *Developmental Neuroscience*, *25*(1), 26–33. doi:10.1159/000071465 PMID:12876428

Kantake, M., Yoshitake, H., Ishikawa, H., Araki, Y., & Shimizu, T. (2014). Postnatal epigenetic modification of glucocorticoid receptor gene in preterm infants: A prospective cohort study. *BMJ Open*, *4*(7), e005318. doi:10.1136/bmjopen-2014-005318 PMID:25023132

Karatsoreos, I. N., & McEwen, B. S. (2013). Resilience and vulnerability: A neurobiological perspective. *F1000prime Reports*, *5*, 13. PMID:23710327

Kember, R. L., Dempster, E. L., Lee, T. H., Schalkwyk, L. C., Mill, J., & Fernandes, C. (2012). Maternal separation is associated with strain-specific responses to stress and epigenetic alterations to Nr3c1, Avp, and Nr4a1 in mouse. *Brain and Behavior*, *2*(4), 455–467. doi:10.1002/brb3.69 PMID:22950049

Keren, M., Feldman, R., Eidelman, A. I., Sirota, L., & Lester, B. (2003). Clinical interview for high-risk parents of premature infants (CLIP) as a predictor of early disruptions in the mother-infant relationship at the nursery. *Infant Mental Health Journal*, *24*(2), 93–110. doi:10.1002/imhj.10049

Kiechl-Kohlendorfer, U., Merkle, U., Deufert, D., Neubauer, V., Peglow, U. P., & Griesmaier, E. (2015). Effect of developmental care for very premature infants on neurodevelopmental outcome at 2 years of age. *Infant Behavior and Development*, *39*, 166–172. doi:10.1016/j.infbeh.2015.02.006 PMID:25867251

Korraa, A. A., El Nagger, A. A., Mohamed, R. A. E. S., & Helmy, N. M. (2014). Impact of kangaroo mother care on cerebral blood flow of preterm infants. *Italian Journal of Pediatrics*, *40*(1), 1–6. doi:10.1186/s13052-014-0083-5 PMID:25391600

Laplante, P., Diorio, J., & Meaney, M. J. (2002). Serotonin regulates hippocampal glucocorticoid receptor expression via a 5-HT7 receptor. *Brain Research. Developmental Brain Research*, *139*(2), 199–203. doi:10.1016/S0165-3806(02)00550-3 PMID:12480134

Latva, R., Lehtonen, L., Salmelin, R. K., & Tamminen, T. (2004). Visiting less than every day: A marker for later behavioral problems in Finnish preterm infants. *Archives of Pediatrics & Adolescent Medicine*, *158*(12), 1153–1157. doi:10.1001/archpedi.158.12.1153 PMID:15583100

Latva, R., Lehtonen, L., Salmelin, R. K., & Tamminen, T. (2007). Visits by the family to the neonatal intensive care unit. *Acta Paediatrica (Oslo, Norway)*, *96*(2), 215–220. doi:10.1111/j.1651-2227.2007.00053.x PMID:17429908

Lee, Y.-H., Malakooti, N., & Lotas, M. (2005). A comparison of the light-reduction capacity of commonly used incubator covers. *Neonatal Network*, *24*(2), 37–44. doi:10.1891/0730-0832.24.2.37 PMID:15835478

Lesch, K. P. (2011). When the serotonin transporter gene meets adversity: The contribution of animal models to understanding epigenetic mechanisms in affective disorders and resilience. *Current Topics in Behavioral Neurosciences*, *7*, 251–280. doi:10.1007/7854_2010_109 PMID:21225411

Lester, B. M., Hawes, K., Abar, B., Sullivan, M., Miller, R., Bigsby, R., & Padbury, J. F. et al. (2014). Single-Family Room Care and Neurobehavioral and Medical Outcomes in Preterm Infants. *Pediatrics*, *134*(4), 754–760. doi:10.1542/peds.2013-4252 PMID:25246623

Lester, B. M., Tronick, E., Nestler, E., Abel, T., Kosofsky, B., Kuzawa, C. W., & Wood, M. A. et al. (2011). Behavioral epigenetics. *Annals of the New York Academy of Sciences*, *1226*(1), 14–33. doi:10.1111/j.1749-6632.2011.06037.x PMID:21615751

Maddalena, P. (2013). Long term outcomes of preterm birth: The role of epigenetics. *Newborn and Infant Nursing Reviews; NAINR*, *13*(3), 137–139. doi:10.1053/j.nainr.2013.06.010

Matricardi, S., Agostino, R., Fedeli, C., & Montirosso, R. (2013). Mothers are not fathers: differences between parents in the reduction of stress levels after a parental intervention in a NICU. *Acta Paediatrica, 102*(1), 8–14.

Meaney, M. J., & Szyf, M. (2005). Maternal care as a model for experience-dependent chromatin plasticity? *Trends in Neurosciences*, *28*(9), 456–463. doi:10.1016/j.tins.2005.07.006 PMID:16054244

Mehta, D., Klengel, T., Conneely, K. N., Smith, A. K., Altmann, A., Pace, T. W., & Binder, E. B. et al. (2013). Childhood maltreatment is associated with distinct genomic and epigenetic profiles in posttraumatic stress disorder. *Proceedings of the National Academy of Sciences of the United States of America, 110*(20), 8302–8307. doi:10.1073/pnas.1217750110 PMID:23630272

Miles, M. S., Holditch-Davis, D., Schwartz, T. A., & Scher, M. (2007). Depressive symptoms in mothers of prematurely born infants. *Journal of Developmental and Behavioral Pediatrics, 28*(1), 36–44. doi:10.1097/01.DBP.0000257517.52459.7a PMID:17353730

Montirosso, R., Del Prete, A., Bellu, R., Tronick, E., & Borgatti, R.NEO-ACquA Study Group. (2012a). Level of NICU quality of developmental care and neurobehavioral performance in very preterm infants. *Pediatrics, 129*(5), e1129–e1137. doi:10.1542/peds.2011-0813 PMID:22492762

Montirosso, R., Fedeli, C., Del Prete, A., Calciolari, G., Borgatti, R., & Mosca, F. et al.. (2014). Maternal stress and depressive symptoms associated with quality of developmental care in 25 Italian Neonatal Intensive Care Units: A cross sectional observational study. *International Journal of Nursing Studies, 51*(7), 994–1002. doi:10.1016/j.ijnurstu.2013.11.001 PMID:24315196

Montirosso, R., & Provenzi, L. (2015). Implications of Epigenetics and Stress Regulation on Research and Developmental Care of Preterm Infants. *Journal of Obstetric, Gynecologic, and Neonatal Nursing, 44*(2), 174–182. doi:10.1111/1552-6909.12559 PMID:25712710

Montirosso, R., Provenzi, L., Calciolari, G., & Borgatti, R.NEO-ACQUA Study Group. (2012b). Measuring maternal stress and perceived support in 25 Italian NICUs. *Acta Paediatrica (Oslo, Norway), 101*(2), 136–142. doi:10.1111/j.1651-2227.2011.02440.x PMID:21827551

Montirosso, R., Provenzi, L., Fumagalli, M., Sirgiovanni, I., Giorda, R., & Pozzoli, U. et al. (2016). Serotonin transporter gene (*SLC6A4*) methylation associates with Neonatal Intensive Care Unit stay and 3-month-old temperament in preterm infants. *Child Development*, 87(1), 38-48. doi:10.1111/cdev.12492

Mörelius, E., Nelson, N., & Gustafsson, P. A. (2007). Salivary cortisol response in mother-infant dyads at high psychosocial risk. *Child: Care, Health and Development, 33*(2), 128–136. doi:10.1111/j.1365-2214.2006.00637.x PMID:17291316

Mörelius, E., Örtenstrand, A., Theodorsson, E., & Frostell, A. (2015). A randomised trial of continuous skin-to-skin contact after preterm birth and the effects on salivary cortisol, parental stress, depression, and breastfeeding. *Early Human Development, 91*(1), 63–70. doi:10.1016/j.earlhumdev.2014.12.005 PMID:25545453

Mueller, A., Brocke, B., Fries, E., Lesch, K. P., & Kirschbaum, C. (2010). The role of the serotonin transporter polymorphism for the endocrine stress response in newborns. *Psychoneuroendocrinology, 35*(2), 289–296. doi:10.1016/j.psyneuen.2009.07.002 PMID:19647944

Oberlander, T. F., Weinberg, J., Papsdorf, M., Grunau, R., Misri, S., & Devlin, A. M. (2008). Prenatal exposure to maternal depression, neonatal methylation of human glucocorticoid receptor gene (NR3C1) and infant cortisol stress responses. *Epigenetics: Official Journal of the DNA Methylation Society, 3*(2), 97–106. doi:10.4161/epi.3.2.6034 PMID:18536531

Own, L. S., Iqbal, R., & Patel, P. D. (2013). Maternal separation alters serotonergic and HPA axis gene expression independent of separation duration in c57bl/6 mice. *Brain Research*, *1515*, 29–38. doi:10.1016/j.brainres.2013.03.032 PMID:23548594

Ozawa, M., Sasaki, M., & Kanda, K. (2010). Effect of procedure light on the physiological responses of preterm infants. *Japan Journal of Nursing Science*, *7*(1), 76–83. doi:10.1111/j.1742-7924.2010.00142.x PMID:20618679

Peng, N., Bachman, J., Jenkins, R., Chen, C.-H., Chang, Y.-C., Chang, Y.-S., & Wang, T.-M. (2009). Stressors and Stress Biobehavioral Responses of Preterm Infants in NICU. *The Journal of Perinatal & Neonatal Nursing*, *23*(4), 363–371. doi:10.1097/JPN.0b013e3181bdd3fd PMID:19915421

Philibert, R. A., Sandhu, H., Hollenbeck, N., Gunter, T., Adams, W., & Madan, A. (2008). The relationship of 5HTT (SLC6A4) methylation and genotype on mRNA expression and liability to major depression and alcohol dependence in subjects from the Iowa Adoption Studies. *American Journal of Medical Genetics*, *147B*(5), 543–549. doi:10.1002/ajmg.b.30657 PMID:17987668

Pillai Ridell, R., Racine, N., Turcotte, K., Uman, L. S., Horton, R., & Osmun, L. D. et al.. (2011). Nonpharmacological management of procedural pain in infants and young children. *Pain Research & Management: The Journal of the Canadian Pain Society*, *16*(5), 321–330. doi:10.1155/2011/489286 PMID:22059204

Provenzi, L., & Barello, S. (2015). Behavioral Epigenetics of Family-Centered Care in the Neonatal Intensive Care Unit. *JAMA Pediatrics*, *169*(7), 697–698. doi:10.1001/jamapediatrics.2015.0367 PMID:26147053

Provenzi, L., Barello, S., & Graffigna, G. (2016). Caregiver engagement in the Neonatal Intensive Care Unit: Parental needs, engagement milestones, and action priorities for neonatal health care of preterm infants. In G. Graffigna, S. Barello, S. Triberti (Eds.), Caregiver Engagement in the Neonatal Intensive Care Unit: Parental Needs, Engagement Milestones, and Action Priorities for Neonatal Healthcare of Preterm Infants (pp. 94-107). Berlin, Germany: De Gruyter.

Provenzi, L., Fumagalli, M., Sirgiovanni, I., Giorda, R., Pozzoli, U., Morandi, F., & Montirosso, R. et al. (2015b). Pain-related stress during the Neonatal Intensive Care Unit stay and SLC6A4 methylation in very preterm infants. *Frontiers in Behavioral Neuroscience*, *9*, 1–9. doi:10.3389/fnbeh.2015.00099 PMID:25941480

Provenzi, L., & Montirosso, R. (2015). Epigenethics" in the Neonatal Intensive Care Unit Conveying Complexity in Health Care for Preterm Children. *JAMA Pediatrics*, *169*(7), 617–618. doi:10.1001/jamapediatrics.2015.43 PMID:25938864

Provenzi, L., & Santoro, E. (2015). The lived experience of fathers of preterm infants in the Neonatal Intensive Care Unit: A systematic review of qualitative studies. *Journal of Clinical Nursing*, *24*(13-14), 1784–1794. doi:10.1111/jocn.12828 PMID:25850518

Ranger, M., Synnes, A. R., Vinall, J., & Grunau, R. E. (2014). Internalizing behaviours in school-age children born very preterm are predicted by neonatal pain and morphine exposure. *European Journal of Pain (London, England)*, *18*(6), 844–852. doi:10.1002/j.1532-2149.2013.00431.x PMID:24318537

Richardson, S. S., Daniels, C. R., Gillman, M. W., Golden, J. L., Kukla, R., Kuzawa, C., & Rich-Edwards, J. (2014). Don't blame the mothers. *Nature, 512*(7513), 131–132. doi:10.1038/512131a PMID:25119222

Roberts, S., Lester, K. J., Hudson, J. L., Rapee, R. M., Creswell, C., Cooper, P. J., & Eley, T. C. et al. (2014). Serotonin transporter methylation and response to cognitive behaviour therapy in children with anxiety disorders. *Translational Psychiatry, 4*(9), e444–e445. doi:10.1038/tp.2014.83 PMID:25226553

Samra, H., McGrath, J. M., Fischer, S., Schumacher, B., Dutcher, J., & Hansen, J. (2015). The NICU Parent Risk Evaluation and Engagement Model and Instrument (PREEMI) for Neonates in Intensive Care Units. *Journal of Obstetric, Gynecologic, and Neonatal Nursing, 44*(1), 114–126. doi:10.1111/1552-6909.12535 PMID:25580952

Scher, M. S., Ludington-Hoe, S., Kaffashi, F., Johnson, M. W., Holditch-Davis, D., & Loparo, K. (2009). Neurophysiologic assessment of brain maturation after an 8-week trial of skin-to-skin contact on preterm infants. *Clinical Neurophysiology, 120*(10), 1812–1818. doi:10.1016/j.clinph.2009.08.004 PMID:19766056

Schinka, J., Busch, R. M., & Robichaux-Keene, N. (2004). A meta-analysis of the association between the serotonin transporter gene polymorphism (5-HTTLPR) and trait anxiety. *Molecular Psychiatry, 9*(2), 197–202. doi:10.1038/sj.mp.4001405 PMID:14966478

Smith, G. C., Gutovich, J., Smyser, C., Pineda, R., Newnham, C., Tjoeng, T. H., & Inder, T. et al. (2011). Neonatal intensive care unit stress is associated with brain development in preterm infants. *Annals of Neurology, 70*(4), 541–549. doi:10.1002/ana.22545 PMID:21976396

Stoll, B. J., Hansen, N. I., Bell, E. F., Shankaran, S., Laptook, A. R., Walsh, M. C., & Higgins, R. D. et al. (2010). Neonatal outcomes of extremely preterm infants from the NICHD Neonatal Research Network. *Pediatrics, 126*(3), 443–456. doi:10.1542/peds.2009-2959 PMID:20732945

Symington, A., & Pinelli, J. (2006). Developmental care for promoting development and preventing morbidity in preterm infants. *Cochrane Database of Systematic Reviews, 2*, CD001814. PMID:16625548

Tsigos, C., & Chrousos, G. P. (2002). Hypothalamic-pituitary-adrenal axis, neuroendocrine factors and stress. *Journal of Psychosomatic Research, 53*(4), 865–871. doi:10.1016/S0022-3999(02)00429-4 PMID:12377295

Vijayendran, M., Beach, S., Plume, J. M., Brody, G., & Philibert, R. (2012). Effects of genotype and child abuse on DNA methylation and gene expression at the serotonin transporter. *Frontiers in Psychiatry, 3*, 55. doi:10.3389/fpsyt.2012.00055 PMID:22707942

Wang, D., Szyf, M., Benkelfat, C., Provencal, N., Turecki, G., Caramaschi, D., & Booij, L. et al. (2012). Peripheral SLC6A4 DNA methylation is associated with in vivo measures of human brain serotonin synthesis and childhood physical aggression. *PLoS ONE, 7*(6), e39501. doi:10.1371/journal.pone.0039501 PMID:22745770

Weaver, I. C. G., Cervoni, N., Champagne, F., D'Alessio, A. C., Sharma, S., Seckl, J. R., & Meaney, M. J. et al. (2004). Epigenetic programming by maternal behavior. *Nature Neuroscience, 7*(8), 847–854. doi:10.1038/nn1276 PMID:15220929

Welberg, L. A., & Seckl, J. R. (2001). Prenatal stress, glucocorticoids and the programming of the brain. *Journal of Neuroendocrinology*, *13*(2), 113–128. doi:10.1111/j.1365-2826.2001.00601.x PMID:11168837

Westrup, B. (2007). Newborn Individualized Developmental Care and Assessment Program (NIDCAP) - family-centered developmentally supportive care. *Early Human Development*, *83*(7), 443–449. doi:10.1016/j.earlhumdev.2007.03.006 PMID:17459617

Witzmann, S. R., Turner, J. D., Meriaux, S. B., Meijer, O. C., & Muller, C. P. (2012). Epigenetic regulation of the glucocorticoid receptor promoter 1(7) in adult rats. *Epigenetics : Official Journal of the DNA Methylation Society*, *7*(11), 1290–1301. doi:10.4161/epi.22363 PMID:23023726

Zwicker, J. G., Grunau, R. E., Adams, E., Chau, V., Brant, R., Poskitt, K. J., & Miller, S. P. et al. (2013). Score for neonatal acute physiology-II and neonatal pain predict Corticospinal tract development in premature newborns. *Pediatric Neurology*, *48*(2), 123–129. doi:10.1016/j.pediatrneurol.2012.10.016 PMID:23337005

KEY TERMS AND DEFINITIONS

Behavioral Epigenetics: Field of research applying the study of epigenetic alterations in relation with phenotypic variations during development.

Caregiver Engagement: Healthcare activities aimed at engage the parents of preterm infants in the daily caregiving activities as well as in providing information and let them participate at different levels in NICU staff interventions.

Developmental Care (DC): DC is an approach that uses a range of interventions addressed to modify the NICU environment in order to minimize the stress experienced by a preterm infant and to allow optimal neurobehavioral development of the infant. DC includes a broad category of interventions such as control of external stimuli (e.g., vestibular, auditory, visual, tactile), parental involvement and the family-centered care (e.g., kangaroo care, policies of NICUs toward parental visiting, promoting infant-parent bonding), developmental activities of daily living (i.e., nesting, swaddling, prone position) and infant pain management.

DNA Methylation: Modification of DNA by the addition of a methyl group to a specific site rich of cytosine (i.e., CpG site) within a specific region of a gene causing gene silencing.

Epigenetics: The study of the chemical modifications of the transcriptional functioning of genes, without structural genes at the level of DNA chain.

Family-Centricity: The belief that family is central to wellbeing and that family members and family issues take precedence over other aspects of life.

Neonatal Intensive Care Unit (NICU): An intensive care facility designed for the care of premature and ill newborn infants.

Preterm Behavioral Epigenetics (PBE): The study of the epigenetic processes associated with preterm birth and the subsequent exposure to NICU-related stressors and caregiving interventions.

Preterm Birth: Live birth before 37 weeks of pregnancy. There are subcategories of preterm birth, based on gestational age: extremely preterm (gestational age < 28 weeks); very preterm (gestational age between 28 and 32 weeks); moderate to late preterm (gestational age between 32 and 37 weeks).

Chapter 7
Why do Patients Protest? Collective Action Processes in People with Chronic Illnesses: A Psychosocial Perspective

Davide Mazzoni
University of Bologna, Italy

Augusta Isabella Alberici
Università Cattolica del Sacro Cuore, Milan, Italy

ABSTRACT

Despite the relevance of the topic, an exhaustive psychosocial reflection on the processes that may facilitate patients' protest is still missing. The chapter provides a theoretical and empirical overview of psychosocial pathways for patients' collective action. Five core factors are reviewed: perceived injustice, group efficacy, group identification, moral convictions and social embeddedness. Each of them provides a different explanation of collective action processes and is examined for its potential impact among patients. The chapter closes suggesting some core elements for a theoretical explanation of patients' collective action and its relationship with patient engagement. Practical and theoretical implications of patients' collective action are discussed to identify new directions for future research and interventions.

Quel che ci accomuna è, soprattutto, la scelta di prendere in mano il nostro destino, di essere noi i protagonisti di questo movimento civile ed umano, senza deleghe in bianco a chicchessia.

[What we share is, most of all, the choice to be protagonists of our fate, to be ourselves the protagonists of this civil and human movement without proxies to anyone.]

– Alberto Damilano, From the homepage of the Italian networkof people with amyotrophic lateral sclerosis (website: http://www.comitato16novembre.org/).

DOI: 10.4018/978-1-4666-9992-2.ch007

INTRODUCTION

Looking at local and national news in many European countries, it is not surprising to see and read about patients taking part in demonstrations, holding flags and posters to defend their own rights. Just to make some examples, we can refer to the pro-Stamina stem cell treatment demonstration that took place on December 2013 in the center of Rome (Italy). The police attempted to block the march and two protesters were stopped by the police. Few months later (June 2014), a group of workers and patients of the Bellvitge University Hospital (Spain) demonstrated against the healthcare budget cuts and blocked a nearby highway for several minutes. Again, on October 2014, a mass protest of patients was hold in Kiev and in some regions of Ukraine. The protest was titled "Black Tuesday". Patients picketed the Cabinet of Ministers, and demanded from the government to procure medicines for critically ill Ukrainians. They brought hundreds of shoe pairs that symbolized the death of the patients in case the government did not procure the necessary medicines.

As suggested by most patient engagement literature, nowadays, patients appear to be increasingly aware of their rights, and more demanding in the fruition of healthcare services. They are concerned with their own needs and preferences, and have become more critical in expressing judgments about the received health services (e.g., Guyatt, Mulla, Scott, Jackevicius, & You, 2014). On the other side, healthcare organizations do not always recognize and accept patients' active role. This may be a source of strain that, under certain circumstances, can result in a real collective mobilization.

Despite the relevance of the question we ask in the title, for patients and society, an exhaustive psychosocial reflection on the processes that may facilitate patients' protest is still missing. The available analyses focused on single groups or episodes (e.g., Rabeharisoa, 2006), while a broader theorization is actually desirable. This echoes Zoller (2005), when she wrote that we are more likely to heardiscussion of AIDS activism or breast cancer activism than we are tohear 'health activism' or other converging terms.

This chapter contributes to the book "Promoting Patient Engagement and Participation for Effective Healthcare Reform" by enlarging the analysis of patient engagement and participation with a group-based perspective, which is distinctive of the social psychology approach. Among the disciplines that were interested on the topic, our chapter focuses on the psychosocial processes at the basis of patients' collective action, conceived as one of the ways through which patients can produce (or resist to) a change in their health care system. Before we proceed to the social psychological answer as to why patients protest, we devote a few words to describe patients' collective action itself.

BACKGROUND: PATIENTS AS ACTIVISTS

In the psychosocial domain, collective action is often defined as a specific form of participation where individuals undertake actions as group members, with the aim to improve the group's conditions (e.g. Wright, Taylor, & Moghaddam, 1990; see also Van Zomeren & Iyer, 2009). According to Wright et al. (1990), collective action is proposed in contrast to individual action, that is specifically directed at improving one's personal conditions rather than group.

A wide range of behaviors can be classified as collective action, ranging from participation in protest demonstrations and strikes to seemingly individualistic acts such as signing a petition (Van Zomeren & Iyer, 2009) or contributing to a cause through an individual donation. More generally, despite some limitations that are discussed in the next paragraphs, patients' participation can potentially cover the broad spectrum of social and political engagement as classified by Ekman and Amnå (2012), including both legal and illegal forms of participation. In all cases, the aim of improving the patients' group conditions coincides with the aim of improving their health by influencing the healthcare system and the society. This influence can be expressed either toward the production of a social change (e.g., a desirable health care reform), and the resistance to an unwanted social change, (e.g., against money cuts for health services).

Moreover, like many other expressions of dissent, patients' collective actions represent the concerted efforts by committed supporters of the cause. Indeed, activists are usually defined as people who actively work for social or political causes. This group includes not only "protesters", that is patients who, for example, concretely march at the front of a demonstration, but also people who recruit for and mobilize people, and sustain the organizational structures that support them (see also Stuart, Thomas, Donaghue, & Russell, 2013; Simon & Klandermans, 2001).

In this sense, we should note that our discourse on patients' collective action must take into account not only the actions concretely run by patients, but also by the community of individuals that support, and sometimes are the only way to make possible, patients' mobilization. Concretely, supporters may include patients' familiars, friends, medical and paramedical professions also with a wide range of actors: researchers (biologists and clinicians), industry, public authorities, institutions, patient organizations, the local communities, etc.

PATHWAYS TO PATIENTS' PROTEST

Why do people protest? Which psychosocial processes are involved in their engagement in collective actions? These questions, despite rarely referred to patients, have occupied social psychologists for at least three decades, and have received diverging answers over the years (see Klandermans, 1997; Van Zomeren, Postmes, & Spears, 2008; Van Stekelenburg, 2013; Van Stekelenburg & Klandermans, 2013; Klandermans & Van Stekelenburg, 2013, for reviews). As suggested by Van Zomeren (2011), the first decade of the 21st century can be rightly called an 'age of integration' for the collective action literature. Before this period, various perspectives on collective action existed side-by-side (Van Zomeren & Spears, 2009; Van Zomeren et al., 2008).

Building on the existing literature, in this chapter we describe the social-psychological motives for undertaking collective action through three 'classical' core variables, such as perceived injustice, group identification, and group efficacy (Gamson, 1992; Klandermans, 1997; Stürmer & Simon, 2004; Van Zomeren et al., 2008; Van Zomeren, 2011). Considering more recent developments, two more factors will be considered: moral convictions (e.g., Van Zomeren, Postmes, & Spears, 2012) and social embeddedness (e.g., Van Stekelenburg & Klandermans, 2013).

Compared to other populations (e.g., migrants, no-global, environmentalist, etc.), patients have not been object of systematic analysis from a psychosocial perspective. In the following sections, we will review each of these psychosocial motives for collective mobilization and we will examine how they can specifically influence collective action processes among patients. Finally, the chapter closes suggesting some core elements for a theoretical explanation of patients' collective action and discussing some lines for further research.

Perceived Injustice

As suggested by some authors (Marwell & Oliver, 1993; Klandermans, 2004), even in view of significant changes in their environment and lives, most people continue to do what they were doing, namely nothing. A consequence of this observation is that, even in contexts of deprivation and cuts to health services, only a minority of patients decide to engage in some forms of collective action.

This is coherent with the idea that (objective) deprivation is neither necessary nor sufficient to determine collective action. At this regard, the study focus should include the subjective experience involved and its presumed connection to objective deprivation. Stouffer and colleagues (Stouffer, Suchman, DeVinney, Star, & Williams, 1949) introduced the concept of relative deprivation to explain why objective deprivation does not always predict peoples' dissatisfactions with their lost. Similar research led to the development of relative deprivation theory (e.g., Folger, 1986, 1987; Pettigrew, 1967; Runciman, 1966; Walker & Smith, 2002), which focused on the subjective experience of unjust disadvantage. Relative deprivation theory proposes that feelings of deprivation develop on the basis of social comparisons, while theory and research have suggested that social inequality in distributions can be perceived as even fair (e.g., Jost & Major, 2001; Major, 1994).

The notion that the subjective experience of inequality has greater weight than its objective, material origins has been considered also in recent developments in the social-psychological literature on fairness judgments, which focuses on how people respond to distributive and procedural fairness and their emotional consequences (e.g., anger, resentment) (Leventhal, 1980; Lind & Tyler, 1988; Miller, 2001; Tyler, Boeckmann, Smith, & Huo, 1997; Van den Bos & Lind, 2002).

Similar conclusions can be found also in patient engagement literature. For example, in a UK qualitative study involving patients who have experienced rationing associated with morbid obesity or breast cancer care, participants had a choice whether to accept that decision, to contest it, or to opt out of the public healthcare system and pay for private care. Results showed that the perception of decision-making being unjust led some patients to contest decisions (Owen-Smith, Coast, & Donovan, 2009). Moreover, among the most important factors affecting how patients reacted to rationing were their sense of entitlement to National Health Service care, and the attitude of the clinical team providing treatment. The importance of perceived fairness of decision-making suggests that it is important to continue to explore the acceptable bases for rationing alongside the accountability of the process of decision making, which has been the focus of much of the recent priority setting literature (Daniels, 2000; Kapiriri, Norheim, & Martin, 2007). In this sense, the authors conclude that patients need to be provided with sufficient information and support to make an informed decision following the revelation of rationing, and that clinicians need training to assist them in communicating rationing decisions.

(Group) Efficacy

In the 1970s, theories like relative derivation were criticized by scholars arguing that grievances do not provide a sufficient reason to participate in protest. In some way, the key question to address was: why do some aggrieved people become mobilized, while others do not? At this regard, in the last decades, personal and group *efficacy* beliefs have become one of the key explanations of collective action. The idea behind group efficacy is that people engage in collective action if they believe this will make it more likely that relevant goals are achieved by the group (e.g., Van Zomeren et al., 2008). Several studies have shown that feelings of efficacy are highly correlated with participation in protest and this relation was confirmed also meta-analytically (Van Zomeren et al., 2008).

In the analysis by Van Zomeren and Spears (2009), efficacy beliefs were grouped together with cost-benefit calculations (Olson, 1965), as motivations of the 'intuitive economists' metaphor. The assumption here about human motivation is that people are individual-based intuitive economists (Edwards, 1962) who make social judgments and decisions by calculating the costs and benefits of a particular action and its consequences. This motivation for collective action is reflected in early sociological work on collective action (e.g., Olson, 1965), which strongly influenced later approaches to collective action in terms of its individual rationality assumption (e.g., Hardin, 1971; Klandermans, 1984; McCarthy & Zald, 1977; Simon et al., 1998). In this sense, the idea that personal commitment depends on expectations that one's group is able to achieve the social change, can be considered an instrumental path to collective action.

It is plausible that similar efficacy beliefs are relevant for patients' collective action. However, we must recognize that efficacy beliefs among patients may be lower than in other populations. As described by Jennings (1999), the effects of pain and loss may reduce efficacy beliefs: people experiencing pain and loss may be disinclined toward political participation because they feel depressed, overwhelmed, and helpless, especially if they also face stigma by others. Even if, in theory, it would be also possible that sometimes pain and loss can "trigger" emotional and cognitive responses that provide incentives and motivations for political action (Jennings, 1999), this is rarely the case. The results of a nationally representative survey in the United States confirmed that several measures of efficacy that help predict-political activity were found to be significantly lower among people with disabilities than among similar people without disabilities (Schur, Shields, & Schriner, 2003).

At this regard, we note that some patients decide to express their dissent and protest against decisions that are hardly possible to modify. For example, it seems unlikely that protests run by patients with amyotrophic lateral sclerosis in Italy, as expressed in the citation we reported at the beginning of this chapter, are moved by instrumental motives only. Even, if it is quite difficult to fully obtain the desirable change, and the costs of the protest for patients are quite high, some people still decide to engage in some forms of collective action. This suggests that also other factors, some of which will be discussed in the next paragraphs, different from efficacy, could be relevant for patients.

However, also the distinction between the individual and the group level of analysis can be useful. Individual efficacy, that is the belief in the achievement of individual goals through one's own actions is an important predictor of such action. Similarly, group efficacy beliefs are important in motivating people to achieve group goals through collective action. Some authors recently suggested that *participative* efficacy, that is the belief that individual's participations matters – i.e., that the individual's participation is seen as having a potential incremental effect on collective action – could be more relevant than group efficacy (Van Zomeren, Saguy, & Schellhaas, 2013).

Group Identity

In the 1980s it become clear to many researchers that instrumental motivation was not a sufficient reason to engage in collective actions. From that time, the literature devoted greater attention to the key-role played also by group identification processes (Tajfel & Turner, 1986; Turner, Hogg, Oakes, Reicher, & Wetherell, 1987). More specifically, some social-psychological studies report consistently that the more people identify with a group, the more they are inclined to protest (e.g., Reicher, 1984; Simon et al., 1998; Stryker, Owens, & Wite, 2000; Mazzoni, Van Zomeren, & Cicognani, 2015). Indeed, identification with others is accompanied by an awareness of similarity and shared fate with those who belong to the same category. When group members perceive a collective disadvantage, they may decide to act as a group to reduce it (Ellemers, 2002).

According to Simon and Klandermans (2001), group identity politicizes when group members become aware of shared grievances and of an opponent who is to blame; when they share a sense of the possibility and normative requirement to act collectively for social change; and when they become aware that the power struggle has to be fought in the public arena, where third parties need to be involved (Simon & Klandermans, 2001). There is strong evidence that politicized identity is a crucial predictor of collective action as it implies that group members, through their struggle, achieve a sense of themselves as being collectively agentic (Blackwood & Louis, 2012; Van Zomeren, Spears, Fischer, & Leach, 2004). Psychosocial research also highlighted that collective identity facilitates beliefs and emotions that, in turn, predict collective action (Van Zomeren at al., 2008). At the same time, collective identity encapsulates beliefs and emotions relevant to action, and mediates their effect on collective action (Thomas, Mavor, & McGarty, 2012).

More recent developments in this area of research pointed out that "dual identity" is particularly important in the collective action processes (e.g., Simon & Grabow, 2010). Social psychology showed that people can hold many different identities at the same time (e.g., as patient, as patient with AIDS, as citizen, as human being, etc.). In the context of collective action, dual identity involves both identification with the aggrieved ingroup (e.g., a group of patients) and identification with a more inclusive group or community (e.g., the same country of residence) that entitles them to societal support for their claims.

Similar processes can be described for patients, where this identification may become even stronger, since, borrowing the term from Rabinow (2002), they are ''biosocially'' linked to one another. Brown et al. (2004) use the term "collective illness identity" to describe the intersection of social constructions of illness and the personal illness experience of a biological disease process. When patients develop a 'cognitive, moral, and emotional connection' with other illness sufferers, a collective illness identity emerges. Moreover, for a politicized collective illness identity to form, the collective illness identity must be linked to a broader social critique that views structural inequalities and the uneven distribution of social power as responsible for the causes and/or triggers of the disease.

Even in case of patients and disabled people, collective action intentions are enhanced by processes of identification (Scotch, 1988). As described by Brown et al. (2004), when "institutions of science and medicine fail to offer disease accounts that are consistent with individuals' experiences of illness, or when science and medicine offer accounts of disease that individuals are unwilling to accept, people may adopt an identity as an aggrieved illness sufferer, and even progress to collective action" (p. 55).

However, the group identity formation presents also some specific features and obstacles for patients. For example, people normally desire to retain an ordinary healthy identity and its value. For this reason, the identification with a group if patients can be initially hindered by feelings of pain and loss (Allsop, Jones, & Baggott, 2004; Kostova, Caiata-Zufferey, & Schulz, 2014). Together with the process of gradual identification, patient engagement is as a multidimensional psychosocial process resulting from the conjoint cognitive, emotional, and behavioral enactment of individuals. The process starts with the "blackout position" that follows the onset of the disease condition. In the "adhesion position" patients start to see him/herself as patient. Only in the last position of the engagement process (i.e., eudaimonic project), patients have fully accepted their condition and their patients' identity is only one of their possible selves (elaboration) (Graffigna, Barello, Riva, & Bosio, 2014).

In this sense, we suggest that is properly in the last position of the engagement (eudamonic) that patients collective action can potentially take place. Indeed, the "adhesion position" is individually characterized by the recognition of him/herself "as a patient", and this is, of course, a prerequisite to identify with the patients' group. However, only in the eudamonic position patient see him/herself "as a person" who can advocate for the health of his/her community (Graffigna et al., 2014). In psychosocial terms, this can be considered the basis for a politicized identity to develop.

Another key point is that communication among group members contributes to the development of group identity. The interactive model of identity formation (IMIF; Postmes, Haslam, & Swaab, 2005) postulates that in interactive groups two different paths are involved in social identity formation: a deductive path and an inductive path (Postmes, Spears, Lee, & Novak, 2005). In the latter case, group identity is inferred via the individual attempts of group members to shape consensus and it is deduced from commonalities at a superordinate group level. Consensus within the group can be obtained through a process through which group members interact with each other and negotiate a common group definition that is more than the sum of the distinctive individual positions. Consistently, Thomas and colleagues (Thomas, Smith, McGarty, & Postmes, 2010) proposed that, to pursue social change, emerging political forces need to consensualize and share their grievances through group interaction.

In a similar way, research on patients' illness narratives has highlighted how some patients can use stories to develop a coherent self, to make sense of their experiences, and to empower their existence (Charmaz, 1991; Frank, 1997; Kleinman, 1988). Moreover, telling stories about one's illness experience may allow both the speaker and the audience to cope with illness, to exchange information, and to reflect and reconstruct their new identities (Dickerson, Posluszny, & Kennedy, 2000; Hsieh, 2004). In this sense, for some patients storytelling may play an important role in the illness identity construction and can be considered a process through which such patients share a common identity potentially linked to social change.

Moral Convictions

Undoubtedly, in many cases, the motivations explained in the above paragraphs are sufficient to explain many people's collective behavior. However, in the last decade, some authors "rediscovered" the importance of moral convictions (e.g. Goodin, 1992), suggesting a special relationship with politicized identities and collective action. More specifically, moral convictions can be defined as strong and absolute stances on moral issues, they do not tolerate any exceptions to the general 'higher-order' principle (Tetlock, 2002). A violation of a moral conviction therefore motivates individuals to actively change that situation (Skitka, Bauman, & Sargis, 2005; Van Zomeren & Lodewijkx, 2005). According to authors, this mechanism would refer not only to moral absolutism - as a distinctly minority position – but could be a motivating factor for many people taking part in collective actions.

Moreover, moral convictions seem to represent a unifying motivation between 'advantaged' and 'disadvantaged' people. Once moral convictions acquire a moral status, they become subjectively universal and thus transcend group boundaries. For example, when moral convictions of 'advantaged' are against social inequality and they are confronted with a disadvantaged group, this constitutes a violation of their moral conviction, which can motivate them to change the situation (Van Zomeren, Postmes, Spears, & Bettache, 2011). Similar processes can be described also in patients' literature.

Moral conviction may also motivate collective action to support universal human rights.Two recent studies showed that the perceived violation of human rights (conceived as moral principles) can motivate activists through their group identity (Mazzoni et al., 2015). Despite its controversial definitions, the right to health is present in many national and international declarations (e.g., Backman et al., 2008). If a detailed review is out of the scopes of the present chapter, what we want to emphasize here is that the right to the highest attainable standard of physical and mental health may represent a strong moral motivator for both patients and supporters who decide to engage in many forms of collective action to defend it.

At this regard, we can refer to the 9th European Patients' Rights Day took place on May 2015, launched by the Active Citizenship Network. That was also the occasion to discuss the European Charter of Patients' Rights to guarantee a "high level of human health protection" (Article 35 of the Charter of Fundamental Rights of the European Union) and to assure the high quality of services provided by the various national health services in Europe.

However, other examples can be found, in which the moral motivation lies behind the manifest behavior, even if it represents an important and strong motivation. Using the metaphor in the classification by Van Zomeren and Spears (2009), "intuitive theologians" are primarily moved by the defense of "sacred" values (like health) then by instrumental motives.

Social Embeddedness

Some sociologists revised previous models of collective action, emphasizing the idea that the decision to take part in protest is not taken insocial isolation (Van Stekelenburg, 2013). On the contrary, individual grievances and feelings are transformed into group-based grievances and feelings within social networks. Networks provide space for the creation and dissemination of a critical discourse toward authorities, and this represents a way for active opposition to authorities to grow (Paxton, 2002). For this reason, being part of a network increases the chances that one will be targeted with a mobilizing message and that people participate (Klandermans & Oegema, 1987).

The literature on new social movements has shown the importance of face-to-face interactions and conflicts in the shaping of a collective reality (Klawiter, 1999; Mueller, 1994). Psychosocial research demonstrated that when people share their opinions within a group, this constitutes a basis for developing new collective identities strictly linked to collective action (e.g. Gee, Khalaf, & McGarty, 2007; Thomas & McGarty, 2009). The underlying idea is that through communication and consensualization people reach agreement upon a shared sense of "we" and, at the same time, crystallize norms for social action (Postmes, Haslam, & Swaab, 2005a).

However, we suggest here that for patients, even if face-to-face interactions are important, web-interactions have a specific value and allows patients to create the necessary network at the basis of mobilization. This is particularly true for patients who experience more difficulties in face to face interactions because of physical impairments. A similar discourse can be true for (but it is not limited to) rare diseases, where a casual meeting is difficult, and for stigmatizing conditions, in which patients show some resistance in showing their condition (e.g., Frohlich & Zmyslinski-Seelig, in press).

There is consensus around the idea that the web 2.0 is deeply changing the health communication paradigm (Laubie & Elie-Dit-Cosaque, 2012). Until the wide adoption of the Internet, health communication was limited to top-down approaches where health professionals and third parties involved were those communicating information to patients. Together with the development of more recent online 2.0 tools, wide connected and bottom-up spaces are opening: patients connect with others by experiencing the same disease, by sharing information about symptoms and treatments and by exchanging ideas about their decision-making processes when coping with the disease (Orizio, Schulz, Gasparotti, Caimi, & Gelatti, 2010). Many have argued that the web is facilitating the creation of health-related virtual communities (Radin, 2006). For example, online communication allows patients to maintain a continuous link with the community members, and to quickly receive information which is understandable and that can be tailored on their personal needs (van Uden-Kraan et al., 2008). Health communication research conceptualized these communities as online support groups, and showed that patients often use these groups to seek informational and emotional support, and to help other patients (e.g. Braithwaite, Waldron, & Finn, 1999; Shaw, McTavish, Hawkins, Gustafson, & Pingree, 2000; Sullivan, 2003; Turner, Grube, & Meyers, 2001; Weinberg, Schmale, Uken, & Wessel, 1996; Wright, 2002; Mazzoni & Cicognani, 2014). Moreover, online patient groups are often aimed at calling the attention of the public opinion and at mobilising consensus around health-related topics. In this sense, online groups may become a kind of collective action itself as well as a basis of other online/offline forms of collective mobilization.

Psychosocial research on collective action has recently showed that online interaction stimulates collective action (Brunsting & Postmes, 2002; Shah, Cho, Eveland, & Kwak, 2005). Online communication facilitates place- and time-independent interaction making it easier for members of less powerful groups to exchange uncensored and dissenting opinions. Furthermore, some have shown that communicating online within social movements shapes the effect of the psychosocial predictors of collective action (Alberici & Milesi, 2013). For example, discussing online frequently enhances the predicting effect of collective efficacy on willingness to act collectively, probably because activists become aware and believe in the potential of the web as a tool for mobilising social support; this in turn empowers users and stimulates collective action (Postmes, 2007). Some studies have consistently found that participating in online support groups empowers patients as they have the chance to exchange knowledge and share experiences. Unwanted isolation is one of the most significant psychosocial stressors that patients face when they receive the diagnosis of a chronic illness. It has been shown that online support groups can help to reduce these stressors, and can enhance collective empowerment especially because of the presence of other participants who have been through similar experiences (Høybye et al., 2010; van Ulden- Kraan et al., 2008). A qualitative analysis of messages posted in an online support group for breast cancer sufferers, survivors and supporters showed that information-gathering became one of the main strategies to reduce uncertainty and produced feelings of control and hope (Radin, 2006).

Online interactions have also a positive influence on well-being. For example, consistent with work showing the benefits of public action (e.g., Putnam, 2000; Freund & McGuire, 1999; Foster, 2015), tweeting actively about a common discrimination increases well-being and decreases negative affect among participants (Foster, in press). Similarly, a study involving activists of web-based social movements found that the more users interacted online, the less it was likely that group-based anger was a driver to collective action (Alberici & Milesi, 2013). Indeed, while angry messages may go viral on online discussions, it has been shown their real influence on participants' behaviour may be much less than one might expect (Choi, 2014). Certainly, the peculiar way in which patients' share their emotions online (e.g., without non-verbal cues), and the consequent influence on collective behaviour is an under-researched point that deserves to be systematically investigated by future studies.

On the whole, in psychosocial terms, these results show that online interactions can be considered as a communication context where psychosocial drivers to collective action are affected and transformed. This seems especially true for group identity. Grounded in the social identity theory, the Social Identity model of De-individuation Effects (SIDE; Reicher, Spears, & Postmes, 1995; Spears & Lea, 19 94) postulates that that group identity can become especially salient during computer-mediated communication. Empirical findings support the idea that group norms become group-defining in online contexts thanks to the anonymity of CMC (e.g., Spears, Lea, Corneliussen, Postmes, & Ter Haar, 2002). Following this perspective, it has been found that participating in online political discussions affects the way in which activists gradually build the meaning of their group politicized identity (i.e., "who we are" and "what we do"), and this indirectly makes collective action more likely. For example, interacting online in an encouraging and 'safe' context makes participants feel that many others support the same cause; sharing these empowering beliefs makes participants understand what it means to be a group member and this in turn stimulates collective action (Alberici & Milesi, in press). A study conducted among patients participating in an online breast cancer online community revealed that sharing group norms was a driver to collective action. Patients reported that when browsing on the forum, they realized they shared the same vision with other patients. Although they were surrounded by their family, they said they needed to talk to people, to women sharing the same disease (Laubie & Elie-Dit-Cosaque, 2012). This collective self-definition was a psychological determinant of patients' willingness to mobilize around the disease-related issues. Thus, on the one hand perceiving a homogeneity of experiences and sharing a common point of view may strengthen the patients' sense of collective identity and empowerment when coping with the disease. On the other hand, however, interacting online with like-minded others may shift to extreme and polarized positions during discussions. In psychosocial terms, polarization is a function of social identity salience and it has to be understood as the convergence of group members upon a group prototypical position or norm (Turner, 1982; Turner et al., 1987). Groups use polarization to signal their consensual and distinctive position, hence comparing themselves with one or more out-groups. Some studies have shown that during online interactions, people are more likely to polarize their opinions (Lee, 2007; Postmes et al., 2005b). Although the weak-ties nature of most online networks may provide people with diverse and non-redundant views, some evidence suggests that online communication encourages self-segregation into homogenous groups (e.g., Wojcieszak, 2011). Consistently, the Internet is often perceived to be an ideal medium for radicalized groups (Back, 2002; Douglas, 2007) because the support of like-minded others can lead to heightened expression of in-group extremist views (Douglas & McGarty, 2002). As a consequence, online interactions may in some cases favor patients' support of polarized and inflexible points of view, challenging medical views. For example, it was found that exposure to vaccine-critical Websites increases perceptions of the risks of vaccinations and decreases perceptions of their benefits (Betsch, Renkewitz, Betsch, & Ulshöfer, 2010). Some of these alternative movements may have positive effects in the long run, but others may not (see the polarization of the online vaccination debate). However, some have suggested that social media technologies may provide patients with novel opportunities for advocating for particular treatments: for example, the chance to combine efficacious narrative-based content (e.g., personal experience diaries posted online or via You Tube) with scientific and medical knowledge (e.g., posting historical statistics about the impact of a vaccine) represents a promising communication strategy which future research should investigate (Witteman & Zikmund-Fisher, 2012; Mazanderani, O'Neill, & Powell, 2013).

On the whole, the effects of perceived similarity among patients sharing via the web the experience of a same disease/treatment certainly represents a critical point which deserve to be better investigated by future research. Psychosocial studies highlighted that similarity forms the basis for the development of a collective (and politicized) identity on the one hand, but on the other it was found that the more members of a group feel the pressure to group norms and standards, the greater they may support polarized points of view. Adopting a psychosocial perspective would enrich research on patients' engagement, for example, by focusing on how the peculiarities of online interactions among patients (e.g., anonymity, lack on non verbal cues) shape perceptions of similarity, and how this would indirectly influence the meaning they give to their collective/politicized identity.

Another critical point regards the quality of online discussions and their effects on mobilization. Online deliberation may be both positively and negatively related to political engagement (Halpern & Gibbs, 2013). On the one hand, the written and asynchronous character of online interactions may stimulate more reflexive, rational and argumentative conversations (Stromer-Galley & Wichowski, 2010). On the other hand, computer-mediated communication (CMC) has been historically regarded as an impersonal phenomenon that deindividuates participants, encouraging uncivil political discourse (e.g., flaming). A recent study found that when online discussions are perceived as being constructive (e.g., with a high conversational coherence), a sense of moral responsibility to act stimulates collective action. On the contrary, when online discussions are unproductive, intention to act collectively is discouraged (Alberici & Milesi, 2015). By extending this line of research to health-care online communication contexts, the psychosocial perspective could help to understand why the effectiveness of online support groups on collective behavior may often be limited, especially on the long term. Indeed, it seems that online interactions have mobilizing effects for some patients, but not for others who are more hard to mobilize. We claim that, besides investigating the role that patients' individual differences may play in stimulating vs. discouraging online collective action, future studies could focus on individuating the peculiar online deliberative practices that can sustain an enduring patients' collective engagement with online health-related communities.

Discussion

This chapter presented a theoretical and empirical overviewof important factors that can influence patients' potentially strong collective action. Among the disciplines who are interested in studying such process, we based on psychosocial literature to draw five most important pathways toward collective action. They include perceived injustice, efficacy, group identity, moral convictions and social embeddedness. Paraphrasing them in simple terms, they provide different possible answers to the question in the title (why do patients protest?): because of a perceived injustice, because they believe that their efforts matter, because they belong to a group they identify with, because they want to defend a threatened moral principle, and because they are embedded in on-line and off-line social networks.

We separately discussed each of these concepts, but obviously, in practice they are all connected. These factors act jointly to propel collective action among patients. As anticipated in the introduction, the last years are sometimes called "age of integration" for collective action literature and many attempts have been done to integrate different factors in more complex models of collective action.

For example, in the famous meta-analysis by Van Zomeren et al. (2008), identity was the key factorthat bridged the injustice and efficacy explanations of collective action. Subsequent attempts tried to integrate in a similar model also moral convictions: in this case, the moral convictions have a special relationship with politicized identities and collective action because of their potentiallystrong normative fit with the action-oriented content of politicized identities (Van Zomeren et al., 2012).

In other models, shared identity was placed before other factors. For example, the model by Van Stekelenburg and Klandermans (2009) combined grievances, efficacy, identity and emotions. This model, that assigns a central and integrating role to processes of identification, suggests that in order to develop the shared grievances and shared emotions a shared identity is needed (Van Stekelenburg

& Klandermans, 2009). More recent developments of such model combine important predictors in a model comprising two routes: an efficacy route steered by social embeddedness and a grievances route (Van Stekelenburg, 2013).

Some limitations of these research approaches must be recognized also in terms of the opportunity of deriving practical implication. Indeed, in the attempt to develop general models, they lose part of the explanatory power of concrete and contextualized situations. Patients represent an heterogeneous population that shares some common concrete experiences and needs. For example, we do not sustain that to make the unfairness go away, all we have to do is to change patients' perception of injustice. Collective action models must be necessarily applied with some cautions and considering the specific context and situation.

At this regard, more research is needed to provide more evidence of the underlying process that may guide patients' collective action. We must recognize, for example, that collective action may assume meanings that are not so relevant for other populations. For example, protests may represent a specific stigma-reduction strategy by diminishing negative attitudes about mental illness (Corrigan & Penn, 1999). On the other side, as we showed in this chapter, it is possible that other factors, like group efficacy, may be less important for patients' motivation.

In this chapter, we focused on factors that can have an impact on patients' collective action. However, this relationship is necessarily more complex, and other outcomes then collective action could be considered. For example, it is possible to sustain that collective action processes may have a more or less direct effect also on patients' health and well-being. For example, identifying with a group can impact (positively) upon group members' health, and this can be explained (in part) through the social relations that a shared identity allows (Khan et al., 2014). To this regard, some authors have recently defined shared social identity in terms of a "social cure" showing that the sense of "we-ness" with other group members results in better health and well-being (Jetten, Haslam, & Haslam, 2012). Moreover, in a study by Brashers and colleagues, activists with HIV or AIDS perceived that their collective behaviors impacted also on the physician-patient communication. Differences between activist and nonactivist individuals showed that activists used more problem-focused coping (and less emotion-focused coping), had a greater knowledge of treatment information sources, and had a greater HIV social network integration (Brashers, Haas, Klingle, & Neidig, 2000). All these positive effects of collective action could serve also as soft incentives (Olson, 1965; Opp, 1986) for patients that, in turn, can sustain their future participation.

FUTURE RESEARCH DIRECTIONS

In our chapter, across the five concepts we discussed, we also suggested some critical points which future research on patients' engagement could investigate. A first point regards the importance to include the examination of subjective experience of injustice and its presumed connection to objective deprivation. For example, future research will clarify how objective deprivation is perceived by patients, and which factors discriminate between mobilization from non-mobilization.

A second point regards the study of patients' perceived efficacy. Here we stressed the opportunity to distinguish the efficacy level of analysis (from the individual to the group). Indeed, patients could be motivated by the perception that their participation can have a potential incremental effect on the group effort, rather than to obtain a real change in the status quo.

As regards patients' collective identity, we argue the focus should be more on the processes and barriers through which patients can build and develop a politicized identity. To do this, it would be interesting to investigate how the other motivations interact with patients' collective identity and their intention to act collectively.

For example, future research will examine the specific role played by moral convictions. Indeed, the defense of an important moral principle could represent a strong motivator, also for other people, to overcome group boundaries and to support patients' collective action.

Moreover, the investigation of the role of patients' collective action could be enriched by the analysis of the ways though which patients consensualize and share their experiences through group interaction, both offline and online. As regards online interactions, we suggested that more research is needed to understand how the peculiarities of online interactions (e.g., anonymity) shape patients' motivations to adhere to collective actions. For example, we stressed the importance to better understand the effects of online perceived homogeneity/similarity on attitudes polarization, as well as the deliberation practices that can sustain or discourage collective mobilization.

CONCLUSION

On the whole, we argue that the study of patients' collective action can strongly enrich the existing research on patient engagement, as it helps to develop practices aimed at making patients/clients co-producers of their health, thus enhancing their collective responsibility in both care and prevention (Graffigna et al., 2014). It is already known that, through their engagement, patients gain a positive approach to health management and recapture an active role in the society. We emphasize here that patients have even more chances to influence their health care system if they are prompted to think and act collectively. A recent and notable result in this direction is the news that in May 2010, the Canadian Agency for Drugs and Technologies in Health (CADTH) added patient group input to its Common Drug Review (CDR) process. This initiative helps ensure that health outcomes and issues important to patients are incorporated into the CDR process in a formal and meaningful way.

Finally, we must also recognize that patients' collective action, as defined the beginning of this chapter (see Wright et al., 1990; Van Zomeren & Iyer, 2009) is not a synonymous and it does not necessarily includes all the features of patient engagement as defined in the literature (see Barello, Graffigna, Vegni, & Bosio, 2014). According to some definitions of patient engagement, it usually requires an alliance, a partnership among patients and health care providers. This alliance is useful to obtain better clinical outcomes as it contributes to foster a collaborative approach to the symptoms' cure and supports the development of effective coping strategies for disease management. On the other hand, collective action often represents an expression of dissent. When patients' collective action take place, from patients' point of view, 'something was not going in the right direction' and a social change is desirable. In this case, health care providers may become close allies for the cause or, alternatively, part of the system to challenge.

In this sense, the value of studying patients' collective action is twofold. From one side, it may represent a good example of patients' empowerment, in which they become able to perceive themselves as patients and citizens, and are consequently able to join together to reach a common goal. For example, as we showed in the paragraph about identification, collective action requires an acceptance of the disease that usually characterized the last positions of the engagement process.

From the other side, collective action may sometimes represent an example in which the alliance between patients and health care system manifests some problems. In this case, collective action is a symptom of a break in patients' trust, that should be carefully considered.

Our suggestion is that further research to better understand processes at the basis of patients' collective action is strongly needed. This could give important insights about how to promote a constructive group-based patients' involvement in the healthcare system. At the same time, it would provide instruments to better understand and prevent radicalization of behaviours, in an even more sustainable exchange between healthcare services and demand.

REFERENCES

Alberici, A. I., & Milesi, P. (2013). The influence of the internet on the psychosocial predictors of collective action. *Journal of Community & Applied Social Psychology*, *23*(5), 373–388. doi:10.1002/casp.2131

Alberici, A. I., & Milesi, P. (2015, July 7-10). "The right thing to do": discussing online and the moral pathway to collective mobilization. *Paper presented at The 14th European Congress of Psychology*, Milan (Italy).

Alberici, A. I., & Milesi, P. (in press). Online discussion, politicized identity, and collective action. *Group Processes & Intergroup Relations*. doi:10.1177/1368430215581430

Allsop, J., Jones, K., & Baggott, R. (2004). Health consumer groups in the UK: A new social movement? *Sociology of Health & Illness*, *26*(6), 737–756. doi:10.1111/j.0141-9889.2004.00416.x PMID:15383039

Back, L. (2002). Aryans reading Adorno: Cyber-culture and twenty-first century racism. *Ethnic and Racial Studies*, *25*(4), 628–651. doi:10.1080/01419870220136664

Backman, G., Hunt, P., Khosla, R., Jaramillo-Strouss, C., Fikre, B. M., & Rumble, C. et al. (2008). Health systems and the right to health: An assessment of 194 countries. *Lancet*, *372*(9655), 2047–2085. doi:10.1016/S0140-6736(08)61781-X PMID:19097280

Barello, S., Graffigna, G., Vegni, E., & Bosio, A. C. (2014). The challenges of conceptualizing patient engagement in health care: A lexicographic literature review. *Journal of Participatory Medicine, 6*.

Betsch, C., Renkewitz, F., Betsch, T., & Ulshöfer, C. (2010). The influence of vaccine-critical websites on perceiving vaccination risks. *Journal of Health Psychology*, *15*(3), 446–455. doi:10.1177/1359105309353647 PMID:20348365

Blackwood, L. M., & Louis, W. R. (2012). If it matters for the group then it matters to me: Collective action outcomes for seasoned activists. *The British Journal of Social Psychology*, *51*(1), 72–92. doi:10.1111/j.2044-8309.2010.02001.x PMID:21294752

Braithwaite, D. O., Waldron, V. R., & Finn, J. (1999). Communication of social supportin computer-mediated groups for people with disabilities. *Health Communication*, *11*(2), 123–151. doi:10.1207/s15327027hc1102_2 PMID:16370973

Brashers, E., Haas, M., Klingle, S., & Neidig, L. (2000). Collective AIDS activism and individuals' perceived self-advocacy in physician-patient communication. *Human Communication Research*, *26*(3), 372–402. doi:10.1111/j.1468-2958.2000.tb00762.x

Brown, P., Zavestoski, S., McCormick, S., Mayer, B., Morello-Frosch, R., & Gasior Altman, R. (2004). Embodied health movements: New approaches tosocial movements in health. *Sociology of Health & Illness*, *26*(1), 50–80. doi:10.1111/j.1467-9566.2004.00378.x PMID:15027990

Brunsting, S., & Postmes, T. (2002). Social movement participation in the digital age: Predicting offline and online collective action. *Small Group Research*, *33*(5), 525–554. doi:10.1177/104649602237169

Charmaz, K. (1991). *Good days, bad days: The self in chronic illness and time*. New Brunswick, NJ: Rutgers University Press.

Choi, S. (2014). Flow, diversity, form, and influence of political talk in social-media-based public forums. *Human Communication Research*, *40*(2), 209–237. doi:10.1111/hcre.12023

Corrigan, P. W., & Penn, D. L. (1999). Lessons from social psychology on discrediting psychiatric stigma. *The American Psychologist*, *54*(9), 765–776. doi:10.1037/0003-066X.54.9.765 PMID:10510666

Daniels, N. (2000). Accountability for reasonableness. *BMJ (Clinical Research Ed.)*, *321*(7272), 1300–1301. doi:10.1136/bmj.321.7272.1300 PMID:11090498

Dickerson, S. S., Posluszny, M., & Kennedy, M. C. (2000). Help seeking in a support group for recipients of implantable cardioverter defibrillators and their support persons. *Heart & Lung*, *29*(2), 87–96. doi:10.1067/mhl.2000.104138 PMID:10739484

Douglas, K. M. (2007). Psychology, discrimination and hate groups online. In A. N. Joinson, K. Y. A. McKenna, T. Postmes, & U. D. Reips (Eds.), *The Oxford handbook of Internet psychology* (pp. 155–163). Oxford: Oxford University Press.

Douglas, K. M., & McGarty, C. (2002). Internet identifiability and beyond: A model of the effects of identifiability on communicative behavior. *Group Dynamics*, *6*(1), 17–26. doi:10.1037/1089-2699.6.1.17

Edwards, W. (1962). Dynamic decision theory and probabilistic information processings. *Human Factors: The Journal of the Human Factors and Ergonomics Society*, *4*(2), 59–74.

Ekman, J., & Amnå, E. (2012). Political participation and civic engagement: Towards a new typology. *Human Affairs*, *22*(3), 283–300. doi:10.2478/s13374-012-0024-1

Ellemers, N. (2002). Social identity and relative deprivation. In I. Walker & H. Smith (Eds.), *Relative deprivation: Specification, development and integration* (pp. 239–264). Cambridge, UK: Cambridge University Press.

Folger, R. (1986). A referent cognitions theory of relative deprivation. In J. M. Olson, C. P. Herman, & M. P. Zanna (Eds.), *Relative deprivationand social comparison: The Ontario symposium* (Vol. 4, pp. 217–242). Hillsdale, NJ: Erlbaum.

Folger, R. (1987). Reformulating the conditions of resentment: A referent cognition model. In J. C. Masters & W. P. Smith (Eds.), *Social comparison, social justice, and relative deprivation* (pp. 183–215). London: Erlbaum.

Foster, M. D. (2015). Tweeting about sexism: The well-being benefits of a social media collective action. *The British Journal of Social Psychology, 54*(4), 629–647. doi:10.1111/bjso.12101 PMID:25639601

Frank, A. W. (1997). Enacting illness stories: When, what, and why. In H. L. Nelson (Ed.), *Stories and their limits: Narrative approach to bioethics* (pp. 31–49). New York: Routledge.

Freund, P., & McGuire, M. (1999). *Health, illness, andthe social body: A critical sociology*. Upper Saddle River, NJ: Prentice Hall.

Frohlich, D. O., & Zmyslinski-Seelig, A. N. (in press). How Uncover Ostomy challenges ostomy stigma, and encourages others to do the same. *New Media & Society*. doi:1461444814541943

Gamson, W. A. (1992). The social psychology of collective action. In A. D. Morris & C. M. Mueller (Eds.), *Frontiers in social movement theory* (pp. 53–76). New Haven, CT: Yale University Press.

Gee, A., Khalaf, A., & McGarty, C. (2007). Using group-based interaction to change stereotypes about people with mental disorders. *Australian Psychologist, 42*(2), 98–105. doi:10.1080/00050060701280581

Goodin, R. E. (1992). *Motivating political morality*. Oxford: Wiley–Blackwell.

Graffigna, G., Barello, S., Riva, G., & Bosio, A. C. (2014). Patient Engagement: The key to redesign the exchange between the demand and supply for healthcare in the era of active ageing. In G. Riva, P. Ajmone Marsan, & C. Grassi (Eds.), *Active Ageing and Healthy Living* (pp. 85–95). Amsterdam, The Netherlands: IOS Press; doi:10.3233/978-1-61499-425-1-85

Guyatt, G. H., Mulla, S. M., Scott, I. A., Jackevicius, C. A., & You, J. J. (2014). Patient engagement and shared decision-making. *Journal of General Internal Medicine, 29*(4), 562. doi:10.1007/s11606-013-2727-3 PMID:24464283

Halpern, D., & Gibbs, J. (2013). Social media as a catalyst for online deliberation? Exploring the affordances of Facebook and YouTube for political expression. *Computers in Human Behavior, 29*(3), 1159–1168. doi:10.1016/j.chb.2012.10.008

Hardin, R. (1971). Collective action as an agreeable "n"-Prisoners' dilemma. *Behavioral Science, 16*(5), 472–481. doi:10.1002/bs.3830160507

Høybye, M. T., Dalton, S. O., Deltour, I., Bidstrup, P. E., Frederiksen, K., & Johansen, C. (2010). Effect of Internet peer-support groups on psychosocial adjustment to cancer: A randomised study. *British Journal of Cancer, 102*(9), 1348–1354. doi:10.1038/sj.bjc.6605646 PMID:20424614

Hsieh, E. (2004). Stories in action and the dialogic management of identities: Storytelling in transplant support group meetings. *Research on Language and Social Interaction, 37*(1), 39–70. doi:10.1207/s15327973rlsi3701_2

Jennings, M. K. (1999). Political responses to pain and loss. *The American Political Science Review, 93*(1), 1–15. doi:10.2307/2585757

Jetten, J., Haslam, C., & Haslam, S. A. (2012). *The social cure: Identity, health, and well-being*. London, UK: Psychology Press.

Jost, J. T., & Major, B. (2001). *The psychology of legitimacy: Emerging perspectives on ideology, justice, and inter-group relations*. New York: Cambridge University Press.

Kapiriri, L., Norheim, O. F., & Martin, D. K. (2007). Priority setting at the micro-, mesoandmacro-levels in Canada, Norway and Uganda. *Health Policy (Amsterdam)*, *82*(1), 78–94. doi:10.1016/j.healthpol.2006.09.001 PMID:17034898

Khan, S. S., Hopkins, N., Reicher, S., Tewari, S., Srinivasan, N., & Stevenson, C. (2014). Shared identity predicts enhanced health at a mass gathering. *Group Processes & Intergroup Relations*, *18*(4), 504–522. doi:10.1177/1368430214556703

Klandermans, B. (1984). Mobilization and participation: Social-psychological expansions of resource mobilization theory. *American Sociological Review*, *49*(5), 583–600. doi:10.2307/2095417

Klandermans, B. (1997). *The social psychology of protest*. Oxford: Basic Blackwell.

Klandermans, B. (2004). The demand and supply of participation: Social-psychological correlates of participation in social movements. In D. A. Snow, S. A. Soule, & H. Kriesi (Eds.), *The Blackwell Companion to Social Movements* (pp. 360–379). Blackwell Publishing; doi:10.1002/9780470999103.ch16

Klandermans, B., & Oegema, D. (1987). Potentials, networks, motivations, and barriers: Steps toward participationin social movements. *American Sociological Review*, *52*(4), 519–531. doi:10.2307/2095297

Klandermans, B., & Van Stekelenburg, J. (2013). Social movements and participation in collective Action. In D. O. Sears, L. Huddy, & R. Jervis (Eds.), *Oxford handbook of Political psychology* (pp. 774–812). Oxford: University Press; doi:10.1093/oxfordhb/9780199760107.013.0024

Klawiter, M. (1999). Racing for the cure, walking women, andtoxic touring. Mapping cultures of action within the BayArea terrain of breast cancer: Programs and organizationalprocesses. *Social Problems*, *46*(1), 104–126. doi:10.2307/3097164

Kleinman, A. (1988). *The illness narrative: Suffering, healing, and the human condition*. New York: Basic Books.

Kostova, Z., Caiata-Zufferey, M., & Schulz, P. J. (2014). The process of acceptance among rheumatoid arthritis patients in Switzerland: A qualitative study. *Pain Research & Management*, *19*(2), 61–68. doi:10.1155/2014/168472 PMID:24527466

Laubie, R., & Elie-Dit-Cosaque, C. (2012, December 16-19). Exploring and predicting online collective action on patients' virtual communities: a multi-method investigation in France. *Research Paper presented at ICIS12*, Orlando, Florida, USA.

Lee, E. J. (2007). Deindividuation effects on group polarization in computer-mediated communication: The role of group identification, public-self-awareness, and perceived argument quality. *Journal of Communication*, *57*(2), 385–403. doi:10.1111/j.1460-2466.2007.00348.x

Leventhal, G. S. (1980). What should be done with equity theory? Newapproaches to the study of fairness in social relationships. In K. Gergen, M. Greenberg, & R. Willis (Eds.), *Social exchanges: Advances in theoryand research* (pp. 27–55). New York: Plenum. doi:10.1007/978-1-4613-3087-5_2

Lind, E. A., & Tyler, T. R. (1988). *The social psychology of proceduraljustice*. New York: Plenum.

Major, B. (1994). In M. P. Zanna (Ed.), *From social inequality to personal entitlement: The role of social comparisons, legitimacy appraisals, and group membership* (Vol. 26, pp. 293–355). Advances in experimental social psychology San Diego, CA: Academic Press.

Marwell, G., & Oliver, P. (1993). *The critical mass in collective action: A micro-social theory*. Cambridge: Cambridge University Press. doi:10.1017/CBO9780511663765

Mazanderani, F., O'Neill, B., & Powell, J. (2013). "People power" or "pester power"? YouTube as a forum for the generation of evidence and patient advocacy. *Patient Education and Counseling*, *93*(3), 420–425. doi:10.1016/j.pec.2013.06.006 PMID:23830239

Mazzoni, D., & Cicognani, E. (2014). Sharing experiences and social support requests in an Internet forum for patients with Systemic Lupus Erythematosus (SLE). *Journal of Health Psychology*, *19*(5), 689–696. doi:10.1177/1359105313477674 PMID:23479300

Mazzoni, D., Van Zomeren, M., & Cicognani, E. (2015). The motivating role of perceived right violation and efficacy beliefs in identification with the Italian Water Movement. *The Journal of Positive Psychology*, *36*(3), 315–330. doi:10.1111/pops.12101

McCarthy, J. D., & Zald, M. N. (1977). Resource mobilization and social movements: A partial theory. *American Journal of Sociology*, *82*(6), 1212–1241. doi:10.1086/226464

Miller, D. T. (2001). Disrespect and the experience of injustice. *Annual Review of Psychology*, *52*(1), 527–553. doi:10.1146/annurev.psych.52.1.527 PMID:11148316

Mueller, C. (1994). Conflict networks and the origins of women's liberation. In H. Johnston, E. Larana, & J. R. Gusfield (Eds.), *New Social movements. From ideology toidentity* (pp. 234–263). Philadelphia: Temple University Press.

Olson, M. (1965). *The logic of collective action: public goods and the theory of groups*. Cambridge, MA: Harvard University Press.

Opp, K. D. (1986). Soft incentives and collective action. Participation in the Anti-Nuclear Movement. *British Journal of Political Science*, *16*(01), 87–112. doi:10.1017/S0007123400003811

Orizio, G., Schulz, P., Gasparotti, C., Caimi, L., & Gelatti, U. (2010). The world of e-patients: A content analysis of online social networks focusing on diseases. *Telemedicine Journal and e-Health*, *16*(10), 1060–1066. doi:10.1089/tmj.2010.0085 PMID:21070131

Owen-Smith, A., Coast, J., & Donovan, J. (2009). "I can see where they're coming from, but when you're on the end of it ... you just want to get the money and the drug.": Explaining reactions to explicit healthcare rationing. *Social Science & Medicine*, *68*(11), 1935–1942. doi:10.1016/j.socscimed.2009.03.024 PMID:19375210

Paxton, P. (2002). Social capital and democracy: An interdependentrelationship. *American Sociological Review, 67*(2), 254–277. doi:10.2307/3088895

Pettigrew, T. F. (1967). Social evaluation theory. In D. Levine (Ed.), *Nebraska symposium on motivation* (pp. 241–315). Lincoln: Nebraska University Press.

Postmes, T. (2007). The psychological dimensions of collective action, online. In A. N. Joinson, K. Y. McKenna, T. Postmes, & U. D. Reips (Eds.), *The Oxford handbook of Internet psychology* (pp. 165–184). Oxford: Oxford University Press.

Postmes, T., Haslam, S. A., & Swaab, R. I. (2005). Social identity and social influence in small groups: Communication, consensualization and socially shared cognition. *European Review of Social Psychology, 16*, 1–42. doi:10.1080/10463280440000062

Postmes, T., Spears, R., Lee, A. T., & Novak, R. J. (2005). Individuality and social influence in groups: Inductive and deductive routes to group identity. *Journal of Personality and Social Psychology, 89*(5), 747–763. doi:10.1037/0022-3514.89.5.747 PMID:16351366

Putnam, R. (2000). *Bowling Alone: The Collapse and Revival of American Community*. New York: Simon and Schuster. doi:10.1145/358916.361990

Rabeharisoa, V. (2006). From representation to mediation: The shaping of collective mobilization on muscular dystrophy in France. *Social Science & Medicine, 62*(3), 564–576. doi:10.1016/j.socscimed.2005.06.036 PMID:16051407

Rabinow, P. (2002). Artificiality and enlightnment: From sociobiology to biosociality. In M. Biagioli (Ed.), The Science Studies Reader. New York: Routledge.

Radin, P. (2006). "To me, it's my life": Medical communication, trust, and activism in cyberspace. *Social Science & Medicine, 62*(3), 591–601. doi:10.1016/j.socscimed.2005.06.022 PMID:16039031

Reicher, S. (1984). The St Paul's riot: An explanation ofthe limits of crowd action in terms of a socialidentity model. *European Journal of Social Psychology, 14*(1), 1–21. doi:10.1002/ejsp.2420140102

Reicher, S., Spears, R., & Postmes, T. (1995). A social identity model of deindividuation phenomena. *European Review of Social Psychology, 6*(1), 161–198. doi:10.1080/14792779443000049

Runciman, W. G. (1966). *Relative deprivation and social justice: A study of attitudes to social inequality in twentieth-century England*. Berkeley: University of California Press.

Schur, L., Shields, T., & Schriner, K. (2003). Can I make a difference? Efficacy, employment, and disability. *Political Psychology, 24*(1), 119–149. doi:10.1111/0162-895X.00319

Scotch, R. K. (1988). Disability as the basis of a social movement: Advocacy and the politics of definition. *The Journal of Social Issues, 44*(1), 159–172. doi:10.1111/j.1540-4560.1988.tb02055.x

Shah, D. V., Cho, J., Eveland, W. P., & Kwak, N. (2005). Information and expression in a digital age: Modeling Internet effects on civic participation. *Communication Research, 32*(5), 531–565. doi:10.1177/0093650205279209

Shaw, B. R., McTavish, F., Hawkins, R., Gustafson, D. H., & Pingree, S. (2000). Experienceso f women with breast cancer; Exchanging social support over the CHESS computer network. *Journal of Health Communication*, *5*(2), 135–159. doi:10.1080/108107300406866 PMID:11010346

Simon, B., & Grabow, O. (2010). The politicization of migrants: Further evidence that politicized collective identity is a dual identity. *Political Psychology*, *31*(5), 717–738. doi:10.1111/j.1467-9221.2010.00782.x

Simon, B., & Klandermans, B. (2001). Politicized collective identity: A social psychological analysis. *The American Psychologist*, *56*(4), 319–331. doi:10.1037/0003-066X.56.4.319 PMID:11330229

Simon, B., Loewy, M., Stürmer, S., Weber, U., Freytag, P., & Habig, C. et al. (1998). Collective identification and social movement participation. *Journal of Personality and Social Psychology*, *74*(3), 646–658. doi:10.1037/0022-3514.74.3.646

Skitka, L. J., Bauman, C. W., & Sargis, E. G. (2005). Moral conviction: Another contributor to attitude strength or something more? *Journal of Personality and Social Psychology*, *88*(6), 895–917. doi:10.1037/0022-3514.88.6.895 PMID:15982112

Spears, R., & Lea, M. (1994). Panacea or panopticon? The hidden power of computer-mediated communication. *Communication Research*, *21*(4), 427–459. doi:10.1177/009365094021004001

Spears, R., Lea, M., Corneliussen, R. A., Postmes, T., & Ter Haar, W. (2002). Computer mediated communication as a channel for social resistance - The strategic side of SIDE. *Small Group Research*, *33*(5), 555–574. doi:10.1177/104649602237170

Stouffer, S. A., Suchman, E. A., DeVinney, L. C., Star, S. A., & Williams Jr, R. M. (1949). Adjustment during army Me. In *Studies in social psychology in World War II* (Vol. 1, pp. 379-387).

Stromer-Galley, J., & Wichowski, A. (2010). Political discussion online. In R. M. Burnett, M. Consalvo, & C. Ess (Eds.), *The handbook of Internet studies* (pp. 168–187). Chichester, UK: John Wiley & Sons.

Stryker, S., Owens, T. J., & White, R. W. (2000). *Self, identity, and social movements* (Vol. 13). Minneapolis: University of Minnesota Press.

Stuart, A., Thomas, E. F., Donaghue, N., & Russell, A. (2013). "We may be pirates, but we are not protesters": Identity in the Sea Shepherd Conservation Society. *Political Psychology*, *34*, 753–777. doi:10.1111/pops.12016

Stürmer, S., & Simon, B. (2004). The role of collective identification in social movement participation: A panel study in the context of the German gay movement. *Personality and Social Psychology Bulletin*, *30*(3), 263–277. doi:10.1177/0146167203256690 PMID:15030619

Sullivan, C. F. (2003). Gendered cybersupport: A thematic analysis of two online cancersupport groups. *Journal of Health Psychology*, *8*(1), 83–104. doi:10.1177/1359105303008001446 PMID:22113903

Tajfel, H., & Turner, J. (1986). The social identity theory of intergroup behaviour. In S. Worchel & W. G. Austin (Eds.), *Psychology of intergroup relations* (pp. 33–47). Chicago: Nelson.

Tetlock, P. E. (2002). Social functionalist frameworks for judgment and choice: Intuitive politicians, theologians, and prosecutors. *Psychological Review*, *109*(3), 451–471. doi:10.1037/0033-295X.109.3.451 PMID:12088240

Thomas, E. F., Mavor, K. I., & McGarty, C. (2012). Social identities facilitate and encapsulate action-relevant constructs: A test of the social identity model of collective action. *Group Processes & Intergroup Relations*, *15*(1), 75–88. doi:10.1177/1368430211413619

Thomas, E. F., & McGarty, C. (2009). The role of efficacy and moral outrage norms in creating the potential for international development activism through group-based interaction. *The British Journal of Social Psychology*, *48*(1), 115–134. doi:10.1348/014466608X313774 PMID:18534045

Thomas, E. F., Smith, L. G. E., McGarty, C., & Postmes, T. (2010). Nice and nasty: The formation of prosocial and hostile social movements. *Revue Internationale de Psychologie Sociale*, *23*(2), 5–43.

Turner, J. C. (1982). Towards a cognitive redefinition of the social group. In H. Tajfel (Ed.), *Social identity and intergroup relations* (pp. 15–40). Cambridge: Cambridge University Press.

Turner, J. C., Hogg, M. A., Oakes, P. J., Reicher, S. D., & Wetherell, M. S. (1987). *Rediscovering the social group: A self-categorization perspective*. Oxford: Basil Blackwell.

Turner, J. W., Grube, J. A., & Meyers, J. (2001). Developing an optimal match withinonline communities: An exploration of CMC support community and traditional support. *Journal of Communication*, *51*(2), 231–251. doi:10.1111/j.1460-2466.2001.tb02879.x

Tyler, T. R., Boeckmann, R. J., Smith, H. J., & Huo, Y. J. (1997). *Social justice in a diverse society*. Oxford, England: Westview Press.

Van den Bos, K., & Lind, E. A. (2002). In M. P. Zanna (Ed.), *Uncertainty management by meansof fairness judgments* (Vol. 34, pp. 1–60). Advances in experimentalsocial psychology San Diego, CA: Academic Press.

Van Stekelenburg, J. (2013). The political psychology of protest: Sacrificing for a cause. *European Psychologist*, *18*(4), 224–234. doi:10.1027/1016-9040/a000156

Van Stekelenburg, J., & Klandermans, B. (2009). Social movement theory: Past, present and prospect. *Movers and shakers: Social movements in Africa, 8*, 17.

Van Stekelenburg, J., & Klandermans, B. (2013). The social psychology of protest. *Current Sociology Review*, *61*(5-6), 886–905. doi:10.1177/0011392113479314

van Uden-Kraan, C. F., Drossaert, C. H., Taal, E., Shaw, B. R., Seydel, E. R., & van de Laar, M. A. (2008). Empowering processes and outcomes of participation in online support groups for patients with breast cancer, arthritis, or fibromyalgia. *Qualitative Health Research*, *18*(3), 405–417. doi:10.1177/1049732307313429 PMID:18235163

Van Zomeren, M. (2011). Four core social-psychological motivations to undertake collective action. *Social and Personality Psychology Compass*, *7*(6), 378–388. doi:10.1111/spc3.12031

Van Zomeren, M., & Iyer, A. (2009). Introduction to the social and psychological dynamics of collective action. *The Journal of Social Issues*, *65*(4), 645–660. doi:10.1111/j.1540-4560.2009.01618.x

Van Zomeren, M., & Lodewijkx, H. F. M. (2005). Motivated responses to 'senseless' violence: Explaining emotional and behavioural responses through person and position identification. *European Journal of Social Psychology*, *35*(6), 755–766. doi:10.1002/ejsp.274

Van Zomeren, M., Postmes, T., & Spears, R. (2008). Toward an integrative social identity model of collective action: A quantitative research synthesis of three socio-psychological perspectives. *Psychological Bulletin*, *134*(4), 504–535. doi:10.1037/0033-2909.134.4.504 PMID:18605818

Van Zomeren, M., Postmes, T., & Spears, R. (2012). On conviction's collective consequences: Integrating moral conviction with the socialidentity model of collective action. *The British Journal of Social Psychology*, *51*(1), 52–71. doi:10.1111/j.2044-8309.2010.02000.x PMID:22435846

Van Zomeren, M., Postmes, T., Spears, R., & Bettache, K. (2011). Can moral convictions motivate the advantaged to challenge social inequality? Extending the social identity model of collective action. *Group Processes & Intergroup Relations*, *14*(5), 735–753. doi:10.1177/1368430210395637

Van Zomeren, M., Saguy, T., & Schellhaas, F. M. H. (2013). Believing in "making a difference" to collective efforts: Participative efficacy beliefs as a unique predictor of collective action. *Group Processes & Intergroup Relations*, *16*(5), 618–634. doi:10.1177/1368430212467476

Van Zomeren, M., & Spears, A. (2009). Metaphors of protest: A classification of motivations for collective action. *The Journal of Social Issues*, *65*(4), 661–680. doi:10.1111/j.1540-4560.2009.01619.x

Van Zomeren, M., Spears, R., Fischer, A. H., & Leach, C. W. (2004). Put your money where your mouth is!: Explaining collective action tendencies through group-based anger and group efficacy. *Journal of Personality and Social Psychology*, *87*(5), 649–664. doi:10.1037/0022-3514.87.5.649 PMID:15535777

Walker, I., & Smith, H. J. (2002). *Relative deprivation: Specification, development, and integration*. Cambridge, England: Cambridge University Press.

Weinberg, N., Schmale, J. D., Uken, J., & Wessel, K. (1996). Online help: Cancer patients participate in a computer mediated support group. *Health & Social Work*, *21*, 24–29. doi:10.1093/hsw/21.1.24 PMID:8626154

Witteman, H. O., & Zikmund-Fisher, B. J. (2012). The defining characteristics of Web 2.0 and their potential influence in the online vaccination debate. *Vaccine*, *30*(25), 3734–3740. doi:10.1016/j.vaccine.2011.12.039 PMID:22178516

Wojcieszak, M. E. (2011). Computer-mediated false consensus: Radical online groups, social networks and news media. *Mass Communication & Society*, *14*(4), 527–546. doi:10.1080/15205436.2010.513795

Wright, K. (2002). Social support within an online cancer community: An assessment of emotional support, perceptions of advantages and disadvantages, and motives for usingthe community from a communication perspective. *Journal of Applied Communication*, *30*(3), 195–209. doi:10.1080/00909880216586

Wright, S. C., Taylor, D. M., & Moghaddam, F. M. (1990). Responding to membership in a disadvantaged group: From acceptance to collective protest. *Journal of Personality and Social Psychology*, *58*(6), 994–1003. doi:10.1037/0022-3514.58.6.994

Zoller, H. (2005). Health activism: Communication theory and action for social change. *Communication Theory*, *15*(4), 341–364. doi:10.1111/j.1468-2885.2005.tb00339.x

KEY TERMS AND DEFINITIONS

Active Citizenship Network: An umbrella association of about 100 civic organizations from 30 countries aimed towards developing a European Active citizenship.

Collective action: A specific form of participation where individuals undertake actions as group members, with the aim to improve the group's conditions. It is proposed in contrast to individual action, that is specifically directed at improving one's personal conditions rather than group.

European Charter of Patients' Rights: Drafted in 2002 by Active Citizenship Network in collaboration with 12 citizens' organizations from different EU countries, it states 14 patients' rights that together aim to guarantee a "high level of human health protection" and to assure the high quality of services provided by the various national health services in Europe.

Moral convictions: Strong and absolute stances on moral issues, they do not tolerate any exceptions to the general 'higher-order' principle.

Participative efficacy: The belief that individual's participations matters – i.e., that the individual's participation is seen as having a potential incremental effect on collective action.

Self-efficacy: Individual's belief in his/her ability to execute behaviors necessary to reach goals and to produce specific performance attainments.

Social Psychology: The scientific field that seeks to understand the nature and causes of individual behavior in social situations.

Section 3

Reforming Healthcare Organizations and Practices in the Light of Patients Participation and Engagement

Chapter 8
The Patient Centered Organizational Model in Italian Hospitals:
Practical Challenges for Patient Engagement

Mara Gorli
Università Cattolica del Sacro Cuore, Milan, Italy

Elisa G. Liberati
Università Cattolica del Sacro Cuore, Milan, Italy

Laura Galuppo
Università Cattolica del Sacro Cuore, Milan, Italy

Giuseppe Scaratti
Università Cattolica del Sacro Cuore, Milan, Italy

ABSTRACT

The concepts of patient-centered care and patient engagement are often used interchangeably in health policy debates. In fact, it is frequently – and implicitly – assumed that putting patients at the centre of care will more or less spontaneously lead to fully engaged patients. This chapter questions these assumptions. By focusing on the hospital's patient-centered reform in Italy, the chapter discusses the overlaps but also the discrepancies between the practices of putting patients at the centre and those of engaging patients. Discrepancies may appear at three levels: the new hospital model may challenge the establishment of a close alliance between patients and professionals, the new hospital spaces may not be perceived as a catalyst for improving patients' experiences, and the inter- and intra- professional struggles derived from the new configuration of hospital teams at an early stage may hinder patient care delivery. The chapter proposes some strategies for patient-centered hospitals to increase their capacity to engage patients and families in the management of their care plan.

DOI: 10.4018/978-1-4666-9992-2.ch008

INTRODUCTION

Today, patient centeredness is considered an essential dimension of the quality of healthcare and a central element of the mission of healthcare organizations (Berwick, 2009; Institute of Medicine [IOM], 2001). Patient centeredness is an approach to health care that emphasizes the limitations of a disease-centered model and calls for an exploration of patients' needs, preferences, values, and concerns with the aim of increasing patients' involvement in the management of their care plan (International Alliance of Patients Organizations [IAPO], 2007).

In a recently published article (Liberati et al., 2015), a narrative review was conducted on the concept of patient-centered care, which showed how this research field could be broadly classified into two main streams. The first and more traditional stream, which is labelled 'dyadic', addresses patient centeredness at a micro level and focuses on the relationship and interaction between individual clinicians and patients (Levenstein, Mccracken, Mcwhinney, Stewart, & Brown, 1986; Bensing, 2000; Stewart et al., 2000), a second stream of research includes more recent publications with a shared aim of identifying organizational facilitators and system-level barriers to patient-centered care. This organizational stream addresses patient centeredness at the macro level and looks at the structural, cultural, and procedural dimensions of healthcare organizations that can help achieve a patient-centered approach (Bergeson & Dean, 2006; Greene, Tuzzio, & Cherkin, 2012; Hernandez, Conrad, Marcus-Smith, Reed, & Watts, 2013; Luxford, Safran, & Delbanco, 2011; Shaller, 2007). This chapter leans on this organizational stream to address the specific challenge of improving healthcare services in the direction of patient centeredness, and it specifically considers the distinction between the concepts of "centered" and "engagement." In fact, despite the overlap in recent debates of the terms "patient centeredness" with the concept of "patient engagement," we argue that, when considering both the literature and the concrete practices through which healthcare services are designed and managed, the two terms may inform very different improvement plans.

Indeed, "patient centeredness" has become a *buzzword* that serves a variety of purposes and is interpreted according to a variety of meanings. Within the broader philosophy of patient centeredness, the concept of patient engagement has pushed further the idea that patients can experience different degrees of participation in their health care experience, thus affecting the cure process itself. In this scenario, it is often assumed that putting patients at the centre automatically leads to a condition of full patient engagement, whereby patients become participants and co-constructors of their health and are capable of improving their quality of life (Barello et al., 2015).

The concept of patient engagement qualifies the type of relationship that the patients establish with their healthcare system of reference (the provision of medical services) at different levels (Carman et al., 2013; Graffigna, Barello, Riva, & Bosio, 2014). The notion of engagement refers both to patient activation (namely the patient's knowledge, skills, ability, and willingness to manage his or her own health and care, e.g., by adopting measures of preventive care, following a balanced diet, or exercising regularly) and to a broader set of interventions designed to increase patients' participation in designing and managing the healthcare delivery systems themselves.

Focusing on the hospital's patient-centered reform, the issue tackled in this chapter is whether or not designing and managing a hospital according to the philosophy of putting the patient at the centre implies active engagement and participation from the patient in his or her care and healing process.

The patient-centered hospital model, as it is commonly known within the academic community, represents an attempt to reshape the care delivery according to the needs of the patients and their care processes, moving away from the traditional physician-centered view (Lega & DePietro, 2005; McKee & Healy, 2002), thus resulting in a rather disruptive cultural change. The patient-centered model (henceforth PCM) requires reshaping hospitals' organizational structure, social and professional practices, and care delivery processes and the modification of hospitals' relative positioning in the healthcare ecosystem. These changes are considered to have consequences on the patients' care experience.

This chapter explores specifically how patient centeredness has been translated into practice through the Italian hospital reform, and it critically discusses the overlaps but also the discrepancies between the practices of putting patients at the centre and of engaging patients. By referring both methods to the literature and to several case studies, the pursued argument is that the new, practiced hospital model on patient centeredness might not guarantee *per se* the process of patients' full engagement (Gorli, Galuppo, & Liberati, 2015a). This analysis is particularly significant in contexts such as Italy, where the patient-centered hospital reform is in its initial stage and has not yet crystallized in a formal and standardized model. In such a context, it is possible to determine in rich detail how the macro-level shift affects the daily experience of patients and healthcare professionals, resulting in the expected and desired changes and giving rise to unexpected challenges. The chapter concludes the analysis by highlighting some possible steps and solutions that could bring the renewed hospitals towards a full process of patient engagement.

PATIENT-CENTERED HOSPITALS: RESHAPING CARE DELIVERY PROCESSES AROUND THE NEEDS OF THE PATIENT

National Healthcare Systems (NHS) worldwide are confronted with increasing challenges, for example, the rising social needs and economic obligations. Patients' increased health literacy and awareness of their rights are leading to new, legitimate public expectations for healthcare service renewal. The increasing demand for homecare, patients' requests for access to their own health records from home, and patients' requests for more engaging and equal access to health care provide further evidence of this changing scenario.

Patient centeredness has become one of the most frequent solutions to such demands and has inspired several hospital reforms (Lega & DePietro, 2005; McKee & Healy, 2002), both in Europe and the United States. In this chapter, we refer to this organizational paradigm as the Patient-Centered Model (henceforth PCM). Evidence of the trends towards the PCM is offered by some landmark studies recently published in this field. Lega and DePietro's extensive literature review (2005) suggests that hospitals worldwide "have started converging patterns of change toward a common paradigm: the care-focused organization.... Emerging trends seem to drive the reshaping of the hospital delivering processes around the needs of care processes and patients and away from the traditional physician-centered view" (pp. 267-268). The review comprises both European and US hospitals; specific references are made to the following countries/regions: France, UK, Italy, Germany, Spain, the United States, and Latin America. In their book, "Hospitals in a Changing Europe", McKee and Healy (2002) also describe the general trend toward the PCM. The authors suggest that "the patient-focused hospital concept represents an attempt to redesign or re-engineer the care delivery process... [which] is now evident in many European countries, including England (Hurst, 1995), the Netherlands (Bainton, van der Steeg, & Weeda, 1995), Spain (Coulson-Thomas, 1996), and Sweden (Brodersen & Thorwid, 1997)" (p. 233). This kind of reorganization is expected to increase the efficiency of care delivery and also to contribute to lower costs and expenses.

To innovate towards a patient-centered approach, hospitals usually go through a process of reorganization that encompasses several restructuring actions, both in the organizational structure and in the building. The entire hospital system is affected by the patient-centered model and by what follows; i.e. some converging patterns of processes and system restructuring (Lega & DePietro, 2005). The central idea of patient-centered restructuring is that organizing a hospital around care processes, rather than medical specialties, increases the effectiveness of care, reduces cost, and improves the quality of patients' experience (Vera & Kunz, 2007).

Although it is self-evident that care should address the need and centrality of patients, in reality, many hospitals are traditionally run with more consideration for the convenience of staff. Thus, in the traditional hospital model, patients are admitted under individual specialist clinicians who can either keep them or transfer them to the care of another clinician. In organizational terms, these mechanisms reflect a *functional* structure in which specialists with a similar area of expertise are grouped into independently controlled departments, thus defining patients' location on the basis of their prevalent pathology. Conceptually, the functional model mirrors a professional-centered culture, whereby patients are organized and managed according to the medical specialties rather than to an assessment of their overall care needs, which might be different from patients affected by the same pathology. This system has in fact shown some shortcomings, such as the many patients' internal transfers within the same hospital structure, associated with an increasing need to control the workflow across departments and thus the coordination of the care activities within a patient care trajectory. Moreover, in the functional organization, resources tend to be duplicated, leading to waste, and the autonomy in using the specialty's resources often prevails over accountability, in some cases reducing the effectiveness of treatments (Vos et al., 2011; Villa, Barbieri, & Lega, 2009; Lega & DePietro, 2005). As a solution to this problem, the core principle of the PCM includes the delivery of the adequate amount of cure and care to patients in the most suitable setting according to their health conditions. Patients are grouped in multi-specialty units (that substitute the traditional specialty-based units) differentiated by the level of patients' clinical and nursing care needs (high, medium, or low intensity of care need) instead of their specific pathologies. In this way, patients' pathways and hospital personnel are organized according to the severity of the conditions of different groups of patients.

Moreover, hospitals have to create a different use of resources such as beds, operating rooms, and equipment, which have to be aggregated and shared by all functional specialties and which require a centralized logistical regulation. The goal is to cease transferring patients across different units or departments; instead, physicians and technologies move to the patients' bedside.

This often entails a redesign of hospital internal functioning, organizational structure, and processes. Such major changes concern first the redesign of the organizational model, which shifts from a functional model to a process-oriented model, and second the care and recovery processes put in place by clinicians (McKee & Healy, 2002). From the standpoint of health professionals, in fact, the new criteria for patients' placement demand that single-specialty units and their staff be regrouped or merged into bigger, multi-specialty units. Such units integrate different specialties and clinicians' competences while sharing the same head nurse and nursing group. Moreover, doctors may treat patients who are physically located in different units, and nurses have to assist patients with different pathologies.

Such a broad innovation is facilitated by its accompaniment with a new physical restructuring of the hospital building, which may enable the new management of wards, ward interconnection, and flow of patients and personnel. In order to produce an effective function, the new "house" must then be inhabited by new professional roles and responsibilities. Integration of care, collaboration, supply coordination, bed management, and case management (for establishing patients' location) are new essential functions that must be safeguarded with profound implications on personnel.

The published studies on PCM (e.g. Lega & De Pietro, 2005; McKee & Healy, 2002; Villa et al., 2009) suggest that this hospital model is designed to meet the needs of patients and their families in several ways:

1. The criteria for patient placement and resource allocation increasingly consider the patient as a whole person rather than a "sick organ", which is acknowledged as one of the keystones of the patient-centered paradigm (Berwick, 2009; Mead & Bower, 2000; Stewart et al., 2000). Moreover, the patient-centered hospital is based on the principle that personnel and technologies, rather than the patients, are the ones that should move inside the hospital. While this shift could appear trivial, it must be considered that the functional hospital model – developed around the growth of medical specialties – has characterized the history of the modern hospitals in several countries and contributed to the establishment of a doctor-centered formal and informal organization, which is often very resistant to change. For this reason, the shift toward an organizational model that shifts the focus of attention from the needs of professionals to the overall care needs of the patients can be regarded as a rather disruptive cultural change.
2. The focus of the new organizational paradigm is on the care process rather than on single treatments; this perspective calls for increased attention to vertical and horizontal integration among providers and for enhanced inter-professional and inter-disciplinary collaboration among health practitioners. In fact, patients should not be burdened any longer with the responsibility of linking and integrating different providers and should not experience inconsistencies of opinions and decisions. Rather, the organization must be in charge of integrating and coordinating the different care actors, thus also safeguarding the care process quality.
3. Once the new hospital starts working properly, the model should ensure shorter hospitalization time, better integration, and shorter waiting lists for operations, among other care services.

DISCREPANCIES BETWEEN THE PATIENT-CENTERED HOSPITAL MODEL AND THE CONCEPT OF PATIENT ENGAGEMENT

The aspects of the PCM certainly bear some clear benefits with respect to the previous organizational model. However, when considering not only the *political narratives* around PCM – namely, how the shift towards a PCM appears in official discourses – but also the *practical narratives* – i.e., how this shift is described and practiced in patients and professionals' mundane activities (Liberati et al., 2015; Liberati, Gorli, & Scaratti, in press) – some discrepancies may arise.

Such discrepancies may include the ways in which both patients and health professionals actually experience the newly organized hospital and whether the practices generated within a PCM hospital are connected to the patients' engagement in their care plan.

First, PCM is assumed to inform a disruptive cultural change; however, how is this change "inhabited" by patients in their everyday experience of healthcare services? What do patients think of such a change? Do patients and families appreciate it as an effective strategy to enhance their engagement and participation in their care management?

Second, it should be considered that the concept of engagement involves both the patient's engagement in his/her care process and also professionals' engagement in providing high-quality health services (their work engagement). The ways professionals perceive the new hospital configuration has an impact on the ways they will engage with one another and with their patients. How does PCM affect inter-professional and inter-disciplinary collaboration? Do integration and coordination come linearly with the planned change? The literature recommends consideration of this issue with a prudential attention, suggesting, for example, that coordination does not happen as per top-down decision (Okhuysen & Bechky, 2009; Wenger, 1998; Braithwaite, Runciman, & Merry, 2009).

The above questions help to approach the PCM with a critical eye, reflecting on possible consequences and potential discrepancies of this approach, if compared with the patient engagement perspective.

In this section, these arguments are proposed and illustrated throughout insights derived from organizational theories and studies applied to the field of healthcare innovation (i.e. Øvretveit, 2011; Ferlie, Fitzgerald, Wood, & Hawkins, 2013; Braithwaite et al., 2009) as well as through examples derived from our own research experience. The context and methods of the two case studies that inform our discussion are summarised in Table 1.

The examples that follow show that the PCM, as conceptualized at an organizational level, may contrast with patients' and providers' expectations and needs, may focus on aspects that they do not consider important or central, or may actually hinder patients' chance of having input and being engaged in their care. These misalignments appear related to: 1) the new challenges posed by the PCM to the relationships between patients and health professionals, 2) patients' experience of the new hospital spaces and environments, 3) the effects of the change on previously established healthcare teams.

Table 1. Methods and context of the case studies

The first case study focuses on a large multispecialty hospital in northern Italy that was recently relocated to a new building, which was designed according to the patient-centered organizational model. Data for this case are drawn from three main sources: 1) 14 semi-structured qualitative interviews (Silverman, 2010) conducted with senior management members (Directors of nursing Staff and Chief of Medical Staff) between June and December 2013. The interviews included questions on the patient-centered innovation philosophy and care principles (e.g. *What are, in your opinion, the aims of this innovation?*), on the actions adopted locally to implement the patient centered model (e.g. *How is the new model developed in your hospital? Which spaces, structures, and activities have been affected and how?*), and on how the new hospital model affected the experiences of patients. 2) Regular ethnographic observations in the new hospital spaces conducted between January 2014 and May 2015. 3) Informal conversations with frontline nurses and frontline doctors working in different hospital wards in the newly built patient-centered hospital. These were aimed at capturing clinicians' understanding of the patient-centered model and the effects of its introduction on their work life. Whenever possible, the researchers also engaged in brief conversations with patients in order to gather their opinion with respect to the inquired issues. The relocation happened around one year before data collection. This timing allowed capturing experiences and meanings developing in the process of reorganizing. The second case study focuses on patient centered organizational innovations on a smaller scale: it looks at a physical medicine hospital ward that was recently renovated according to patient-centered principles. Ethnographic data for this case were gathered between September 2011 and April 2012 and involved the collection of data of three data types: 1) 8 documents drawn from the hospital's official regulation and the patient documentation of the hospital ward. 2) 80 hours of observations of selected areas of the ward (nurses' station, doctors' offices, the rehabilitation gymnasium, the ward hallways, the team meeting room) and shadowing of frontline clinicians. 3) 5 ethnographic interviews with various members of the ward staff. In this case, we were interested in understanding both how patient centeredness became visible in the ward place and throughout the ward material arrangements, official policies, and internal documents and how patient centeredness was practiced by frontline clinicians in their daily working activities.

The PCM and the Challenges to the Patient-Professional Relationship

As discussed in the previous session, the formal aim of the PCM is to re-organize hospitals around the needs of patients and their care (and away from a professional-centered view) to provide patients with high-quality care in the most suitable care setting (Villa et al., 2009; Lega & DePietro, 2005). However, inquiries into patient-centered hospitals reveal that the new patient-centered hospital sometimes fails to improve the quality of patient-professional relationships and, in the end, to sustain a mutual process of engagement.

For example, several doctors interviewed in the research, believed that the new criteria for patients' placement do not adequately take into account patients' specific clinical needs, thus undermining the importance of the medical specialties. Consequently, care quality and safety were perceived to be at risk. Nurses expressed very similar opinions; they believed that, if the patients grouped in the same unit had clinical needs that differed too much, nurses might lack the specialised competences to treat them properly.

Excerpt 1. [Interview with head nurse, medical ward]

I did not sleep at night for a long time! I feared that something could have happened to the patients... We (nurses) are experienced, but we are also specialised... We are not prepared to assist every kind of patient.

Doctors and nurses also believed that the new criteria for patients' placement might disorient patients rather than improve their care process; clinicians suggested that patients and caregivers' main psychological need is to identify their care provider (the medical specialist) rather than to be placed in the "most adequate care setting".

Excerpt 2. [Interview with a ward manager]

In the previous model we were used to another kind of relationship with our patients. And, you know, I am aware that times have changed and we have to deal with many more patients, with less resources, etcetera. But patients haven't change: they need a unique point of reference, they need to identify "their" doctor, to know where they can find us.... I believe that this new model does not really allow us to be close to the patients as we should. We have to see patients that are spread all over the hospital. The least it can happen is that some of them receive less attention. (...) They (patients) see an awful lot of different providers now, many of whom are not well informed about patients' history, they might give them contradictory information... Maybe I am just a nostalgic old man, but I think that sometimes we should stop this urge of innovating at all costs and reflect a little more on what do we really want to change.

Whereas many patients involved in the study had not experienced the previous (traditional) hospital model (thus being unable to compare it with the new model), their comments often resonated with the opinions of frontline clinicians: they were provided with few occasions to meet their doctors, with obvious consequence on the construction of a trust relationship and therapeutic alliance.

Excerpt 3. [Conversation with a patient, surgical ward]

Doctors are frenetic: they always run, it seems they don't have much time to stop and ask patients how they feel. Nurses, however, they are always here with us. I see them updating doctors constantly, for example in the corridor or whenever they have an occasion to do so. It's not that I don't trust nurses, but sometimes it would be nice to have a more direct contact with doctors.

The excerpts show that the possibility of relying on the physical proximity between doctors and their regular patients is regarded by both actors as an important component of the care experience and therapeutic alliance, despite the broader organizational benefits of creating new groups of patients with the aim to shorten the length of stay and the number of patients' transfers across wards.

Therefore, when attempting to reshape the role of patients and providers in care delivery, standardized improvement principles (no matter how valuable in theory) need to be connected with the expectations and priorities perceived by its main protagonists.

The Experience of New Hospital Spaces: Patients at the Centre of "Someone Else's Space"

The implementation of the PCM often comes as a result of the restructuring of hospital spaces; new (multi-specialty) wards are created to welcome greater numbers of patients and new technology, and other resources are centralized rather than distributed within the wards. This requires hospital managers to invest resources in large-scale restructuring projects. Nevertheless, the need to ensure the success of the overall project may divert hospital managers' attention from patients' everyday experience of the newly built spaces of care. In this way, top-level managers may fail to test whether the philosophy of patient centeredness has taken root beyond the mere physical structure.

Excerpt 4. [Interview with hospital manager]

One of our greater successes is the new organization of the hospital spaces: now all the operating rooms are on the same floor, and day-hospital services are located in the same areas. This means for us a much more efficient organization, and it is an advantage for many patients as well: for example, if they need a blood test plus other medical exams, they can have them performed in one unique area, rather than having to travel around the different specialized wards.

Excerpt 5. [Interview with patient, medical ward]

We have kept reading in the newspaper (for ages!) that the reorganization was ongoing. Now here it is. This is so distant from our old loved hospital! You see: it is a giant monster at the periphery of our city centre. Access and parking costs so much! And when you come here you get lost in one second: they seem to take for granted that we should know where to go… But if you look for a unit, say cardiology… you don't find it anywhere! (…) When my wife came to visit me yesterday, I spent ten minutes on the phone trying to explain to her where to go.

Excerpt 6. [Interview with patient, medical ward]

Okay, I get that the central block is the emergency, and the operating rooms are at the first floor. But where is the inpatients unit? How can I distinguish them? It seems that this hospital has been designed by an architect, rather than by a pool of hospital experts and citizens. It's our money in the end. I think they should have given us a say in how our new hospital was to be built.

Excerpt 7. [Interview with nurse, surgical ward]

This is a very impersonal structure; every building is identical to the other. You cannot imagine how much time I spend guiding patients and caregivers throughout the wards, while addressing patients' complaints about their difficulty identifying their doctor.

These discrepancies resonate with other studies analysing the interpretation and enactment of patient-centered hospitals in other countries. For example, Bromley and colleagues observed that the designers and planners of a hospital interpret patient centeredness in ways that challenge the roles of medical professionals and conflict with nurses' implicit and explicit understanding of their work (Bromley, 2012; Mikesell & Bromley, 2012).

Moreover, in-depth observations inside newly constructed hospitals uncovered other, more subtle, discrepancies between the interpretation and the enactment of 'patient centered spaces' and the daily experiences of patients. For instance, despite practitioners' declared and honest commitment to 'put the patient at the centre' (see Excerpt 8), patients experienced a limited freedom of movement, limited access to space and information, and limited possibilities to manage their own time (see Excerpt 9).

Excerpt 8. [Interview with a head nurse]

We try to improve many aspects of the quality of the hospitalization experience... I think what we try to do is to make patients and their families feel like they were at home. That is why we are constantly thinking about new little things that could make this place comfortable and cozy. For example, we had the living room restructured and provided with a ward library where patients and families could borrow books and magazines. There is a fridge there, dedicated to patients and families, together with a small cart with hot coffee or water, teabags and snacks, which we call the cuddle corner.

Excerpt 9. [Note from the shadowing of a nurse]

A patient's wife accompanies her husband to the toilet and closes the door after them. A nurse tries to get in but the door has been locked. The nurse: "You don't have to lock yourself in!" The wife: "But I am in here with him!" The nurse: "It doesn't matter! Don't you know that one time someone remained locked in there for a week?!" he jokes. The patient's wife looks upset.

As is commonly known, one sees the devil in the details. These excerpts, derived from an ethnographic study on the practice of patient care, teach that the sole attention to the structural side of hospital spaces may not be sufficient to embrace the many different layers of patients' experiences within them. Hospitals spaces, as spaces in any organization, are composed of two intertwined elements: on the one hand, there is a manifest and declared dimension constituted by architectures, structures, materiality, rules, and policies; on the other, there is a tacit – although highly operative – dimension made by the practices and relationships that shape and actively construct those spaces. These two dimensions are expressed in the distinction between the concepts of *place* and *space*. Place indicates a proper space in which the elements that constitute it are organized and controlled by organizational institutions and power relations in a stable form (De Certeau, 1990, pp. 172-173). Space, in contrast, consists of the *practiced* place, namely the arrangement resulting from the many ways in which individuals inhabit the place, position themselves within it, and re-create their own borders. What is of interest for the debate here is that these distinctions make visible the discrepancy between a place *thought* of as being patient centered, and a space *practiced* in ways such as patient cannot feel at the centre of personnel's consideration. Rather, one can imagine that the patient, by experiencing intrusion on privacy and denied intimacy with his/her caregiver, will perceive himself/herself at the periphery of the process of care, with direct consequences on his/her perceived level of engagement.

Struggles in the New Healthcare Teams and Effects on the Delivery of Patient Care

Conceptually, the PCM aims to overcome a professional-centered culture and to address more adequately patients' recovery and caring needs. In practical terms, this implies the establishment of different criteria for patient placement and the consequential re-organization of healthcare teams, which pass from being mono-disciplinary to multi-disciplinary. Despite the potential for competence and skill integration provided by the new teams, social science studies by healthcare professionals show that the mere juxtaposition of professionals with different disciplinary expertise (i.e. multidisciplinary teams) does not guarantee effective collaboration towards the delivery of integrated patient care (i.e. interdisciplinary work) and may affect patients' perceived care quality. Effective care may be hindered by professionals' attempts to protect their jurisdictions, their specialised knowledge, and pre-existent practices (Atwal & Caldwell, 2002; Oborn & Dawson, 2010). Resonating with other studies, our observations in patient-centered hospitals show that health providers differed in their clinical approaches; in their views on what constitutes evidence, safety, and patient centeredness; and in the importance attributed to autonomy or teamwork. These disciplinary boundaries hindered both intra-professional and inter-professional collaboration, with consequences on the delivery of integrated care.

Excerpt 10. [Surgical nurse in a newly created multi-specialty ward]:

... It's like there is a virtual wall separating us. (…) We (neurosurgery) treat the brain, we're a sterile ward, while they (otolaryngology) treat dirty patients, if you know what I mean… They treat the nose, the mouth. It's impossible to work together. They never try to help us. And every time we want to help them it seems that we are doing something wrong... They say to us that they don't do the IV [intravenous] that way, they don't do a bladder wash that way… But seriously, from a clinical point of view, who says that things in the otolaryngology work better than in neuro-surgery? It has become so difficult to work together that someone has even put on a sign on the rooms' door to signal to whom the patients inside them belong.

As the following excerpt shows, these conflicts can have disruptive consequences on the delivery of patient care. Indeed, rather than integrating their complementary skills to deliver better patient care, professionals who are not used to working together may compete over the "ownership" of patients or, on the other hand, may fail to provide the needed attention to patients that are "owned" by others professionals (Dixon-Woods, 2010; Mackintosh & Sandall, 2010; Nugus, Greenfield, Travaglia, Westbrook, & Braithwaite, 2010).

Excerpt 11. [Observational notes from participant observation in a multi-specialty ward]:

A neurologist and a neurology nurse are doing the ward round visit of neurologic patients. A patient's relative (R.) keeps asking whether his beloved is going to be discharged during the day, but nobody is able to answer him. R. goes to the neurology nurse and asks her the same thing. The neurologist intervenes and says: "I'm sorry sir, but we are in the neurologic ward, whilst the patient you are looking for must be in the neuro-surgery. I know we are on the same floor but we are all another clan, we don't know anything about them...

In conclusion, if multi-disciplinary work is not strengthened in practice in the patient-centered hospitals, formal multidisciplinary teams remain more abstract than effective and may include little collaborative activity. As in the previous traditional hospital model, patients may still be seen as "owned" by individual professionals; patients may perceive inconsistencies among the information received, and members of different medical disciplines can make decisions and take actions in ways that substitute (rather than integrate) previous ones.

This section has illustrates three types of potential discrepancies between the way in which PCM is implemented and the outcome of a patient fully engaging in his/her care, capable of activating and managing important aspects of it. The PCM may challenge the establishment of a close alliance and trust relationship between patients and professionals; the new hospital spaces may not be perceived as a catalyst for improving patients' experiences; the inter- and intra- professional struggles derived from the new configuration of hospital teams at an early stage may hinder patient care delivery.

Moreover, a common element emerging from our cases and literature studies is that PCM is usually designed and implemented top-down, following broad policy instruction. While the patient-centered hospital is created to better address patients' expected needs, taking into account both their clinical treatment and their overall health conditions, in the cases reported, patients themselves did not have a say in managing their hospitalization experience. Whereas overcoming a strict focus on patients' pathology, the new hospitals may not explicitly consider patients' social belonging, cultural differences, and potential divergent expectations in the care delivery process. This patient-centered perspective mirrors an image of the patient as a rather standardized subject, and it might fail to account for the complexities introduced by the specific familiar, social, and cultural contexts of the patients. Patients and families carry specific expectations and worldviews, which must be considered and included in the dialogue with the healthcare providers and organizations in order to achieve patient engagement.

FILLING THE GAP AMONG DISCREPANCIES: SOME POSSIBLE DIRECTIONS

The visible discrepancies found by analysing the research and field data are potential problems that patients encounter when facing a new model of hospital care based on the patient-centered philosophy. What does emerge is that the two concepts of patient centeredness and patient engagement in the process of care do not always overlap and do not spontaneously sustain one another.

One reason for this misalignment can be due to the different meanings and scopes of the two labels.

The paper suggests that *centeredness* and *engagement* lean on two slightly different concepts: while the former stresses the idea of having a central place, the latter puts more emphasis on the idea of taking position. The centre can be represented as a symbolic and physical place, affecting motivation, goals, and missions, but the centre is an ambiguous concept itself. It can be regarded as the point around which everything rotates (the vertex of a circumference) or as the point that has to be addressed, the target that has to be hit. Considering somebody as a vertex may mean valuing her/his active participation and power. On the other hand, the image of a target brings the representation of an undesired and unrequested exposure. Being put at the centre can suggest a paternalistic perspective, where who is at the centre is seen as harmless and passive, needing to be anticipated in her/his requests, rather than to be listened and activated.

The concept of engagement, on the other hand, refers to an active positioning of the one who is engaged. It suggests the possibility of being listened to and given space, depending on the resources and powers at play. Sometimes occupying a lateral position may be more functional and attuned to patients' desires rather than a central position. Being engaged may therefore suggest a process of progressive participation in a system of activity. Regardless the place where somebody is positioned, what it is important here is being given the possibility to choose the proper place to take a position that is suitable with ones' desires, capabilities, and perceived autonomy.

Reorienting health organizations towards either patient centeredness or patient engagement, therefore, can generate very different practices.

The mismatches between the actual experiences of frontline clinicians and patients in PCM hospitals and what is needed for sustaining an effective patient engagement illustrates that it is necessary to refine our lenses and to critically reflect on which interpretation of centeredness and engagement are put in practice in any organizational reform. These two terms may in effect inform a variety of organizational solutions, depending on the given interpretations, perspectives, and interests at play in specific contexts, cultures, and histories.

The possibility of considering patient centeredness as the viaticum of patient engagement should therefore not be taken for granted, since it requires a delicate balance between patients' and professionals' expectations and organizational configurations. It requires placing value on the patient as the point around which everything rotates in a way that makes him or her feel listened to regarding his or her own specific needs and positioning preferences.

The recent international literature offers some examples of how PCM hospitals can address the complex challenges posed by the need to engage patients by putting them at the centre. Several practices and many different engaging settings can be promoted in this direction. First, hospitals may increase patients' and families' participation in the direct care. Second, they can systematically monitor patients' experience and gather feedback and suggestions for improving the organization of the care delivery. Finally, they can enhance the professional capacity for reflexivity.

Patients and Families' Participation in Direct Care

This form of engagement refers mainly to patients' active role in decision-making practices (Barry & Edgman-Levitan, 2012; Charles, Gafni, & Whelan, 1997; Coulter, 1997) and to other initiatives that allow patients and providers to co-manage the decision involving their treatment and care delivery process. One example is the implementation of formal programs in which decision aids (leaflets, books, videos, websites, and other interactive media) are used to give patients information on the risks and benefits of various treatment options and to help them make a choice consistent with their expectations. Similarly, hospitals can sustain the development of peer support programs, aimed at empowering their members through information exchange, orientation, and mutual support. A final example is patients' and families' activation and involvement directly in points of care; for instance, by facilitating families' access or by sustaining their inclusion in the hand-off process (Luxford et al., 2011), namely the set of communication and knowledge transfers required to transfer patients from one caregiver to another. Another level of engagement consists of creating meaningful part-time or full-time paid positions for patients and family leaders to facilitate their systematic participation in strategic decision-making and to promote hospitals' connection with the local communities. These procedures help patients and families become partners in care (Luxford et al., 2011), making their voices heard in different moments of the care delivery.

Systematic Monitoring of Patients and Families' Experience and Collection of Feedback

Monitoring and measuring hospitals' performance from the point of view of patients is another strategic asset that contributes to the engagement of patients and their families in the organizational design and management. Some studies (Greene et al., 2012; Luxford et al., 2011) have for instance shown as best practices the activation of regular surveys on patients' care experience, the results of which are used to identify opportunities for improving the organizational structures and work systems as well as single professional performances. In other cases, the monitoring of patients' experience from a practice-based perspective (Liberati et al., 2015) is proposed for identifying care contradictions, patient and caregiver needs, or unmet opportunities, which could help rethink and improve hospitals' capabilities. This approach may allow patients and caregivers to be active co-evaluators and co-producers (Sorrentino, Guglielmetti, Gilardi, & Marsilio, 2015) of their own healthcare system of reference. All of these procedures allow hospitals to become learning organizations (Luxford et al., 2011), willing and able to redesign both their care practices and their overall organizational functioning and layout to increase their capacity for engaging patients.

Enhancing Professionals' Capacity for Reflexivity

Finally, another possibility for PCM hospitals to address the complex challenges posed by the need to engage patients is the activation of reflexive learning settings for healthcare professionals, aimed at promoting awareness and critical views on the different meanings and possible interpretation of the patient centeredness and patient engagement philosophies.

The assumption behind reflexive learning settings is that healthcare practitioners have many more resources to improve care services than are usually recognized. Such resources can be better exploited by providing care professionals with opportunities to question issues that are taken for granted (Cunliffe, 2003) using first-hand accounts of patient experiences within healthcare services as well as rich ethnographic descriptions of daily care practices and interactions.

During the reflexive learning programs, participants are temporarily not involved in their daily working practices and agree to observe their work from a different perspective. Specifically, when working reflexively on the concepts of patient centeredness and patient engagement, healthcare practitioners might be encouraged to collect and discuss data related either to patients' experience or to their care practices. Sharing these data and interpretations may help professionals generate insights into how health-care services, processes, and facilities can be modified to better respond to patients' needs. Reflexive learning settings might reveal that different professionals understand patient centeredness in different and possibly contrasting ways (Liberati et al., 2015). These settings offer opportunities to assume and discuss differences and contradictions in order to explore their pragmatic effects and to promote more coherent practices. Reflexivity can then help trigger collective explorations of knowledge, values, and meanings that inform everyday care practices (Ripamonti, Galuppo, Gorli, Scaratti, & Cunliffe, 2015; Gorli, Nicolini, & Scaratti, 2015b; Cunliffe, 2003; Scaratti, Gorli, & Ripamonti, 2009), thus providing possibilities for enriching the concept of patient centeredness and engagement and for internal service development.

CONCLUSION

This chapter argued that the two concepts of patient centeredness and patient engagement are not spontaneously and mutually sustained throughout the process of care. Rather, they require specific attention to work as complementary aspects surrounding the same vision: improving the quality of healthcare by giving value to patients' and caregivers' agenda and needs.

By focussing on hospital contexts, this contribution debated that many innovation programs pursue a patient-centered model although risking overlooking the specificities of local contexts or of single voices, even sometimes contradicting patients and providers' needs for full engagement. These healthcare reforms do not always address how practitioners interpret and enact patient centeredness in their local context or capture what patients perceive as actually significant along their overall care path.

From a patient engagement perspective, it is fundamental not only to guarantee that the patient is positioned in a valuable place, but also that he or she is allowed an active re-positioning with respect to the care process. In other words, it is essential to consider organizational solutions for making the patient a *participant* in such processes.

The question is how to get started with such an ambitious plan. One suggestion is that, in order to keep the two concepts of patient centeredness and patient engagement connected, hospitals should follow the logic of co-production of knowledge. In co-production, actors and stakeholders jointly contribute to frame setting and aspects of the service (Gilardi, Guglielmetti, Casati, & Monti, 2014; Dunston, Lee, Boud, Brodie, & Chiarella, 2009).

Participation in this process concerns both patients and patients' families, professionals, hospital managers and external stakeholders, since every actor is a carrier of his or her own views from specific angles. In order to construct more effective healthcare and hospital reforms, these views become necessary as they highlight potential problems and possible conflicts, and at the same time, they can offer innovative solutions and interpretations.

Patient orientation, which refers to listening to the specific needs and engaging with active and mutual repositioning, implies the capacity to reflect on the care practices in use and on the opportunity to rethink and to regenerate them. This is the challenge that involves every level and every stakeholder of the healthcare systems, who should be available to reconsider taken-for-granted arrangements, values, and implicit assumptions, thus opening the way to an actual change toward more participative healthcare services.

REFERENCES

Atwal, A., & Caldwell, K. (2002). Do multidisciplinary integrated care pathways improve interprofessional collaboration? *Scandinavian Journal of Caring Sciences*, *16*(4), 360–367. doi:10.1046/j.1471-6712.2002.00101.x PMID:12445105

Bainton, D., van der Steeg, H., & Weeda, L. (1995). Restructuring. Building blocks. *The Health Service Journal*, *105*(5445), 26–27. PMID:10141857

Barello, S., Graffigna, G., Vegni, E., Savarese, M., Lombardi, F., & Bosio, A. C. (2015). 'Engage me in taking care of my heart': A grounded theory study on patient–cardiologist relationship in the hospital management of heart failure. *BMJ Open*, *5*(3), e005582. doi:10.1136/bmjopen-2014-005582 PMID:25776041

Barry, M. J., & Edgman-Levitan, S. (2012). Shared decision making – The pinnacle of patient-centered care. *The New England Journal of Medicine*, *366*(9), 780–781. doi:10.1056/NEJMp1109283 PMID:22375967

Bensing, J. (2000). Bridging the gap: The separate worlds of evidence-based medicine and patient-centered medicine. *Patient Education and Counseling*, *39*(1), 17–25. doi:10.1016/S0738-3991(99)00087-7 PMID:11013544

Bergeson, S. C., & Dean, J. D. (2006). A systems approach to patient-centered care. *Journal of the American Medical Association*, *296*(23), 2848–2851. doi:10.1001/jama.296.23.2848 PMID:17179462

Berwick, D. M. (2009). What a "Patient-Centered" should mean: Confession of an extremist. *Health Affairs*, *28*(4), 555–565. doi:10.1377/hlthaff.28.4.w555 PMID:19454528

Braithwaite, J., Runciman, W. B., & Merry, F. (2009). Towards safer, better healthcare: Harnessing the natural properties of complex sociotechnical systems. *Quality & Safety in Health Care*, *18*(1), 37–41. doi:10.1136/qshc.2007.023317 PMID:19204130

Brodersen, J., & Thorwid, J. (1997). Enabling sustainable change for healthcare in Stockholm. *British Journal of Healthcare Computing and Information Management*, *14*, 22–25.

Bromley, E. (2012). Building patient-centeredness: Hospital design as an interpretive act. *Social Science & Medicine*, *75*(6), 1057–1066. doi:10.1016/j.socscimed.2012.04.037 PMID:22703887

Carman, K. L., Dardess, P., Maurer, M., Sofaer, S., Adams, K., Bechtel, C., & Sweeney, J. (2013). Patient and family engagement: A framework for understanding the elements and developing interventions and policies. *Health Affairs*, *32*(2), 223–231. doi:10.1377/hlthaff.2012.1133 PMID:23381514

Charles, C., Gafni, A., & Whelan, T. (1997). Shared decision-making in the medical encounter: What does it mean? (Or it takes, at least two to tango). *Social Science & Medicine*, *44*(5), 681–692. doi:10.1016/S0277-9536(96)00221-3 PMID:9032835

Coulson-Thomas, C. (1996). Re-engineering hospitals and health care processes. *British Journal of Health Care Management*, *2*(6), 338–342.

Coulter, A. (1997). Partnerships with patients: The pros and cons of shared clinical decision-making. *Journal of Health Services Research & Policy*, *2*, 112–121. PMID:10180362

Cunliffe, A. L. (2003). Reflexive inquiry in organizational research: Questions and possibilities. *Human Relations*, *56*(8), 983–1003. doi:10.1177/00187267030568004

De Certeau, M. (1990). *L'invention du quotidien. 1. Arts de faire*. Paris: Gallimard.

Dixon-Woods, M. (2010). Why is patient safety so hard? A selective review of ethnographic studies. *Journal of Health Services Research & Policy*, *15*(Suppl. 1), 11–16. doi:10.1258/jhsrp.2009.009041 PMID:20075122

Dunston, R., Lee, A., Boud, D., Brodie, P., & Chiarella, M. (2009). Co-Production and Health System Reform–From Re-Imagining To Re-Making. *Australian Journal of Public Administration*, *68*(1), 39–52. doi:10.1111/j.1467-8500.2008.00608.x

Ferlie, E., Fitzgerald, L., Wood, M., & Hawkins, C. (2013). The Nonspread of Innovations: The Mediating Role of Professionals. *Academy of Management Journal*, *48*(1), 117–134. doi:10.5465/AMJ.2005.15993150

Gilardi, S., Guglielmetti, C., Casati, S., & Monti, P. (2014). Promuovere l'engagement dei pazienti con malattie croniche: un percorso di ricerca collaborativa. *Psicologia della salute, 3*(3), 58-79.

Gorli, M., Galuppo, L., & Liberati, E. G. (2015a). Hospital innovations in the light of patient engagement. Insights from the organizational field. In G. Graffigna, S. Barello, & S. Triberti (Eds.), *Patient engagement: a consumer-centered model to innovate healthcare* (pp. 120–137). Warsaw, Poland: Gruyter Open. doi:10.1515/9783110452440-011

Gorli, M., Nicolini, D., & Scaratti, G. (2015b). Reflexivity in practice. Tools and conditions for developing organizational authorship. *Human Relations*, *68*(8), 1347–1375. doi:10.1177/0018726714556156

Graffigna, G., Barello, S., Riva, G., & Bosio, C. (2014). Patient Engagement: The Key to Redesign the Exchange Between the Demand and Supply for Healthcare in the Era of Active Ageing. In *G. Riva, P. Ajmone Marsan & C. Grasso, Active Ageing and Healthy Living* (pp. 85–95). Amsterdam: IOS Press.

Greene, S. M., Tuzzio, L., & Cherkin, D. (2012). A framework for making patient-centered care front and center. *The Permanente Journal*, *16*(3), 49–53. PMID:23012599

Hernandez, S. E., Conrad, D. A., Marcus-Smith, M. S., Reed, P., & Watts, C. (2013). Patient centered innovation in healthcare organizations: A conceptual framework and case study application. *Health Care Management Review*, *38*(2), 166–175. doi:10.1097/HMR.0b013e31825e718a PMID:22669050

Hurst, K. (1995). *Progress with Patient Focused Care in the United Kingdom*. United Kingdom: NHS Executive.

Institute of Medicine. (2001). Crossing the quality chasm: a new health system for the 21st century. In *Committee on Quality of Health Care in America*. Washington: National Academies Press.

International Alliance of Patients Organizations. (2007). *What is patient-centered healthcare? A review of definition and principles*. Retrieved from http://iapo.org.uk/sites/default/files/files/IAPO%20Patient-Centred%20Healthcare%20Review%202nd%20edition.pdf

Lega, F., & DePietro, C. (2005). Converging patterns in hospital organization: Beyond the professional bureaucracy. *Health Policy (Amsterdam, Netherlands)*, *74*(3), 261–281. doi:10.1016/j.healthpol.2005.01.010 PMID:16226138

Levenstein, J. H., Mccracken, E. C., Mcwhinney, I. R., Stewart, M. A., & Brown, J. B. (1986). The patient-centered clinical method. A model for the doctor-patient interaction in family medicine. *Family Practice*, *3*(1), 24–30. doi:10.1093/fampra/3.1.24 PMID:3956899

Liberati, E. G., Gorli, M., Galuppo, L., Moja, L., Scaratti, G., & Ripamonti, S. (2015). Exploring the practice of patient centered care: The role of ethnography and reflexivity. *Social Science & Medicine*, *133*, 45–52. doi:10.1016/j.socscimed.2015.03.050 PMID:25841094

Liberati, E. G., Gorli, M., & Scaratti, G. (in press). Reorganising hospitals to implement a patient-centered model of care: The effects on clinical practice and professional relationships in the Italian NHS. *Journal of Health Organization and Management*. PMID:26556155

Luxford, K., Safran, D. G., & Delbanco, T. (2011). Promoting patient-centered care: A qualitative study of facilitators and barriers in healthcare organizations with a reputation for improving the patient experience. *International Journal for Quality in Health Care*, *23*(5), 510–515. doi:10.1093/intqhc/mzr024 PMID:21586433

Mackintosh, N., & Sandall, J. (2010). Overcoming gendered and professional hierarchies in order to facilitate escalation of care in emergency situations: The role of standardised communication protocols. *Social Science & Medicine*, *71*(9), 1683–1686. doi:10.1016/j.socscimed.2010.07.037 PMID:20850919

McKee, M., & Healy, J. (2002). *Hospital in a changing Europe*. Buckingham: Open University Press.

Mead, N., & Bower, P. (2000). Patient-centeredness: A conceptual framework and review of the empirical literature. *Social Science & Medicine*, *51*(7), 1087–1110. doi:10.1016/S0277-9536(00)00098-8 PMID:11005395

Mikesell, L., & Bromley, E. (2012). Patient centered, nurse averse? Nurses' care experiences in a 21st-century hospital. *Qualitative Health Research*, *22*(12), 1659–1671. doi:10.1177/1049732312458180 PMID:22923388

Nugus, P., Greenfield, D., Travaglia, J., Westbrook, J., & Braithwaite, J. (2010). How and where clinicians exercise power: Interprofessional relations in health care. *Social Science & Medicine*, *71*(5), 898–909. doi:10.1016/j.socscimed.2010.05.029 PMID:20609507

Oborn, E., & Dawson, S. (2010). Knowledge and practice in multidisciplinary teams: Struggle, accommodation and privilege. *Human Relations*, *63*(12), 1835–1857. doi:10.1177/0018726710371237

Okhuysen, G. A., & Bechky, B. A. (2009). Coordination in organizations: An integrative perspective. *The Academy of Management Annals*, *3*(1), 463–502. doi:10.1080/19416520903047533

Øvretveit, J. (2011). Understanding the conditions for improvement: Research to discover which context influences affect improvement success. *BMJ Quality & Safety*, *20*(Suppl. 1), 18–23. doi:10.1136/bmjqs.2010.045955 PMID:21450764

Ripamonti, S., Galuppo, L., Gorli, M., Scaratti, G., & Cunliffe, A. L. (2015). Pushing action-research towards reflexive practice. *Journal of Management Inquiry*. doi:10.1177/1056492615584972

Scaratti, G., Gorli, M., & Ripamonti, S. (2009). The power of professionally situated practice analysis in redesigning organisations: A psychosociological approach. *Journal of Workplace Learning*, *21*(7), 538–554. doi:10.1108/13665620910985531

Shaller, D. (2007). Patient-centered care: What does it take?. *The Commonwealth Fund* N. 1067.

Silverman, D. (2010). *Doing Qualitative Research: A Practical Handbook* (4th ed.). SAGE.

Sorrentino, M., Guglielmetti, C., Gilardi, S., & Marsilio, M. (2015). Health Care Services and the Co-production Puzzle: Filling in the Blanks. *Administration & Society*. doi:10.1177/0095399715593317

Stewart, M., Brown, J. B., Donner, A., McWhinney, I. R., Oates, J., Weston, W. W., & Jordan, J. (2000). The impact of patient-centered care on outcomes. *The Journal of Family Practice*, *49*(9), 796–804. PMID:11032203

Vera, A., & Kuntz, L. (2007). Process-based organization design and hospital efficiency. *Health Care Management Review*, *32*(1), 55–65. doi:10.1097/00004010-200701000-00008 PMID:17245203

Villa, S., Barbieri, M., & Lega, F. (2009). Restructuring patient flow logistics around patient care needs: Implications and practicalities from three critical cases. *Health Care Management Science*, *12*(2), 155–165. doi:10.1007/s10729-008-9091-6 PMID:19469455

Vos, L., Chalmers, S. E., Dückers, M. L., Groenewegen, P. P., Wagner, C., & Van Merode, G. G. (2011). Towards an organisation-wide process-oriented organisation of care: A literature review. *Implementation Science; IS*, *6*(1), 8. doi:10.1186/1748-5908-6-8 PMID:21247491

Wenger, E. (1998). *Communities of Practice: Learning, Meaning and Identity*. Cambridge, UK: Cambridge University Press. doi:10.1017/CBO9780511803932

KEY TERMS AND DEFINITIONS

Functional Hospital Model: The functional hospital model is one where individuals with a similar area of expertise are grouped into independently controlled units, thus defining patients' location according to their prevalent pathology.

Healthcare Professionals: Medical professional involved in the healthcare delivery (physicians, nurses).

Organizational Model/Organizational Structure: An organizational structure defines how activities such as task allocation, coordination, control and supervision are directed towards the achievement of organizational aims.

Patient Centered Care: is an approach to healthcare that emphasizes the limitations of a disease-centered model and calls for an exploration of patients' needs, preferences, values and concerns with the aim to increase patients' involvement in the management of their care plan.

Patient Centered Organizational Model: The patient-centered hospital model, as it is commonly known within the academic community, represents an attempt to reshape the care delivery according to the needs of the patients and their care processes, moving away from the traditional physician-centered view, thus resulting in a rather disruptive cultural change. The patient-centered model (henceforth PCM) requires reshaping hospitals' organizational structure, social and professional practices, and care delivery processes and the modification of hospitals' relative positioning in the healthcare ecosystem. These changes are considered to have consequences on the patients' care experience.

Practice/Practice-Based View: Assuming a practice-based view to the study of organizations means considering that the work practices are key analytical elements through which to consider how individuals organize, know, perform and learn in their work contexts. Through the practices it is possible to look at given interpretations of work, perspectives and interests at play.

Reflexivity: The notion of reflexivity stems from the concept of meditative thinking – that is, the active 'turning back on oneself' to question ourselves as subjects and the accuracy and objectivity of our knowledge. Reflexivity can be seen as a dialogical and relational activity that is undertaken to unsettle conventional practices, to examine the habitual ways of seeing the world, to evaluate consolidated habits of perceiving, thinking, remembering, resolving problems and feeling.

Space/ Organizational Space/ Hospital Space: Organizational spaces are made by two intertwined elements. On the one hand, there is a manifest and open dimension, constituted by architectures, structures, materiality, rules and policies; on the other, there is a tacit and unexposed dimension– although highly operative –made by the practices and relationships that shape and actively construct those spaces. It is possible to distinguish between *place* - as a proper space in which the elements that constitute it are organized and controlled by organizational institutions and power relations in a stable form - and *space* - as the practiced place, namely the arrangement resulting from the many ways in which individuals inhabit the place, position themselves within it, and re-create their own borders.

Chapter 9
No Entry:
Prohibitions and Violations in Organizational Spaces across the Patient-Staff Interface in Hospital

Livia Bruscaglioni
University of Florence, Italy

ABSTRACT

The chapter investigates the dynamic of encounters between staff and patients in two case studies on hospital organisation, taking special account of the emotional and psychological aspects associated with practices in the use of organisational space. By drawing on two empirical cases set in different hospital contexts (the waiting rooms of two outpatients wards and an emergency unit), analysis is made of two examples of practices which represent express violations of the rules on the use of space by patients and their relatives. Violations that could be analysed as demand of engagement - by patients and relatives - in the process of care. In these empirical cases the governance defensive reaction strategies used by hospital staff in their interaction with waiting patients is shown in light of the rules that define the behaviour acceptable for patients and relatives. The study is based on a qualitative methodological approach using the techniques of observation and in-depth interviews with hospital staff, patients and relatives.

INTRODUCTION

The objective of the chapter is to analyse the spatial elements of hospital setting that hinder or foster patient engagement. Through the analysis of two empirical cases set in different hospital contexts, examples are provided of how both hospital's configuration and hospital's norms on use of spaces may influence the dynamic of encounters between staff, patients and relatives. The research takes into account the patient's perspective, in particular considering one of the components of the development of patient engagement, that is to say the importance of building a trusted relationship between patient and health staff (Graffigna, Barello, Riva, & Bosio, 2014). In the paper we take into account the relational aspects in using organizational space in the first phase of the process of care, that is to say when the patient

DOI: 10.4018/978-1-4666-9992-2.ch009

and his/her relatives enter the hospital. We highlight two cases in which practices of non-compliance with hospital norms on use of spaces are observed. The paper presents a reflection upon the interaction between the individual and the relational dimensions of patient engagement, in particular the relation patient-health providers and patient-caregivers. The study takes into account the role of spatial elements in the patient's perception of access and continuity of care process, looking at the patient as a subject involved into a relational context. We take into account not only the perspective of the patient but also the point of view of the caregiver, considering the dyad patient-care giver as representing the consumer in the service offered by the hospital organization. The perspective of health staff (in particular of front office nurses) is analysed as well.

BACKGROUND

Space in Organisation Studies and Territoriality

Organizational space is becoming everyday more an object of analysis in organization studies, so that several scholars have talked about a "spatial turn" (Hernes, 2004; Clegg & Kornberger, 2006; Taylor & Spicer, 2007; Dale & Burrell, 2008; Warf & Arias, 2009; Van Marrewijk & Yanow, 2012).

The lack of attention at spatial setting in previous organization studies was linked to a vision of organizations as decorporealized and dematerialised entities. In the past decades many organization theories focused on cognitive aspects and on dynamic character and time, rather than on space (Clegg & Kornberger, 2006), while now that organising is connected with spatial organization we can reintroduce its materialization and embodiment. Space and architecture are taken into account in organisation as *social object creating social space whose forms provide implicit answer to crucial question of power, order, classification, control and function, while simultaneously implying theories of aesthetic, creativity innovation and freedom* (Clegg & Kornberger, 2006, p. 12)

According to Chanlat (2006) organisational space *is best thought as simultaneously divided, controlled, imposed and hierarchical, productive, personalised, symbolic and social* (p. 18). Organisation space is a social space where different people are organized in a social system where the division of labour and power relations between social actors structure space configuration. Spatial division through *physical boundaries* is also personalised by territorial limit: workers and employees invest the work place with personal meaning through a process of appropriation.

Partially inspired by Lefebvre (1991), Taylor and Spicer (2007) propose an integrated framework for studies on space in organization and management approaches, by conceptualizing space as a *pattern of distance which is interpreted by actors within materialization of the relation of power* (p. 341).

Organisation space could be seen like a socio-material, performative process (Hernes, 2004; Beyes & Steyaert, 2012). The "recursive view" of space is an analytical framework that studies how space emerges, evolves and transforms. While *space is what shapes action and interaction it is reshaped by action and interaction in turn* (Hernes, 2004, p. 44), space is a basic concept to understand the stabilisation and change processes occurring in organisation. *Stabilisation takes place through space formation and reproduction* (Hernes, 2004, p. 46).

The socio-spatial conceptualization of space distinguishes between "place", meant as an orthodox geometric view of space, an arrangement of formal elements (Kearn & Joseph, 1993; Liberati et al., 2015), and "place" meant as both experienced and re-produced by organisational actors.

If organisational space is crucial to establish and maintain relations of power, workers often do not conform to the rational plans of it. *Rather, they use and experience these controlled spaces in deviant ways, people move around in ways that do not follow prescribed paths* (Taylor & Spicer, 2007, p. 331), using tactics of spatial transgression (Wilton & Cranford, 2002).

Goffman (1961) has analysed territoriality in psychiatric hospitals, taking into exam the spaces that are off-limits to patients (such as the supervisor's office and the area adjacent to it), and the "free places" considered the back-stage for the staff-patient interaction, such as the staff coffee bar. Goffman (1961) also considers what he calls "personal territory", where an individual feels at ease and protected, to the extent the system permits him or her to be; his conclusion is that in the case of psychiatric hospitals "freedom has its own geography".

By introducing the concept of territoriality into organizational research, Brown et al. (2005) claim that territorial behaviours are used to construct, communicate, maintain, and restore territories.

Marking a territory involves the social construction of spaces, as workers negotiate to whom the territories belong, as well as their boundaries (Brown, Lawrence, & Robinson, 2005) through patterns of spatial practice such as social interaction.

The social nature of boundaries sometimes implies conflicts or differing interpretations about informal norms and formal rules about who is entitled to use spaces.

Adjacent territories may have overlapping perceptual boundaries and infringements could take place. To recover their territory, social actors then react with defensive actions, connoted by emotional reactions towards the infringement (Brown et al., 2005). Conceptual categories such as free places, group territories and personal territory (consider, for example, the concept of privacy and confidentiality) may be considered useful for the analysis of spaces in hospitals

Liminality

Notwithstanding the new recent perspective, introduced by the "spatial turn", to understand organisational life, in the last two decades the majority of social scientists have continued to analyse mainly dominant spaces in organisations, neglecting the so-called liminal spaces (Shortt, 2014).

On the contrary liminal space is not less important, as it is also a space where the process of development of workers' emotions and identity take place (Dale & Burrel, 2008).

The concept of liminality derives from the Latin word *limen*, meaning a threshold or a boundary. In anthropology (Van Gennep, 1960) liminality refers to the period of time in-between during a rite of passage, when participants experience a disorientation at the moment of losing their pre-ritual status but yet not starting the transition to the new status. During the liminal stage of a ritual, participants stand at the threshold between their previous way of structuring their identity, time, or community, and the new way established by the ritual.

Turner (1974) re-discovered the concept of liminality extending it to the transition from a social position or identity. *Liminality is a movement between fixed points and is essentially ambiguous, unsettled, and unsettling* (Turner, 1974, p. 274). Liminal is *betwixt and between the positions assigned and arrayed by law, custom, convention and ceremonial* (Turner, 1969, p. 95).

The concept of liminality has been used in organization studies (Beech, 2011), for example in the de/construction of liminal identities in relation to translocal patterns of work (Daskalki, Butler, & Petrovic, 2015). Shortt (2014) extends the concept of liminality, focusing on the workers' construction of liminal spaces in their everyday routines, so that liminal spaces become *transitory dwelling spaces* (p. 22). In his visual study about a hairdresser's workspace in a hair saloon, the Author argues that liminal space is *where arguably a more autonomous non-corporate identity can be created and permitted to emerge* (Shortt, 2014, p. 21).

If workspace literature has analysed dominant space in organizations and how it embodies corporate culture, liminal spaces could instead become fundamental for privacy, for the creation of informal territories reserved for the staff, and for creativity and inspiration.

While observing the practices of a clinical team in an Australian metropolitan hospital, Iedema, Long and Carroll (2012) found that the corridor performed a central role. Important conversations took place in the corridor space, perceived to be a 'liminal space', that is to say a space where hierarchy and specialization may be suspended, and where people can bypass fixed rules. Hospital's corridors therefore seem to be a space where tasks and positioning become sufficiently flexible and negotiable to enable hospital staff to face the complexities of a multi-disciplinary practice.

Hospital Space

A hospital is a complex organisation where spatial design reflects and reinforces contemporary concepts of patient-hood and caring (Bromley, 2012). Osmond (1957) highlighted the relationship between the configuration of spaces in hospital and social relations. A space can be defined socio-fugal if it is able to inhibit social relationships, or socio-petal if on the contrary it is able to foster them. Osmond (1957) observed as relatives and patients arranged chairs to form centre of relations during their visits in hospital. Every morning the hospital staff repositioned the chairs by changing the configuration created by patients and relatives, thus highlighting a conflict between the ways of using space by different organizational actors in hospital organization. The focus on these conflicting elements brings us to the central point of the rules on the use of the space of hospital organisation. A growing body of health literature focused on spatial elements in hospital (Andrews, 2002; Markus & Cameron, 2002; Gilmour, 2006; Bromley, 2012). Bromley (2012) analysed the design strategies to implement the patient-centeredness in a new hospital in the USA, claiming that a patient-centeredness design may challenge medical professionals' roles and may distance patients from the realities of medical care. Markus and Cameron (2002) analysed the spatial configuration of a homeopathic hospital in Glasgow stressing the importance of self-care patients and therapeutic community, with the general goal to be alternative to the orthodox care vision. A conflict arises from their analysis, between the *radical breaking boundary aspiration* (ivi, p. 57) of the hospital's institutional logic and the way the hospital space has been arranged in practice. For instance, *a 'therapeutic community' might imply that the space for education been not labelled as "patient education room" with the implications not only the conventional division between patients and the professional staff, but also between patient and the community from which they come. Such a space would need to attract patient, friends and relatives and professional staff, meeting during the day or in the evenings with the access to the computer terminals (Markus & Cameron, 2002, p. 58).*

This study focused on the importance of a proper hospital space organization to promote patient and relatives' engagement. It also stressed the difficulty to embody and reflect new values and vision of care in the spatial structure of the hospital, because the conventional way of dividing hospital spaces is often not questioned,

Patient centeredness is a *process that interlaces with the professional identities and with well-established balances of "spaces", positions and roles that involve different health practitioners* (Liberati et al., 2015, p. 50). It may collide with multi-professional regulations of power and legitimation. In particular a growing research interest focused on the dynamic between nurses' practice and place in hospital (Andrews, 2002; Halford & Leonard, 2003; Gilmour, 2006; Andrews & Shaw, 2008; Mikesell & Bromley, 2012), recognizing the impact of space on the process of nursing working routine (Walston, Lawton, & Kimberly, 2000). Original insights into nurses' working conditions as well as into inter-professional relations are provided by researches focused on space (Halford & Leonard, 2003). Several aspects of the dynamic between nurses and hospital spaces are to be taken in account: the degree of nurses' access to the different hospital spaces, with respect to gender and professional differences (male? doctors for example have much greater freedom to move around the hospital and have more private space); bodily movement in space as highly differentiated by profession and gender; different meanings and perceptions of spaces impacting on nurses' styles of performance and identity (Halford & Leonard, 2003).

Gilmour (2006) examined hospital settings where nurses constructed the hospital as a home space for patients. Using the geographic notion of therapeutic landscape (Gesler, 1992) and the concept of "hybrid space", the Author signalled that *the meaning hierarchies and power relations that shape space and places of hospital and the home permeate nurse's constitution of the hospital as home space* (Gilmour, 2006, p. 20). Nurses' practices imply a greater freedom of movement, a more personal choice, and a closer emotional nurse-patient relationship than in more medically centred hospital design.

The constitution of hospital as patient's home deals with the conventional use of professional use of space, with some risks for nurses' working routine. *Spatial vulnerability* (Gilmour, 2006, p. 20) is produced by the inclusion of nurses' space into patient's space. The consequence is the loss of personal space for nurses despite its importance to ameliorate their stressful working conditions.

A study on the waiting room of the emergency unit of a large hospital in Italy (Donnini & Lumini, 2008) revealed conflicting points of view between nurses and relatives regarding access to internal spaces in the emergency unit: on the one hand, nurses expressed their fear of being judged by the presence of relatives who enter spaces perceived as work areas, and which therefore became visible, while on the other hand, relatives expressed the fear that they would not be present at moments crucial for the choice of treatment for their relative. Mikesell and Bromley (2012) investigated nurses' experiences in a hospital designed to be patient-centered, with the aim to improve patients' experience and comfort with features such as private rooms and special customer service.

The centered model of care, embedded in the physical space, change the articulation of the routine work of nurses bringing a number of nurses' tasks "under the eyes of everyone", making them much more visible than before. In Mikesell and Bromley's research (2012) nurses' needs appeared in opposition to patients' needs and many nurses reported that the customer service orientation interfered with the reciprocity of nurse-patient relationship. The visibility of customer service's features changed the role of the patient and the perceived role of nurses (Mikesell & Bromley, 2012). Nurses reported feelings of abandonment and neglect about not being considered in the design decisions, suggesting a *more holistic conceptualization of patient centeredness in which the perspectives of both patients and staff are considered* (Mikesell & Bromley, 2012, p. 1660). Studies focused on nurses' experience and practice reveal how processes of transformation and development towards a more patient-centered model deeply involve spatial settings, and how hospital spatial configuration might have an impact on the process of construction of working routine and identity of hospital staff.

Space and Relations in Hospital

The possibility to facilitate or inhibit the relationship provided by a specific space is particularly interesting in our reasoning, as it focuses on whether the spatial configuration of the hospital may facilitate or inhibit the relationships between patients, relatives and hospital staff.

One of the central elements of the patient engagement is the chance to build a trusted relationship with doctors and hospital staff. Spatial elements linking the healthcare system and the socio-cultural frame in which the patient is involved may influence the development of patients' engagement in their care process.

Focusing on patient engagement in healthcare organizations is today a priority. *Giving (back) a role to patients and allowing them to become protagonists of their care have become a priority to promote the sustainability of healthcare. In this framework, the goal of engaging patients in their health management appears to be the key. Precisely, the concept of engagement may be conceived as a qualifier of the exchange between supply and demand of healthcare services. The English verb "to engage" is polysemous from the point of view of language. It refers to the ability to attract someone's attention, but also to emotionally binding a person to a contract that is long lasting and strongly affective, and finally to "take over" someone to "get him on board," that is, to make someone part of something* (Graffigna et al., 2014, p. 87). In a multifaceted definition of patient engagement (Graffigna & Barello, 2015) individual dimensions should be related to relational and organizational dimensions, like healthcare settings and admission process. Spatial elements in the hospital can promote or inhibit the process of building relationships both between patients and health providers, and between patients and patients (Bruscaglioni, 2013).

ORGANIZATIONAL SPACE IN HOSPITAL: THE WAITING AREA AS INTERFACE BETWEEN STAFF AND PATIENTS

Issues, Controversies, Problems

In the "consumer sovereignty" society (Bauman, 2007), organisational analysis can only be performed from a standpoint that acknowledges the triadic nature of contemporary work and organization, in which the consumer plays a central role. Together with the traditional dyad that comprises workers and managers, in contemporary organisations consumers enter the organisational arena in such a decisive manner that they influence the rules governing working practices. Also in the health sector, consumerism has brought about significant changes in an organization like a hospital, where the power relations between members of the powerful medical profession and 'patient-consumers' have for many years been imbalanced by very clearly-defined rules and procedures (Freidson, 1988; Marzano, 2002).

Further actors inhabit a hospital organisation: not only staff and patients, but also patients' relatives, who experience the space for longer or shorter periods of time.

The concept of engagement tries to describe the process of demand and supply of services that occurs between the patient, together with his/her peers and family support system, and the health system (Graffigna, Barello, & Triberti, 2015).

The spaces between users and operators are not always kept rigorously separate, unlike other organisations where users only have access to certain limited external spaces. The work of hospital staff is therefore carried out under the gaze of relatives and other patients, and becomes visible, public and exposes workers to forms of control.

It has been stated (Stein, 2007) *that an excessive permeability of border areas leads to unconscious feelings of toxicity on the part of the workers. The boundary region is governed by implicitly agreed norms specific in the employee relationship and an excessive boundary permeability and lack of control over it may lead front-line workers to have the unconscious fantasy that they have resulting in their being polluted by toxic substance* (Stein, 2007).

While many contributions focus on the spaces in hospitals, empirical studies on the liminal spaces are less frequent and reflections on the waiting room as a social space are missing from the available literature. The waiting space and the access to the hospital and to its procedures are an important moment of transition from "citizen" to "patient". Waiting rooms are the space where the patient first encounters hospital rules, and they contribute to his or her overall perception of the quality of care (Arneil & Devlin, 2002; Becker & Douglass, 2008). For hospital staff, waiting rooms are where they first encounter the consumer-patient. The waiting room, the first place where the relationship between patient and hospital organization is established, may represent as a whole an important occasion in the process of patient engagement.

According to the *Patient Health Engagement Model (PHE)* (Graffigna & Barello, 2015, p. 27), patient engagement is a dynamic process where building a trusted relationship between patients, relatives and health professional is an important element in the first phase. A more in-depth patient engagement may be defined as *a multidimensional psychosocial process resulting from the conjoint cognitive, emotional, and behavioural enactment of individuals towards their health condition and its management* (Graffigna et al., 2014, p. 87).

A hospital is simultaneously the place where patients and relatives receive care and the workplace of the hospital staff; and the waiting room is the 'interface' between staff and patients and their relatives.

While there are important contributions that consider the perspective of the hospital staff on the transformation of the hospital space, less frequent studies take into account the needs of both hospital staff and patients in the same hospital space. Hospital organisation expresses the spatial borders of the patient's role through its procedures and rules: those who enter a hospital are faced with a set of procedures, which frequently differ according to the context, that govern access, the order in which care is provided, and the spaces within which the patient can move.

The subject of the "distance" from the place where care services are provided is an issue to be considered not so much in terms of absolute distance, from an external point of view, but in terms of relative distance according to patients' perceptions based on the processes and the activities carried out within the space (Murdoch, 1998).

Methodology

The following sections analyse two empirical cases of use of the space in places where that was expressly prohibited. The fieldwork was conducted through both observation and semi-structured interviews with patients, relatives and hospital staff.

The study is based on a qualitative methodological approach using the techniques of observation and in-depth interviews.

Data Collection

The research, which lasted for over a year, moved through three phases. A first phase of encounters with the Heads of health departments in the hospital involved in the research, to prepare the access to the field and present the research tools, also to the hospital Ethics Committee.

A second phase of non-participatory observation of spaces in the two case studies: waiting rooms, reception spaces, circulation areas and transition thresholds between one space and another. The observation technique (Cellini, 2008) used enabled the researcher watch patient, relatives and hospital staff's practices under natural conditions, with the intention to minimize our interference in all these actors' behaviour. The researcher, waiting like a patient in waiting and transition areas, observed practices of use of the spaces and behaviours of patients, relatives and staff. The researcher carried out 64 hours of non-participatory observation. This phase allowed to reconstruct the psychosocial processes applied in the observed spaces. Ethnographic notes, according to Gobo scheme (2001) that divides observational, theoretical, methodological and emotional notes, were the outcome of this phase.

In the third phase, in-depth interviews were conducted with patients, relatives and hospital staff (admission staff, nurses and doctors) in order to analyse the point of views of patients and relatives on one hand, and on the other hand the point of view of staff about the practices observed. Twenty interviews were conducted for each case study (ten patients and relatives, ten health staff – including seven nurses, two admission staff, one doctor –).

Each interview lasted between 45 to 90 minutes, was recorded and then transcribed. The first interviews started with general questions and gradually focused on specific topics according to the approach of Grounded Theory.

The overall fieldwork was driven by Grounded Theory approach (Glaser & Strauss, 1967; Strauss & Corbin, 1990, 1994; Charmaz, 2006). Grounded Theory is a research approach proposed by Glaser and Strauss in their methodological monograph "The Discovery of Grounded Theory", as *a general method of comparative analysis and set of procedures designed to generate theory from data systematically obtained from social research* (Glaser & Strauss, 1967, p. VIII).

Theorizing in Grounded Theory is an emergent process generated by continuous cycling of the integrated processes of collecting, coding and conceptual analysis with the results written up constantly in memos (Glaser, 2004, para. 3). Grounded Theory approach requires that concepts and hypotheses be not defined a priori. Rather, a grounded theory is driven by concepts derived from data and not from preconceived concepts, making use of abductive thinking (Bruscaglioni, 2015). Only later concepts are integrated with the conceptual categories and hypotheses previously validated by the literature. Concerning that, Strauss and Corbin (1990, p. 23) state that *data collection, analysis and theory stand in reciprocal relationship with each other*. One does not begin with a theory, then prove it. Rather, one begins with an area of study and what is relevant to that area is allowed to emerge.

The Grounded theory method *is open ended and relies on emergent processes, and the researcher's emerging constructions of concepts shape both process and product* (Charmaz, 2006, p. 178). In the present study the topic of violations of the rules on the use of space was not considered a priori: it emerged during the fieldwork.

The two case studies were a medium-sized hospital in a rural area of Central Italy, and a medium-sized public hospital in a city of Central Italy. Data collection started in the first case study (the outpatient unit) selected for the characteristic of its waiting area (its large dimension and the spatial configuration of the waiting area in relation to the treatment area and the contact area), and then continued in the second case site, which was selected following non-random, theoretical sampling (Glaser & Strauss, 1965, 1967; Strauss & Corbin, 1990) in order to include in the analysis the relationship between patients and relatives during the waiting experience. *The aim of theoretical sampling is to sample events, incidents and so forth, that are indicative of categories, their properties and dimensions, so that you can develop and conceptually relate them* (Strauss & Corbin, 1990, p. 177).

In order to clarify the notion of theoretical sampling here is an example from an empirical study by Glaser and Strauss (1965). *Visits to the various medical services were scheduled as follows: I wished first to look at services that minimized patient awareness (and so first looked at premature baby service and then at a neurosurgical service where patients were frequently comatose). I wished next to look at dying in a situation where patients were expectancy of staff and often patients were great and dying was quick, so I observed on an Intensive Care Unit. Then I wished to observe on where staff expectation of terminality was great but where the patient's might or might not be, and where dying tended to be slow. So I looked at a cancer service. (…) While we were looking at some different types of services, we also observed the above types of services at other type of hospitals* (Glaser & Strauss, 1965, p. 89).

Data Analysis

Textual qualitative analysis of ethnographic records and interview materials and data collection were conducted concurrently. They were followed by coding phases as envisaged by the Grounded Theory approach: open, focused and theoretical (Strauss & Corbin, 1990).

The analysis of the cases focuses on the following elements:

- The spatial configuration of the waiting area in relation to the treatment area and the contact area.
- The organizational rules on the use of the space.
- The infractions of the rules by patients and relatives.
- The reactions of staff and organization to infractions of the spatial rules, and their strategies to ensure compliance with the rules.
- The perception of patients and relatives regarding access and continuity of care process, as a central element of patient's engagement.
- The perception of health staff, and in particular of nurses, regarding patients' infractions of the spatial rules

The Waiting Room of the Outpatient Unit: Spatial Elements, Patients' Perspective and Staff's Reactions

The first empirical case concerns the waiting area of the outpatient ward of a medium-sized hospital in a non-urban area in Tuscany. The outpatient ward was located in an area of the hospital made up of a number of adjacent corridors, many of which did not provide seats for waiting patients. The outpatient ward had a centralised waiting room connected to one of the sides of the area, in a position where the waiting patients did not have visual access to the rooms in the outpatient ward. Our observational sessions revealed the presence of numerous notices attached to the doors of the outpatient rooms stating: 'Please do not wait in the corridor. Wait in the waiting room to be called'. These notices were repeated at various points along the corridor, and contained the same prohibition in various forms: do not wait near the doors or in the corridors. The rule expressed by the written prohibition therefore indicated that patients could wait in the space next to the consulting rooms: the central waiting room, which was about ten metres from the doors of the consulting rooms. Observation revealed the presence of repeated infractions of the rules. In particular, couples in which the woman was pregnant were observed standing outside the obstetrics unit. Considering the distance from seating, people chose not to use it, but to stand and wait so they could be near the consulting room doors, even in special circumstances such as pregnant women. The use practices were also socially constructed on the basis of the behaviour of the other actors: couples arriving at the consulting rooms and seeing other couples standing at the doors imitated their behaviour.

Patients' Point Of View

Later in the investigation, the points of view of both waiting patients and staff were studied by means of targeted interviews. A patient who was nine months pregnant explained that if she had to wait somewhere distant from the door of the laboratory her behaviour was 'to be neither seen nor heard'. She told us that she was willing to stand and wait, at considerable cost in terms of personal comfort, because otherwise she felt that the staff had forgot her.

Did You Wait There Standing Up?

Yes, I waited there on my feet because if you stay here they forget you have an appointment. That's the truth. If you stand there in front of the door, they remember you have an appointment and you wait. The fact is that I'm nine months pregnant and I have to give birth in ten days, and when. Why people wait outside the outpatient unit on their feet? They were all there, you find the seats empty because in some way they remember that you are there waiting too. I'm sorry, but that's the truth [Patient of the obstetrics out-patients department, pregnant].

Another patient stated:

There's a waiting room there. Did you know? Yes, I saw it. There's a Madonna. I've been there, I even said a prayer. But there's the fear that they will not call you. You never know when your turn will be – the schedule is never followed [Patient at the ear, nose and throat out-patients department].

The interviews showed that patients sought the maximum amount of spatial continuity between waiting areas and areas where the medical services were furnished in cases where there was the lack of a perception of continuity in being assisted. Where the spatial configuration did not make this spatial proximity possible, violations of the rules were observed. In this case the perception of being followed by the healthcare system is strongly compromised, and the relationship between patient and healthcare begins with a gap that will likely affect the promotion of patient engagement during the waiting stage, and then again before the therapeutic encounter.

Health Staff's Point of View

The interviews with health workers also raised the problem of the spatial configuration of the outpatient unit and the consequences for the relations between patients and staff. At issue were overcrowding and use of waiting areas by patients, who were seen as being too 'invasive' in the health workers' space. The staff's point of view focused on pressure from patients who were 'too close', who 'entered' the place where care was delivered. It evidenced the staff's need to have a protected working space. The health workers saw the need for treatment and the waiting areas as separated by a buffer zone: the 'correct' distance, in the opinion of the staff. Privacy was framed as an explicit rule to be complied with. As a further dimension of the interpretative scenario of the two cases, the privacy and confidentiality of patients receiving treatment should also be considered. In this case, when the doors were opened, if waiting patients were outside the consulting rooms, they had visual access to what was happening inside, and patient confidentiality was therefore compromised.

There is a curtain, but the women know that when the door is opened, there are three people waiting outside, and it is natural for them to glance in. Even though there's a curtain, I don't think a patient will feel relaxed [Out-patient unit nurse].

This showed the problems encountered by staff working under conditions where waiting patients made their presence felt to such an extent. The work of the nurses and doctors in the outpatient unit consulting rooms *became public*, and could be seen by everyone.

And then above all these people make a hubbub, noise, confusion, and working with this noise every morning is something you get used to; it's like the trains you don't hear any more, you understand? There's this train, there's this hubbub and over time you get irritated. When I finish my work in the outpatient unit I can't stay at work five minutes more. I need silence, and this means there's too much noise. It's an indicator for me [Out-patient unit nurse].

Partly, there's a lack of space because there's too much going on. There are twenty-nine consulting rooms. There are four people for each consulting room, so do the maths. There are sixty people out in the corridor, and you have to get through 'Excuse me. Excuse me'. You can't work like this [Out-patient unit nurse].

Sometimes you can't even close the door properly because of how everyone ... is crammed in. Crammed in. Sometimes, if I go to make a photocopy, to get in you have to leave and then shout! They're intrusive. They treat us badly sometimes; they talk in loud voices and blab to each other. Sometimes you really have to shut them up [Out-patient unit nurse].

Encounters between patients anxious about their illnesses and health practitioners who have to work in a context that is stressful by definition risked to become critical: the workers 'on the front line with patients' on the one hand, and the patients on the other developed an interaction with negative connotations. Some patients showed aggression, to which the worker was unable to respond suitably. As the interviews with the staff underlined, there was therefore a risk that the encounter may become explosive due to the stress of the two parties.

Patients are often aggressive; this is normal because they're ill, they're already ill and they have to wait for three, four hours, if I don't understand or if they haven't got the report ready. People who work in contact with patients: it's tiring. Just try to be in that box for six hours ... those poor nurses all crammed together. They're in the front line with the patients. B. and I hear patients shouting and screaming 'I'll report you'. So you work shut up in that box, which I think is awful, and you suffer aggression, and so it's also hard to be nice and kind all the time. It's like what happens at the Post Office, but here there's illness in the mix, anxiety and stress. There's no space for the professionals that might let you be nicer. So basically you have a patient who asks you ten thousand questions, but you are stressed as well. And so you have two stressed-out people meeting up. [Doctor, laboratory head]

Infractions of explicit rules by patients signal the presence of a dualism existing between patients and hospital staff.

This was a case of contrasting interpretation of the use function of a space between staff and patients: for patients, even though there may be no seats, the corridor was seen as a waiting area; for the staff, on the other hand, it was seen as a free space not intended for waiting, a sort of buffer zone between the health practitioners' working space (the consulting rooms) and the patients' waiting area.

The Waiting Room of the Emergency Unit: Spatial Elements, Relatives' Engagement and Staff's Reactions

The second empirical case concerns the waiting room of an emergency unit of a city centre hospital in a large Italian city, and it links with an emerging topic in the literature on hospital experience: the relationship between patients and relatives during the treatment experience.

In this hospital the internal premises of the emergency unit and the waiting rooms are the result of a recent rebuilding programme.

The restructuring plan envisaged a reorganisation of space to provide an external waiting room for relatives, which does not communicate directly with the internal area of the emergency unit, and an internal waiting room reserved for patients. The institutional logic was to provide different waiting areas for patients and relatives but linked by a "hinge" space with a reception desk, where administrative staff welcomed patients and relatives and also informed relatives about patient process of triage. The idea was to provide a more patient-centred service that ensured both patient privacy and prompt information for relatives.

The observation sessions shed light on some critical issues in the management of the reception desk, as that was in many cases totally unattended.

With this special configuration, a patient arriving at the emergency unit undergoes triage admission with his or her relative, and then the procedure requires the two to be separated: the patient waits in the internal room in the case of less urgent codes, or is taken to the consultation rooms in the event of more urgent ones. The relative waits in the external waiting room.

From the very first sessions observed in the emergency unit spaces, repeated violations of this procedure were apparent. Family members were observed approaching their waiting relatives by repeatedly entering the internal space of the emergency unit.

How did the hospital staff react?

When faced with this behaviour, the hospital staff vigorously reacted: they sought to enforce compliance with the spatial limits of the waiting area, by intervening directly and very explicitly with verbal reminders or more forceful methods to move the relatives.

A security guard entered the waiting room and said 'All relatives must move into the external waiting room'. The relatives were a little surprised, but took their things and moved into the external area, which until then had been empty. We were struck by the case of two young men (a foreign patient and his relative) who had to separate because of this: the relative in the external waiting room and the patient in the internal waiting room. The relative watched the patient in the internal waiting room through the glass door (which had opaque and transparent strips) from the external room. A woman who had also been moved said 'This is crazy'.

After about half an hour, some of the relatives again began to move into the internal room to be with the patients. After a while, a nurse appeared and told them to move, and the relatives moved into the external room once again. The patients with less urgent codes remained in the internal waiting room, and were gradually called to go through the doors of the outpatient area. After a while, however, the flow of relatives entering the emergency unit continued anyway, and they waited in the internal waiting room and the corridors. [Observation notes, waiting room Emergency Unit]

Once inside the internal space of the emergency unit, there was no separation between the internal waiting room and the area for patients with more urgent codes, who were often on stretchers: the space was entirely open, and relatives felt that they were authorised to move around, and also to enter this area. This behaviour constituted a further, and one might say more serious, violation of spatial boundaries.

From the privileged viewpoint of the admissions staff, who could observe the arrivals and departures of patients and their relatives, the interviews clarified the dynamics of approach to, and entry into, the spaces of the emergency unit and infractions of the rules.

If a patient arrives with a relative, what happens? In theory, the ideal process: they do the admission to triage together, and then they should separate. But often, the relatives sit in the patients' waiting room. So we go in and try to explain, and they leave, but it's hard to manage. It's not that the relatives and friends agree to stay out willingly. And so they go back in? Yes. Sometimes on the sly. You see them slink in [Worker at the admissions desk, Emergency Unit].

Once relatives entered the internal space, they found it difficult to comply with the staff's requests to leave and separate from their relatives during the waiting period.

People stop here and ask how to do the admission procedure, we send them inside, and often we lose them. They sit down inside. Then it depends on internal management: when there are greater flows and more confusion, we try to divide them [Worker at the admissions desk Emergency Unit].

Violations of the rules were linked to the anxiety created by the spatial division from relatives, by separation at an emotionally important moment such as that lived in an emergency unit, above all in the case of especially fragile patients like the elderly.

Some relatives complain. Many can't accept the separation, the anxiety it creates. This separation makes them very nervous. Often, they are the sons and daughters of very elderly parents. A lot of them come to me and say, my mother is eighty-six and is in there alone, above all in the case of many elderly people [Worker at the admissions desk, Emergency Unit].

In emergency unit areas in particular a greater need for relational continuity between relatives and patients was evident, since uncertainties about the diagnosis increased anxiety and emotionality.

In these cases the infraction of explicit rules signalled the presence of a conflict between different organisational actors, i.e. relatives and hospital staff. The search for spatial continuity between patients and their relatives clashed with the prohibition on use of the space, which was codified according to the biomedical model based on the dyadic relationship between doctor and patient, the model of the 'absent family' (Simoni, 2001).

In this case study, our observation of the practices of rules infringement allowed us to raise the issue of relatives' difficulties of respecting the internal 'territory' of the emergency unit and the spatial borders of waiting areas as codified by the hospital organisation. At the same time, our empirical study highlighted the extremely intense reaction of the staff, who, when faced with the permeability of the internal territory of the emergency unit and the visible entry of relatives into the internal working area, even resorted to security staff in order to move the relatives.

In this case study a non-functional exchange between supply and demand of health services occurred. Here consumers of healthcare were both patients and relatives, in search of increased contacts in the delicate phase of access to the service in an emergency situation.

SOLUTIONS AND RECOMMENDATIONS

Space and Emerging Needs of Patients and Health Providers

From the first impact with the hospital in the waiting room, spatial configuration and rules on use of the organization space may be such to generate a subjective feeling of being neglected in the patient and are thus likely to affect the process of patient engagement from the start of the process of care.

The empirical analysis of patient flows in the two hospital areas has revealed cases of overlaps among the 'territories' of diverse social actors (patients, practitioners and staff), and the presence of behaviours that violate rules and procedures defining spaces.

The waiting area appears as a *liminal space* (Turner, 1974; Sturdy, 2006; Beech, 2011; Shortt, 2014), a *threshold space,* that is to say a space where the person who enters the hospital is in transition from the social position of citizen to the social position of patient. The waiting room, as a liminal space, is an area of transition where the rules regulating distance and separation between the staff's workplace and the waiting spaces for patients and their relatives are sufficiently flexible to be violated.

In the two empirical cases, the governance strategies used by hospital staff in their interaction with waiting patients define the behaviour that is acceptable for patients and relatives.

The analysis of the empirical cases highlights the possibility that there may be 'deviant' patients who stray from the path defined by the procedures, and who follow spatial paths other than those that have been codified. There is the possibility that a patient may not comply with the spatial borders created for the waiting period and may move into 'territories' that hospital procedures deem off-limits, so that the staff considers the permeability of the border area as a problem.

The presence of patients who do not obey the rules signals both an attempt to negotiate the norms on use of the spaces, and an emerging need to be analysed.

According to the Patient Engagement model (Graffigna & Barello, 2015), the relational dimensions play an important role in the first phase of the process of care. In particular a trusted relationship with

Table 1. Case study 1 and Case study 2: elements of analysis

	Case study 1 **Outpatient waiting room**	**Case study 2** **Emergency waiting room**
Spatial configuration of the waiting area	• Waiting space for relatives and patients is distant with no connection (no electronic system for calling) from clinical space.	• The waiting space for relatives is separated from the waiting space for patients.
Organizational norms	• Patients are not allowed to wait near the clinical space.	• Relatives are not allowed to enter the waiting space for patients.
Practice of non-compliance with norms	• Patients and families approaching the clinical space.	• Observed practices of relatives who repeatedly move in the waiting room of patients to wait with them. • The waiting room for relatives/care givers is empty.
Staff's reactions to infractions of the spatial rules	• On the doors of clinics are posted signs with the prohibition to stand in the corridor for privacy reasons.	• Nurses, administrative personnel or security guards moving relatives in the outer room.
Patients and relatives' perception of access and continuity of care	• The physical distance is perceived as relational distance. "If I'm distant I'm not viewed".	• Many relatives can't accept the separation and the anxiety it creates.
Patients and relatives' Emerging needs	• Doctor/nurse-patient relationship to be to be ameliorated- • Better access to information	• Missing space for patient-relatives relationship • Better access to information
Staff's Emerging needs	• Marking a territory	• Marking a territory

the healthcare provider is crucial. An emphatic response is also central. If patients fail to build a solid relationship with the healthcare provider, their emotional behavioural responses may become dysfunctional to the engagement process. If patients feel "to be neither seen nor heard" the relational dimension may be compromised.

The waiting room is a space in which the presence of rules communicated through written or verbal instructions is significant, indicating a need of territoriality of the staff, especially of front line nurses. Health providers marking the territory negotiate to whom the territories belong (Brown, 1987) through patterns of spatial practice such as social interaction.

As shown in Table 1, emerging needs of patients, of relatives, and staff may conflict: on the one hand patients and relatives express a need of a better staff-patient relationship, a better access to information and a specific space for relatives-patient relationship; on the other hand, the hospital staff expresses a need of territoriality that emerges through the reactions to infractions of spatial rules.

The process of access to hospitals can be divided in different phases where the spatial aspects play a crucial role. In the two empirical cases analysed these phases can be summed up as follows:

Phase One: Patient's first contact with health staff. The patient's chance to establish a trusted relationship is also conditioned by several aspects, such as the possibility to access hospital spaces, the perception of distance from the care space and the continuity of care. The rules on use of the space are interpreted subjectively by patients. In this phase for relatives the access to space affects the possibility to have a relational continuity with patients.

Phase Two: Defensive reactions of health staff. Health staff (especially nurses on the front line) reacts to territorial vulnerability, to the invasion of what is perceived as a disrespect of the territoriality of their own work space, by means of defensive strategies (written notices, actions of security staff).

Phase Three: Consequences of defensive reactions on relationships with patients: when faced with reactions of territorial defence, the perception of inadequate care increases in patients and their relatives, and the building of a trusted relationship with health staff is therefore at risk.

FUTURE RESEARCH DIRECTIONS

The above empirical cases have shown how the analysis of the waiting room as liminal space is very fruitful for research. The waiting room is actually a space where patients' and caregivers' needs can emerge more freely than in internal hospital spaces marked by strict and non-negotiable rules on use.

For a future development of the research on patient engagement, the analysis of hospital spaces and waiting rooms seems to be rich of suggestions for a further elaboration on patient engagement. The investigation on interactions between patients, relatives and staff in the waiting room should be included in the research agenda on spatial factors favouring patient engagement in the initial phase of the care process. In the two cases taken into consideration the processes of social construction and spatial appropriation of patients and staff intersect and conflict, with staff using territorial boundaries to appropriate their own work space.

Both processes are fluid and dynamic and the rules on use of the space define the relationship between staff, relatives and patients. Along with the conceptual passage from patient to customer of health service, the relationship moves towards a greater decision autonomy for the patient also in the definition of the rules on use of the space.

CONCLUSION

How does staff react when faced with an invasion of the border area by patients and relatives?

Through the rules on the use of hospital spaces, hospital staff seeks to reduce contacts between waiting patients and their relatives and the hospital staff within the waiting area. The defensive strategies (Brown et al., 2005) used by staff in order to have the rules obeyed – for example, as we have seen, by using written notices or more actively moving people away – attempt to channel patients and relatives within the boundaries of the role of "patient" as perceived by hospital staff.

Spaces are regulated, and there is an attempt at 'spatial interface regulation' in order to manage the encounter between staff and consumers within the hospital organisation through spatial borders.

But in liminal non dominant spaces a more autonomous non-corporate identity could emerge.

In the waiting room, as interface between patient and hospital staff, two processes can be analysed in future research directions: the process of emerging of patient's identity and the process of construction and re-construction of the professional identity of hospital staff, like front-line nurses, through working routines. Both processes go through the social construction of hospital space and the negotiation of the rules on use and access of space, and start in the liminal space of the waiting room.

The process of emerging of patient's identity is based on spatial aspects, such as the access and free movement of patients and relatives in the areas of hospital and the negotiation of the rules on use of space.

Regarding the example in the first case study, we may consider the pregnant woman as a patient, even if she is not necessarily ill, as she established a relationship with the hospital staff for medical exams and treatments. The process of construction and re-construction of the professional identity of health staff, and in particular of nurses, is based on maintaining the territoriality of their working space.

For health staff the spatial division through *physical boundaries* permits to personalise spaces with *territorial limit.* The process of appropriation of space (Chanlat, 2006) defines professional identities.

The two processes intermingle with the relationship between patient and hospital staff and are also related to the power relationship of access and movement within the hospital (Mikesell & Bromley, 2012).

For a further development of patient engagement the analysis has highlighted the importance of design in hospital spaces, as a key factor to promote a balance between different needs of staff and patients. The institutional view shaping space design should necessarily take into consideration two levels of analysis:

hospital space as social space structured by routines of hospital staff and hospital space structured by patient and relatives who express a need of care continuity and positive relationship with the hospital from the very first moment of entering its doors.

On one hand, the effort towards the model of patient engagement must consider spatial aspects promoting a positive relationship with hospital staff.

Some aspects in particular should be examined. In the case of separation of waiting spaces from care spaces, a particular attention at communication with patients in the phase of access, so to avoid the patient to feel "neither seen nor heard".

Moreover, a special attention must be paid to a common waiting room for both relatives and patients in some phases of their access to the hospital.

On the other hand, to promote patient engagement it is essential not to neglect the process of construction of staff's professional identity, which passes also through space territoriality, provided there are no defensive reactions obstructing their capacity of listening to patients' needs. It is fundamental to promote and safeguard health staff's territoriality, especially of front line nurses, by designing specific spaces for decompression and protection of labour rights. A private reserved space, inaccessible to patients, must be guaranteed to health staff (dedicated room).

The interpretation of the territoriality conflicts risen in the two empirical cases has emphasised how a model of greater patient engagement, with a stronger focus on the patient allowed to have greater freedom of movement, more personal choice and closer emotional nurse-patient relationship (*hospital as a home*, Gilmour, 2006), is not possible without the consideration of territoriality needs of staff, who otherwise develops defensive reactions obstructing the development of patient engagement.

A greater attention to patient engagement requires a transformation of patient's identity that necessarily implies also a transformation of staff's professional identity where the concept of *spatial vulnerability* plays a crucial role.

Hospital space, because of its nature of socially constructed space, is a privileged point of view to observe and highlight the conflicts and dualisms emerging from those health services aimed at promoting patient engagement.

REFERENCES

Andrews, G. J. (2002). Towards a more place-sensitive nursing research: An invitation to medical and health geography. *Nursing Inquiry*, *9*(4), 221–238. doi:10.1046/j.1440-1800.2002.00157.x PMID:12460418

Andrews, G. J., & Shaw, D. (2008). Clinical geography: Nursing practice and the (re) making of institutional space. *Journal of Nursing Management*, *16*(4), 463–473. doi:10.1111/j.1365-2834.2008.00866.x PMID:18405263

Arneil, A. B., & Devlin, A. S. (2002). Perceived quality of care: The influence of the waiting room environment. *Journal of Environmental Psychology*, *22*(4), 345–360. doi:10.1006/jevp.2002.0274

Bauman, Z. (2007). *Consuming life*. Cambridge: Polity Press.

Becker, F., & Douglass, S. (2008). The Ecology of the Patient Visit. Physical Attractiveness, Waiting Times, and Perceived Quality of Care. *The Journal of Ambulatory Care Management*, *31*(2), 128–141. doi:10.1097/01.JAC.0000314703.34795.44 PMID:18360174

Beech, N. (2011). Liminality and the practices of identity reconstruction. *Human Relations*, *64*(2), 285–302. doi:10.1177/0018726710371235

Beyes, T., & Steyaert, C. (2012). Spacing organization: Non-representational theory and performing organizational space. *Organization*, *19*(1), 45–61. doi:10.1177/1350508411401946

Bromley, E. (2012). Building patient-centeredness: Hospital design as an interpretative act. *Social Science & Medicine*, *75*(6), 1057–1066. doi:10.1016/j.socscimed.2012.04.037 PMID:22703887

Brown, B. B. (1987). Territoriality. In D. Stokols & I. Altman (Eds.), *Handbook of environmental psychology* (pp. 505–531). New York: Wiley.

Brown, G., Lawrence, T. B., & Robinson, S. (2005). Territoriality in organizations. *Academy of Management Review*, *30*(3), 577–594. doi:10.5465/AMR.2005.17293710

Bruscaglioni, L. (2013). Rapporto sulle evidenze emerse durante la fase di ricerca sul campo - flusso ambulatoriale. In A. Simoncini, M. C. Torricelli, L. Chiesi, & S. Surrenti (Eds.), Lo Spazio dei Diritti. L'effettività del diritto alla salute nelle strutture ospedaliere (pp. 116–144). Firenze: Edi Toscana.

Bruscaglioni, L. (2015). Theorizing in Grounded Theory and creative abduction. *Quality & Quantity*, 2015, 1–16. DOI 10.1007/s11135-015-0248-3

Cellini, E. (2008). *L'osservazione nelle scienze umane*. Milano: Franco Angeli.

Chanlat, J. F. (2006). Space, organization and management thinking: a socio-historical perspective. In S. Clegg & M. Kornberger (Eds.), *Space, Organization and Management Theory* (pp. 17–43). Copenhagen: Copenhagen Business School Press.

Charmaz, K. (2006). *Constructing Grounded A Practical Guide through Qualitative Analysis*. Rohnert Park: Sonoma State University.

Clegg, S. R., & Kornberger, M. (2006). *Space, Organizations and Management Theory*. Frederiksberg: CBS Press.

Dale, K., & Burrell, G. (2008). *The Spaces of Organization and the Organization of Space: Power Identity and Materiality at Work*. Basingstoke: Palgrave Macmillan.

Daskalki, M., Butler, G. L., & Petrovic, J. (2015). Somewhere In-Between: Narratives of Place, Identity, and Translocal Work. *Journal of Management Inquiry*, *7*(3).

Donnini, M., & Lumini, E. (2008). Non aprite quella porta. Le percezioni e i bisogni dei familiari in sala di attesa. *Paper presented at 27' Aniarti Conference/3rd EfCCNa Congress: Influencing Critical Care Nursing in Europe*, Florence.

Freidson, E. (1988). *Profession of Medicine. A Study of sociology of applied knowledge*. Chicago: The University of Chicago Press.

Gesler, W. M. (1992). Therapeutic landscapes: Medical issues in light of the new cultural geography. *Social Science & Medicine*, *34*(7), 735–746. doi:10.1016/0277-9536(92)90360-3 PMID:1376497

Gilmour, J. A. (2006). Hybrid space: Constituting the hospital as a home space for patients. *Nursing Inquiry*, *13*(1), 16–22. doi:10.1111/j.1440-1800.2006.00276.x PMID:16494663

Glaser, B. G. (2004). Remodeling Grounded Theory. *Forum Qualitative Social Research*, 5(2). Retrieved from http://nbn-resolving.de/urn:nbn:de:0114-fqs040245

Glaser, B. G., & Strauss, A. L. (1965). *Awareness of Dying*. Chicago, IL: Aldine Pub. Co.

Glaser, B. G., & Strauss, A. L. (1967). *The Discovery of Grounded Theory: strategies for qualitative research*. Chicago: Aldine de Gruyter.

Gobo, G. (2001). *Descrivere il mondo. Teoria e pratica del metodo etnografico in sociologia*. Roma: Carocci.

Goffman, E. (1961). *Asylums: Essays on the Social Situation of Mental Patients and Other Inmates*. New York: Doubleday Anchor.

Graffigna, G., & Barello, S. (2015). Modelling Patient Engagement in Healthcare: Insight for Research and Practice. In G. Graffigna, S. Barello, & S. Triberti (Eds.), *Patient Engagement: a consumer-centered model to innovate healthcare* (pp. 27–43). Warsaw, Poland: De Gruyter Open. doi:10.1515/9783110452440-004

Graffigna, G., Barello, S., Riva, G., & Bosio, A. C. (2014). Patient engagement: the key to redesign the exchange in between the demand and supply for healthcare in the era of active ageing. In G. Riva, P. Ajmone Marsan, & C. Grassi (Eds.), *Active Ageing and Healthy Living: A Human Centered Approach in Research and Innovation as Source of Quality of Life* (pp. 85–95). Amsterdam: IOS Press.

Graffigna, G., Barello, S., & Triberti, S. (2015). *Patient Engagement: a consumer-centered model to innovate healthcare*. Warsaw, Poland: De Gruyter Open. doi:10.1515/9783110452440

Halford, S., & Leonard, P. (2003). Space and place in the construction and performance of gendered nursing identities. *Journal of Advanced Nursing*, *42*(2), 201–208. doi:10.1046/j.1365-2648.2003.02601.x PMID:12670387

Hernes, T. (2004). *The Spatial Construction of Organization*. Amsterdam: John Benjamin. doi:10.1075/aios.12

Iedema, R., Long, D., & Carroll, K. (2012). Corridor communication, spatial design and patient safety: enacting and managing complexities. In A. Van Marrewijk & D. Yanow (Eds.), *Organizational Spaces. Rematerializing the Workaday World* (pp. 41–57). Northampton, Massachusetts, USA: Edward Elgar Publishing.

Kearns, R. A., & Joseph, A. E. (1993). Space in its place: Developing the link in medical geography. *Social Science & Medicine*, *37*(6), 711–717. doi:10.1016/0277-9536(93)90364-A PMID:8211286

Lefebvre, H. (1991). *The Production of Space*. Oxford: Blackwell.

Liberati, E. G., Gorli, M., Moja, L., Galuppo, L., Ripamonti, S., & Scaratti, G. (2015). Exploring the practice of patient centered care: The role of ethnography and reflexivity. *Social Science & Medicine*, *133*, 45–52. doi:10.1016/j.socscimed.2015.03.050 PMID:25841094

Markus, T. A., & Cameron, D. (2002). *The Words Between the Spaces: Buildings and Language*. Psychology Press.

Marzano, M. (2002). La medicina, la morte e la modernità: Un'analisi sociologica. *Rassegna Italiana di Sociologia*, *43*(2), 267–294.

Mikesell, L., & Bromley, E. (2012). Patient Centered, Nurse Averse? Nurses' Care Experiences in a 21st-Century Hospital. *Qualitative Health Research*, *22*(12), 1659–1671. doi:10.1177/1049732312458180 PMID:22923388

Murdoch, J. (1998). The Spaces of Actor-Network Theory. *Geoforum*, *29*(4), 357–374. doi:10.1016/S0016-7185(98)00011-6

Osmond, H. (1957). Function as Basic Psychiatric Ward Design. *Psychiatric Services (Washington, D.C.)*, *8*(4), 23–27. doi:10.1176/ps.8.4.23

Shortt, H. (2014). Liminality, space and the importance of 'transitory dwelling places' at work. *Human Relations*, 2014, 1–26.

Simoni, S. (2001). Salute e Cultura organizzative. In M. Bucchi & F. Neresini (Eds.), *Sociologia della salute* (pp. 122–138). Roma: Carocci.

Stein, M. (2007). Toxicity and the unconscious experience of the body at the employee-customer interface. *Organization Studies*, *28*(8), 1223–1241. doi:10.1177/0170840607079527

Strauss, A. L., & Corbin, J. (1990). *Basics of qualitative research*. Thousand Oaks: Sage.

Strauss, A. L., & Corbin, J. (1994). Grounded theory methodology: an overview. In N. K. Denzin & Y. S. Lincoln (Eds.), *Handbook of qualitative research*. London: Sage.

Sturdy, A. (2006). *Knowledge Evolution in Action: Consultancy-Client Relationships*. Economic & Social Research Council.

Taylor, S., & Spicer, A. (2007). Time for space: A narrative review of research on organizational spaces. *International Journal of Management Reviews*, *9*(4), 325–346. doi:10.1111/j.1468-2370.2007.00214.x

Turner, V. W. (1969). *The Ritual Process: Structure and Anti-structure*. Chicago: Aldine.

Turner, V. W. (1974). *Dramas, Fields, and Metaphors: Symbolic Action in Human Society*. London: Cornell University Press.

Van Gennep, A. (1960). *The rites of Passage*. Chicago: University of Chicago Press. (Original work published 1909)

Van Marrewijk, A., & Yanow, D. (2012). *Organizational Spaces. Rematerializing the Workaday World*. Northampton, Massachusetts, USA: Edward Elgar Publishing.

Walston, S. L., Lawton, R. B., & Kimberly, J. R. (2000). Does reengineering really work? An examination of the context and outcomes of hospital reengineering initiatives. *Health Services Research*, *34*(6), 1363–1388. PMID:10654836

Warf, B., & Arias, S. (2009). *The spatial turn. Interdisciplinary perspectives*. Abingdon, New York: Routledge.

Wilton, R., & Cranford, C. (2002). Toward an understanding of the spatiality of social movements: Labor organizing at a private university in Los Angeles. *Social Problems*, *49*(3), 374–394. doi:10.1525/sp.2002.49.3.374

KEY TERMS AND DEFINITIONS

Grounded Theory: A methodological approach proposed by Glaser and Strauss as a general method of comparative analysis and set of procedures designed to generate theory from data systematically obtained from social research.

Health Staff: The personnel of the hospital (doctors, nurses and administrative staff).

Liminal Space: A transitory space in organizations like a corridor and a waiting room. Liminal space become important for privacy and for the creation of informal territories reserved for the staff.

Organizational Rule: A norm set up by the organization to regulate the behavior of staff and consumers

Practice of Non-Compliance: A practices which represent express violations of the organisation rules.

Spatial Setting: The layout of spatial elements in organisation like spaciousness of rooms and furniture arrangement.

Territoriality: A behaviour used by workers to construct, communicate and maintain territories in organization.

Chapter 10
The Value of Measuring Patient Engagement in Healthcare:
New Frontiers for Healthcare Quality

Guendalina Graffigna
Università Cattolica del Sacro Cuore, Milan, Italy

Serena Barello
Università Cattolica del Sacro Cuore, Milan, Italy

ABSTRACT

The concept of patient engagement offers a unique opportunity to inform our understanding of patients' ability to be active in managing their care. However, unless promoting the active role of patients is today identified as a priority to promote care quality, a wide debate still exists on how to translate this principle into practice and how to assess initiatives aimed at increasing the level of patient participation in their care. Measuring patient engagement along the care course might ensure that the medical care truly serves patients' needs, priorities, and preferences. Unless the measurement of patient engagement is today a big issue for policy makers and healthcare practitioners, only few scientifically validated assessment tools currently exist to identify patients' level of involvement in their healthcare. In this chapter authors review the main validated tools currently available in the scientific community devoted to assess the patients' ability and availability to be actively engaged in their care, with a particular focus on the recently developed Patient Health Engagement Scale, specifically designed to assess the emotional and psychological adaptation of patients along their care process and their level of engagement in the healthcare management.

INTRODUCTION

Western healthcare systems are today facing some of the greatest challenges of their history. Population growth, breakthroughs in the treatment and management of chronic disease conditions and changes concerning the levels of patients' health needs and expectations have led to a system that is increasingly under pressure and financially unsustainable (Beaglehole et al., 2008; Blinded et al.,

DOI: 10.4018/978-1-4666-9992-2.ch010

2013; Wiederhold et al., 2013). In considering how best to develop an effective system that delivers quality care and value for health consumers – and one that is able to meet future care demand – the role that patients play has become ever more important: giving them back a starring role is today a priority for health policies both at an ethical and pragmatic levels.

Indeed, increasing evidence has demonstrated that patients' engagement in their health and healthcare is a key solution for leading innovative actions in the complex and mutable context of healthcare delivery and organization (Graffigna et al., 2015a). The term patient engagement encompasses a number of related concepts, including patient-centered care and shared decision-making, all of which build on the idea of involving patients as full partners in their care and health-related decisions. Patient engagement, indeed, aims at giving (back) a leading role to patients and taking them on board for a more efficient and effective process of care delivery. Under this broad umbrella term, there is evidences that patient engagement is linked with fewer adverse events, better patient self-management, fewer diagnostic tests, decreased use of healthcare services and shorter lengths of stay in hospitals. Particularly, researches have showed that those patients who are more active and engaged in their care more frequently reports better clinical outcomes (Hibbard & Greene, 2013), higher quality of life (Barello & Graffigna, 2014a), higher satisfaction with their care relationships (Becker & Roblin, 2008; Alegría et al., 2009), healthier behaviors (Hibbard et al., 2007), more effective self-management skills (Skolasky et al., 2008) and treatment adherence (Green & Hibbard, 2012). Furthermore, empirical researches have demonstrated how patient engagement may contribute to a reduction of healthcare costs and to better economically sustainable organizational processes (Coulter & Ellins, 2007; Berwick et al., 2008; Hibbard et al., 2013).

In this chapter, moving from a review of current literature about the healthcare requirements to face the ongoing societal and economic challenges, we shall introduce the concept of "person-centered care", such as a new approach to healthcare organization able to acknowledge the complex psycho-social needs and identities representation of care recipients. We shall also discuss how this broader vision – which encompass that one merely focused on "patients" such as healthcare clients – is crucial in the context of integrated care.

Adopting a multifaceted definition of patient's engagement is in this light very important, to acknowledging not only the cognitive and behavioral components of this patients' attitude to healthcare, but also to become aware of the role that the patients' emotional adjustment to their diagnosis and to the new medical regimen may play in fostering or hindering patients' ability to accomplish self-management. Another crucial aspect to move steps forward towards the effective reform of healthcare is adopting procedures to assess the needs of engagement of the patients: currently, only a few dedicated assessment tools exist to help clinicians in diagnosing the level of engagement of their patients, and thus their needs and expectations in order to manage their care in a more satisfactory and effective way. The chapter reviews the principal ones and then deepens the feature of a new tool dedicated to measure the patients' ability to psychologically adjust to their disease and to engage in its management: the Patient Health Engagement Scale (PHE-s; Graffigna et al., 2015a). The chapter concludes with some concrete advices to assess patients' engagement in the clinical setting and use this "diagnosis" to improve the care process.

BACKGROUND: CULTURAL AND ORGANIZATIONAL IMPLICATIONS OF PATIENT ENGAGEMENT

To adequately address the challenges related to chronic care processes, questioning current care models is today required. Present healthcare processes are more often designed to respond to the acute needs of individuals, rather than to anticipate and shape patterns of care for long-term chronic conditions (Berwick et al., 2008). The long-term treatment of chronic conditions requires a revision of classical models of care in order to guarantee sustainable care services. To address this requirement, and consequently to successfully manage patients and their own care, a better synergy between healthcare organizations and territorial services is necessary. Acute conditions are primarily treated within the traditional hospital or clinical settings for short period of time. On the contrary, chronic conditions need long-term approach to care: this should result in a more synergic connection between services (inside and outside the hospital settings) by taking advantage of all the resources (psychological, social and pragmatic) that are present in the territory the patients belong to. Integrated care and home-based care models are currently considered as a potential solution to improve quality and sustainability of healthcare services, particularly when the management of chronic conditions is concerned (Kodner & Spreeuwenberg, 2002). However, to achieve the goal of an integrated system of care, the role of the patients and the lenses through which healthcare actors look at them, need to be questioned and revised. Indeed, in this context, patients have to become main actors in the care environment by acquiring the needed motivation, knowledge and skills to face the medical course in partnership with a proactive care team. Furthermore, an integrated model of chronic care implies the systematic consideration of all the potential resources or hindrances to care management that are present in the territory. Moving towards an effective integrated care model requires the previous assessment of all the organizational, social and human factors that are implied in the complex system of care, both inside and outside the classical institutional boundaries of the hospital. Thus, not only it is important to achieve a fluid synergy among all the healthcare services dislocated on the territory in order to improve their effective communication and collaboration; but it becomes also crucial to sustain the fruitful interdisciplinary collaboration among all the different healthcare professionals involved along the patients' care journey management. Furthermore, extremely important is acknowledging the role that unformal network of caregivers may play along the care process. Peers may offer important support to patients both at the pragmatic and at the affective level and they should be considered healthcare partners in the spectrum of an integrated model of care. Thus, their presence, their action and their role should be questioned in order to contribute to healthcare systems innovation, in the direction of a really systematic and fruitful dialogue between healthcare organizations and the territory they belong to.

In the practice, linking healthcare services (as well as hospital and primary care organizations) means considering whose missions are overlapping across the spectrum of care delivery. This requires a coordinative behavior among health service suppliers and actively engaged patients to work as a system for gaining health goals. In this scenario promoting patients' engagement appears crucial: if empowered and made aware of the importance of their active role along their care journey, patients may become a fundamental ingredient to favoring the achievement of an effective and efficient integrated model of care.

TOWARDS A "PERSON-CENTERED" APPROACH TO HEALTH AND CARE

As stated above, the idea of engagement expresses the goal of a maximum acknowledge of the patients' role in the care process. However, in the practice, this is still far to be realized. Curious to be noticed, the words we use to advocate for engagement are still anchored to a "*passivizing*" approach of medical care. We still speak of "*patients*", and we argue that "*they have to be engaged*" in the care process. These linguistic expressions are a sort of paradox (and very often our language and the terms we choose to indicate concept and practices tell us a lot of our implicit conventions and assumptions!).

The word patient originally meant 'one who suffers'. This English noun comes from the Latin word patients, the present participle of the deponent verb, *patior*, meaning 'I am suffering,' and akin to the Greek verb *πάσχειν* (= *paskhein*, to suffer) and its cognate noun *πάθος* (= *pathos,* to feel). As a matter of fact, today the most recurrent conceptualizations and use of the patient engagement concept implicitly evoke an asymmetric relationship between an "*expert*" (i.e. the healthcare professionals) and a "*lay*" person who have to be changed in some extent, namely made more responsive, more adherent to prescriptions, more activated in the care management, etc. Conceptualizations, thus, that appear a reparatory answer to the still "passivizing" approach of medical care, within a healthcare system that has not yet succeeded in the concretization of a real patient-centered approach to medicine. A part from the rhetoric claims that we share with the literature, in the practice the patient is still often considered "*a disease carrier*", and the focus is still on the illness treatment, rather than on the person in its whole.

Given the scenario of integrated care highlighted above, to circumscribe the representation of recipients of care to the mere identity of patients appears reductive. The concept of patients, well advocated by the patient centered movement in medicine, refers to the prominent consideration of all the manifestations of the disease that the individual is carrying and to its psychosocial correlates (i.e., the "illness", Leventhal et al., 1997). However, in an integrated model of care, where the individuals who need and receive care are not only registered in an institutional context of care but they are back in their social context and integrated in their community, this representation needs to be revised. Indeed, along their chronic management of care, such "patients" need to find a new balance between their healthcare requirements and their previous roles, commitments and life routines. In other words, in order to become effective and sustainable, integrated model of care have to acknowledge that the recipients of the healthcare services are often *also* workers, partners, family members, community members, sons, daughters, and so on. Recipients of care are thus *persons*, not only patients. They are individuals who play several social roles, and the patient role is only one of them. Thus, referring to healthcare clients in the terms of "persons" better acknowledges the psycho-social complexity of their health needs and expectations: this acknowledgement is a fundamental precursor of the translation of patient's engagement from a mere claim to a real guidance of practice. Persons that are more complex than "patients". Persons incarnate different social roles, different desires, different aspirations in their public and private life. Roles that have to be acknowledged and sustained even after the occurrence of a diagnosis, even after that an individual is labelled "patient", in a very passivizing medical language. Thus, passing a sense of control on one own disease and cure process – not only at the behavioral level, but foremost at the cognitive and emotional levels – appears to be crucial for guaranteeing a true engagement of people towards their health and care.

Given an integrated care scenario, thus, a new paradigm shift in medicine has to be advocate: that one towards a "person-centered care". Speaking about "person centered care", in sum, means adopting a more holistic, critical and ethical approach to medical care and to the recipient of such interventions: it means to become aware of the complex and fluid identity projects that patients are carrying and to understand how a changed health status may impact on such life projects. The claim for a broader and more positive conceptualization of patient engagement would lead to a more genuine consideration of "patients" as "persons", who are carrier of histories, desires, needs, preferences and projects for their present and the future life: projects that – at least at the emotive levels – shouldn't made impossible by the disease, but – at the maximum – reconfigured and reoriented, in the *eudaimonic* development of a new self-representation.

In the practice, realizing a "person-centered" vision of care requires to adopt a holistic approach towards individuals: this vision deeply challenge the past dominant bio-medical paradigm, by refocusing healthcare organizations from a doctor-centered practice – where the health practitioner is considered the knowledge holder –, to a model of care where listening to the "persons' voice" and making them main actors of their medical course is fundamental to align health services provisions and care expectations. The shift towards person-centered sensibility in healthcare should re-oriented medicine's objectives: in this perspective, taking care of persons means not only dealing with disease treatment and technical procedures but also implies a full consideration of the whole person's life projects and illness experience – that is the emotional and relational patient's needs concerning his/her own care. In other words, a person-centered care approach advocates for a more comprehensive understanding of care recipients, not only as carriers of organic dis-functionalities, but as whole persons involved in a sociocultural context and featured by unique life histories, experiences, and expectations of health and care.

PROMOTING PATIENTS ENGAGEMENT: THE KEY TO ACHIEVE A PERSON CENTERED MODEL OF CARE

Currently, several definitions of patient engagement exist, addressing different aspects of such experience (Barello et al, 2014a).

Some scholars focused on the analysis of the organizational and cultural elements that may hinder or sustain patients' engagement, mainly addressing the role of doctor-patient relationship in the process. For instance, Dearing and colleagues (2005) states that developing engagement means to foster a client-therapist working alliance that may help the client gaining a more realistic understanding of the nature, process, and expected outcomes of treatment. Other scholars pointed at the shared decision making strategies as a crucial asset to enhance patients' engagement in their care. Davis and colleagues (2007), for instance, agree that patient's engagement is the result of patients becoming informed partners in their care, including a recasting of the care relationship where clinician enact the role of adviser, and patients - or designated surrogates for incapacitated patients - serving as the locus of decision making. Other scholars adopted a more holistic analysis of the organizational and contextual factors in play in the patients' engagement process. Mahmud (2004), for instance, sees engagement as an organizational process that leads to a revision of the healthcare priorities in the direction of empowering people to provide input in decisions that affect their lives encourages support for those decisions, which in turn improves the public's trust and confidence in the healthcare system. Finally, Mc Bride and colleagues (2007) also point at the importance of informal care and define engagement as the element that will allow, at different levels, the wider community to have a say in the future direction of their health.

These definitions of patients' engagement have the value of systematizing some of the relational and organizational dynamics that happen in the management of chronic care and that may result in important levers for patients' engagement. However, on the other side, these definitions tend to oversimplify the experience of engagement itself, by representing it as an "on-off" status, that may be present or absent, instead of acknowledging the dynamic and complex psycho-social roots of such patients' experience.

In this light, other authors, neglected the analysis of organizational and contextual factors that contribute to the development of engagement to primarily focus on the inter-individual components of patients' engagement experience. These authors, thus, advocated that understanding how the illness experience influences the way patients feel and function in their daily lives is essential for developing appropriate care pathways. Authors interested in the inter-individual dimensions of patient engagement tended to problematize the dynamic development of such experience, by pointing at engagement as a complex psycho-social process which develops in time according to specific stages or experiential positions.

According to these scholars, promoting patient active participation in healthcare presupposes to have a holistic vision of the individual. Effective disease management implies to consider that multiple experiential dimensions interact when a patient faces his/her illness course. These dimensions could be synthetized as follows:

- **Behavioral Dimension:** Connected to all the activities the patient acts out to face the disease, basing on its emotional and cognitive reaction.
- **Cognitive/Knowledge Dimension:** Connected to the need to know, understand and make sense of the disease, its treatments, its possible developments, its monitoring;
- **Emotional Dimension:** Connected to the need to psychologically and emotionally manage (and adjust to) the onset of the disease and new life condition linked to it.

However, scholars often tended to address only one of this psycho-social components of engagement in their definition, by neglecting the others.

For instance, Légaré and colleagues (2013) mainly focused on the cognitive dimensions of engagement. They detected in patients' level of knowledge and literacy about their health status and their medical prescriptions, the most important resources for patients' engagement. The ability of searching for health information, of decoding such information and of using them, thus, is considered by this authors the essence of engagement.

Gruman and colleagues (2010) and Hibbard and colleagues (2009), further than patients' health literacy, focused on their behavioral abilities to enact effective self-care behaviors. The ability to manage health and healthcare, throughout conscious and "consumeristic behaviors" is considered by these authors such an indicator of patients' ability to self-determinate their health status, and thus, of them being well engaged in their care. Particularly Hibbard and colleagues (2009) developed the concept of "activation" to underline the importance of addressing patients' ability to enact engagement conducts and to participate in their care management. Hibbard also stated that patient activation is a function of the patients' confidence in their own knowledge and ability to participate in the care process.

PROMOTING PATIENTS' ENGAGEMENT: THE ROLE OF THE EMOTIONAL ELABORATION OF THE DISEASE

The emotive and psychodynamic component of engagement has been less addressed so far, although scholars agree on the role of patients' emotions in hindering or sustaining patients' engagement (Street et al., 2005; Hibbard & Mahoney, 2010; Meglic et al., 2010; Barello et al., 2014a). Graffigna and colleagues

(2014a) try to address this component of engagement by stating that engagement is a "*process-like and multi-dimensional experience, resulting from the conjoint cognitive, emotional and conative enactment of individuals towards their health management. In this process patients go through four subsequent phases (blackout, arousal, adhesion and eudaimonic project). The unachieved synergy among the different subjective dimensions (think, feel, act) at each stage of the process may inhibit patients' ability to engage in their care*". Theses authors exemplified the role of emotions as a fundamental component of patients' engagement in some specific pathological areas such as diabetes (Graffigna et al., 2014b) and cardiovascular diseases (Barello et al., 2015a). Patients' experience of their illness(es) and the emotional elaboration of the health condition is recognized to affect the patients' strategies for dealing with their health care experience. Promoting patient active participation healthcare means fostering the patient's advancement in the process of emotional elaboration and adjustment of his/her own illness condition (i.e. patient engagement). Only supporting this aspect, the patient will be able to enhance his/her disease management skills (i.e. patient activation).

The interaction among these three dimensions impact the patients' attitudes toward the disease condition and the ways of disease management. The failure of this interaction might explain patients' resistance and barriers in effectively managing their disease condition. Each dimension, indeed, allows to discover specific unmet needs that patients might experience in several domains of their daily life. Addressing those needs might enhance the level of patient engagement in the disease care and positively impact on clinical outcomes.

For instance, in the diabetic patient lack of health literacy and behavioral skills for managing treatments associated to the emotional burden related to the diagnosis might affect the capacity of individuals of effectively coping with the diabetes care process.

MEASURING PATIENT ENGAGEMENT: A FUNDAMENTAL FOR PROMOTING HEALTHCARE QUALITY

The fast pace of change in the healthcare system requires patients to be more and more aware of their care options and be active agents in evaluating options about where and when to seek care. Patients are no longer passive recipients of care; instead, they are empowered consumers of medical products and services and are recognized to be real partners in the process by which those products/services are developed. Patients increasingly act as advocates for new treatments, and many be fully engaged in making decisions about their care. In this context, patients strongly require clinicians to be helped in meeting their health goals (Stewart, 2001).

However, unless promoting the active role of patients is today identified as a priority to promote care quality, a wide debate still exists on how to translate this principle into practice and how to assess initiatives whose goal is to increase the level of patient participation in their care (Coulter & Dunn 2002).

If we want patient engagement to mean real partnership between patients and health providers on mutually-agreed health plans, healthcare systems need to find effective ways to measure the quality and the effect of this collaborative process. These interventions should work towards medical outcomes and care procedures that the patient understands and has had an opportunity to help determine. Measuring patient engagement along the care course might ensure that the medical care truly serves the patient's needs, priorities, and preferences.

Measuring patient engagement in healthcare is a crucial step for improving patient's care experience and outcomes. In this contexts patient-reported experience measures (PREMs), might support this process. This kind of measures is important because we should not assume that every individual in a specific socio-demographic group is the same when engaging with taking decision about heath and treatments, acquiring new health information, participating in health-promoting behaviors, following treatment prescriptions, or even interacting with the health professional during a clinical consultation. To assume that all patients will respond to these situations in the same way is counterproductive. That's why it is important to measure the level of patient engagement to understand these differences. Particularly, measuring patient engagement might have different aims and is a fundamental condition for:

- Population segmentation and risk stratification to target interventions;
- Designing customized care pathways according to the unique patient's needs;
- Evaluating the quality and quantity of intervention to support the active role of patients in their care process;
- Measuring the performance of health care systems and evaluating the effectiveness of care interventions.

From a strategical point of view, it is fundamental to establish not only why administering assessment for patient engagement, by also to reason about when and which patients have to be included. Indeed, the timing of patient engagement measurement might vary depending on the patients' disease and illness history, the setting of care, the socio-cultural context the patient belongs to and the patients' ability to self-report.

Moreover, clinicians should consider that assessing the level of patient engagement could follow two main logics (Figure 1):

- On the one hand, a "*linear logic*" might suggest to administrate measures for patient engagement in crucial turning points of the care process (i.e. diagnosis, treatment decision making, hospital discharge, clinical follow-ups...);
- On the other hand, a "*processual logic*" might encourage clinicians to administrate patient engagement measures when critical events occur in the disease course. These events could be both clinical-related (i.e. new symptoms, disease relapse, unexpected new diagnosis…) and patients' context-related (i.e. caregivers' disease or death, changes in the patients' psychological status,

Figure 1. Linear vs. processual logics in patient engagement measurement

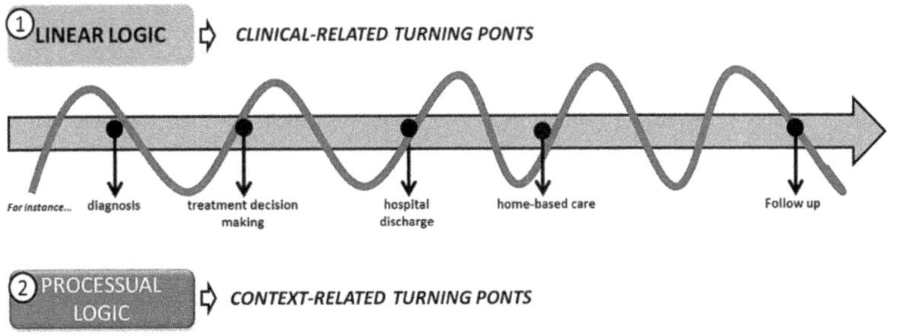

changes in the patients' social context…). These events might deeply impact on the ability of patients to be active participants of their care and on their availability in engaging in treatment/care decisions.

THE CURRENT MEASUREMENT TOOLS FOR ASSESSING PATIENT ACTIVE ENGAGEMENT IN THEIR CARE

Unless the measurement of patient engagement is today a big issue for policy makers and healthcare practitioners and the need for defining criteria to assess interventions devoted to meaningfully include individuals in their care constitutes a priority for healthcare, only few scientifically validated assessment tools currently exist to help identify patients' level of involvement in their healthcare.

More in depths, the scientific literature provides practitioners of very few instruments specifically developed to assess these crucial aspects in the patients' care experience. The following paragraphs are aimed at offering readers a brief overview of the main assessment tools - currently available in the scientific community – devoted to assess the patients' ability and availability to be actively engaged in their care, with their main characteristics and psychometric properties. These instruments can be grouped into two main categories: some instruments collapse in the group of measures aimed at assessing the patients' ability to self-manage the health condition; another category is, on the other hand, constituted by instruments dedicated to assess the patients' engagement experience along their care management journey. Let's see them in more details.

MEASURING THE PATIENTS' ABILITY TO SELF-MANAGE THEIR HEALTH AND HEALTHCARE

The Patient Activation Measure (PAM)

Developed by Hibbard and colleagues (2005; 2012) and recently validated in Italy (Graffigna et al., 2015b), the 13-item Patient Activation Measure is an interval-level, unidimensional Guttman-like measure that contains items measuring self-assessed knowledge about chronic conditions, beliefs about illness and medical care, and self-efficacy for self-care. The PAM focused on physical conditions, and it was designed to measure activation as a broad construct. PAM can be a valuable instrument when the aim of assessment is to evaluate the current patients' behavioral skills in managing the disease and the care prescriptions.

The Altarum Consumer Engagement (ACE) Survey

ACE (Duke et al., 2015) is a 15-question survey measures consumer behavior in managing their own health and making health care decisions. This instrument consists of four valid subscales (commitment, informed choice, navigation, ownership) each indicative of a unique aspect of engagement. According to these premises, ACE is an insightful tool when clinicians need to evaluate the ability of patients in facing current health decision making processes basing on their knowledge and skills for care management

The Partners in Health (PIH) Scale

Developed by Battersby and colleagues (2003), the PIH is a generic assessment scale for patients managing their chronic medical conditions, that is relevant to the primary health care setting. The scale consists of 11 items aimed at measuring the patients' features regarding the following dimensions: (1) Knowledge of the condition and various treatment options; (2) Ability to negotiate a plan of care; (3) Engagement in activities that protect and promote health; (4) Monitoring and management of the symptoms and signs of the clinical condition(s). Both patients and health professionals judged the scale as acceptable and easy to use, and the health professionals endorsed its clinical utility

The Patient Enablement Instrument (PEI)

The Patient Enablement Instrument (PEI) – developed by Howie and colleagues (1998) is designed to capture the patients' ability to understand the nature of their problems and cope with their illness. The PEI was developed to be used in primary care and is to be completed by the patient after consultation. This tool addresses six questions regarding a patient's recent visit, and, assess the following areas: how much they felt able to (1) cope with life, (2) understand their illness, (3) cope with their illness, (4) keep healthy, (5) felt confident about their health, and (6) able to help themselves. The scale was found to be reliable (Cronbach's $\alpha = 0.897$). Scores were categorized to indicate low (0–4), medium (score 5–9), and high enablement (10–12)

The Self-Management Ability Scale (SMAS)

Developed by Cramm and colleagues (2012) and based on the self-management of well-being (SMW) theory (Steverink et al., 2005), the 30-item Self-Management Ability Scale (SMAS) measures self-management abilities (SMA). The 30-item SMAS consists of six five-item subscales. Each sub-scale assesses one of the six core abilities to form the composite construct of self-management: (1) to take initiatives (be instrumental or self-motivating in realizing aspects of well-being); (2) to invest in resources for long-term benefits; (3) to maintain variety in resources (achieve and maintain various resources for each dimension of well-being); (4) to ensure resource multi-functionality (gain and maintain resources or activities that serve multiple dimensions of well-being simultaneously and in a mutually reinforcing way); (5) to self-efficaciously manage resources (gain and maintain a belief in personal competence to achieve well-being); and (6) to maintain a positive frame of mind. Each of these abilities directly relates to the dimensions of well-being specified in the SPF theory: physical well-being (comfort and stimulation) and social well-being (affection, behavioral confirmation, and status)

MEASURING PATIENTS' ENGAGEMENT PSYCHOLOGICAL EXPERIENCE: THE PATIENT HEALTH ENGAGEMENT SCALE (PHE-s*)*

These different assessment tools described above are widely used to measure patients' health literacy and level of behavioral competence in self-management. They are thus mainly oriented towards the cognitive and behavioral components of patients' self-management. However, as stated above, growing acknowledgement is played to the emotional and psychodynamic components of the patients' illness experience that appears to be the first movers of patients' confidence and ability to acquire information about their health status and to master self-management behaviors. The emotional component of engagement, conceived as the patients' process of elaboration and adjustment to the disease, has also been demonstrated to be a crucial mediator of patients' activation and adherence (Graffigna et al., 2015c; Graffigna et al., in press).

The patient's illness experience is recognized to be mutable and unstable across time. This aspect impacts on the patient's both availability and ability to actively engage in his/her process of care management. Although healthcare professionals and scholars agree in recognizing the importance of the emotional elaboration of the patients' illness journey in the chronic care management process (Barello et al., 2015), so far validated tools to assess this aspect have been neglected.

To our knowledge an original contribution in this direction is given by the recently developed Patient Health Engagement scale (PHE-s). The PHE-s developed by Graffigna and colleagues (2015a) is a measure of patient engagement psychological experience that is grounded in rigorous conceptualization and appropriate psychometric methods. The scale consists of 5 ordinal items and was developed based on the authors' conceptual model of patient engagement (PHE model), which features four evolutionary stages along a continuum of engagement (Figure 2).

The PHE model, offers clinicians a general picture of the patients' global attitudes toward their health conditions and treatment management. Particularly, it describes an evolutionary process of patient engagement featuring four subsequent phases (i.e. *blackout*; *arousal*; *adhesion*; *eudaimonic project*). According to this model, patient engagement appears to be a function of the patients' emotional elaboration toward their health and care management.

According to this model, patient engagement is a dynamic and evolutionary psychological process that involves the recovery of life projectuality - even with the disease. This process also features peculiar ways of interaction and decisional negotiation between the patient and the healthcare that depends strongly on the phase of the process through which the patients is passing. This evolutionary view of the patient engagement process suggests that a fully engaged patient results from a series of psychological reframing of his/her health condition and that the success of the patient in advancing along the process

Figure 2. The process of patient engagement as described in the PHE model (Graffigna et al., 2014a)

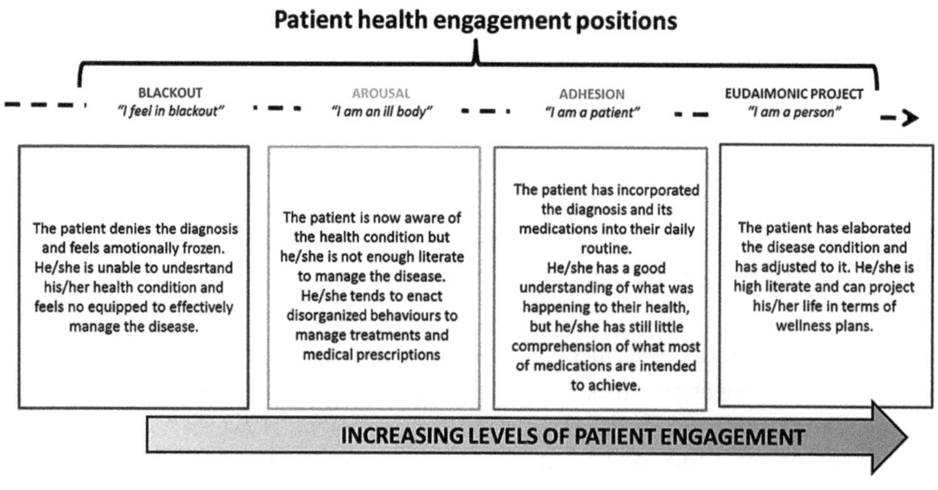

depends on how he/she succeeded in the previous phases. The last position of the engagement process (i.e., eudaimonic project) culminates in a patient that has gained a positive approach to health management and has recaptured an active role in society by re-establishing plans for wellness. Such patient has succeeded in incorporating disease management into his/her life. In particular, the four positions of engagement featured by the PHE model may be summarized as it follows.

Blackout

This position is typical of patients at the beginning of their care journey, usually at the moment of the diagnosis or in the occurrence of a relapse or worsening of their clinical condition. The urgency and perceived drama of these moments creates in patients a state of emotional, behavioral, and cognitive blockage ("*blackout*"). Patients describe themselves as psychologically frozen, shocked by the disease, unable to face and manage it. Patients thus perceive the disease and its management out of their control. They feel like "in suspension," as they are looking forward to obtain a ruling from someone. In this phase patients tend to be passive and to delegate their cure to their reference healthcare professional. Patients are disengaged in this moment, but the emotional elaboration of their condition start from this, thus this initial experience is crucial to then evolve in the journey of engagement.

In this initial position patients describe their diagnosis as distressing and unacceptable. They perceive strongly negative emotions and tend whether to refuse the disease (by denying the symptoms and their recurrence) or to depressively experience it, as the end of their positive trajectory of life. Patients in this stage cannot easily elaborate the received information about the disease (cognitive blindness) and as a consequence they also feel blocked in acting (behavioral freezing) and managing their disease. Patients in this phase tend to be completely absorbed in their illness experience and often experience difficulty attending to the needs of their private and social life due to a focus on the management of their disease and its treatment. In this phase, the patients' quality of life strongly depends on the effectiveness in controlling/reducing the side effects connected to treatments and clinical stability.

Arousal

In the position of *"arousal"*, patients have acquired and initial understanding of their health condition and of the medical requirements to manage them. They have also elaborate a first adjustment to their disease, although if they are still far from having accepted it. At the emotional level patients still appear distressed and very preoccupied for their health condition: as a result they are hyper-attentive to every signal in their bodies (emotional alert) that they tend to overestimate and to refer to their diagnosis, even when this is not appropriate. Patients in this position perceive symptoms as an "alarm" that worries the patient and may cause overwhelming emotional reactions. Patients are equipped with more information about their health condition compared to the previous phase, although their health literacy is still superficial and fragmented (superficial knowledge). Moreover, they feel behaviorally unable to manage their disease and treatment prescriptions effectively (behavioral disorganization).

Adhesion

In this position patients have moved some progress along their emotional elaboration of the disease. This position of engagement is often experienced by patients in a more advanced stage of their medical journey and it appears function of the broader spectrum of health knowledge (cognitive adhesion) which the patients have acquired from their reference healthcare professional or autonomously searching for health information. Patients in this position have accepted their disease and their new identity of "patient". They also have developed the basic behavioral skills (formal adherence) to effectively comply with medical prescriptions. They also feel sufficiently confident in their own emotional strength to cope with their disease. Although already manifesting a satisfactory level of activation, patients in this position are not really autonomous in managing the rules necessary to be healthy (i.e., healthy life style and correct medication regimen). The ability of these patients to cope with their disease and its management is challenged when some change happens in their daily routine (i.e., when going to holiday, when travelling for work…). Since patients in this position have not fully elaborated and integrated their disease condition yet, they find also difficult to completely accept the rationale behind the medical requests of changing their lifestyle or of their new medication regimen. Accordingly, patients revealed the need to continuously hang on their reference healthcare professionals' authority, which they conceive as a «life-line», waiting for the time when they will be able and self-confident to self-manage.

According to the specificities of this status, the patient's quality of life depends mainly on the fulfillment of the patient's healthcare needs and on the responsiveness of the healthcare provider. The patient's wellness is closely associated with the experience of a healthcare system that is truly attuned to the care expectations of the patient.

Eudaimonic Project

Finally, in the "*eudaimonic project*" position, patients have fully accepted their health condition and the successfully integrated their new identity of "patients" in a more complex and broader self-representation. They have elaborated the idea that the disease occurrence has impacted greatly on their life routines but that it is still possible (and legitimate) to maintain some sort of positive self-realization in their private life (elaboration). Patients in this experiential position became able to recognize internal resources that are useful for acquiring a positive approach to life and to health, despite the diagnosis, and that become the base for a full engagement in their self-management. Patients gradually become co-constructors of their health and capable of enacting a meaningful health management, which allows them to improve their quality of life. Patients are able to effectively search for appropriate information about their disease conditions and medications. This allows them to give full sense to their health experience (sense making) and effectively enact healthy behaviors, in due time, even when contexts change (situated practices). Patients have also developed a new perspective about their disease, which can now be thoughtful and integrated in a wider life project. They also become able to make some reasonable but still satisfactory plan for their near feature, in the light of the new health condition and maybe despite shorter expectations of life. According to this experiential position, patients are the managers of their own care, and they can mobilize healthcare services proactively when there is a need. Moreover, they can advocate for the health of their community (e.g., raising concerns to policymakers, helping others navigate the health care system, and advancing healthcare quality and equity). The patient in this phase becomes an experienced testimonial of good self-care practice who is able to become a caregiver of others similar to him/her. Given the patients' reconquered possibility to consider themselves as whole persons despite their disease condition, their quality of life depends strongly on their renewed ability to make realistic life decisions that are consistent with the influence of their disease on their life. This position of the model is considered as the full realization of patients' engagement, also at the level of the emotional elaboration and acceptation of the disease. This is the position to which patients should tend along their emotional journey of disease management and adjustment to their illness.

APPLICATION OF THE PHE-S IN CLINICAL SETTINGS

The Patient Health Engagement Scale (PHE-s), based on this model, allows to briefly and easily assess the level of emotional elaboration of a patient concerning his/her health condition by simply asking five straight forward questions. This set of questions — and the alternative of answers that the model offers — may orient clinicians, managers, and other professionals in dealing with interventions aimed to sustain patients' self-care abilities in assessing primary psychological needs and care expectations. Basically, the PHE-s questions the patients' stage of psychological elaboration about the changed health condition and of their engagement needs (way of "feeling" when reflecting on health status). This instrument is today the only one specifically dedicated to assess the degree of emotional elaboration and adjustment reached by the patient concerning his/her own health condition when engaging in health management. The specificity of this scale lays in the fact that it allows not only to assess the current patient's attitude towards his/her health condition, but also to forecast the patient's risk for disengagement in health management and thus to design preventive targeted intervention to optimize care pathways.

Figure 3. Instruction form for introducing the PHE-s to the patient (Graffigna et al., 2015a)

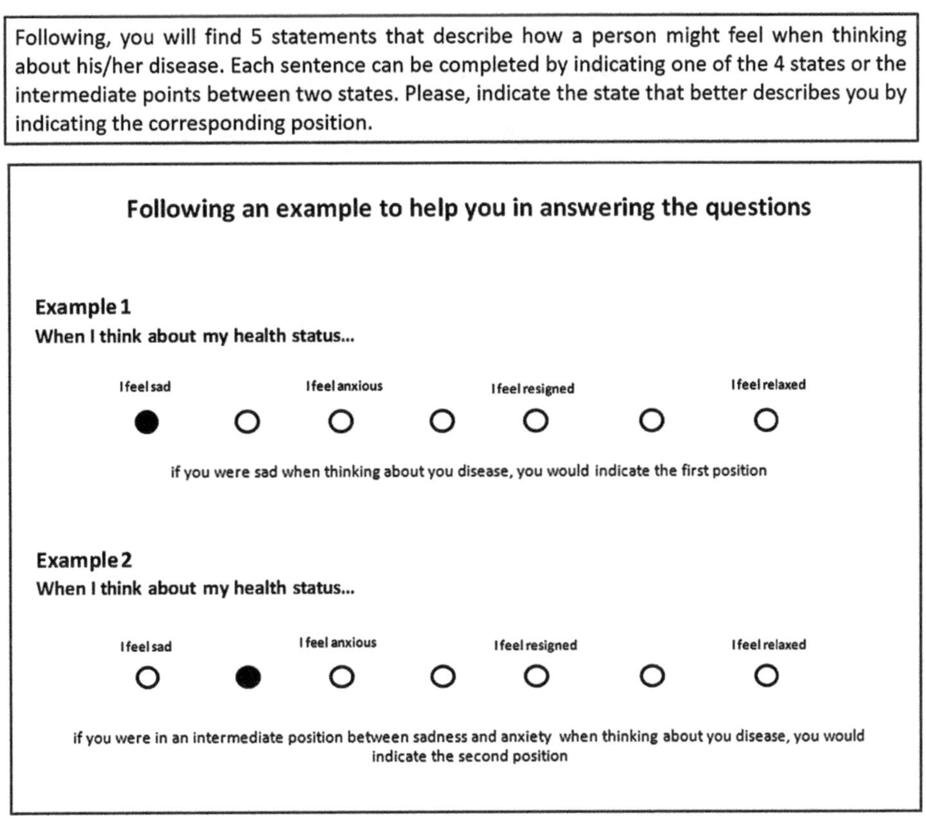

Following, you will find 5 statements that describe how a person might feel when thinking about his/her disease. Each sentence can be completed by indicating one of the 4 states or the intermediate points between two states. Please, indicate the state that better describes you by indicating the corresponding position.

Following an example to help you in answering the questions

Example 1
When I think about my health status...

I feel sad — I feel anxious — I feel resigned — I feel relaxed

if you were sad when thinking about you disease, you would indicate the first position

Example 2
When I think about my health status...

I feel sad — I feel anxious — I feel resigned — I feel relaxed

if you were in an intermediate position between sadness and anxiety when thinking about you disease, you would indicate the second position

Figure 4. The PHE-s (Graffigna et al., 2015a)

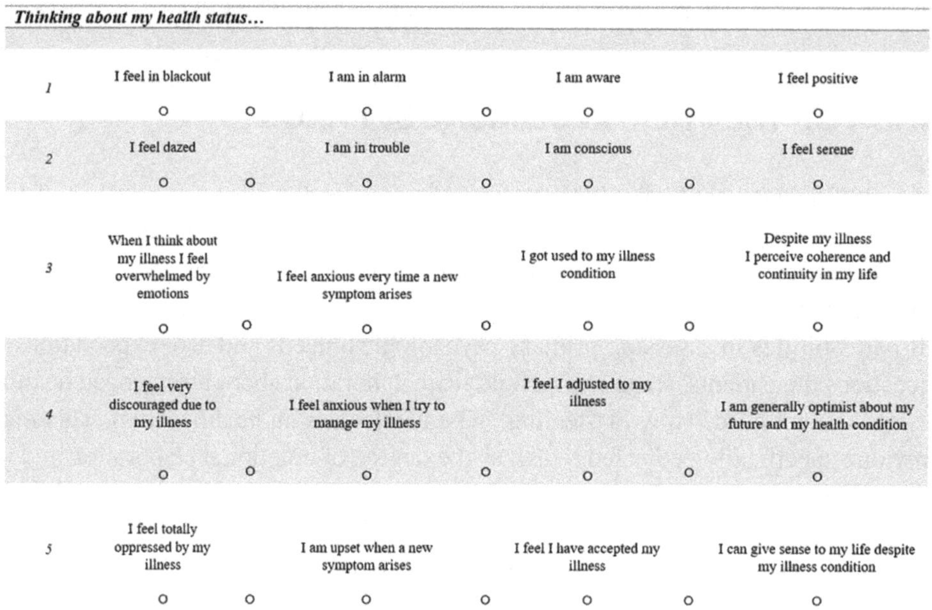

Thinking about my health status…							
1	I feel in blackout		I am in alarm		I am aware		I feel positive
	o	o	o	o	o	o	o
2	I feel dazed		I am in trouble		I am conscious		I feel serene
	o	o	o	o	o	o	o
3	When I think about my illness I feel overwhelmed by emotions		I feel anxious every time a new symptom arises		I got used to my illness condition		Despite my illness I perceive coherence and continuity in my life
	o	o	o	o	o	o	o
4	I feel very discouraged due to my illness		I feel anxious when I try to manage my illness		I feel I adjusted to my illness		I am generally optimist about my future and my health condition
	o	o	o	o	o	o	o
5	I feel totally oppressed by my illness		I am upset when a new symptom arises		I feel I have accepted my illness		I can give sense to my life despite my illness condition
	o	o	o	o	o	o	o

Figure 5. Conversion table for calculating the PHE-s score

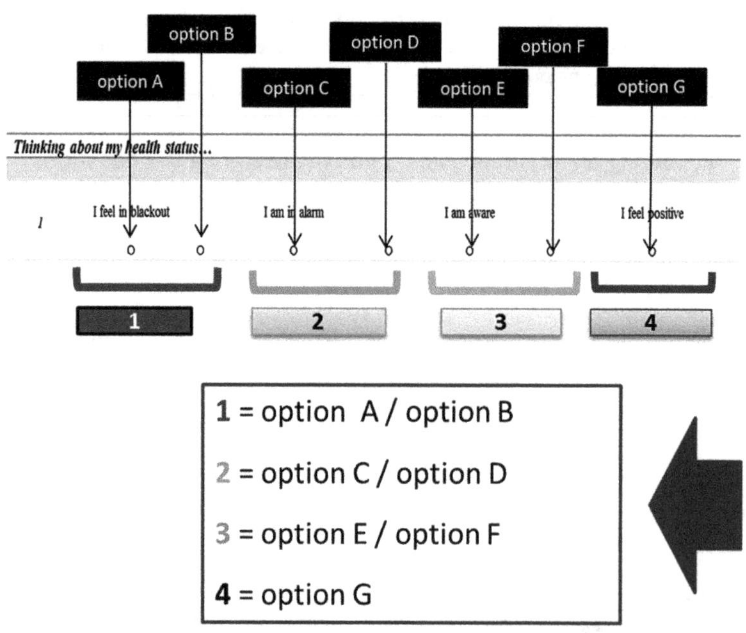

The PHE-s is a patient self-administrable questionnaire developed with the aim of diagnosing the level of patient engagement in their healthcare process that is function of his/her degree of emotional elaboration of the new health condition. This tool allows clinicians to move from a style of interaction that is clinician-directed and focuses on patients' adherence to treatments, to one that supports patients' motivation and autonomy in the care process, matches patients' level of engagement, and ultimately increases engagement. The information from the PHE-s might help guide the discussion and the action plan for care. Figure 3 shows the instruction form to be presented to the patient before asking him/her to fill out the questionnaire. Figure 4 shows the complete PHE-s.

The clinician who is in charge when administering the scale to the patient has to introduce and explain to the subject the aim of the questionnaire by specifying that to be effective in answering the proposed questions, the patient should refer to how he/she is currently living/experiencing his/her health status; The response options featuring this instrument (i.e. ordinal scale) allow patients to easily mirror with the current emotional states related to their disease condition. The ordinal structure of the response options also allows subjects to position themselves along an experiential continuum. Finally, the 7 response options for each item allow patients to position themselves in "intermediate" points (also for avoiding the social desirability mechanism). These 7 positions can be easily converted into a "patient engagement" scoring by following the instructions offered by the conversion table (Figure 5).

Finally, the clinician has to support the patient during the administration of the instrument in order to clarify possible doubts when filling out the questionnaire. The PHS-s has been constructed moving from 5 items with points (rang) of an ordinal categorical nature, instead of a quantitative-metric logic as usually adopted in psychometrics scales. The final scoring, thus, have to keep into account the ordinal origin of items answers. In order to calculate the PHE score, the most correct choice at the methodological level would be considering the metrical factor resulting from the not-linear analysis of principal components (CATPCA). This statistical technique requires an advanced knowledge of data-mining procedures and the use of dedicated software. This would not be possible in the applied clinical settings and during the daily clinical practices. Thus, during scale validation procedures, a simpler approach was used, in order

Figure 6. Procedure to calculate the PHE-s level

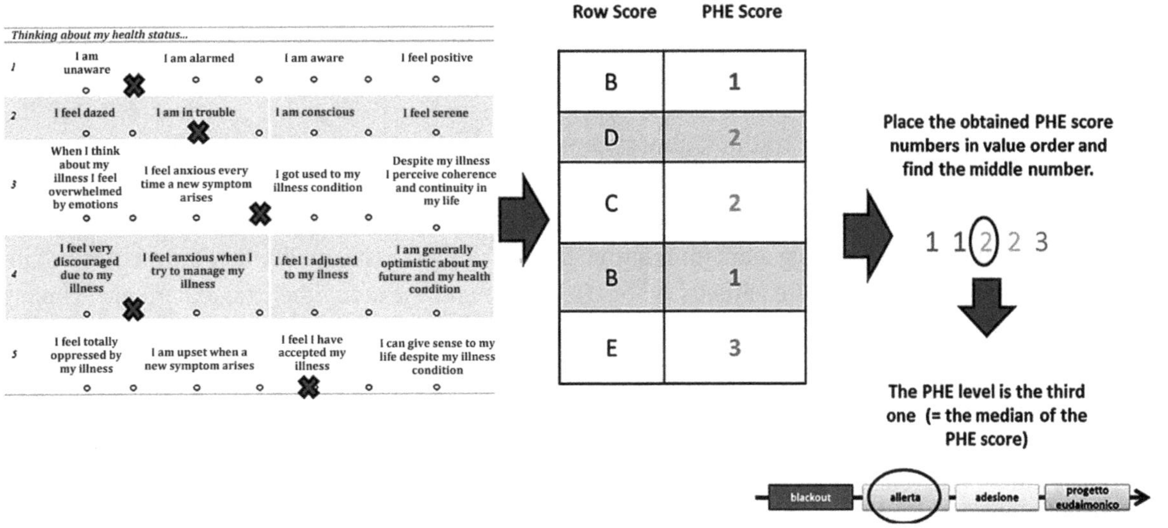

to make the PHE-s usable from the larger group of patients and healthcare professionals interested in assessing the emotional adjustment of patients along their engagement process. The two best adequate indexes to synthetize ordinal data are the median and the mode. In the PHE-s validation study (Graffigna et al., 2015a) the linear correlation between the metric factor of CAPTCA and, respectively, mode and median have been calculated. Both correlations resulted high (i.e. correlation with mode=.91; correlation with median= -96). For ordinal data, the median score is considered a more robust and reliable index and, differently from the mode, it is always univocally defined. Thus the median has been adopted as the index to calculate the PHE-s score. To obtain the PHE-s level, the median of the row PHE-s scores should be calculated. And with a simple conversion it is possible to transform the row PHE-s scores in the corresponding patient's engagement position (Figure 6).

THE PHE SCALE AS A GUIDELINE FOR CLINICAL ACTIONS

When clinicians have to face a diagnostic process, they might proceed according to different logics. On the one hand, they can follow a "top-down" approach where the diagnosis determines an intervention (i.e. clinical, pharmacological…). In this case the diagnosis is based on predetermined criteria which are part of the clinician's expertise. Diagnosing patient engagement following this logic means to administrate the questionnaires and collect data and information in order to plan an intervention aimed at "correcting" dysfunctional behaviors or knowledge which might hinder the active role of patients in the care process.

On the other hand, another logic might guide the clinician's action when assessing the patient engagement level. In this case, the clinician and the patients are considered both expert actors of the care process. Diagnosis and intervention are guided by a circular logic which results in the definition of a therapeutic and relational contract between the patient and the provider. The diagnosis represents - in this case - a starting point for guiding the clinical encounter and establishing a shared plan for care. It is conceivable as a moment of patient's self-awareness (and empowerment) concerning his/her capacity and availability to actively engage in the care process. The diagnostic phase is a first occasion to promote the patients' change. In this sense, we can say that the assessment has a therapeutic value *per sé* (Provenzi et al., 2016). However, it is important to consider the diagnostic moment as the first step for planning a shared plan for intervention basing on the information collected by administering the questionnaires.

In particular, when defining a shared plan of intervention basing on the level of patient engagement assessed in the diagnostic moment, means questioning different strategical aspects:

- First of all, clinicians have to think about the style of interaction more suitable for each level of engagement. This means reflecting upon the best way of relationship with each patient in order to better fine tune with his/her illness experience and role expectation in the care process.
- Second, effective patient engagement requires to carefully plan the quality and the quantity of information and knowledge the patients is able to receive and use along the care experience. Having in mind the level of patient engagement and activation might orient clinicians in selecting the most effective information to be provided to improve the patients' active management of the care prescriptions.
- Finally, planning a co-constructed intervention for patient engagement, also implies to define the best timing for intervening and the frequency of interaction with the patients to effectively support them.

The PHE-s allows to evaluate patients in a holistic way by collecting multiple information regarding all the experiential dimensions involved in the patient engagement experience. However, by combining this with the other instruments today available, practitioners might obtain a comprehensive overview about the patient's level of skills, knowledge and emotional acceptance of his/her health condition. In particular, the adoption of the PHE-s (alone or in combination with the other tools) may guarantee to have not only a superficial measure of what patients do or know when dealing with the disease management, but also a deeper understanding of the emotional dynamics underlining the adjustment of patients to the disease condition and the acceptance of his/her new patient identity. Catching this last aspect – that is the patient illness experience – should be considered as a reading key for health practitioners to fine tune with their patients when taking decisions about healthcare (Barello & Graffigna, 2015b).

For instance, when patients receive a PHE-s score of "*Blackout*", the clinicians should be aware that, in order to improve their level of engagement, patients need to overcome the emotional confusion connected to the disrupting critical event. In this scope, a trusted relationship with the healthcare provider is crucial for overcoming the blackout phase. The healthcare professional is asked to scaffold patients in this phase and offer solidarity by making an empathic response and educating them about their health. This informative action is expected from the referential healthcare professional who becomes, since the moment of the diagnosis, the privileged spokesperson for the patient along the care process. If patients fail to build a solid relation with the healthcare provider, their emotional behavioral responses may become dysfunctional, often leading to patients' dropout.

In other cases, when patients receive a PHE-s score of "*Arousal*", they manifest to have acquired a basic understanding of their diagnosis and of their health status, but they are still overwhelmed by negative emotions linked to the diagnosis. Patients in this phase, in order to move forward in their engagement journey, need to be supported in emotionally and pragmatically copying with the change related to the health condition. With patients in this PHE-s positions, healthcare professionals have to legitimate patients in asking for help and be open to answer all the questions and doubts they may have. Furthermore, healthcare professional should provide a "how to do" list with practical situations and ways to face them in the daily management of health for planning an reminding screenings.

When patients receive a PHE-s score of "*Adhesion*" they have reached a good adjustment to their disease, although they are not able to approach it in a positive light and thus they do not have enough personal resources to completely mange medical prescriptions. At this stage, healthcare professionals are claimed to train problem-solving skills and sustain patients' motivation towards self-management. They also should promote a therapeutic alliance aimed to sustain patients' initiatives and motivation to be autonomous. Empowering sessions are also welcome with patients tailored healthy behavior tracking.

The PHE-s score of "*Eudaimonic Project*" indicates patients who fully accomplished their engagement journey: they have successfully elaborated their new healthcare conditions and adjusted to it. They learned the information and the skills necessary to cope with the disease and the medical prescriptions. They also matured a positive approach to health and life, recognizing how the "patient role" is only referring to a new identity of the individual, additional to previous role and commitment. These patients need to be sustained in this positive approach to healthcare, they need support for succeed in this renewed balance between healthcare needs and quality of life needs. Healthcare professionals are claimed to health coaching, goal setting and support these patients in planning and achieving positive health plans. Healthcare systems should promote at distance relationship and remote communication with a referential healthcare professional. Patients and caregivers' participation to make their voice reflected in healthcare organizations governance should also be accomplished at this stage.

CONCLUSION

From what we defined a "person-centered" approach to integrated care, assessing the level of patient engagement is an essential component of a successful strategy for improving patients' experience. Eliciting feedback from patients regarding their attitudes towards their health status affords an opportunity to highlight and address aspects of care that need improvement and to monitor performance with regard to meeting patient expectations in the delivery of care. Furthermore, being able to assess the level of emotional elaboration of the disease and the patient psychological adjustment to its management is crucial to sustain not only effective clinical interventions but also to allow patients to maintain positive and satisfactory life trajectories and their successful engagement in care management.

At present few dedicated tools exist to assess the level of patients' engagement. Although the emotional and psychodynamic component of the engagement experience is recognized by health scholars to play an important role in sustaining or hindering patients' ability to managing their disease, so far only one dedicate tool exists to diagnose the emotional mindset of patients along their engagement journey. In this chapter we have described and discussed the specificities of the Patients Health Engagement Scale (PHE-s), developed in order to assess patients' engagement also in its emotional component. Since previous empirical study have showed how the level of patients' elaboration of the disease is an antecedent and mediator of patients' activation towards self-management, becoming able to assess it may help in forecasting patients' ability in improving their skills to cope with the disease and the medical prescriptions in daily life. This may lead to the planning of better personalized and, thus, more effective healthcare interventions. However, the PHE-s may be useful also when used to measure the effectiveness of clinical interventions. Particularly, measuring the level of patient engagement after an educational session, after a medical consultation, or even after service delivery reorganization may be an important asset to account for the made changes and achieved goals.

Furthermore, if combined with other validated tools, the PHE-s may contribute to the deeper and more complete assessment of patients' healthcare needs and priorities, together with their quality expectations towards the healthcare systems.

Moving steps forwards in the practice of measuring healthcare effectiveness in engaging patients should be envisaged as a crucial goal to concretely reform services and to make them better effective and sustainable at the economic level.

REFERENCES

Alegría, M., Sribney, W., Perez, D., Laderman, M., & Keefe, K. (2009). The role of patient activation on patient–provider communication and quality of care for US and foreign born Latino patients. *Journal of General Internal Medicine*, *24*(3), 534–541. doi:10.1007/s11606-009-1074-x PMID:19842003

Barello, S., & Graffigna, G. (2014b). Engaging patients to recover life projectuality: An Italian cross-disease framework. *Quality of Life Research: An International Journal of Quality of Life Aspects of Treatment, Care and Rehabilitation*, *24*(5), 1087–1096. doi:10.1007/s11136-014-0846-x PMID:25373927

Barello, S. & Graffigna, G. (2015b). Patient engagement in healthcare: pathways for effective medical decision making. *Neuropsychogical Trends,* 2015, 53.

Barello, S., Graffigna, G., Savarese, M., & Bosio, A. C. (2014a). Engaging patients in health management: Towards a preliminary theoretical conceptualization. *Psicologia della Salute*, *3*(3), 11–33. doi:10.3280/PDS2014-003002

Barello, S., Graffigna, G., Vegni, E., Savarese, M., Lombardi, F., & Bosio, A. C. (2015a). 'Engage me in taking care of my heart': A grounded theory study on patient–cardiologist relationship in the hospital management of heart failure. *BMJ Open*, *5*(3), e005582. doi:10.1136/bmjopen-2014-005582 PMID:25776041

Battersby, M. W., Ask, A., Reece, M. M., Markwick, M. J., & Collins, J. P. (2003). The Partners in Health scale: The development and psychometric properties of a generic assessment scale for chronic condition self-management. *Australian Journal of Primary Health*, *9*(3), 41–52. doi:10.1071/PY03022

Becker, E. R., & Roblin, D. W. (2008). Translating primary care practice climate into patient activation: The role of patient trust in physician. *Medical Care*, *46*(8), 795–805. doi:10.1097/MLR.0b013e31817919c0 PMID:18665059

Berwick, D. M., Nolan, T. W., & Whittington, J. (2008). The triple aim: Care, health, and cost. *Health Affairs*, *27*(3), 759–769. doi:10.1377/hlthaff.27.3.759 PMID:18474969

Coulter, A., & Dunn, N. (2002). After Bristol: putting patients at the centre. Commentary: Patient centered care: timely, but is it practical? *British Medical Journal*, *324*(7338), 648–651. doi:10.1136/bmj.324.7338.648 PMID:11895824

Coulter, A., & Ellins, J. (2007). Effectiveness of strategies for informing, educating, and involving patients. *BMJ: British Medical Journal*, *335*(7609), 24–27. doi:10.1136/bmj.39246.581169.80 PMID:17615222

Davis, R. E., Jacklin, R., Sevdalis, N., & Vincent, C. A. (2007). Patient involvement in patient safety: What factors influence patient participation and engagement. *Health Expectations*, *10*(3), 259–267. doi:10.1111/j.1369-7625.2007.00450.x PMID:17678514

Dearing, R. L., Barrick, C., Dermen, K. H., & Walitzer, K. S. (2005). Indicators of client engagement: Influences on alcohol treatment satisfaction and outcomes. *Psychology of Addictive Behaviors*, *19*(1), 71–78. doi:10.1037/0893-164X.19.1.71 PMID:15783280

Duke, C. C., Lynch, W. D., Smith, B., & Winstanley, J. (2015). Validity of a New Patient Engagement Measure: The Altarum Consumer Engagement (ACE) Measure™. *The Patient-Patient-Centered Outcomes Research*, *8*(6), 559–568. doi:10.1007/s40271-015-0131-2 PMID:26097010

Graffigna, G., Barello, S., Bonanomi, A., & Lozza, E. (2015a). Measuring patient engagement: Development and psychometric properties of the Patient Health Engagement (PHE) scale. *Frontiers in Psychology*, 2015, 6. PMID:25870566

Graffigna, G., Barello, S., Bonanomi, A., Lozza, E., & Hibbard, J. (2015b). Measuring patient activation in Italy: Translation, adaptation and validation of the Italian version of the patient activation measure 13 (PAM13-I). *BMC Medical Informatics and Decision Making*, *15*(1), 1. doi:10.1186/s12911-015-0232-9 PMID:26699852

Graffigna, G., Barello, S., Bonanomi, A., Menichetti, J. (in press). The Motivating Function of Healthcare Professional in eHealth and mHealth Interventions for Type 2 Diabetes Patients and the Mediating Role of Patient Engagement, *Journal of Diabetes Research.*

Graffigna, G., Barello, S., Libreri, C., & Bosio, C. A. (2014b). How to engage type-2 diabetic patients in their own health management: Implications for clinical practice. *BMC Public Health, 14*(1), 648. doi:10.1186/1471-2458-14-648 PMID:24966036

Graffigna, G., Barello, S., Riva, G., & Bosio, A. C. (2014a). Patient Engagement: The Key to Redesign the Exchange Between the Demand and Supply for Healthcare in the Era of Active Ageing. *Active Ageing and Healthy Living: A Human Centered Approach in Research and Innovation as Source of Quality of Life, 203*, 85

Graffigna, G., Barello, S., & Triberti, S. (2015c). *Patient Engagement: A Consumer-Centered Model to Innovate Healthcare.* Berlin: DeGruyter Open. doi:10.1515/9783110452440

Greene, J., & Hibbard, J. H. (2012). Why does patient activation matter? An examination of the relationships between patient activation and health-related outcomes. *Journal of General Internal Medicine, 27*(5), 520–526. doi:10.1007/s11606-011-1931-2 PMID:22127797

Gruman, J., Rovner, M. H., French, M. E., Jeffress, D., Sofaer, S., Shaller, D., & Prager, D. J. (2010). From patient education to patient engagement: Implications for the field of patient education. *Patient Education and Counseling, 78*(3), 350–356. doi:10.1016/j.pec.2010.02.002 PMID:20202780

Hibbard, J. H. (2009). Using systematic measurement to target consumer activation strategies. *Medical Care Research and Review, 66*(1 Suppl.), 9S–27S. doi:10.1177/1077558708326969 PMID:19052169

Hibbard, J. H., & Greene, J. (2013). What the evidence shows about patient activation: Better health outcomes and care experiences; fewer data on costs. *Health Affairs, 32*(2), 207–214. doi:10.1377/hlthaff.2012.1061 PMID:23381511

Hibbard, J. H., Greene, J., & Overton, V. (2013). Patients with lower activation associated with higher costs; delivery systems should know their patients' scores. *Health Affairs, 32*(2), 216–222. doi:10.1377/hlthaff.2012.1064 PMID:23381513

Hibbard, J. H., & Mahoney, E. (2010). Toward a theory of patient and consumer activation. *Patient Education and Counseling, 78*(3), 377–381. doi:10.1016/j.pec.2009.12.015 PMID:20188505

Hibbard, J. H., Mahoney, E. R., Stock, R., & Tusler, M. (2007). Do Increases in Patient Activation Result in Improved Self-Management Behaviors? *Health Services Research, 42*(4), 1443–1463. doi:10.1111/j.1475-6773.2006.00669.x PMID:17610432

Howie, J. G., Heaney, D. J., Maxwell, M., & Walker, J. J. (1998). A comparison of a Patient Enablement Instrument (PEI) against two established satisfaction scales as an outcome measure of primary care consultations. *Family Practice, 15*(2), 165–171. doi:10.1093/fampra/15.2.165 PMID:9613486

Kodner, D. L., & Spreeuwenberg, C. (2002). Integrated care: Meaning, logic, applications, and implications–a discussion paper. *International Journal of Integrated Care*, 2002, 2. PMID:16896389

Légaré, F., & Witteman, H. O. (2013). Shared decision making: Examining key elements and barriers to adoption into routine clinical practice. *Health Affairs*, *32*(2), 276–284. doi:10.1377/hlthaff.2012.1078 PMID:23381520

Leventhal, H., Benyamini, Y., Brownlee, S., Diefenbach, M., Leventhal, E. A., Patrick-Miller, L., & Robitaille, C. (1997). Illness representations: theoretical foundations. In *Perceptions of health and illness* (Vol. 2, pp. 19-46).

Mahmud, S. (2004). Citizen participation in the health sector in rural Bangladesh: Perceptions and reality. *IDS Bulletin*, *35*(2), 11–18. doi:10.1111/j.1759-5436.2004.tb00116.x

McBride, T., & Korczak, V. (2007). Community consultation and engagement in healthcare reform. *Australian Health Review*, *31*(5), 13–15. doi:10.1071/AH070S13 PMID:17402899

Meglic, M., Furlan, M., Kuzmanic, M., Kozel, D., Baraga, D., Kuhar, I., & Brodnik, A. et al. (2010). Feasibility of an ehealth service to support collaborative depression care: Results of a pilot study. *Journal of Medical Internet Research*, *12*(5), e63. doi:10.2196/jmir.1510 PMID:21172765

Provenzi, L., Menichetti, J., Coin, R., & Aschieri, F. (2016). (in press). Psychological assessment as an intervention with couples: Single case application of collaborative techniques in clinical practice. *Professional Psychology*.

Rask, K. J., Ziemer, D. C., Kohler, S. A., Hawley, J. N., Arinde, F. J., & Barnes, C. S. (2009). Patient activation is associated with healthy behaviors and ease in managing diabetes in an indigent population. *The Diabetes Educator*, *35*(4), 622–630. doi:10.1177/0145721709335004 PMID:19419972

Skolasky, R. L., Mackenzie, E. J., Wegener, S. T., & Riley, L. H. III. (2008). Patient activation and adherence to physical therapy in persons undergoing spine surgery. *Spine*, *33*(21), E784–E791. doi:10.1097/BRS.0b013e31818027f1 PMID:18827683

Steverink, N., Lindenberg, S., & Slaets, J. P. J. (2005). How to understand and improve older people's self-management of wellbeing. *European Journal of Ageing*, *2*(4), 235–244. doi:10.1007/s10433-005-0012-y

Stewart, M. (2001). Towards a global definition of patient centered care: The patient should be the judge of patient centred care. *British Medical Journal*, *322*(7284), 444. doi:10.1136/bmj.322.7284.444 PMID:11222407

Street, R. L. Jr, Gordon, H. S., Ward, M. M., Krupat, E., & Kravitz, R. L. (2005). Patient participation in medical consultations: Why some patients are more involved than others. *Medical Care*, *43*(10), 960–969. doi:10.1097/01.mlr.0000178172.40344.70 PMID:16166865

KEY TERMS AND DEFINITIONS

Illness Experience: Disease refers to a specific clinical entity characterized by a disturbance in the structure or function of any part, organ, or system of the body. Illness is a broader concept that refers to any condition that a person views as sickness (Eisenberg, 1977). Leventhal and colleagues identified five dimensions of the illness experience: 1) identity of the illness – connecting the symptoms with the illness and having an understanding of the illness; 2) timeline – duration and progression of the illness; 3) causes – perceived reason for the illness; 4) consequences – what will be the physical, psychosocial and economic impact of the illness; 5) controllability – can the disease be controlled or cured?

Measuring Patient Experience: Ensuring that care is person-centered is one of six essential aims for achieving high-quality health care. The use of assessment measures to query patients about their experiences of health and healthcare management is the best and often only way to examine whether the experiences deemed essential for high-quality, person-centered care actually take place.

Patient Activation Measure: Developed by Hibbard and colleagues, the 13-item Patient Activation Measure is an interval-level, unidimensional Guttman-like measure that contains items measuring self-assessed knowledge about chronic conditions, beliefs about illness and medical care, and self-efficacy for self-care. The PAM focused on physical conditions, and it was designed to measure activation as a broad construct.

Patient Activation: Patient activation can be defined as the degree of patient baheviour as an active agent in the management of his/her own health including developmental stages: 1) believing the patient role is important, 2) having the confidence and knowledge necessary to take action, 3) actually taking action to maintain and improve one's health, and 4) staying the course even under stress.

Patient Engagement: Process-like and multidimensional experience, resulting from the conjoint cognitive (think), emotional (feel) and conative (act) enactment of individuals towards their health management. Patient engagement can be characterized by how much information flows between patient and provider, how active a role the patient has in care decisions, and how involved the patient or patient organization becomes in health organization decisions and in policy making.

Patient Health Engagement Scale: developed by Graffigna and colleagues, this is a measure of patient engagement that is grounded in rigorous conceptualization and appropriate psychometric methods. The scale consists of 5 ordinal items and was developed based on the authors' conceptual model of patient engagement (PHE model), which features four positions along a continuum of engagement (i.e., blackout; arousal; adhesion; eudaimonic project).

Patient Participation: Patient participation means to involve patients in the decision making process regarding health issues and also it is a strategy aimed at encouraging patients to participate in improving patient safety

Chapter 11
Accountability and Public Reporting:
Publication of Performance to Improve Quality

Maria Tanzariello
Università Cattolica del Sacro Cuore, Rome, Italy

Sabina Bucci
Università Cattolica del Sacro Cuore, Rome, Italy

Walter Ricciardi
Università Cattolica del Sacro Cuore, Rome, Italy

Antonio Giulio de Belvis
Università Cattolica del Sacro Cuore, Rome, Italy

ABSTRACT

Patient engagement is based on the assumption that making patients co-producers of their health might enhance their satisfaction and responsibility with the healthcare system and it strictly linked with the health provider choice. Making patients active participants in their healthcare is considered a crucial component of high-quality healthcare services. Quality of care is a central concern for health systems: accountability, transparency, and public reporting are some key factors in promoting healthcare improvement. In the healthcare field, public reporting is one of the major tools in supporting patients' decisions making process, by providing structure, process and outcome measures. We performed a web-based analysis of the major initiatives of public reporting in order to highlight their main characteristics: properties (public or private), data source (health providers, ad hoc surveys, etc.), general information reported (i.e. size, language spoken, amenities), doctors' information, patients' ratings (satisfaction / experience), clinical indicators.

DOI: 10.4018/978-1-4666-9992-2.ch011

INTRODUCTION

In this chapter, moving from the link between quality in healthcare and patient/consumer engagement, as driving concept, we deeply explain interactions between some challenging topics in the healthcare sector: quality of health care, accountability, transparency and public reporting.

In the first part of the chapter, more theoretical, we provide a synthesis of the literature about the topics.

Patient engagement – borrowed from the marketing conceptualization of consumer engagement – is based on the assumption that making patients/clients co-producers of their health might enhance their satisfaction and responsibility with the healthcare system, by improving positive clinical outcomes and reducing health delivery costs (Graffigna, Barello, & Triberti, 2015).

A recent report on patient engagement in health care, identifies an Engagement Behavior Framework, as a qualitative description of the behaviors that individuals must perform to optimally benefit from their care, based on ten types of tasks, that deals with the healthcare process as a whole, from the choice to the payment of providers, from health promotion and prevention to the end of life planning (Center for Advancing Health, 2010).

Making patients active participants in their healthcare is considered a crucial component of high-quality healthcare services. Since 2001, the Institute of Medicine's report "Crossing the Quality Chasm" (2001) has been recognizing patient-centered care as an essential dimension of high-quality care (Clancy, 2011). In 2006, the World Health Organization indicates patients and the population engagement as one of the six domains of quality interventions (World Health Organization [WHO], 2006).

Wide definition of quality and quality improvement and a focus on quality measurement are proposed.

Several formulations of quality definition are both possible and legitimate: all the stakeholders involved in the healthcare sector consider different aspects of quality of care depending on where they are located in the systems of care and on the nature of their responsibilities.

Avedis Donabedian, known as the founder of the theory of quality in healthcare stated that "quality of care is the kind of care that is expected to maximize an inclusive measure of patient welfare after one has taken into account the balance of expected gains and losses that attend the process of care in all its parts" (Donabedian, 1980). His definition can be synthetized by this quote: "Do only what is useful (effective theory), in the best way (effectiveness) with the least cost (efficiency), for who (accessibility), and only to those who really need (appropriateness), making do care who is competent to do it (competence), obtaining the best results considered (satisfaction)" (Donabedian, 1980).

Quality of healthcare has been one of the most challenging issues for researchers for many years. Taking part from quality of healthcare definition, other streams of research emerged: quality assessment or measurement, quality improvement, measurement of quality improvement approaches, and many other still appears. Furthermore, quality of healthcare dominates and leads public policy agenda, so that it has been defined as a process for making strategic choices in health systems, as World Health Organization stated in the subheading of a report published in 2006 (WHO, 2006). Thus, quality of healthcare connects with one of the most important Public Health movement of the last decades, the Clinical Governance, that promotes continuous quality improvement by creating an environment in which excellence in clinical care will flourish (Scally & Donaldson, 1998) and many other current concept, such as accountability and transparency, that encompasses procedures and processes by which healthcare organizations try to reach their goals in terms of quality improvement.

On the patient side, this reflects on better clinical experiences, greater appropriateness of care, increased trust in the patient-physician relationship. Moreover, patients own more information that make they able to choose the providers that better meet their needs, aware about the care they receive and involved in their health plans, becoming engaged in their health and care. Public reporting has a great role in this frame, as it refers to the publication of information and reports on the quality of care delivered by providers, that could support patient choices.

Patients have to decide whether and when to seek care, which plans and providers meet their needs, how to manage their health (Clancy, 2011). Provider choice is one of the most important patient engagement pillar. But, are patients informed about the best care that they could receive? Do they know how to choose hospitals, health plans or professionals to address their healthcare needs? Are there tools able to support and guarantee aware choices?

Usually patients choose providers who meet criteria such as geographic access, personal style, often advised from friends or family. Preferences for characteristics vary across patient, and they also vary depending on the type of provider to choose (e.g. hospitals, primary care doctors, home care or care home providers) (Kumpunen, Trigg, & Rodrigues, 2014). It would be better if patients will use also comparative performance information, from public reporting initiatives, to identify the provider that better meets their need.

In the second part of the chapter, moving from this theoretical frame, we will present the result of a web based analysis aimed at comparing major initiatives of public reporting, classified by the following characteristics: properties (public or private), data source (health providers, ad hoc surveys, etc.), general information reported (i.e. size, language spoken, amenities), doctors' information, patients' ratings (satisfaction /experience), clinical indicators.

PATIENT ENGAGEMENT AND QUALITY IN HEALTHCARE

Western societies are facing some changes of scenario at the economic, social, and environmental levels that reflects also on the healthcare sector calling for revisions in policies and interventions (Graffigna et al., 2015). The economic crisis, the ageing of populations and the rise of chronic conditions are just some of these challenges that every country should take on in order to improve systems sustainability. Promoting patients engagement in healthcare management, by supporting them in the decision-making and in enacting healthy behaviors, is one of the actionable intervention for achieving such goals.

Why "engagement"? The word engagement derives from the verb "to engage" that "implies a dynamic and relational context, in which two parties agree on the goals of an action and on the phase of its process" (Graffigna et al., 2015). It has been introduced in the healthcare field not long ago to indicate a renewed partnership between different actors and institutions involved in health and care management (Hibbard, Stockard, Mahoney, & Tusler, 2004). The expression patient engagement has been borrowed from the marketing conceptualization of consumer engagement that refers to the (potentially positive) attitude of a consumer toward brands, products, services, or even media events (Gambetti & Graffigna, 2010).

The concept of patient engagement is based on the assumption that making patients/clients co-producers of their health might enhance their satisfaction and responsibility with the healthcare system, by improving positive clinical outcomes and reducing health delivery costs (Graffigna et al., 2015). It can be seen as a key qualifier of the exchange between the demand (i.e. citizens/patients) and the supply (i.e. healthcare system) of healthcare services in the different phases of the care processes. Understand

and manage the strategic levers that sustain patient engagement is crucial to innovate healthcare systems and to improve their sustainability (Graffigna et al., 2015).

It seems that patients engaged in their health and care may reach better quality of care and patient/health provider relationship, thus improving patient's clinical indicators and compliance to recommended treatments; on the contrary, patient not engaged in their health and care may cause waste of resources and poor clinical outcomes (Greene & Hibbard 2012; Graffigna et al., 2015).

The concept of patient engagement can be seen as an evolution of Patient Centered Medicine.

Patient Centered Medicine replaced the historical dominant bio-medical paradigm, bringing back "patients' voices" at the center of the healthcare processes. Even though it has been shown that Patient Centered Medicine contributes to clinical effectiveness improvements and psychological sustainability of care practices, it has not always been translated into real practice, usually as a resistance to organizational change. Nevertheless, if involvement and participation of consumers/clients of healthcare services have to be seen as a priority, patient engagement could be useful, as a qualifier in the exchange between the "demand" and "supply" of healthcare (Graffigna, Barello, Riva, & Bosio, 2014).

A recent report on patient engagement in health care, identifies an Engagement Behavior Framework, as a qualitative description of the behaviors that individuals must perform to optimally benefit from their care, based on ten types of tasks, that deals with the healthcare process as a whole, from the choice to the payment of providers, from health promotion and prevention to the end of life planning (Center for Advancing Health [CFAH], 2010). Making patients active participants in their healthcare is considered a crucial component of high-quality healthcare services.

The World Health Organization identifies patients and population engagement as one of the six domains of quality interventions. It is defined as critical to quality improvement, because individuals and communities play many roles within health systems. In fact, directly or indirectly, they finance care, work in partnership with health workers to manage their own care, they are sometimes the arbiter of what is or is not acceptable across all the dimensions of quality. Thus, ensure patients and population engagement is seen as a challenge, the heart of all policies and strategies for quality improvement. Policies and strategies to this end are likely to improve health literacy, self-care, and patients' experience with the health system. Patients and population would be involved in the governance of the health system, influencing decision-making trough their views and preferences and sharing responsibility for their own health. New interventions in quality must take into account these strategic fundamentals (WHO, 2006).

QUALITY IN HEALTHCARE

Quality in Healthcare: Definitions, Dimensions, Measurement

Quality of patient care is a central concern for health systems, especially in an era of unprecedented financial constraints, and rising demand and expectations. Thus, the focus on quality has intensified because of the concern that healthcare is costly, may sometimes be dispensed inappropriately and inequitably, and varies unduly among physicians and location.

The gap between the quality of healthcare possible and that currently provided has been referred to as a chasm. The reason way health systems globally frequently fail to provide patients with quality healthcare have been proposed as follows: an increase in chronic conditions, poorly organized systems for healthcare delivery, limited use of information technology, and the increased complexity of care as a result of medical advances (Institute of Medicine [IOM], 2001).

What is quality of care? How can it be defined? Quality is a complex and multi-faceted concept which have been defined in many different ways for the last decades. Several formulations of quality definition are both possible and legitimate: all the stakeholders involved in the healthcare sector consider different aspects of quality of care depending on where they are located in the systems of care and on the nature of their responsibilities. For example, doctors may consider medical outcomes or processes; economists may focus on social welfare, including features that consumers happen to care about, but that clinicians do not (i.e. appearance and size of hospital rooms); health plans may reflect on concepts of preventive care or organizational efficiencies (Wong, McNamara, & Greenberg, 2004; Cantù & Tzannis, 2011).

Firstly, quality can be referred both to healthcare and health systems. First of all, it reflects the extent to which an healthcare service or product produces a desired outcome (Runciman, Merry, & Walton, 2007). Furthermore, quality can be defined as a principle to assess if health system is performing well in its mission to improve health (National Health Performance Committee [NHPC], 2001). Avedis Donabedian, known as the founder of the theory of quality in healthcare, defined "Quality of care" in 1966 in its article, "Evaluating the Quality of Medical Care" (Donabedian, 1966) that has been cited by 4428 authors during the last 50 years. His revised definition stated that "quality of care is the kind of care that is expected to maximize an inclusive measure of patient welfare after one has taken into account the balance of expected gains and losses that attend the process of care in all its parts" (Donabedian, 1980). His quality definition can be synthetized by this quote: "Do only what is useful (effective theory), in the best way (effectiveness) with the least cost (efficiency), for who (accessibility), and only to those who really need (appropriateness), making do care who is competent to do it (competence), obtaining the best results considered (satisfaction)" (Donabedian, 1980). Furthermore, Donabedian highlights three principal quality dimensions:

- The structure (organizational quality), the static part of the system, the equipment
- The process (professional quality), the behaviors of personnel and customers on a scientific, ethic and social basis (diagnostic procedures, continuity of care, professional standards, comfort, privacy, etc.)
- The outcome (perceived quality) that is the evolution of the patient's health due to the care process (Donabedian, 1988; Cantù & Tzannis, 2011).

In the following years several authors gave highlighting definitions across a continuum of more or less operational and generalizable dimensions, such as: "excellence" (Samuel, Grant, & Irvine, 1994), "expectations" or "goals which have been met" (Ellis & Whittingham, 1993; Steffen, 1988), "zero defects" (Crosby, 1979) and "fitness for use" (Juran, 1988; Campbell, Roland, & Buetow, 2000). Nevertheless, the "Hippocratic Oath" seems to be one of the link between all the definitions of quality in healthcare provided, surely the oldest and the most complete one.

It was 1990 when the US Institute of Medicine, by assuming that healthcare ought to be safe, effective, patient centered, timely, efficient and equitable, introduced the well-known definition of quality: "the degree to which health services for individuals and populations increase the likelihood of desired health outcomes and are consistent with current professional knowledge" (IOM, 1990).

The Institute of Medicine's definition relates quality to the goals of the healthcare system. Quality of care is often defined trough individual dimensions or components that allows recognizing its complexity:

Table 1. Quality in healthcare: main classifications through dimensions (Modified by Campbell et al., 2000)

Donabedian (1990)	Maxwell (1992)	HSRG (1992)	O'Leary and O'Leary (1992)	Campbell et al. (2000)	WHO (2006)
	Accessibility	Accessibility	Accessibility	Accessibility	Accessibility
		Patient centredness	Patient perspectives		Patient centredness
Effectiveness	Effectiveness	Effectiveness	Effectiveness	Effectiveness	Effectiveness
Efficiency	Efficiency	Efficiency	Efficiency		Efficiency
		Continuity/ Co-ordination	Continuity		
Efficacy			Efficacy		
Acceptability	Acceptability				
Equity	Equity				Equity
Legitimacy					
		Comprehensiveness			
	Relevance				
					Safety

when viewed in combination the dimensions offer more specific definitions of quality (Campbell et al., 2000). Table 1 shows main dimensions according to some of the most important definitions of quality of care (Campbell et al., 2000).

For the World Health Organization quality is made by six areas or dimensions:

- Effectiveness, as adherence to evidence base medicine and improvement of health outcomes for individuals and communities, based on needs;
- Efficiency, as maximization of resources use and reduction in wastes;
- Accessibility, as the ability to face medical needs in a timely and geographically reasonable manner, provided in a setting where skills and resources are appropriate;
- Patient-centeredness, taking into account preferences and aspirations of individual service users and cultures of their communities;
- Equity, avoiding discrimination because of personal characteristics such as gender, race, ethnicity, geographical location, or socioeconomic status;
- Safety, minimization of risks and harm to service users (WHO, 2006).

Appropriateness is another important quality dimension. The UK Department of Health, introducing appropriateness, defined the quality of care as: "doing the right things (what); to the right people (to whom); at the right time (when); and doing things right the first time. Such a document also stressed on patient centeredness in quality appraisal, thus including the degree to which healthcare interventions are delivered responsive to patients' needs and preferences" (Department of Health, 1998).

Quality definition is preparatory to quality measurement: it is essential to reach an agreement on the element that constitute it before starting quality assessment, otherwise the risk is to court disaster (Donabedian, 1988).

The relevance of healthcare quality measurement is well-known for a long time. Famous is the quotation attributed to Florence Nightingale: "The ultimate goal is to manage quality. But you cannot manage it until you have a way to measure it, and you cannot measure it until you can monitor it" (Eagle & Davies, 1993).

At present, measurement and evaluation of the quality of health systems/ organizations is aimed mainly at determining the degree to which health systems successfully pursue the objectives of maintaining and increasing the health status of the population and how the health system respond, both in structural and organizational terms, to the expectations of all those who benefit. At national and international level, it should be noted that the emergence of problems related to the restructuring of health systems must be framed within the broader context of crisis in welfare states.

Quality of care refers to the level of performance that characterizes the healthcare provided. Such a quality can be assessed with quantitative measures, where delivered healthcare is compared with the healthcare that is expected/ought to be delivered, sometimes referred to indicate care or quality standards. Measures of quality of care would encompass, for example, measures of effectiveness and patient satisfaction or patient-centeredness. Mortality, morbidity, and patient satisfaction were identified as key criteria for assessing the quality of care (Hinshaw, 1992).

Patient satisfaction is both a dependent variable of quality of care and a predictor of subsequent health related behaviour, since satisfied and dissatisfied health care consumers behave differently (Ware, Davies-Avery, & Stewart, 1978; Pascoe, 1983; Ware & Davies, 1983; Tzannis & Nadin, 2011). Satisfied patients lead to higher levels of profitability, market share and, likely, to higher levels of clinical outcomes (Greenwich, 1993).

As quality measurement is a costly and time consuming activity, indicators must be selected that contribute to an aggregate understanding of health-care quality is imperative. Sources of information would include administrative/clinical data collected by healthcare providers and patients' reports collected through population or patient surveys, the so-called patient reported outcome measures (Streiner & Norman, 2008).

Quality Improvement

It seems dramatically clear that healthcare will not realize its full potential unless change making becomes an intrinsic part of everyone's job, every day, in all parts of the system. John Øvretveit defined quality improvement in healthcare as a better patient experience and outcomes achieved through changing provider behavior and organization through using a systematic change method and strategies (Øvretveit, 2009). Such a combined and unceasing efforts of everyone -healthcare professionals, patients and their families, researchers, payers, planners and educators- is important to make changes that will lead to better patient outcomes, better system performance and better professional development (Batalden, 2007).

Actually multiple strategies and tools to improve quality exist but which one works?

Groene, Kringos and Sunol on behalf of the DUQuE Project (2014) identified seven ways to improve quality in hospitals:

- Align organizational processes with external pressure
- Put quality high on the agenda
- Implement supportive organization-wide systems for quality improvement
- Assure responsibilities and team expertise at departmental level
- Organize care pathways based on evidence of quality and safety interventions
- Implement pathway-oriented information systems
- Conduct regular assessment and provide feedback.

In most reports emphasis is placed on crosscutting issues such as oversights and leadership, building support systems for quality improvement and providing the necessary resources for high quality care to be provided. Approaches on quality improvement has been developing into a major strand of research during the last decades.

Common approaches to quality improvement (Boaden, Harvey, Moxham, & Proudlove, 2008) came from industrial approaches:

- Total Quality Management, defined as a participative, systematic approach to planning and implementing a continuous organizational improvement process (Kaluzny, McLaughlin, & Simpson, 1992)
- Business Process Reengineering that is the redesign of systems and processes used to produce, deliver and support patient care in order to achieve improvements in organizational performance within a short period of time (Carmichael, 1994)
- Plan- Do- Study- Act (PDSA) cycles, small tests of change in which a change practitioner will plan a test of change (plan), carry out the change (do), study the results (study) and act on them in the next cycle of change (act) (Deming, 1986)
- Lean Thinking that is an integrated system of principles, practices, tools and techniques focused on reducing waste, synchronizing work flows, and managing variability in production flows (Joosten, Bongers, & Janssen, 2009)
- Six Sigma defined as "an organized and systematic method for strategic process improvement and new product and service development that relies on statistical methods and the scientific method to make dramatic reductions in customer defined defect rates (Linderman, Schroeder, Zaheer, & Choo, 2003)
- Statistical process control, that leads to quality improvement by learning through data and is based on the theory of variation (Carey, 2003).

But, which approaches are likely to really improve quality of care? Unfortunately, no clear evidences still exist on this topic. A systematic review synthetizes existing evidence on interventions to improve quality of care in an hospital based setting. It shows that that despite the very large volume of literature on quality of care improvements, only a few hospital interventions have a theoretically based design or implementation. Studies varied from small scale improvements for specific patient groups to large scale quality improvement programs across multiple settings. Interventions were usually divided into two categories: interpersonal and technical. Interpersonal interventions sought to improve patient satisfaction and tended to be implemented by nursing staff while technical interventions were generally implemented by physicians and reported measurable improvements in medical outcomes for patients with specific illnesses (Conry et al., 2012).

Towards a Clinical Governance Approach

Quality of healthcare is not only one of the major strand of research of the last decades but also on important topic for the government all over the world. It dominates and leads public policy agenda, so that it has been defined as a process for making strategic choices in health systems, as World Health Organization stated in the subheading of a report published in 2006 (WHO, 2006). Thus, quality of healthcare connects with one of the most important Public Health movement of the last decades, the Clinical Governance, that promotes continuous quality improvement by creating an environment in which excellence in clinical care will flourish. The introduction of clinical governance aimed at improving the quality of clinical care at all levels of healthcare provision (Scally & Donaldson, 1998).

Each intervention aimed at improving Clinical Governance is likely to positively influence healthcare quality and consequently appropriateness of care (Specchia et al., 2015). Quality of care permeates many other current concept, such as accountability and transparency, moreover linked to Clinical Governance, that encompasses procedures and processes by which healthcare organizations try to reach their goals in terms of quality improvement.

ACCOUNTABILITY AND TRANSPARENCY

Measuring quality of healthcare is a key factor to promote improvements in the delivery of care and to increase accountability and transparency (Chassin, Loeb, Schmaltz, & Wachter, 2010). On the other hand, implementing public health policies based on accountability and transparency of the actions can encourage quality improvement and the ability for people to make informed choices.

Over the years, various definitions of accountability in healthcare have been given. It has been defined as the activity of "taking into account and responding to political, commercial, community, and clinical/ patient interests and expectations" (American Hospital Association Board of Trustees, 1999). Furthermore, it may be defined as the process by which health leaders pursue the objectives of efficiency, quality, and access to meet public interests and expectations (AHA Board of Trustees, 1999). In general, accountability is the obligation of individuals or agencies to provide information about, and/ or justification for, their actions to other actors (Brinkerhoff, 2003). Therefore, a subject is accountable if he reports, explains, or justifies something on which he is responsible and has the duty to answer (AHA Board of Trustees, 1999).

Given the relevant role of the healthcare organizations for the society as a whole, expectations on their activities and capability to provide good quality healthcare services and to be performant is very high and not only limited to specific legal and regulatory standards. Healthcare organizations are responsible for a broad range of activities including patient care, community services, and business functions and have to be accountable for a series of activities. First of all they have to taking into account the expectations and interests of their different stakeholders. Furthermore, of great relevance, they have to measure and evaluate their performance in multiple areas, including quality, access, efficiency and finance, continuously improving their performance in each of these areas. Finally, they have to communicate their performance to the stakeholders (AHA Board of Trustees, 1999).

Individuals and institutions that have interest in healthcare providers' accountability are many: purchasers and payers of healthcare services, patients, advocacy groups, regulators, stockholders and lending institutions, health policy makers, practitioners, hospital staff/employees, media, and generally the community. They expect that the institutions that provide healthcare services will act in the best interests of the people who need its services and provide safe, effective and high quality care (AHA Board of Trustees, 1999).

In this perspective, accountability could represent a fundamental issue to implementing health reforms and improving health systems performance (Brinkerhoff, 2003).

In all the health systems there are different types of relationships among different actors, that may partially vary according to the healthcare system type. Principal speakers of these relationships are health ministries, insurance agencies, health services' public and private providers, legislatures, finance ministries, regulatory agencies (Brinkerhoff, 2003), exercising a mutual role of control, cooperation and reporting. In the healthcare area, main domains of accountability are: professional competence, legal and ethical conduct, financial performance, adequacy of access, public health promotion, and community benefit (Emanuel & Emanuel, 1996).

The most relevant element of accountability is answerability, according to the idea that to be accountable means to have the obligation to answer questions regarding decisions and actions. There are two levels of accountability: the first deals with the need to be informed, the second deals with the need to know and understand the reason of a choice and its implementation. The need to be informed implies a one-way transmission of information from the accountable actor to the actor who needs to be informed. The need to know and understand the reason implies a two-way transmission of information, requiring a dialogue between the accountable actor and the overseer actor.

In these terms, the informing aspect of answerability that characterized accountability, deals with the idea of transparency in a democratic government (Brinkerhoff, 2003). To be transparent mean give access to public data and information, building the capacity of civil society to monitor the management of resources, and on the other side the capacity of government to implement effective policies.

Accountability refers to three different areas: financial accountability, performance accountability and political/democratic accountability. Financial accountability concerns laws, rules and regulations regarding financial control and management, focusing on allocation, disbursement and utilization of financial resources. Performance accountability concerns performance measurement and evaluation, focusing on healthcare services, outputs, and results. It is linked to financial accountability because of financial resources are essential to product services for citizens. Political/democratic accountability deals with mechanisms to ensure that government plans are realized and respond to citizens' interests (Brinkerhoff, 2003).

These three specification of accountability are linked with its objectives. Control of use and abuse of public resources is directly related to financial accountability. Support and promote improved healthcare services delivery and management is linked with performance accountability. Finally, belonging to all accountability's specification, is the assurance that resources are used and authority is exercised according to appropriate and legal procedures, professional standards and societal values (Brinkerhoff, 2003).

Transparency is considered a driver of public service reform worldwide. It derives from theories of civic responsibility of the 1980s. Though there is a growing interest in transparency in healthcare sector, as it may be a predictor for services and productivity improvement, transparency is not yet widely implemented (Henke, Kelsey, & Whately, 2011).

The IOM (2011) defines healthcare transparency as "making available to the public, in a reliable and understandable manner, information on the healthcare system's quality, efficiency and consumer experience with care, which includes price and quality data, so as to influence the behavior of patients, providers, payers and others to achieve better outcomes".

The American College of Physician (2010) identifies eight major domains of healthcare transparency:

- Clinical quality and safety, that deals with structure, process and outcome measures;
- Resource use, expressed as episode of care, yearly and per capita costs, number of hospital bed days, etc;
- Efficiency, measured as clinical quality outcome related to resource utilization;
- Patient experience of care, typically relived by ad hoc survey;
- Professionalism, measured as qualifications, professional standing and training;
- Healthcare system/ facility recognition accreditations for meeting national standards, that deals with accreditation;
- Financial relationship between physicians, other healthcare professionals and industry, measured by public reporting of relationship;
- Health insurance company processes, expressed in terms of medical loss ratio, efficiency of claims processing, criteria for preferred provider status.

Transparency might impact on six areas: accountability, patients' choices, productivity, quality of services delivered, social innovation and economic growth (Henke et al., 2011). In fact transparency forces healthcare regulators to be accountable; guides informed choices thanks to the availability of comparative and complete information; drives providers to efforts effective and cost-effective services, encourages patients to be more informed, transforming the relationship between patients and providers; opens new opportunities for public and private providers, stimulating competitiveness.

Many potential benefits from increased healthcare transparency emerged both for patients and health systems, like improving availability of information needed to make informed healthcare choices, increasing trust in the patient-physician relationship and improving quality, safety and efficiency due to competition and availability of clinical benchmarks (Colmers, 2007; Collins & Davis, 2006; Snyder & Leffler, 2005). Furthermore, above all in publicly funded and administered healthcare systems, transparency is considered a main value: professionals and the other health sector employees must behave professionally and ethically, avoiding to commit fraud, accept bribes, or leak confidential information.

In the early part of the twentieth century, Codman (1975) promoted the importance of publicly reporting the results of hospitals activity in order to promote quality improvement, physician learning and patient choice, inspiring the current healthcare transparency movement.

The most recurring information showed about hospitals performance are: clinical quality as adherence of services provided to evidence-based, structured, clinical process or positive health outcomes benchmarks or guidelines), resource use (both structural and human resources) and experience of care (patients' view of the care received from providers). Even though it's well known that transparency could increase healthcare quality, many hospitals aren't ready to face the transparency challenge, staying reluctant to disclose their performance data.

Transparency is more than access to healthcare data: information to be effective must be shown in a way that reflects different users' abilities to understand and use information. Data should be not too much detailed and complex, not too much aggregate (IOM, 2010).

Moreover, transparency can encourage the practice of results based management in healthcare. In particular, there are three primary aspects of transparency relevant to management practice: information disclosure, clarity and accuracy

Finally, it's useful not to confuse transparency for knowledge: transparency causes an increase in knowledge, it may facilitate knowledge, but it's not knowledge itself (Schauer, 2011).

PUBLIC REPORTING IN HEALTHCARE

Definitions and Objectives

In the healthcare field, a well-trodden path to provide transparency and to be accountable is the public reporting. There is growing interest in public reporting of information on the quality of healthcare delivered by different providers (i.e. physicians, hospitals, health plans), as it is strictly linked to the accountability of health systems and transparency of information and processes. It has become an increasingly common health policy tool (Faber, Bosch, Wollersheim, Leatherman, & Grol, 2009), both in publicly and privately funded systems.

Public reporting of performance information and feedback to providers is one of the major approaches to improve quality of care, because on the one hand allows to evaluate your own performance, on the other pushes the comparison with other providers; moreover, allowing patients to make informed choices stimulates competition. Furthermore, information supports patients' and users' decision making process, facilitating choices in selecting providers that best meet needs and preferences (Rice, 2001; Kumpunen et al., 2014), by comparing differences across them. Information on the quality of providers should be accurate and timely accessible (Victoor, Delnoij, Friele, & Rademakers, 2012).

Many author and national agency provide definitions of public reporting.

Public reporting refers to the publication of information and reports on the quality of care delivered by providers. Information is made available on the internet, on paper and in other formats for use by patients and users (Kumpunen et al., 2014).

It is defined as the way to promote high quality and efficient healthcare delivery and to increase the transparency of quality information enabling disparities in access to such information (Cacace, Ettelt, Brereton, Pedersen, & Nolte, 2011). It is also a strategy to address quality and cost making available to consumers, payers and healthcare providers information about performance and insurance plans and it should provide information on patient's satisfaction (James, 2012).

Actually, the Agency for Healthcare Research and Quality public reporting definition is the most widespread: "Public Reporting is data, publicly available or available to a broad audience free of charge or at a nominal cost, about a healthcare structure, process or outcome at any provider level (individual clinician, group, organization)" (Totten et al., 2012). The main objective of Public Reporting is to help actors of the health system to be accountable by spreading information about their performance in order to enable their stakeholders to make informed decisions and to support patients in choosing their own provider. Furthermore, it should promote healthcare quality improvement encouraging providers' competition and behavioral change (Cacace et al, 2011).

A Theoretical Framework: The Berwick Model

In public health field, information systems involve three kind of actors: patients or users, providers and regulators. Given the relationship between these three types of subjects, the main lever to induce quality improvement is providers behavioral change (Berwick, James, & Coye, 2003). This behavioral change could be induced acting on the side of demand for health services or on the side of production of health services, linking the processes of measurement pathways to the processes of improvement. According to Berwick's framework, exist two principals through which measurement and reporting can induce providers behavioral change: improvement through selection and improvement through selection (Berwick et al., 2003). The first pathway is based on the assumption that information on healthcare services' quality enables patients or users to select providers according to quality criteria, making informed decisions on their providers. Furthermore, regulators may use the information on quality to make decisions on payment, activating incentive mechanisms such as reward for high quality performance or penalty for low quality performance. In the second pathway, healthcare services' quality information is used by providers themselves to identify underperformance or good performance areas in order to stimulate competition on services quality and to act an organizational behavioral change.

These pathways may stimulate behavioral changes only if there is providers' intention to compete and maintain or increase their reputation (Cacace et al., 2011). The will to be competitive with other providers and to maintain a good reputation to attract patients should stimulate behavioral changes aimed at improving performance.

It is also important to observe that providers have two different kind of functions on two different levels. First of all, they are information users in order to make decisions about their operative strategy and organization, on the other side they are the main information providers and target audience of information systems and their capacity to produce information is decisive to healthcare quality. On the second level, in more operative terms, providers do not only react to the output of information systems, such as outcome indicators, they also produce information to make possible these comparisons and stimulate competition and quality improvement (Cacace et al., 2011).

Furthermore, it is relevant to note that the literature has suggested that patients choose their healthcare providers considering a wide range of services' characteristics: in addition to the quality of care or positive evaluations of the outcomes, could also affect other non-clinical elements such as the proximity of the provider, good ancillary services (food, cleanliness, etc.) or a previous experience (Kumpunen et al., 2014). A relevant aspect is the measurement of patient expectations and perceptions. This represent a valuable dimension of the process by which the quality of health care service is evaluated. Administrators should understand the areas in which expectations are particularly high so that the service delivery process can be tailored to meet those expectations (Babakus & Mangold, 1992).

Main Characteristics of Public Reporting: Indicators and Availability

A public reporting system is based on a set of indicators through which provide information to different stakeholders. The first important step to take when building a system of public reporting is to identify a set of indicators suitable for measuring the activity. In healthcare, public reporting of services' quality is strictly linked and influenced by the multidimensionality of quality, so it is necessary to identify different indicators able to measure all the quality dimensions. Usually, three types of indicators are used in order to monitoring quality of healthcare services: structural measures, process measures and outcome measures (Donabedian, 2005).

Structural indicators monitoring structural, technological, organizational and professional resources of healthcare providers, measuring tangible aspects, such as number of physician for patients, bed's occupancy rate or operating rooms' utilization rate. They are easy to measure and probably are the more easily to understand for patients. Process indicators measure the appropriateness of the care process and usually are classified into organizational process indicators that measure volumes (i.e. number of admissions; length of stay), waiting times for services and continuity of care, and professional process indicators that measure appropriateness of care decisions, correctness of execution and timeliness of care. Outcome indicators measure the health status of a patient resulting from care process, highlighting a change of health status, for example in terms of mortality or morbidity, but also in terms of quality of life or satisfaction. Often it is too difficult to link both structural and process indicators outcomes measures, making an integrated interpretation.

Data can be reported at different levels of care: physician level, measuring the quality of care provided by a single healthcare professional; hospital ward or specialty level, measuring a team performance; hospital level, measuring the entire organization performance.

The use of public reporting could encourage physicians or providers to adopt opportunistic behaviors, in terms of selecting services or patients in order to obtain better results, or to focusing on the clinical care that are monitored, omitting provision of other important care. A solution to try to avoid these behaviors is the utilization of risk and case-adjustment methods in calculating indicators (Kumpunen et al., 2014).

Generally, the data used to public reporting may come from three kind of sources: administrative, surveillance and *ad hoc* (Kumpunen et al., 2014).

Health administrative databases are information flows for monitoring the delivery of health services in which data are routinely collected to produce administrative reports. Despite their goal was predominantly the accounting, they have proved to be the best sources available as regards the aspects of monitoring accessibility and completeness of care. Health surveillance databases aims to routinely collect to detect anomalies or changes in providers activities or performance.

Health *ad hoc* databases are realized to collect specific information about an event that needs to be monitored, so data are collected specifically to monitor some aspects of quality and performance. Intervals for collecting data may vary according to the kind of information to provide: routine collection, regular intervals collection or ad hoc collection (Kumpunen et al., 2014).

Always more frequently a source of healthcare quality information is represented by patients or users themselves. In fairly recent times it occurred the development of a number of sites or blogs where patients give information, exchange opinions and make ratings. These kind of initiatives have both many vantages and disadvantages. For example, patients who directly received care can comment many aspect of care process, also not included in conventional surveys. On the other side, patients may not have technical or specific knowledge on some complex aspects of care and it is very difficult to verify identity and credibility of those who write a comment. Furthermore, given the complexity of understanding statistical information, it may happen that anecdotal personal information are favored in making choices (Trigg, 2011).

One of the most common and easily available source on healthcare quality information is Internet that makes possible a direct and fast access to information. This way of access allows to have ever up to date information, being able providers to timely updates them. Furthermore it is possible to create web sites customized to the users' preferences and easy to consult. However, the use of Internet could exclude to the access of healthcare quality information people without internet availability or unable to use it (Kumpunen et al., 2014).

The Evolution of Public Reporting In Healthcare

The great interest in quality management and improvement in healthcare induced systematic assessment and international benchmarking of quality of care provided. Many quality or performance assessment frameworks implemented at national, regional or local level have been developed as quality or performance improvement is possible only if measurement is fulfilled (Cacace et al., 2011). Measurement allows for monitoring effectiveness, guarantee patient safety, support decision-making and insurance value for money among other things (Smith, Mossialos, & Papanicolas, 2008).

Moreover, data on the quality of healthcare, compared between healthcare providers, has been publicly widespread producing the public reporting phenomenon. The first important public reporting initiatives date back to the 1980s and were developed in the United States: the publication of mortality rates by the Health Care Financing Administration (today Centers for Medicare and Medicaid Services) in 1986 and the New York State and Pennsylvania's Cardiac Reporting Systems in 1989 and 1992 (Schneider & Epstein, 1998; Shahian et al., 2011). Afterward, many other high-income countries, especially in the West, have experienced public reporting in their healthcare systems (Faber et al., 2009).

The effects of the first implementation of public reporting varied widely among providers: many sustained that data did not take into account some patients' characteristics (i.e. age, comorbidities) that might influence their performance (James, 2012).

Actually, though there is a great number of public reporting websites they differ in many characteristics. First of all, websites should be managed at local, regional or national levels and should be operated by different stakeholders (i.e. governments, insurers or commercial organizations). Websites should be targeted at purchasers, regulators, providers or patients. Even the contents vary: not only performance information, that are the most common from waiting times to more complex clinical and patient experience indicators, but also information about structure, facilities and so on (Kumpunen et al., 2014).

There are, additionally, significant differences between public reporting due to healthcare system model. In example, in some insurance funded systems some data must be published (e.g. hospital admissions in Germany) and those are used at national level, regional or insurance level. In private insurance systems, like the United States one, where there is an high fragmentation of public reporting initiatives, a larger quantity of administrative and quality data are available, that makes the use of information more complex for all the stakeholders (Marshall, Shekelle, Davies, & Smith, 2003; Kumpunen et al., 2014).

Effects of Public Reporting In Healthcare

Which are the real effects of public reporting since its implementation? Is it able to support stakeholders' decision making and patients in choosing their own provider? Does it allow healthcare quality improvement?

Public reporting is supposed to: support and empower consumers/ patients to choose their provider and/ or to share their opinions or preferences; help purchasers in their decision making processes, choosing providers that create value reaching population health goals; increase self-regulation among providers (Leatherman & McCarthy, 1999).

How should public reporting improve healthcare quality?

At first public reporting might help patients and referring physicians select high-quality providers. This happens if patients access the information, are able to understand the quality rankings and believe them and act on the information itself or if referring physicians use it. Even though patients and referring physicians don't use it, purchasers should use public reporting data in order to select or establish providers' contracts. Then rated providers should react to public reporting by improving the quality of the delivered care in three different ways: remediation (providers change their practices to improve quality); restriction (providers stop supplying care for which they rated poorly); removal (low-quality providers exit the healthcare market). It might also encourage quality competition, so that providers might compete on quality to maintain or improve their market share. Finally, public reporting might improve providers' accountability (Werner & Asch, 2005).

How Does Public Reporting Improve Healthcare Quality?

The growing interest in public reporting leads many authors to investigate the use and impact of publicly released performance data. Conflicting results emerged. A recent systematic review highlighted that outcomes' heterogeneity and moderate evidence's strength make it difficult to draw definitive conclusions. Particularly, public reporting seems to have a positive impact on quality measures, although quality varies across plans or patients' subgroups. As regards harms or unintended negative effects, more evidence of no harm than evidence of harm emerged, especially on access. Providers seems to react to public reporting by changing positively their behavior, though evidences are scant and not available for all settings. Regardless of the setting, public reporting appears to little or no influence the selection of health services providers by patients, usually because they do not know that quality information is available, the information do not meet their needs or are not available when needed or are not understandable. It determines an effect if it is used by some subgroup of patients (i.e. younger, more educated patients). There is a few evidence about which report characteristics affected the impact of public reporting on any outcome. Some evidences show that public reporting is more effective in competitive markets and if referred to providers with initial lower scores (Totten et al., 2012). Intermediate and ultimate healthcare outcomes could be influenced by the way in which healthcare data are publicly reported. There are some specific examples of report characteristics that seems to be associated with public reporting effects:

- Acceptable/ appropriate: data should be believable, high quality and accurate
- Accessible: reports should be understood by target populations; it deals both with format, language, and graphics and advertising and promotion
- Actionable: on the patient side reports should help in keeping a decision; on the provider side (individuals or organizations) reports are related to factors they can influence (Totten et al., 2012).

The cost-effectiveness evaluation of a public reporting initiative is difficult, because a comparison between public reporting and other quality improvement intervention in terms of costs, benefits and risks is needed. The costs of public reporting typically include development of measures, methods and information systems, data collection and preparation, analysis and auditing, and public dissemination and education (Leatherman & McCarthy, 1999). More detailed analysis is needed to address this issue.

Analysis of the Major Initiatives of Public Reporting

The concept of patient engagement is based on the assumption that making patients co-producers of their health might enhance their satisfaction and responsibility with the healthcare system (Graffigna et al., 2015) and it strictly linked with the health provider choice. In the healthcare field, public reporting is one of the major tools in supporting patients' decisions making process, by providing structure, process and outcome measures. Nowadays, many public reporting initiatives exist that differ in some characteristics such as: the management that can be at local, regional or national levels, the property that can be public or private (i.e. governments, insurers or commercial organizations), the target (i.e. purchasers, regulators, providers or patients), main contents (i.e. performance information, waiting times patient satisfaction), the healthcare system model.

A web-based analysis of the major initiatives of public reporting was performed in order to highlight their main characteristics: properties (public or private), data source (governmental, not governmental, ad hoc surveys) and type of data reported (general information, doctors' information, patients' satisfaction). Two independent reviewers searched public reporting websites. The information was collected in an *ad hoc* database. The reviewers solved disagreements through discussion to reach a final consensus. Only public reporting websites in English or Italian were searched, as the languages spoken by the reviewers. Furthermore, public reporting initiatives if they did not allow comparison between providers.

Forty-one public reporting websites were identified, but only 18 were searched because in English or Italian. The excluded one were public reporting initiatives from Netherland, Denmark, Germany, Finland, Sweden and Norway. This is one of the major limit of our analysis as they could add further information about different items considered.

Seven out of 18 websites were subsequently excluded as they did not allow comparison between providers.

The analysis was conducted on 11 public reporting websites: 8 from the United States, 2 from Great Britain and 1 from Italy. Table 2 shows main characteristics of public reporting initiative investigated. Nine out of 11 were private initiatives, 2 were public. The property did not influence the data source utilized: 8 out of the 11 websites used governmental data, of which 5 combined governmental data and other data source (not governmental or ad hoc surveys), 2 websites used only ad hoc surveys and 1 website used only not governmental data.

Regarding the type of data reported, all the public reporting websites investigated showed general information about providers such as structural and/ or processes indicators, 5 reported also information about doctors, 2 reported data also about patients' satisfaction /experience ratings and 6 reported also clinical indicators. Only the NHS Choices website showed all the type of data searched. The California Nursing Home Search and Quality Check reported only general information about providers.

As regard the aim of the public reporting initiatives searched, the interest in supporting patients choices showing providers information emerged as a common feature.

CONCLUSION

As a result of what was discussed, it emerged that involving patients in decisions about their health is a crucial component for the quality improvement of healthcare services. As previously mentioned, the IOM's report "Crossing the Quality Chasm" has been recognizing patient-centered care as an essential dimension of high-quality care (Clancy, 2011). In 2006, the World Health Organization indicates patients and the population engagement as one of the six domains of quality interventions (WHO, 2006).

Being patient involved and engaged, strictly connected with healthcare quality improvement, is important to stimulate strategies to make informed patients and able to take informed decisions about their health.

Table 2. Main characteristics of public reporting initiative investigated

Public reporting website	State	Web-site	Properties	Data source	Aim
United States: Medicare.gov	USA	http://www.medicare.gov/	Public	Governmental data	To find providers and compare the quality of their care
Leapfrog	USA	http://www.leapfroggroup.org	Private	Ad hoc surveys	To promote transparency through data collection and public reporting initiatives
U Compare Healthcare	USA	http://www.ucomparehealthcare.com/	Private	Governmental data. Ad hoc surveys	To help people make better decisions about their healthcare choices
California Nursing Home Search	USA	http://www.nursinghomeguide.org/NHG/nhg_txt_home.lasso	Private	Governmental data. Ad hoc surveys	To help people search for a nursing home in California
National Committee for Quality Assurance (NCQA)	USA	http://www.ncqa.org/HomePage.aspx	Private	Ad hoc surveys	To help people select a health plan or physician
US News Health	USA	http://health.usnews.com/	Private	Governmental data	To provide consumer guides that include rankings of hospitals, nursing homes, health plans
The American Hospital Directory	USA	https://www.ahd.com/	Private	Governmental data. Not governmental data	To provide information about hospitals
Quality Check	USA	http://www.qualitycheck.org/consumer/searchQCR.aspx	Private	Not governmental data	To providing meaningful information about the comparative performance of accredited organizations
NHS Choices	GB	http://www.nhs.uk/Pages/HomePage.aspx	Public	Governmental data. Ad hoc surveys	To create a new information, feedback, transactions and participation service delivered through mobile apps, SMS, phone lines and online channels
Dr. Foster	GB	http://myhospitalguide.drfosterintelligence.co.uk/	Private	Governmental data	To use information to improve lives
Doveecomemicuro	IT	http://www.doveecomemicuro.it/	Private	Governmental data. Not governmental data	To find providers and compare the quality of their care

A well-recognized strategy to inform patients is the public reporting of health care information. This kind of strategy is relevant on a side to allow patients to take informed decisions on healthcare services according to their needs, on the other hand to guarantee accountability and transparency in provision.

As mentioned, accountability have to represent a fundamental issue to improving health systems performance and transparency increases benefits both for patients and health systems, improving availability of information needed to make informed healthcare choices, increasing trust in the patient-physician relationship and improving quality, safety and efficiency due to competition and availability of clinical benchmarks.

Public reporting of performance information and feedback to providers is recognized as one of the major approaches to improve quality of care, thanks to the possibility for providers to evaluate your own performance and to make a comparison with other providers and for patients to make informed choices. Furthermore, well designed public reports help patients making informed choices. Public reports seem to improve citizens and health consumers empowerment (Totten et al., 2012; Silenzi et al., 2013).

Because of the relevance of public reporting in improving quality of care and stimulating patient engagement, there are many public reporting initiatives, across different countries, that differs for many characteristics. In this chapter we reported the results of a web based analysis aimed at comparing major initiatives of public reporting, classified by the following characteristics: properties (public or private), data source (health providers, ad hoc surveys, etc.), general information reported (i.e. size, language spoken, amenities), doctors' information, patients' ratings (satisfaction /experience), clinical indicators. The results show that main common feature is the declared aim of all the initiatives analyzed: to support patients' choices showing providers information, despite consistent differences in properties of the initiatives or data sources.

In conclusion we believe that a good strategy aimed at informing patients about providers' performance through initiatives like public reporting websites could represent a way to improve healthcare quality, stimulating accountability of providers and transparency of decisions and making patients co-producers of their health.

REFERENCES

American College of Physicians. (2010). *Healthcare Transparency-Focus on Price and Clinical Performance Information*. Philadelphia.

American Hospital Association Board of Trustees. (1999). *Accountability – the pathway to restoring public trust and confidence for hospitals and other health care organizations.*

Babakus, E., & Mangold, W. G. (1992). Adapting the SERVQUAL scale to hospital services: An empirical investigation. *Health Services Research*, *26*(6), 767–786. PMID:1737708

Batalden, P., & Davidoff, F. (2007). What is quality improvement and how it can transform healthcare. *Quality & Safety in Health Care*, *16*(1), 2–3. doi:10.1136/qshc.2006.022046 PMID:17301192

Berwick, D. M., James, B., & Coye, M. J. (2003). Connections between quality measurement and improvement. *Medical Care*, *41*(Suppl. 1), I30–I38. doi:10.1097/00005650-200301001-00004 PMID:12544814

Boaden, R., Harvey, G., Moxham, C., & Proudlove, N. (2008). *Quality improvement: theory and practice in healthcare*. National Health Service Institute for Innovation and Improvement/ University of Manchester Business School.

Brinkerhoff, D. (2003). *Accountability and Health Systems: Overview, Framework, and Strategies.* Bethesda, MD: The Partners for Health Reformplus Project, Abt Associates Inc.

Cacace, M., Ettelt, S., Brereton, L., Pedersen, J., & Nolte, E. (2011). *How health systems make available information on service providers. Experience in seven countries*. United Kingdom: RAND and London School of Hygiene and Tropical Medicine.

Campbell, S. M., Roland, M. O., & Buetow, S. A. (2000). Defining quality of care. *Social Science & Medicine, 51*(11), 1611–1625. doi:10.1016/S0277-9536(00)00057-5 PMID:11072882

Cantù, C., & Tzannis, A. (2011). *From health service quality to health system quality. A network innovation adoption and diffusion* (Working paper). Retrieved from http://www.impgroup.org/uploads/papers/7696.pdf

Carey, R. G. (2003). *Improving healthcare with control charts: basic and advanced SPC methods and case studies*. Milwaukee: ASQ Quality Press.

Carmichael, B. D. (1994). Business process reengineering: A remedy for health care. *Healthcare Management Forum, 7*(4), 44–50. doi:10.1016/S0840-4704(10)61077-0 PMID:10140167

Center for Advancing Health. (2010). *A New Definition of Patient Engagement: What is Engagement and Why is it Important?* Retrieved from http://www.cfah.org/pdfs/CFAH_Engagement_Behavior_Framework_current.pdf

Chassin, M. R., Loeb, J. M., Schmaltz, S. P., & Wachter, R. M. (2010). Accountability Measures - Using Measurement to Promote Quality Improvement. *The New England Journal of Medicine, 363*(7), 683–688. doi:10.1056/NEJMsb1002320 PMID:20573915

Clancy, C. M. (2011). Patient Engagement in Health Care. *Health Services Research, 46*(2), 389–393. doi:10.1111/j.1475-6773.2011.01254.x PMID:21371026

Codman, E. A. (1975). *A Study of Hospital Efficiency: As Demonstrated by the Case Report of the First Five Years of a Private Hospital*. Joint Commission.

Collins, S. R., & Davis, K. (2006). *Transparency in Health Care: The Time Has Come*. The Commonwealth Fund.

Colmers, J. M. (2007). *Public Reporting and Transparency*. The Commonwealth Fund.

Conry, M. C., Humphries, N., Morgan, K., McGowan, Y., Montgomery, A., Vedhara, K., & Mc Gee, H. A. et al. (2012). A 10 year (2000-2010) systematic review of interventions to improve quality of care in hospitals. *Health Services Research, 12*(1), 275. doi:10.1186/1472-6963-12-275 PMID:22925835

Crosby, P. B. (1979). *Quality is free: The art of making quality certain*. New York: McGraw Hill.

Deming, W. E. (1986). *Out of the crisis*. Cambridge, MA: Centre of Advanced Engineering Study, MIT.

Department of Health. (1998). *A first class service: quality in the new NHS*. London: HMSO.

Donabedian, A. (1966). Evaluating the quality of medical care. *The Milbank Memorial Fund Quarterly, 44*(3), 166–206. doi:10.2307/3348969 PMID:5338568

Donabedian, A. (1980). The Definition of Quality and Approaches to Its Assessment (Vol. 1). *Explorations in Quality Assessment and Monitoring*. Ann Arbor, MI: Health Administration Press.

Donabedian, A. (1988). The Quality of Care How Can It Be Assessed? *Journal of the American Medical Association, 260*(12), 1743–1748. doi:10.1001/jama.1988.03410120089033 PMID:3045356

Donabedian, A. (1990). The seven pillars of quality. *Archives of Pathology & Laboratory Medicine, 114*, 1115–1118. PMID:2241519

Donabedian, A. (2005). Evaluating the quality of medical care. *The Milbank Quarterly, 83*(4), 691–729. doi:10.1111/j.1468-0009.2005.00397.x PMID:16279964

Eagle, C. J., & Davies, J. M. (1993). Current models of "quality" – an introduction for anaesthetists. *Canadian Journal of Anaesthesia, 40*(9), 851–862. doi:10.1007/BF03009257 PMID:8403179

Ellis, R., & Whittington, R. (1993). *Quality assurance in health care: A handbook*. London: Arnold.

Emanuel, E. J., & Emanuel, L. L. (1996). What Is Accountability in Health Care? *Annals of Internal Medicine, 124*(2), 229–239. doi:10.7326/0003-4819-124-2-199601150-00007 PMID:8533999

Faber, M., Bosch, M., Wollersheim, H., Leatherman, S., & Grol, R. (2009). Public reporting in health care: How do consumers use quality-of-care information? A systematic review. *Medical Care, 47*(1), 1–8. doi:10.1097/MLR.0b013e3181808bb5 PMID:19106724

Gambetti, R. C., & Graffigna, G. (2010). The concept of engagement. *International Journal of Market Research, 52*(6), 801–826. doi:10.2501/S147078531020166

Graffigna, G., Barello, S., Riva, G., & Bosio, A. C. (2014). Patient Engagement: The Key to Redesign the Exchange Between the Demand and Supply for Healthcare in the Era of Active Ageing. *Studies in Health Technology and Informatics, 203*, 85–95. PMID:26630515

Graffigna, G., Barello, S., & Triberti, S. (2015). *Patient Engagement: A consumer-centered model to innovate healthcare*. De Gruiter Open. doi:10.1515/9783110452440

Greene, J., & Hibbard, J. H. (2012). Why does patient activation matter? An examination of the relationships between patient activation and health-related outcomes. *Journal of General Internal Medicine, 27*(5), 520–526. doi:10.1007/s11606-011-1931-2 PMID:22127797

Greeneich, D. (1993). The link between new and return business and quality of care: Patient satisfaction. *ANS. Advances in Nursing Science, 16*(1), 62–72. doi:10.1097/00012272-199309000-00008 PMID:8311426

Groene, O., Kringos, D., Sunol, R. (2014). *Seven ways to improve quality and safety in hospitals. An evidence-based guide.* DUQuE Collaboration.

Health Services Research Group. (1992). Quality of care. *Canadian Medical Association Journal, 146*, 2153–2158. PMID:1611571

Henke, N., Kelsey, T., & Whately, H. (2011). Transparency the most powerful driver of healthcare improvement? *Health International, 11*, 65–73.

Hibbard, J. H., Stockard, J., Mahoney, E. R., & Tusler, M. (2004). Development of the Patient Activation Measure (PAM): conceptualizing and measuring activation in patients and consumers. *Health services research,* 39(4 Part 1), 1005-1026.

Hinshaw, A. (1992). *Welcome Patient outcomes research conference, In Patient Outcomes Research Examining the Effectiveness of Nursing Practice Proceedings of the state of the science conference sponsored by the National Center for Nursing Research.* Rockville, MD: National Institutes of Health Publication.

Institute of Medicine. (1990). *Medicare: a strategy for quality assurance*. Washington, D.C.: National Academy Press.

Institute of Medicine. (2001). *Crossing the Quality Chasm: A New Health System for the Twenty-First Century*. Washington, D.C.: National Academies Press.

Institute of Medicine (US) Roundtable on Evidence-Based Medicine. (2010). The Healthcare Imperative: Lowering Costs and Improving Outcomes. In P. L. Yong, R. S. Saunders, & L. Olsen (Eds.), *Washington (DC)*. US: National Academies Press.

James, J. (2012). Health Policy Brief: Public Reporting on Quality and Costs. *Health Affairs*.

Joosten, T., Bongers, I., & Janssen, R. (2009). Application of lean thinking to health care: Issues and observations. *International Journal for Quality in Health Care*, *21*(5), 341–347. doi:10.1093/intqhc/mzp036 PMID:19696048

Juran, J. M. (1988). *Juran on planning for quality*. New York: McGraw-Hill.

Kaluzny, A. D., McLaughlin, C. P., & Simpson, K. (1992). Applying total quality management concepts to public health organizations. *Public Health Reports*, *107*(3), 257–264. PMID:1594734

Kumpunen, S., Trigg, L., & Rodrigues, R. (2014). *Public reporting in health and long-term care to facilitate provider choice*. Denmark: WHO Regional Office for Europe and European Observatory on Health Systems and Policies.

Leatherman, S., & McCarthy, D. (1999). Counterpoint. Public disclosure of health care performance reports: Experience, evidence and issues for policy. *International Journal for Quality in Health Care*, *11*(2), 93–98. doi:10.1093/intqhc/11.2.93 PMID:10442837

Linderman, K., Schroeder, R. G., Zaheer, S., & Choo, A. S. (2003). Six Sigma: A goal-theoretic perspective. *Journal of Operations Management*, *21*(2), 193–203. doi:10.1016/S0272-6963(02)00087-6

Marshall, M. N., Shekelle, P. G., Davies, H. T., & Smith, P. C. (2003). Public reporting on quality in the United States and the United Kingdom. *Health Affairs*, *22*(3), 134–148. doi:10.1377/hlthaff.22.3.134 PMID:12757278

Maxwell, R. J. (1992). Dimensions of quality revisited: From thought to action. *Quality in Health Care*, *1*(3), 171–177. doi:10.1136/qshc.1.3.171 PMID:10136859

National Health Performance Committee. (2001). *National Health Performance Framework report*. Canberra: AIHW.

O'Leary, D. S., & O'Leary, M. R. (1992). From quality assurance to quality improvement. The Joint Commission on Accreditation of Healthcare Organizations and Emergency Care. *Emergency Medicine Clinics of North America*, *10*, 477–492. PMID:1628555

Øvretveit, J. (2009). *Does improving quality save money? A review of the evidence of which improvements to quality reduce costs to health service providers*. London: the Health Foundation.

Pascoe, G. C. (1983). Patient satisfaction in primary health care: A literature review and analysis. *Evaluation and Program Planning*, *6*(3), 185–210. doi:10.1016/0149-7189(83)90002-2 PMID:10299618

Rice, T. (2001). Should consumer choice be encouraged in health care? In J. B. Davis (Ed.), *The social economics of health care* (pp. 9–39). London: Routledge. doi:10.4324/9780203459898.pt1

Runciman, B., Merry, A., & Walton, M. (2007). *Safety and Ethics in Healthcare: A Guide to Getting it Right*. Burlington, VT: Ashgate.

Samuel, O., Grant, J., & Irvine, D. (1994). *Quality and audit in general practice: Meanings and definitions*. London: Royal College of General Practitioners.

Scally, G., & Donaldson, L. J. (1998). Clinical governance and the drive for quality improvement in the new NHS in England. *British Medical Journal, 317*(7150), 61–65. doi:10.1136/bmj.317.7150.61 PMID:9651278

Schauer, F. (2011). Transparency in Three Dimensions. *University of Illinois Law Review, 4*, 1339–1342.

Schneider, E. C., & Epstein, A. M. (1998). Use of public performance reports: A survey of patients undergoing cardiac surgery. *Journal of the American Medical Association, 279*(20), 1638–1642. doi:10.1001/jama.279.20.1638 PMID:9613914

Shahian, D. M., Edwards, F. H., Jacobs, J. P., Prager, R. L., Normand, S. L., Shewan, C. M., & Grover, F. L. et al. (2011). Public reporting of cardiac surgery performance: Part 1--history, rationale, consequences. *The Annals of Thoracic Surgery, 92*(Suppl. 3), S2–S11. doi:10.1016/j.athoracsur.2011.06.100 PMID:21867789

Silenzi, A., Falvo, R., Lazzari, A., Marino, M., Pelone, F., Basso, D., & Ricciardi, W. (2013). Health systems reviews and policy. Quality in public reporting: where do we go? An overview of systematic reviews. *The European Journal of Public Health,* 23(Suppl. 1).

Smith, P., Mossialos, E., &, Papanicolas, I. (2008). *Performance measurement for health system improvement: experiences, challenges and prospects.* Copenhagen: World Health Organization on behalf of the European Observatory on Health Systems and Policies.

Snyder, L., & Leffler, C. (2005). Ethics and Human Rights Committee, American College of Physicians, Ethics manual: fifth edition. Annals of Internal Medicine, 142(7), 560-82.

Specchia, M. L., Poscia, A., Volpe, M., Parente, P., Capizzi, S., Cambieri, A., & De Belvis, A. G. et al. (2015, December). Does clinical governance influence the appropriateness of hospital stay? *Health Services Research, 15*(1), 142. doi:10.1186/s12913-015-0795-2 PMID:25889675

Steffen, G. E. (1988). Quality medical care: A definition. *Journal of the American Medical Association, 260*(1), 56–61. doi:10.1001/jama.1988.03410010064036 PMID:3379723

Streiner, D. L., & Norman, G. R. (2008). *Health Measurement Scales: A Practical Guide to Their Development and Use* (4th ed.). Oxford, UK: Oxford University Press. doi:10.1093/acprof:oso/9780199231881.001.0001

Totten, A. M., Wagner, J., Tiwari, A., O'Haire, C., Griffin, J., & Walker, M. (2012). *Public Reporting as a Quality Improvement Strategy. Closing the Quality Gap: Revisiting the State of the Science*, Evidence Report No. 208. AHRQ Publication No. 12-E011-EF, Rockville, MD, Agency for Healthcare Research and Quality. Retrieved from http://www.effectivehealthcare.ahrq.gov/ehc/products/343/1199/EvidReport208_CQGPublicReporting_FinalReport_20120724.pdf

Trigg, L. (2011). Patients' opinions of health care providers for supporting choice and quality improvement. *Journal of Health Services Research & Policy*, *16*(2), 102–107. doi:10.1258/jhsrp.2010.010010 PMID:20870690

Tzannis, A., & Nadin, G. (2011, September 1-3). Elderly and health care services: the elements characterizing the patient satisfaction. *Proceedings of the 14th Toulon-Verona Conference "Organizational Excellence in services"*, University of Alicante & University of Oviedo (pp. 1201-1017).

Victoor, A., Delnoij, D. M. J., Friele, R. D., & Rademakers, J. J. (2012). Determinants of patient choice of healthcare providers: A scoping review. *BMC Health Services Research*, *12*(1), 272. doi:10.1186/1472-6963-12-272 PMID:22913549

Ware, J. E. Jr, Davies-Avery, A., & Stewart, A. L. (1978). The measurement and meaning of patient satisfaction. *Health & Medical Care Services Review*, *1*(1), 1–3. PMID:10297474

Ware, J. E. Jr, & Davis, A. R. (1983). Behavioral consequences of consumer dissatisfaction with medical care. *Evaluation and Program Planning*, *6*(3), 291–297. doi:10.1016/0149-7189(83)90009-5 PMID:10267257

Werner, R. M., & Asch, D. A. (2005). The unintended consequences of publicly reporting quality information. *Journal of the American Medical Association*, *293*(10), 1239–1244. doi:10.1001/jama.293.10.1239 PMID:15755946

Wong, H. S., McNamara, P., & Greenberg, W. (2004). Provider competition and health care quality: Challenges and opportunities for research. *International Journal of Health Care Finance and Economics*, *4*(2), 99–111. doi:10.1023/B:IHFE.0000032418.86010.5d PMID:15211101

World Health Organization. (2006). *Quality of care, a process for making strategic choices in health systems*. Geneva: WHO Press. Retrieved from http://www.who.int/management/quality/assurance/QualityCare_B.Def.pdf

KEY TERMS AND DEFINITIONS

Accessibility: The opportunity to have access to the care according to our healthcare needs.

Answerability: Responsibility for explaining or justifying one's actions.

Clinical Governance: Systematic approach to maintaining and improving the quality of patient care within a health system.

Disclosure: The act or process of revealing. Public disclosure is a situation in which an organization makes information available by publishing it.

Effectiveness: The capability of producing a desired result. In medicine, effectiveness relates to how well a treatment works in practice.

Efficiency: The ability to do things well, successfully, and without waste. Efficiency in healthcare is the capability to use resources to get the best results in terms of care with the less waste of resources.

Equity: The absence of avoidable or remediable differences among groups of people, whether those groups are defined socially, economically, demographically, or geographically.

Evaluation: Is a systematic determination using criteria governed by a set of standards.

Chapter 12
Could Patient Engagement Promote a Health System Free From Malpractice Litigation Risk?

Massimo Miglioretti
University of Milano-Bicocca, Italy

Francesca Mariani
University of Milano-Bicocca, Italy

Luca Vecchio
University of Milano-Bicocca, Italy

ABSTRACT

In recent decades, medical malpractice litigation experienced a large-scale expansion in the United States as well as in Europe, involving both medical and surgical specialties. Previous studies have investigated the reasons why patients decide to sue doctors for malpractice and highlighted that adverse outcome, negative communication with doctors and seeking compensation are among the major reasons for malpractice litigation. In this chapter, patient engagement is discussed as a possible method for reducing the risks of doctors being sued for medical malpractice. The results of a first qualitative study underline how an active role for patients and their engagement in the treatment definition and execution could be a way to limit the occurrence of malpractice litigations. However, a second study noted that in Italy, many patients are still struggling to become involved in the process of their care. The authors discuss the role of professional education in promoting patient engagement in Italy.

DOI: 10.4018/978-1-4666-9992-2.ch012

INTRODUCTION

The first document presenting a case of medical malpractice litigation dates back to the second half of the 14th century. In 1374, Chief Justice John Cavendish on the Court of King Bench in England ruled on a civil liberty action against a London surgeon for the treatment of the crushed and mangled hand of a woman (Spiegel & Kavaler, 1997). However, it is during the nineteenth century that the number of malpractice suits first substantially increased. In the United States, between 1835 and 1865, the first "malpractice crisis" is documented. At that time, most cases were associated with poorly repaired fractures or were obstetrics problems (Badri, 2014). Some authors attribute the increase in malpractice litigations to the hostility between the law and professional medical practices because medicine is a prospective profession, whereas law is a retrospective one. In this regard, Ficarra (1976) wrote: "When a physician does anything to any patient, he is experimenting or medically speculating. However, if the patient suffers adverse results and sues, then the court applies what is by definition a retrospective judgement of a particular course of treatment" (p. 23). This point of view, used to explain that first increase in malpractice suits, is still valid. However, despite the increased interest in medical malpractice during the second half of the 20th century, updated data on the proportion of physicians who faced malpractice claims are lacking, at least until the last decade of the 1900s. Jena, Seabury, Lakdawalla and Chandra (2011) state that in the United States, from 1991 to 2005, 7.4% of all physicians had a malpractice claim, with many differences between the various medical specialties. Indeed, the proportion of physicians facing a claim each year ranged from 19.1% in neurosurgery to 2.6% in psychiatry.

In the same period, even in Europe, medical malpractice litigation has rapidly expanded (Di Nunno, Vimercati, Viola, & Vimercati, 2005). In Italy, hospitals, doctors and health professionals in general are increasingly subject to patients' complaints and are at risk of facing legal proceedings. As a consequence, current legal actions against physicians number approximately 15,000 per year, and hospitals spend over €10 billion to compensate patients injured by therapeutic and diagnostic errors. (Traina, 2009). Some clinical areas are historically more at risk of legal challenges, as is the case for orthopaedics, obstetrics and gynaecology; however, in recent years, even less traditional areas – such as emergency, radiology, surgery, oncology, etc. – have been subjected to malpractice litigation (Traina, 2009; National Association of Insurance Companies [ANIA], 2014). As an example, for Italian radiologists the risk of incurring a malpractice lawsuit has progressively increased and is now estimated at 44 per 1000. For these professionals, this corresponds to one malpractice claim for every 231 years of activity (Magnavita et al., 2013). The data provided by ANIA (2014) demonstrate that disputes in the medical field in Italy have increased by over 255% from 1994 to 2011 and further increased by 15% in 2011 compared to 2010, while in 2012 they decreased by 5% compared to 2011. This reduction does not necessarily mean a real decrease of malpractice litigations; rather, it can be considered the consequence of a different way of coping with the problem by local health organizations. Indeed, these organizations try increasingly to directly manage the vast majority of claims without giving notice to the insurance system, given the growth of insurance premiums and, often, the refusal of an insurer to willing assume the risk (Norelli, De Luca, Focardi, Giardiello, & Pinchi, 2015; ANIA, 2014). For a more reliable assessment of the extent of medical malpractice suits in Italy, a system able to acquire accurate information on medical litigation and to classify it would be useful. However, to date, a complete and comprehensive database on medical malpractice litigation is not available.

Table 1. Main reasons for patients suing doctors and other health workers

Topic	Study
Negative doctor-patient/family communication and communication failure	- Hickson et al. (1994) - Levinson, Roter, Mullooly, Dull and Frankel (1997) - Moore, Adle and Robertson (2000) - Roter (2006)
Dissatisfaction about care	- Beckman, Markakis, Suchman and Frankel (1994) - Hickson, Clayton, Githens and Sloan (1992) - Levinson et al. (1997)
Desire to protect others from similar problems and to prevent similar incidents in the future.	- Hickson et al. (1992) - Vincent, Young and Philips (1994)
Desire for compensation (monetary or moral).	- Bismark, Dauer, Paterson and Studdert (2006)
Cultural factors (connected with national/race characteristics)	- Chiu (2010) - Fileni and Magnavita (1995)

Among the main reasons that cause the suing of health professionals are diagnostic and therapeutic errors committed in their professional activities. Medicine is certainly not free from errors (Kohn, Corrigan, & Donaldson, 2000). Despite the great efforts made during the last decades to avoid medical errors and their consequences for patients, the number of adverse events caused by medical practice has not been reduced nor have hospitals become safer. Previous studies have highlighted a mutual influence between physicians' errors, adverse events and malpractice litigation risk (Renkema, Broekhius, & Ahaus, 2014). These authors noted that because medicine has become more complex, it is natural that adverse events have also increased.

Facing the increasing risk of litigation to physician behaviour, many physicians respond with more defensive medicine, a peculiar interpretation of medical practice. Defensive medicine includes performing unnecessary medical procedures and tests, deviating from the practice guidelines and avoiding high-risk patients. However, to adopt a defensive approach in medical practice is not the best way to limit medical error. On the contrary, previous studies have underlined the importance of error disclosure by physicians and others health workers, for both organization and patient safety (Kreckler, Catchpole, McCulloch, & Handa, 2009; Waring, 2005). However, error disclosure can be difficult when there is a fear of complaints, so adopting a defensive approach seems to be a simpler response, even if it favours an increase in medical litigation (Renkema et al., 2014).

However, what drives a patient to sue his/her doctor or another health worker? Studies have investigated from various points of view the reasons why patients sue doctors. Table 1 lists the main studies that explore these reasons and categorizes them on the basis of the identified motives. According to these studies, an important role is played by failures in communication among physicians, patients and their family. Other important factors are dissatisfaction about care caused by an adverse outcome, the desire to prevent similar problems for other patients in the future, and the desire for revenge and compensation. Finally, some cultural factors could also have an important role, such as different ways of considering the patient-doctor relationship between Western or Eastern cultures.

Recent studies (Barello & Graffigna, 2014) have shown that increased active patient engagement is associated with better health behaviour, improved health outcomes, and more efficient healthcare utilization. Today, healthcare policies are evolving with a progressive shift in medical practice towards patient-centred care, one aspect of which is the approach known as shared decision-making. Many professionals have assumed that promoting shared decision-making and involving patients in the process of decisions about their care would reduce medical litigation. However, Durand, Moulton, Cockle, Mann and Elwyn (2015), in their systematic review of the relevant literature about this issue, concluded that given the number and heterogeneity of the studies, there is insufficient evidence to confirm this statement. Regardless, they suggested continuing the practice and research in this direction because these approaches could be effective against medical litigation. Indeed, when patients and physicians are engaged in a collaborative medical decision process, the health professional informs patients of the known harms and benefits and seeks to know the patients' preferences; every decision is discussed and documented, and this process should protect against medical litigation. In contrast, if the patient is not engaged in the process of care, the health professional more frequently adopts a defensive medicine approach; he/she orders more tests and diagnostic procedures, neither discussing the harms and benefits nor sharing the decisions with the patients. Thus, if a patient experiences an adverse outcome, there is a high risk of medical litigation.

In this chapter, an increase in patient engagement will be proposed as a way to prevent medical litigation. The first qualitative study will explore the reasons that cause patients or their relatives to sue physicians. Based on the results of this study, the chapter will discuss whether the engagement of patients in the process of care and in the medical decision-making process could be protective against medical litigation in Italy. The second study will analyse whether patients in Italy can be considered ready and willing to be involved in the process of their care. Finally, the implications of both studies for the development of educational programmes for health professionals will be considered.

FIRST STUDY: FACTORS INFLUENCING PATIENTS' DECISIONS TO SUE PHYSICIANS

Aim

As discussed previously, malpractice litigation in Italy has been progressively increasing in the last decades. However, to our knowledge, there are no studies trying to identify the causes of this phenomenon, at least with reference to the situation in Italy. The first study aims to analyse what drives patients or their families to sue health professionals, with particular reference to the specific situation in Italy. In exploring the reasons why patients decide to sue healthcare professionals, attention will be specifically devoted to aspects connected with their professional activities, as well as the impact of medical malpractice lawsuits on patients' and physicians' lives.

Methods

Participants

Nine individuals were involved in this interview-based study: the head of the legal department of an important hospital in Northern Italy, a technical consultant, two lawyers specializing in medical malpractice cases, two physicians, two patients and a family member of a deceased patient.

The physicians, the patients and the family member were directly and personally implicated in cases of medical malpractice. The inclusion criteria for these participants were that the civil lawsuit or criminal proceedings should still be ongoing or should have recently concluded. The two lawyers, the technical

Table 2. Socio-demographics of the participants of Study 1

Participants	Age	Gender	Education	Role in the study and profession	Abbreviation
Participant 1	52	Male	Master Degree	Lawyer	Law 1
Participant 2	32	Female	Master Degree	Patient (Nurse)	Pat 1
Participant 3	76	Male	Master Degree	Lawyer	Law 2
Participant 4	62	Male	Master Degree	Physician	Phy 1
Participant 5	53	Female	Middle school	Patient (Bartender)	Pat 2
Participant 6	70	Female	Master Degree	Physician	Phy 2
Participant 7	48	Male	Master Degree	Head of a legal hospital department	Hld
Participant 8	79	Male	Master Degree	Technical consultant	Tc
Participant 9	54	Female	High school graduation	Family member (Entrepreneur)	Fam

consultant and the head of the legal department of hospital were involved because they have long-term experience with medical litigation and with the judicial process derived from it.

Table 2 illustrates some socio-demographic characteristics of the participants, along with the abbreviations that will be used to identify them later in the text.

Recruitment of the participants was quite difficult, and finding physicians willing to talk about their experiences of medical malpractice was particularly difficult, despite help from some medical professional associations and from AMAMI, an association protecting doctors accused of malpractice. However, those who agreed to participate were generally collaborative and interested in the study. One patient and the family member were happy to be given the opportunity to talk about the illness and their malpractice experience. The other patient was a little worried because the legal suit was particularly delicate and she was afraid that participating in the research could damage the possibility of winning the case and obtaining fair compensation; in any case, despite her concern, she too was collaborative. Even the lawyers, the physicians, the technical consultant and the head of the legal department participated without any particular problems.

Before beginning the study, ethical approval was obtained from the University of Milano-Bicocca, and the appropriate permission and information forms were used. Each participant received an information sheet and a consent form.

Interview

The participants were individually interviewed through a semi-structured interview consisting of previously prepared open-ended questions. The questions were centred on their personal experiences and understanding of medical malpractice and of its impact on their lives. The interview began with very general questions about what happened (e.g.: "Tell me about the experience of your illness and malpractice…"). When trust had been obtained and a good relationship had been established, questions about more focussed issues were asked (e.g.: "Why did you decide to sue your physician?").

The participants were asked to talk as freely as possible about what happened to them and what they considered important to their experience. In this way, the participants were free to orient the contents of the interview, selecting the most relevant aspects of the experience that resulted in the choice to sue, even if the interviewer often requested further details to obtain rich, insightful accounts on the basis of the participants' initial responses. Thanks to the flexibility of semi-structured interviewing, the participants could change the direction of the interview and even introduce new matters that the research team might not have thought of in planning the interview schedule (Smith & Osborn, 2003).

The interviews lasted from 60 to 90 min. and took place in a proper setting, either in the clinic or at the participants' homes or offices, depending on their preference. All of the interviews were audio taped with consent and all of the recordings were transcribed verbatim, ensuring anonymity for each participant. A verbatim transcript of the semi-structured interview served as the raw data for the study. The participants were sent a copy of their interview transcript to verify its accuracy (Lincoln & Guba, 1985). This gave the participants the opportunity to either add things they forgot to say or change what they said. One participant was further interviewed to explicate some of his narrative. This procedure guaranteed the authenticity of the obtained data.

Analysis

The data were analysed using interpretative phenomenological analysis (IPA) (Smith, 1996; Marriott & Thompson, 2008). IPA is an idiographic qualitative methodology that involves the analysis of verbatim transcripts derived from in-depth, semi-structured interviews with participants (Smith, 1995). It is widely used in health psychology to understand the ways in which individuals construe, make a sense of, and talk about their illness or aspects of it (Smith, Flowers, & Osborn, 1997). The aim of IPA is to explore in detail the participants' point of view about the topic under investigation; in this case, the experience linked with malpractice litigation. For IPA, a detailed analysis of each case is important, and it isn't necessary to have a consistent number of participants; therefore, sample sizes are usually small (Dickson, Allan, & O'Carroll, 2008). The results, of course, represent only this particular group of individuals and cannot be considered to be representative of the experiences of all patients and of all physicians.

Each transcript was read by every author thoroughly and repeatedly so that he/she could become familiar with the story and also obtain new insights about the issue explored. Then, one researcher made a close interpretative analysis of each case: while reading, she recorded her initial notes in the text in one margin; then she re-read her notes, translating them into emergent themes at a higher level of abstraction; finally, she wrote these themes in the other margin of the text, using key words or phrases to capture the essence of the content. A second researcher reviewed and examined the themes identified by the first reader to ensure that they were well represented in the transcripts. Many themes emerged within each individual transcript; when the same themes appeared in at least half of the transcripts, they were categorised as being recurrent. The recurrent themes were then clustered into a consolidated list of super-ordinate themes.

Results

The analysis of the interviews with patients, physicians and lawyers demonstrated that medical litigation is the result of a process of care with many problems, particularly when it is considered from the patient's point of view. The respondents often spoke about the problematic relationship among patients and doctors during the process of care. They also underlined the difficulties in the relationship among physicians and the conflicts that originated from that situation. Sometimes it is very difficult for the patients to understand their disease and the real possibility of care and healing. Another aspect indicated by the respondents as a source of medical litigation concerned problems in the organization of the health facilities, which are often neglected and mismanaged by health workers but can lead to making errors. The physicians and lawyers also indicated that underlying the medical litigation was the desire for economic compensation by the patients or their relatives; this appears as a desire for partial compensation of the damage suffered by the patient.

Difficulties Concerning the Relationship between Patients and Doctors

There is consolidated evidence that the doctor-patient relationship plays a fundamental role in patient satisfaction (for a recent review, see Velasco, Miglioretti, Strada, & Vecchio, 2014). The (poor) quality of this relationship has also been identified as an important issue in most medical lawsuits. Indeed, in the cases considered in our study, it is possible to note that many malpractice suits are brought neither because of malpractice nor as a consequence of the poor quality of medical care but mainly as an expression of resentment about some aspect of the patient-doctor relationship and communication.

As the technical consultant says:

In many cases - I can't say what the exact percentage is, but in a large percentage - there's always been at least a disagreement between the family members and the doctor. (Tc)

And again:

Often doctors are arrogant. For example: a doctor couldn't get out from a critical care unit, and when he met relatives asking after their beloved's health, he made the sign that he flew to heaven. It happened! There are doctors who have behaved extremely rudely, even irritatingly. (Tc)

Even the two lawyers are of the same opinion:

Sometimes I observed that the inhumanity of the physician was behind a certain hatred towards him, and it had a part in determining the course of events, independent of the liability of the physician. (Law 1)

And:

Not infrequently, doctors are quite brusque with patients, and this is the worst mistake they can make. Quite frequently – I notice, from what I hear –there are patients or relatives who ask for information and aren't treated by doctors with due courtesy; doctors neither give adequate explanations of what they are doing nor what they should have done, and so on. And this is really important! So, the more the doctor tries to explain and to be present towards patients or family, that often are objectively boring, the better it is, since if things don't go well, the memories that these people have will be much more positive than if they were treated in a different way. The doctors are sometimes quite arrogant! (Law 2)

That's just what happened to one of the patients interviewed:

Meanwhile, he [the doctor] gave me a really exaggerated scolding in the hospital ward: he started banging, screaming and he took my wheelchair and threw it! He behaved this way in front of other patients, saying it was me that didn't want to walk and that my pains were not real. (Pat 1)

The feeling of not being considered as a person seems to also have a great influence on the decision to sue. This is what the family of the deceased patient says:

NO ONE at the hospital has ever deigned to make at least a phone call! This arrogance! This hauteur! They wanted to feel more powerful than medicine because probably if they had done what they had to do, such as medical checks, they would have noticed! And instead! Instead he passed on. (Fam)

...It was a place...a place where you aren't considered as a person, there isn't a smile, there isn't a word, there isn't a time when one feels comforted! (Fam)

However, above all, what seems to be the most unbearable for a patient is not to be heard:

He asked for help because he couldn't breathe, and after taking a deep breath, he said: 'I can't, I can't do it, please go to ask someone for an oxygen mask or something else because I can't breathe'; and so I went all around the ward to look for the doctor, and they always told me: wait lady, just a moment, this moment has to pass in a minute, he is just out of surgery! So I have to say that I did not feel cared for by physicians of the hospital. (Fam)

Doctors behaving in such a way also become an easy target of the anger that patient and their relatives already feel due to the disease and its consequences.

The doctor-patient relationship has also become more and more difficult in recent years because patients have raised their expectations. Indeed, in some cases, the cause of medical litigation is the refusal of the complications of the disease: patients not only want to heal, but they want to return to their previous lives. As one of the doctors interviewed highlights:

After the boom of the wellness, the patient claims to be healed, and he takes for granted that the doctor cured him of his problem. But now he asks not only to be recovered from his illness but also to be healed from alcohol, obesity, ugliness, and drugs, and these requests can cause increasing conflicts with doctors. The patient no longer hangs on to every word of the doctor... he continuously presents demands that are quite impossible to satisfy...Science, especially surgery, has made great strides, but we have not yet become taumaturgi." (Phy 1)

So there are a growing number of complaints and malpractice lawsuits involving physicians who are less prone to listening and discussing with patients. In this regard, the experience reported by the head of the hospital legal department who participated in our research is notable:

The relationship that the doctor has with the patient, based on: "I am the doctor, you are the patient, and you have to accept what I say," surely causes a damage claim, even only to punish the doctor and to be told that the patient was right. I have noticed that some doctors, especially for character profiles, establish such a relationship and then almost always take a claim. (Hld)

Given the problematic nature of the doctor-patient relationship in these circumstances, some doctors seem to experience a professional crisis in reference to their role. One of the doctors interviewed believes that:

Nowadays, the relationship with the patient has become too technical, we have lost that previous "golden charm"...that is, when I enter into a clinic to visit a patient I don't find there someone who hangs on my every word...I find one who thinks, 'let's see what he is going to tell me,' maybe he has heard other opinions; it's almost a symmetric confrontation, that is, I have to explain to this patient why he must come to me or why he has to do what I say rather than what he thinks, or what my other colleagues have said, or what he read in the literature or on the internet! It is a job; it isn't a pleasure any more, like offering a gift; now, fundamentally I solve a problem, there is a problem and I'll solve it; before, to solve this same problem, it was enough to say: "Yes, ok, I'll do it, trust me." (Hld)

Trust is fundamental for a good doctor-patient relationship, in particular the trust of the patient towards his doctor:

It was a bad experience because I really trusted her...I trusted her and instead...and then, before I trusted another dentist, it took a bit of time...but this doctor put me at ease, he is so cute... (Pat 2)

All this involves inevitable negative experiences for the doctors who feel they have been betrayed:

She lost trust in us because she got worse and probably they thought that the surgery that I did was maybe too aggressive or that the full dentures should not have been made; what bothered me is that she asked to be re-operated on in another structure near our hospital by a doctor who did not know more than me, and so I felt betrayed. (Phy 1)

Another possible reason for suing, linked to the doctor-patient relationship, concerns transmission of information. If doctors do not speak clearly, there is a risk that lawsuits can be initiated to know exactly what happened. Physicians who are empathic towards their patients and can respond properly to their emotional needs and those of their families are less likely to be sued. According to one of the interviewed:

The physician must treat not only the patient, he must also assist relatives, since the doctor's presence is noticed by the relatives. When a patient is serious, relatives stay in the hospital from morning to night and even meet the doctors, maybe in the hallway, and saying a word is useful. I think this is the point to avoid...to reduce a lot the conflict. (Tc)

In addition to dealing with the patients in an honest and direct way, treating them as if they were a family member reduces risk. When things go wrong, if the physicians are honest and try to do everything possible to remedy the situation, the patient or his/her family will almost always give them the benefit of the doubt when they are in a critical situation. Listening, assuming responsibility, apologizing for situations where physicians or their team were responsible, and, finally, doing everything they can possibly do to resolve the situation manages the patient's (or family members') anger and reduces the risk of a malpractice lawsuit. Here is the experience of one of the interviewed physicians:

Once, we left gauze in a patient's belly, and we pulled it out. The patient laughed the matter off; he could sue us. This man was a patient who underwent surgery, and he had seven thousand gauzes inside him, and one of them remained there. It must not happen! But it can happen! This isn't a distraction, it is that a surgeon who was in the operating room for seven hours, to be careful here... to be careful there, the poor girl who is there and who has a row of gauze...it sometimes can happen. The surgeon was desperate, this was a very critical case, when I called his wife to tell her: 'Look, a terrible thing happened,' his wife almost died, and when I said it was a piece of gauze, she started to laugh, 'Just for that?' He came here with a great spirit, he went through his minor surgery…we had a good relationship with them, they were here a while, we joked when the surgery went well. (Phy 2)

Difficulties Concerning the Relationships between Physicians and Between Physicians and Other Health Workers

Another reason for medical litigation originates in difficulties in communication and in the relationship among colleagues, in particular among physicians and between physicians and nurses. These difficulties often cause a lack of trust among health professionals. In this case, doctors prefer to work alone but this can lead to an incomplete view of the patient's condition and can affect the quality of care. About this point, a doctor says:

I don't ever look at the medical records of nurses because these records are always written a little superficially: they see a parameter and write it, they don't think about the parameter. (Phy 2)

Sometimes, conflicts can also be caused by the desire to hoard as many patients as they can. Today, the physicians are increasingly in competition with each other to have many patients. In Italy, this is certainly caused by the diffusion of private healthcare, which has increased in the last two decades. About this phenomenon, a doctor says:

One of the causes of medical litigation are our colleagues, since to grab the customer, the colleague is ready to fire on his colleague's work; but he doesn't say anything directly, just a little phrase or just not to say something, and so they instil doubts, and the patient asks for information or consults a lawyer. (Phy 1)

When a lawsuit is pending, conflicts among physicians can adversely affect the physician involved in the process; if in the past, he had some conflicts with other colleagues, it is possible that his actions can be judged more negatively than they actually are.

For a long period, a doctor hardly dared to explicitly blame another colleague. Now, the situation in some way has reversed, in the sense that forensic medicine has often become a fierce opponent of the doctor. Unfortunately, in the medical world, there is also strong friction between schools and even between individuals: "I had to become the primary, he became the primary," and sometimes, especially in the provinces where there is a smaller community, I have been in situations where, when my client knew who was the consultant chosen by the judge, he said: 'Alas, I'm in trouble because this doctor is my enemy.' And so it was! In spite of everything. (Law 2)

Problems in the Organization of Health Facilities

Even the organizational aspects may play a role in increasing the amount of medical litigation. In the last decade, in Italy, to diminish the costs, many health facilities reduced their personnel while trying to maintain the same quality in the service provided. In some cases, technological progress and an increase in efficiency compensated for personnel reduction. In other cases, the personnel reduction enhanced the risk of mistakes. Organizational chaos, tight schedules and work overload may drive the occurrence of mistakes both by the medical staff and by other health care professionals and may even be an obstacle for a good doctor-patient relationship.

Here are the views of one of the lawyers interviewed:

In the emergency ward anything can happen; one has to make quick, very quick decisions, in tremendous chaos, so these doctors are actually undergoing very considerable stress and therefore can make mistakes. (Law 2)

Difficulties of working under certain conditions are also recognized by one of the patients who participated in the research. She underlines that the nurses:

...experienced three shift changes in two and a half days (afternoon, morning, night). So I knew that the staff that I saw in the morning would have remained even through the night, and of course, this personnel won't be rested, since they are coming from a heavy round...and surely the shifts affected the availability of the nurses.

...The nurses were understaffed: if you called for a painkiller, no one came, nobody reached me. I called for ice because I had a big haematoma, and no one brought me ice, I remember, my relatives went to pick it up. (Pat 1)

Another problem underlined by patients is the lack of properly trained personnel in some health facilities, especially among nurses. The problem is attributed to the nationality of the nurses, and, in some cases, to their difficulties in speaking in Italian. This may adversely affect the relationship with the patient and also with other components of the care team. Regarding this aspect, a patient says:

The service was not good, the nurses gave you drugs without telling you the name, and so I said, 'What are these drops? You must tell me what you're giving to me!' 'No, just drink.' Then, the nurses were mostly foreigners. Nothing against a foreigner who has the right educational qualifications, but a Russian who comes to me and doesn't speak Italian, honestly how he can explain a drug? He can't because he can't speak to me. (Pat 1)

Sometimes patients can be frustrated by the lack of medical equipment. One of our interviewed patients declared:

They did not have the appropriate equipment to take you to the X-rays; the beds didn't pass through the doors, and so they had to constantly relocate from a bed to a stretcher, and moving immediately after surgery was already so painful, that is...already the surgery was painful, but some of my pain was probably also due to that issue. (Pat 1)

The Desire for Economic Compensation

According to some people who participated in this research, patients and their family can also sue physicians for economic reasons. One of the interviewed lawyers declared that:

Perhaps we are approaching the American model where people sue a doctor because a doctor is solvent, the doctor has insurance behind him.

... Now, medical negligence is also becoming one of the most desired areas by lawyers. Against a doctor, who is always insured but also against a medical hospital, the possibility for a patient to obtain compensation and for a lawyer to obtain a recompense are very high, and this is the reason why it is a particularly popular specialty. (Law 1)

For this reason, medical malpractice (real or perceived) has become a real business.

In other occasions, physicians themselves incite patients to sue their colleagues:

The person who urges people to make these damage claims or misleads the lawyer to make damage claims is a legal doctor who really misjudges the physician's work, both for lack of professional knowledge and for other reasons and to profit, to get money (to obtain the parcel). (Hld).

Finally, there are friends and acquaintances that advise the patient to sue:

Most requests are often induced by acquaintances, friends, and perhaps these people, after a certain time in years, suggest that the patient proceed with a damage claim because one could get compensation. (Hld)

However, only people who have not suffered real damage are motivated by speculative reasons:

Some people are driven more by speculative reasons, though this happens, in my opinion, mostly to those who haven't suffered a real wrong. Those who have been wronged don't start a lawsuit for that reason. (Law 1)

Discussion

The results we obtained from our interviews are in line with those previously highlighted in the literature of other countries (Hickson et al., 1994; Roter, 2006), in particular with regard to the role of the relationship among patients and health workers as the most relevant reason underlying the origin of medical litigation. Furthermore, to offer other explanations for malpractice complaints, our results also highlight the importance of trust among the different actors in the care team (e.g., physicians and nurses), along with some of the organizational characteristics of the health facilities. Finally, in some cases, the reasons for suing health workers are connected with the expectation of economic compensation of damage.

This study involves only a small group of participants, and so these results are not generalizable to other contexts. However, it is possible to draw some interesting conclusions that could be used as a basis for further studies aimed at exploring the reasons for suing in a wider population.

First, our results underline the importance of the diffusion of the patient-centred approach because certainly this medical approach favours better communication and a better relationship among patients and physicians. The patient-centred approach provides care consistent with the values, needs and desires of patients and is achieved when clinicians involve patients in healthcare discussions and decisions (Constand, MacDermid, Dal Bello-Hass, & Law, 2014). Little et al. (2001) underline three main characteristics of the patient-centred approach that, in the light of the results of the present study, are also relevant for preventing medical litigation: effective communication, partnership and health promotion. Effective communication has been defined as the exploration of the patient's disease and illness to develop an understanding of the patient's health care experiences. Partnership between clinicians and patients occurs to find common ground upon which a healthcare plan can be developed mutually. Finally, health promotion means the development of a health care plan tailored to the history of the patient (Mead & Bower, 2000). These three aspects could combat the effects of bad communication with patients. Moreover, by putting the patients at the centre of the medical process, doctors could also favour the relationship among colleagues and orient the organization of services, another two aspects that may cause medical litigation if they are poorly managed. If physicians adopt the patient-centred approach, they also likely make their decisions regarding care with patients, adopting a shared decision-making approach. This appears important to avoid medical litigation, though the efficacy of shared decision-making in medicine is poorly supported by research. However, even if there isn't any evidence that the patient-centred approach directly reduces medical litigation, this study suggests that this is likely one way to limit defensive medicine and also the possibility of medical litigation (Durand el al., 2015). This approach is also in line with greater patient engagement in the process of care. Graffigna, Barello, Wiederhold, Bosio and Riva (2013) define patient engagement as "a multidimensional psychosocial process resulting from the conjoint cognitive, emotional, and behavioural enactment of individuals towards their disease condition and its management." However, this first study showed that the patients appear not to be engaged in the process of their care; in fact, they complain about not being informed and involved, and they emphasize that the physicians certainly do not adhere to the culture of patient engagement. Thus, patient engagement cannot be taken for granted. The scientific literature shows that the concept of patient participation is still poorly defined. In particular, many terms are used to indicate similar concepts, such as "patient engagement," "patient involvement," "patient collaboration," "patient empowerment," and "patient-centred care." Certainly, if more participation of patients than in the past could be very useful to improve medical practices and to avoid errors and medical litigation, this approach must still be adopted among physicians because they not always favour it.

However, probably this is true also among patients: we know very little about what the patients think about their engagement in the process of care. Considering that, traditionally, the patient was passive and waited for the physician's decision, we can expect that also for patients, there could be some resistance to assuming a more active role in their care due to psychological, educational or cultural reasons.

In the second study presented in this chapter the focus is specifically on this aspect: do patients want to be engaged in the process of care?

SECOND STUDY: PATIENT ENGAGEMENT IN CARE AND SAFETY PROCESSES IN A HOSPITAL SETTING

Background

Patient participation in care is a complex concept developed within the consumer movement since the 1960s. In this period, the idea that the consumer has the right to safety, to be informed, to choose and to be heard emerged (Longtin et al, 2010). In the last decades, patient participation has increasingly become a key component in the process of care, in particular with regard to the safety of care and the process of decision-making and treatment of chronic disease. Indeed, the evidence that underlines the importance of patient participation or patient engagement is abundant.

Our previous study highlighted the role of patient participation to prevent medical litigation. Hall et al. (2010) present some evidence for the effectiveness of interventions designed to promote patient involvement to favour the safety of the medication. In another study, Arnetz et al. (2010) found a significant association between patient involvement and health and behavioural outcomes after acute myocardial infarction. O'Brien et al. (2013), departing from the previous evidence that involvement of patients in therapeutic decision-making is beneficial to patients, have identified facilitators and barriers to the involvement of women with breast cancer in therapeutic decisions.

The core of patient participation and patient engagement is the new definition of the role of patients, where the patient becomes a key player in every process of health care. This new active role for the patient is encouraged not only in the scientific literature but also in the governmental policies of many states (Longtin et al., 2010). However, do the patients want to assume this new role? Previous studies among the US population estimated that approximately half of the respondents prefer to delegate decisions about care to physicians (Levinson, Kao, Kuby, & Thisted, 2005). In another study in the UK, involving patients waiting for a visit by general practitioner, 86% of the participants expressed the desire to determine the course of treatment together with their physician (Little et al., 2001). To our knowledge, there are currently no other studies that explore this aspect in Italy.

Aim

This second study evaluates the level of involvement in the health care process and in safety management in a group of Italian inpatients. Moreover, the study aims to investigate the relationship among the patients' involvement and their social and personal characteristics, their beliefs about the importance of their involvement and their self-efficacy about their involvement.

Method

This study was conducted in two medium-sized hospitals in Northern Italy. An ad hoc questionnaire was developed to investigate patient involvement in the care process and in the management of their safety. The study was proposed to all hospitalized patients, after their informed consent, in the last days before discharge (1 or 2 days before).

Table 3. Demographic characteristics of the participants in Study 2

Age:	59±15
Male:	53.3%
Education:	
– Primary school	37.1%
– Middle school	26.8%
– High school	29.0%
– Degree	7.1%
Profession:	
– Manager	3.6%
– White collar	16.4%
– Blue collar	11.6%
– Self-employer	8.9%
– Student	1.8%
– Retired	52.4%
– Unemployed	5.3%

Participants

Two hundred twenty-five patients participated in the study. Table 3 describes the principal characteristics of the patients. They were hospitalized for a large number of reasons, but for general classification purposes, 25.8% of the patients were hospitalized for diagnostic reasons, 29.8% for surgery and 44.4% for rehabilitation. More than half of the patients were hospitalized for more than seven days.

Questionnaire

The ad hoc questionnaire was developed from an earlier study by Davis, Koutantji and Vincent (2008). These authors analysed the patients' propensity to ask doctors and other health workers two types of questions: i) questions concerning actions regarding their care (factual questions) and ii) intrusive questions (challenging questions) regarding their safety and its management. According to the authors, the propensity of patients to ask these types of questions can be considered a signal of their active participation in the process of care and in the management of safety in the hospital.

The questionnaire was structured in four parts. The first part considered the social and personal characteristics of the participants. The second part (30 items) concerned the involvement of the patients in the process of care and in the management of safety; as an example, this part contained items like: "Have you ever asked doctors or other health workers: How long shall I stay in hospital?" (factual question) or "Have you ever asked doctors or other health workers: Have you washed your hands before this medical procedure?" (challenging question). The responses were given on a five-point Likert scale, ranging from 1= never to 5= very frequently. The third part (17 items) collected the beliefs of the participants about the importance of patient involvement; an example of an item in this category is as follows: "How necessary is it for you to have information about your health?" In this part, the responses were given on a five- point Likert scale, ranging from 1= none to 5= most. The last part (12 items) considered the patients' self-efficacy about their active role in the process of care and in their safety management. Examples of items are: "Are you able to ask information about your health to health workers?" or "Are you able to report the errors of doctors or other health workers?" The responses were given on a five-point Likert scale, ranging from 1= none to 5= most.

Analysis

The mean and standard deviation for each item in the scale was calculated to evaluate the involvement of patients in the process of care and in safety management, the beliefs of patients regarding the importance of their involvement and their self-efficacy in the process of involvement. ANOVA and t-test were used to evaluate whether sex, age and education could be determinants of the differences in the involvement of the patients. All analyses were performed using SPSS v.21.

Results

Table 4 presents the results for the items regarding the involvement of patients in the process of care and in safety management. Generally, the mean for each item was low and highlighted that the patients are not in the habit of asking the physicians about their health or the management of their safety. In particular, patients seem to be reluctant to ask questions that the physicians could evaluate as intrusive, like those regarding their role, the accuracy of the medical procedures performed and safety. However, patients with higher levels of education (degree) are more likely than patients with lower levels of educational (elementary school) to ask questions concerning their health and safety (in Table 4, an asterisk * signals the questions where there was a significant difference in frequency ($p < .05$) based on the level of the education of the respondents). Even the age of the respondents influenced the tendency to ask questions about the process of care and the management of safety. In particular, younger patients (<50 years) ask questions more frequently than others (in Table 4, significant differences ($p < .05$) are signalled by the symbol †).

The third and fourth parts of the questionnaire considered the beliefs of patients regarding the importance of having an active role in the management of disease and their safety and self-efficacy about their involvement in the care process and in safety management. To verify the mono-dimensionality of the scales concerning these issues, two Principal Component Analyses were performed on the data obtained. Both analyses resulted in one factor explaining a consistent proportion of variance: 38% for the beliefs scale and 34% for the self-efficacy scale; in both cases, the reliability of the scales was good, with a Cronbach alfa of 0.89 and 0.83, respectively.

Indices of belief about the importance of patient involvement and self-efficacy about involvement were calculated, based on the average of the items for each factor. Table 5 shows the mean value of each factor for the total sample and for segments identified by gender, age and level of education. While gender does not influence the patients' beliefs about the importance of involvement and their self-efficacy, age influences their beliefs, and the level of education seems to have a role in increasing both of the dimensions. Indeed, younger patients give more importance to patient involvement, and patients with a higher level of education give more importance to patient involvement and also show a higher self-efficacy in their role in the process of care and in the management of safety.

Table 4. Patient involvement in the process of care and in safety management

	All	Difference by age			Difference by scholarity			
		<=50	51-70	>70	Elementary school	Middle school	High school	Master degree
Patient involvement in the process of care. *(response scale: 1-never; 5-very frequent)*								
Have you ever asked physicians:	**Mean; SD**	**Mean; SD**	**Mean; SD**	**Mean; SD**	**Mean; SD**	**Mean; SD**	**Mean; SD**	**Mean; SD**
Can I have more information about my health status?	2.92; 1.2	2.77; 1.2	3.09; 1.2	2.77; 1.2	2.84; 1.2	3.03; 1.2	2.78; 1.2	3.50; 0.7
How long am I in hospital? †*	2.67; 1.4	3.46; 1.3	2.64; 1.4	1.98; 1.3	2.28; 1.4	2.83; 1.4	2.92; 1.5	3.06; 1.4
Shall I be fine after discharge from the hospital? †	2.57; 1.3	2.68; 1.4	2.78; 1.3	2.08; 1.3	2.51; 1.3	2.72; 1.3	2.42; 1.4	2.80; 1.4
Am I ready to go to home? †	2.55; 1.5	3.07; 1.5	2.65; 1.6	1.88; 1.3	2.27; 1.5	2.73; 1.6	2.60; 1.5	3.00; 1.6
Can I have more information about rules that I will have to respect after discharge? †	2.49; 1.3	2.70; 1.3	2.69; 1.4	1.93; 1.3	2.36; 1.4	2.65; 1.4	2.49; 1.3	2.63; 1.4
How long shall I be off from work? *	2.45; 1.4	2.74; 1.5	2.32; 1.4	1.89; 1.2	1.84; 1.1	2.66; 1.4	2.78; 1.5	2.36; 1.4
Which problems shall I have after my return home? †	2.26; 1.3	2.65; 1.3	2.38; 1.4	1.67; 1.2	2.05; 1.4	2.30; 1.4	2.38; 1.3	2.63; 1.3
Do I have to keep taking the medicines I was taking at home along with the treatment that you are giving to me now? †	2.23; 1.3	2.25; 1.1	2.53; 1.3	1.68; 1.2	2.06; 1.3	2.37; 1.3	2.18; 1.2	2.88; 1.1
Do I have to follow a diet? †	1.73; 1.0	1.82; 1.0	1.93; 1.1	1.30; 0.8	1.63; 1.0	1.75; 1.1	1.65; 0.9	2.25; 1.3
Do the drugs prescribed to me have side effects?	1.68; 1.0	1.60; 1.0	1.85; 1.1	1.43; 0.9	1.63; 1.0	1.75; 1.1	1.65; 1.1	1.75; 1.1
What are the possible alternatives of care? †*	1.62; 1.0	1.84; 1.0	1.74; 1.1	1.20; 0.6	1.39; 0.8	1.60; 1.0	1.86; 1.1	1.88; 1.1
Why should I sign the consent form?	1.51; 1.1	1.35; 0.9	1.63; 1.3	1.45; 0.9	1.55; 1.2	1.47; 1.1	1.34; 1.0	1.49; 1.0
What is the consent form?	1.48; 1.0	1.26; 0.7	1.56; 1.1	1.57; 1.0	1.53; 1.0	1.33; 0.9	1.46; 0.9	1.94; 0.3
Why do you use those instruments? †	1.40; 0.9	1.50; 1.0	1.54; 0.9	1.05; 0.3	1.24; 0.7	1.44; 0.9	1.43; 0.8	1.88; 1.3
Can you give me more exams before deciding on my treatment?	1.34; 0.8	1.37; 0.8	1.34; 0.7	1.32; 0.7	1.28; 0.6	1.42; 0.8	1.34; 0.7	1.44; 0.8
Would it not be safe to perform more evaluation before my discharge?	1.29; 0.7	1.32; 0.6	1.32; 0.8	1.22; 0.7	1.16; 0.6	1.50; 0.9	1.28; 0.6	1.31; 0.8
Which role do you have in this unit?	1.17; 0.6	1.26; 0.9	1.17; 0.6	1.10; 0.4	1.18; 0.6	1.23; 0.8	1.09; 0.4	1.25; 0.6
Could you re-check the procedure that you are performing because I do not feel it is correct? *	1.06; 0.3	1.07; 0.3	1.08; 0.3	1.02; 0.2	1.07; 0.3	1.05; 0.3	1.00; 0.0	1.25; 0.6

Table 4. Continued

	All	Difference by age			Difference by scholarity			
		<=50	51-70	>70	Elementary school	Middle school	High school	Master degree
Patient involvement in his safety management. ***(response scale: 1-never; 5-very frequent)***								
Have you ever verified that:	**Mean; SD**	**Mean; SD**	**Mean; SD**	**Mean; SD**	**Mean; SD**	**Mean; SD**	**Mean; SD**	**Mean; SD**
The hospital spaces are clean and healthy †*	2.82; 1.3	3.46; 0.9	3.00; 1.2	1.90; 1.2	2.42; 1.4	3.00; 1.1	3.09; 1.2	3.25; 1.1
Meals are distributed according to the hygiene rules †*	2.69; 1.5	3.56; 1.2	2.91; 1.5	1.50; 1.1	2.24; 1.5	3.17; 1.5	2.79; 1.4	2.88; 1.7
Health workers are always tidy †*	2.58; 1.4	3.49; 1.1	2.71; 1.3	1.47; 0.9	2.05; 1.3	3.05; 1.4	2.72; 1.3	3.00; 1.5
Every medical procedure is performed in a way that is respectful of privacy †*	2.48; 1.3	3.14; 1.2	2.63; 1.3	1.57; 0.9	2.02; 1.3	2.90; 1.3	2.66; 1.3	2.56; 1.4
The medical procedure is performed in a way that is respectful of safety norms. †*	2.48; 1.3	3.11; 1.2	2.67; 1.3	1.57; 1.0	2.02; 1.2	2.85; 1.3	2.69; 1.3	2.75; 1.4
Health workers scrupulously respect the rules and procedures of hygiene and safety †*	2.40; 1.3	3.11; 1.0	2.55; 1.2	1.47; 1.0	1.98; 1.2	2.72; 1.2	2.58; 1.3	2.69; 1.2
Hospital equipment (beds, wheelchairs) are tailored to the needs of the patient †*	2.34; 1.3	2.95; 1.2	2.57; 1.4	1.35; 0.8	1.94; 1.3	2.77; 1.3	2.48; 1.3	2.38; 1.3
In the hospital, there is an office for public relations in which is it possible to make complaints? †	1.52; 1.0	1.65; 1.0	1.68; 1.1	1.12; 0.4	1.37; 0.9	1.53; 1.0	1.69; 1.0	1.56; 1.1
Have you ever asked:	**Mean; SD**	**Mean; SD**	**Mean; SD**	**Mean; SD**	**Mean; SD**	**Mean; SD**	**Mean; SD**	**Mean; SD**
How many times have you performed this kind of procedure (medication)?	1.16; 0.5	1.14; 0.4	1.21; 0.6	1.07; 0.2	1.11; 0.4	1.25; 0.7	1.09; 0.3	1.25; 0.6
Have you checked that the instruments used are clean and sterile? *	1.06; 0.4	1.07; 0.4	1.09; 0.4	1.00; 0.0	1.07; 0.4	1.00; 0.0	1.05; 0.3	1.31; 0.9
Have you washed your hands before starting this procedure? *	1.04; 0.2	1.02; 0.1	1.05; 0.3	1.03; 0.3	1.06; 0.3	1.00; 0.0	1.00; 0.0	1.19; 0.5
Why are you not using gloves for this procedure?	1.01; 0.1	1.02; 0.1	1.01; 0.9	1.00; 0.0	1.00; 0.0	1.02; 0.2	1.02; 0.1	1.00; 0.0

Note: †= significant difference in patients with different ages (p<.05); *=significant difference in patients with different levels of education (p<.05).

Discussion

This second study aimed to verify, in a sample of Italian patients, whether they were interested in being engaged in the process of their care. In particular, it considered the frequency with which the participants posed questions to their physicians about their health and safety management, as a proxy of their active participation in the process of care. The importance for the patients to be involved in their care and their

Table 5. Belief of the importance of patient involvement and self-efficacy about patient involvement

	Belief of the importance of patient involvement	Self-efficacy about patient involvement
All participants	3.86±0.5	2.73±0.5
Sex		
Male	3.84±0.5	2.78±0.5
Female	3.88±0.4	2.68±0.5
Age		
<40	4.00±0.4*	2.81±0.5
41-50	4.02±0.5†	2.80±0.5
51-65	3.95±0.4	2.79±0.5
66-75	3.73±0.4	2.65±0.5
>75	3.64±0.5*†	2.62±0.5
Level of education		
Elementary school	3.73±0.4*	2.57±0.4*†
Middle school	3.91±0.5	2.77±0.5
High school	3.99±0.4*	2.83±0.6*
Master's Degree	3.88±0.5	3.10±0.7†

Note: * and † = significant difference intergroups for age or level of education, Bonferroni test, $p < 0.05$

self-efficacy in assuming an active role in their process of care were also investigated. In this study, an ad hoc questionnaire developed from an earlier study by Davis, Koutantji and Vincent (2008) was used. This is a limit of the study. However, the results show that the participants in the study were minimally involved in the process of care and safety management. Many of them assumed a passive role, giving to the clinician the total control of their care and treatment. As in previous studies, educational level and age seem to affect the level of the patients' engagement, with older and less educated patients assuming a more passive role then others (Haug & Lavin, 1981; Longtin et al., 2010). Participants recognized the importance of having an active role in the process of care, but many of them did not assume this role because they felt unable to participate actively in their care. Indeed, the level of self-efficacy regarding the involvement of care was low in this study. Again, the educational level seems to affect both the level of importance given to patient involvement and the level of self-efficacy, with patients with lower education levels giving less importance to patient engagement and having a low level of self-efficacy. These results are consistent with studies that underline the importance of increasing patients' self-efficacy to improve their engagement. It is possible to do this by promoting reading, understanding and taking action on health information (health literacy), working together with clinicians to select appropriate treatment or management options (shared decision making) and providing feedback on health care processes and outcomes (quality improvement) (Coultier, 2012).

Certainly, from these results, it seems that there is still a long way to go in Italy to engage patients in the process of care.

CONCLUSION

In this chapter, we considered the causes of medical litigation in Italy, and we discussed the promotion of patients' engagement as a way to limit this phenomenon. In recent decades, medical malpractice litigation experienced a large-scale expansion in Europe and also in Italy. Previous studies have highlighted that an important role in determining medical litigation is played by failures in communication among physicians, patients and their family; by dissatisfaction with care; and by the desire for revenge and compensation. The first study of this chapter confirmed that a poor relationship between patients and clinicians is one of the most important causes of medical litigation, together with some organizational aspects, physicians' conflicts and the patients' desire for damage compensation. The patients and the physicians interviewed referred to the communication and relationships among physicians and also to patients assuming a role that is too passive. In the stories we collected, the patients passively accept the physician's decision about the therapeutic process; thus, if there is a problem, the physician remains the principal person responsible. The participants did not report co-participation of patients, and the physicians are the only director of the care, both in positive cases, when the care is successful, and in negative cases, when the care causes damage to the patient. The participants in the first study underline the fact that medicine today often describes itself as foolproof. Patients increasingly claim to have healed and desire to return to the life they led before the onset of the disease; they do not accept the complications or the disease itself. In these situations, the patients could rapidly change their opinions about the physicians, shifting from a state of complete trust to a state where the doctor-patient relationship is characterized by lack of trust, causing conflicts that can contribute to the increase in litigation. Moreover, in the case of a serious chronic illness, the patient may experience a strong sense of helplessness and abandonment. He/she may feel lonely and depressed, and when anger takes over, the physician who accompanied the patient in his/her care can become an easy target for this deep state of uneasiness and resentment, particularly if the physician has not considered the patient in the process of care from the beginning of the disease. The risk decreases significantly when a patient feels that the treatment decisions were shared. In this case, the patient will be better able to accept the negative consequences, without being overwhelmed by anger or thinking poorly of the capability and professionalism of the doctor. The risk of malpractice litigation diminishes if the patient feels that he is co-participating with clinicians in the therapeutic choices. Thus, the promotion of patient involvement and patient engagement seems important to prevent medical litigation.

However, the second study showed that in Italy, many patients continue to have a passive style regarding their care. In particular, older patients and patients with a lower level of education did not discuss their care with their physicians, perhaps because they do not feel capable of doing so. These results highlight an aspect that is little discussed in the literature about patient engagement, specifically regarding the patients' participation. Often, the literature underlines the importance of physicians adopting a less traditional and less paternalistic approach, instead choosing an approach that favours the patient's participation such as the patient-centred approach. However, the results of our two studies show that even if an approach that favours patients' participation is important to avoid medical litigation, it is also necessary that patients change their approach to care. Today, to promote patient engagement means to initiate health education campaigns that help the population, in particular older people and those with a lower level of education, to understand and learn this different approach to their care. Physicians play an important role in this, but they cannot be alone. All health professionals should have a role. Even psychologists, as experts of health education and behavioural change, are important because they help in tailoring the interventions, taking into account the real lives of the patients. This aspect could be useful to help patients manage the different aspects of life in which they are invited to be engaged: work, family, health, etc. This is not simple for the patient, and in different moments of his life, he may refuse an active role in some aspect, including work, family or management of health. Future studies should focus on addressing this problem.

REFERENCES

Arnetz, J. E., Winblad, U., Höglund, A. T., Lindahl, B., Spångberg, K., Wallentin, L., & Arnetz, B. B. et al. (2010). Is patient involvement during hospitalization for acute myocardial infarction associated with post-discharge treatment outcome? An exploratory study. *Health Expectations*, *13*, 298–311. PMID:20579120

Badri, M. (2014). Medical malpractice litigation. *Journal of the American College of Cardiology*, *64*(4), 418–419. doi:10.1016/j.jacc.2014.06.013 PMID:25060379

Barello, S., & Graffigna, G. (2015). Engaging patients to recover life projectuality: An Italian cross-disease framework. *Quality of Life Research: An International Journal of Quality of Life Aspects of Treatment, Care and Rehabilitation*, *24*(5), 1087–1096. doi:10.1007/s11136-014-0846-x PMID:25373927

Beckman, H. B., Markakis, K. M., Suchman, A. L., & Frankel, R. M. (1994). The doctor-patient relationship and malpractice: Lessons from plaintiff depositions. *Archives of Internal Medicine*, *154*(12), 1365–1370. doi:10.1001/archinte.1994.00420120093010 PMID:8002688

Bismark, M., Dauer, E., Paterson, R., & Studdert, D. (2006). Accountability sought by patients following adverse events from medical care: The New Zealand experience. *Canadian Medical Association Journal*, *175*(8), 889–894. doi:10.1503/cmaj.060429 PMID:17030939

Chiu, Y. C. (2010). What drives patients to sue doctors? The role of cultural factors in the pursuit of malpractice claims in Taiwan. *Social Science & Medicine*, *71*(4), 702–707. doi:10.1016/j.socscimed.2010.04.040 PMID:20646806

Costand, M. K., MacDermid, J. C., Dal Bello-Hass, V., & Law, M. (2014). Scoping review of patient-centered care approaches in healthcare. *BMC Health Services Research*, *14*(1), 271. doi:10.1186/1472-6963-14-271 PMID:24947822

Coultier, A. (2012). Patient engagement-What works? *The Journal of Ambulatory Care Management*, *2*(2), 80–89. doi:10.1097/JAC.0b013e318249e0fd PMID:22415281

Davis, R. E., Koutantji, M., & Vincent, C. A. (2008). How willing are patients to question healthcare staff on issues related to the quality and safety of their healthcare? An exploratory study. *Quality & Safety in Health Care*, *17*(2), 90–96. doi:10.1136/qshc.2007.023754 PMID:18385400

Di Nunno, N., Vimercati, L., Viola, L., & Vimercati, F. (2005). Epidemiological case survey of medical malpractice in some medical and surgical specialties. *Forensic Science International*, *149*(2-3), 139–142. doi:10.1016/j.forsciint.2004.06.029 PMID:15749354

Dickson, A., Allan, D., & O'Carroll, R. (2008). Biographical disruption and the experience of loss following a spinal cord injury: An interpretative phenomenological analysis. *Psychology & Health*, *23*(4), 407–425. doi:10.1080/14768320701219136 PMID:25160576

Durand, M. A., Moulton, B., Cockle, E., Mann, M., & Elwyn, G. (2015). Can shared decision-making reduce medical malpractice litigation? A systematic review. *BMC Health Services Research*, *15*(1), 167. doi:10.1186/s12913-015-0823-2 PMID:25927953

Ficarra, B. J. (1976). A history of legal medicine. In C. Wecht (Ed.), *Legal medicine annual*. New York: Appleton Century Crofts.

Fileni, A., & Magnavita, N. (1995). Malpractice lawsuits in Radiology - Comparison of the Italian and American situations. *Radiology*, *197*(2), 548–549. doi:10.1148/radiology.197.2.548-b PMID:7480715

Graffigna, G., Barello, S., Wiederhold, B. K., Bosio, A. C., & Riva, G. (2013). Positive technology as a driver for health engagement. *Studies in Health Technology and Informatics*, *191*, 9–17. PMID:23792833

Hall, J., Peat, M., Birks, Y., Golder, S., Entwistle, V., Gilbody, S., & Wright, J. et al. (2010). Effectiveness of interventions designed to promote patient involvement to enhance safety: A systematic review. *Quality & Safety in Health Care*, *19*, 1–7. PMID:20427301

Haug, M., & Lavin, B. (1981). Practitioner or patient – who's in charge? *Journal of Health and Social Behavior*, *22*(3), 212–229. doi:10.2307/2136517 PMID:7288129

Hickson, G. B., Clayton, E. W., Entman, S. S., Miller, C. S., Githens, P. B., Whetten-Goldstein, K., & Sloan, F. A. (1994). Obstetricians' prior malpractice experience and patients' satisfaction with care. *Journal of the American Medical Association*, *272*(20), 1583–1587. doi:10.1001/jama.1994.03520200039032 PMID:7966867

Hickson, G. B., Clayton, E. W., Githens, P. B., & Sloan, F. A. (1992). Factors that prompted families to file medical malpractice claims following prenatal injuries. *Journal of the American Medical Association*, *267*(10), 1359–1363. doi:10.1001/jama.1992.03480100065032 PMID:1740858

Jena, A. B., Seabury, S., Lakdawalla, D., & Chandra, A. (2011). Malpractice risk according to physician specialty. *The New England Journal of Medicine*, *365*(7), 629–636. doi:10.1056/NEJMsa1012370 PMID:21848463

Kohn, L. T., Corrigan, J. M., & Donaldson, M. S. (2000). *To err is human: building a safer health system*. Washington: National Academic Press.

Kreckler, S., Catchpole, K., McCulloch, P., & Handa, A. (2009). Factors influencing incident reporting in surgical care. *Quality & Safety in Health Care*, *18*(2), 116–120. doi:10.1136/qshc.2008.026534 PMID:19342525

Levinson, W., Kao, A., Kuby, A., & Thisted, R. A. (2005). Not all patients want to participate in decision making: A national study of public preferences. *Journal of General Internal Medicine*, *20*(6), 531–535. doi:10.1111/j.1525-1497.2005.04101.x PMID:15987329

Levinson, W., Roter, D. L., Mullooly, J. P., Dull, V. T., & Frankel, R. M. (1997). Physician-patient communication: The relationships with malpractice claims among primary care physicians and surgeon. *Journal of the American Medical Association*, *277*, 553–559. doi:10.1001/jama.1997.03540310051034 PMID:9032162

Lincoln, Y. S., & Guba, E. G. (1985). *Naturalistic inquiry* (Vol. 75). Sage.

Little, P., Everitt, H., Williamson, I., Warner, G., Moore, M., Gould, C., & Payne, S. et al. (2001). Preferences of patients for patient centered approach to consultation in primary care: Observational study. *British Medical Journal*, *322*(7284), 468–472. doi:10.1136/bmj.322.7284.468 PMID:11222423

Longtin, Y., Sax, H., Leape, L. L., Sheridan, S. E., Donaldson, L., & Pittet, D. (2010). Patient participation: Current knowledge and applicability to patient safety. *Mayo Clinic Protocol*, *85*(1), 53–62. doi:10.4065/mcp.2009.0248 PMID:20042562

Magnavita, N., Fileni, A., Mirk, P., Magnavita, G., Ricci, S., & Cotroneo, A. R. (2013). Malpractice Claims in interventional radiology: Frequency, characteristics and protective measure. *Radiological Medicine*, *118*(3), 504–517. doi:10.1007/s11547-012-0878-7 PMID:22986698

Marriot, C., & Thompson, A. R. (2008). Managing Threat to femininity: Personal and interpersonal experience of living with vulval pain. *Psychology & Health*, *23*(2), 243–258. doi:10.1080/14768320601168185 PMID:25160053

Mead, N., & Bower, P. (2000). Patient-centredness: A conceptual framework and review of the empirical literature. *Social Science & Medicine*, *51*(7), 1087–1110. doi:10.1016/S0277-9536(00)00098-8 PMID:11005395

Moore, P. J., Adler, N. E., & Robertson, P. A. (2000). Medical malpractice: The effects of doctor-patient relationships on medical patient perceptions and malpractice intentions. *The Western Journal of Medicine*, *173*(4), 244–250. doi:10.1136/ewjm.173.4.244 PMID:11017984

National Association of Insurance Companies. (2014). *Malpractice, the hastle. Dossier Ania about medical malpractice* [Malpractice, il grande caos. Dossier ANIA sul tema della malasanità]. Retrieved from http://www.ania.it

Norelli, G. A., De Luca, F., Focardi, M., Giardiello, R., & Pinchi, V. (2015). The claims management committees trial: Experience of an Italian hospital of the National Health System. *Journal of Forensic and Legal Medicine*, *29*, 6–12. doi:10.1016/j.jflm.2014.10.004 PMID:25572077

O'Brien, M. A., Ellis, P. M., Whelan, T. J., Charles, C., Gafni, A., Lovrics, P., & Hodgson, N. et al. (2013). Physician-related facilitators and barriers to patient involvement in treatment decision making in early breast cancer: Perspectives of physicians and patients. *Health Expectations*, *16*(4), 373–384. doi:10.1111/j.1369-7625.2011.00712.x PMID:21923813

Renkema, E., Broekhius, M., & Ahaus, K. (2014). Conditions that influence the impact of malpractice litigation risk on physicians' behavior regarding patient safety. *BMC Health Services Research*, *14*(1), 38. doi:10.1186/1472-6963-14-38 PMID:24460754

Roter, D. (2006). The patient-physician relationship and its implications for malpractice litigation. *Journal of Health Care Law & Policy*, *9*, 304–314.

Smith, J. A. (1995). Semi-structured interviewing and qualitative analysis. In J. A. Smith, R. Hark, & L. Van Langenhove (Eds.), *Rethinking Methods in Psychology*. London: Sage. doi:10.4135/9781446221792.n2

Smith, J. A. (1996). Beyond the divide between cognition and discourse: Using interpretative phenomenological analysis in health psychology. *Psychology & Health*, *11*(2), 261–217. doi:10.1080/08870449608400256

Smith, J. A., Flowers, P., & Osborn, M. (1997). Interpretative phenomenological analysis and the psychology of health and illness. In L. Yardley (Ed.), *Material discourses of health and illness*. London: Routledge.

Spiegel, A. D., & Kavaler, F. (1997). America's first medical malpractice crisis, 1835-1865. *Journal of Community Health*, *22*(4), 283–308. doi:10.1023/A:1025104520383 PMID:9247851

Traina, F. (2009). Medical Malpractice. The experience in Italy. *Clinical Orthopaedics and Related Research*, *467*(2), 434–442. doi:10.1007/s11999-008-0582-z PMID:18985423

Velasco, V., Miglioretti, M., Strada, M., & Vecchio, L. (2014). Patient satisfaction regarding general practitioners: A theoretical model based on patients' experience and engagement in care process. [La soddisfazione dei pazienti rispetto ai medici di medicina generale: Un modello teorico basato sull'esperienza e l'engagement dei pazienti nei processi di cura]. *Psicologia della salute, 2*, 34-57.

Vincent, C., Young, M., & Phillips, A. (1994). Why do people sue doctors? A study of patients and relatives taking legal action. *Lancet*, *343*(8913), 1609–1613. doi:10.1016/S0140-6736(94)93062-7 PMID:7911925

Waring, J. J. (2005). Beyond blame: Cultural barriers to medical incident reporting. *Social Science & Medicine*, *60*(9), 1927–1935. doi:10.1016/j.socscimed.2004.08.055 PMID:15743644

KEY TERMS AND DEFINITIONS

Defensive Medicine: Medical practices designed to avoid the future possibility of malpractice suits. Clinicians may order tests, procedures, or visits, or avoid high-risk patients or procedures primarily to reduce their exposure to malpractice. Defensive medicine causes an unjustified increased of sanitary cost.

Interpretative Phenomenological Analysis (IPA): IPA is an idiographic qualitative methodology that involves the analysis of verbatim transcripts derived, for example, from semi-structured interviews. It is widely used in health psychology to understand the ways in which individuals construe, make a sense of, and talk about their illness or aspects of it. The aim of IPA is to explore in detail the participants' point of view about the topic under investigation.

Medical Error: The deviations from the process of care, which may cause harm to the patients. Reason (1990) talk about the failure of a planned action to be completed as intended (an error of execution) or about the use of a wrong plan to achieve an aim (an error of planning).

Medical Litigation: A lawsuit or legal action moved by a patient or by his/her relatives against medical practitioner in relation to a doubt of medical malpractice.

Medical Malpractice: Medical malpractice occurs when a medical practitioner acts in a negligent manner when treating a medical condition. In particular, the treatment provided is substandard and may cause harm, injury or death to a patient.

Patient Centred Medicine: "Patient-centered medicine" is a form of medical practice, in which the doctors seek to focus attention on the individual patient's needs and concerns, rather than only on the illness.

Patient Engagement: A way to propose the patients' participation into health care systems in which patients and providers work together to improve health.

Patient Involvement: In a lot of cases this term is used as a synonymous of patient engagement to indicate the patients' participation in the process of care and in the decisions about it.

Shared Decision Making: Shared decision making is a collaborative process in which patients and their providers make health care decisions together, taking into account the best scientific evidence available, as well as the patient's values and preferences.

Chapter 13
Engagement in Health and Safety at the Workplace:
A New Role for the Occupational Health Physician

Nicola Magnavita
Università Cattolica del Sacro Cuore, Rome, Italy

ABSTRACT

Dramatic changes in the age structure of the population have led to a rise in the age of retirement. An ageing working population may be a problem for companies and for their health and safety services that must face the long-term management of active, chronically ill workers. For sustainability reasons the discipline of occupational medicine must be replaced by occupational health, which not only combats occupational diseases, but actively works to promote the health of older workers. More in general, occupational health has a strong interest in promoting engagement in professional activities. Shifting from a reactive to a proactive logic will take time and require a big effort on the part of employers, employees and health and safety staff in order to develop participatory ergonomics and best health promotion practices in the workplace.

INTRODUCTION

Over the next few decades, the rapid ageing of populations will be one of the most powerful forces for change in society. The increase of life span, and a lower fertility rate, particularly in industrial nations, have caused a dramatic demographic shift towards an increase in the mean population age: fewer people are being born and people are living longer.

Long-term projections show that although this demographic shift started in developed countries, it is fast becoming a global challenge. Currently 10% of the global population is over 65 years old, but this figure is expected to jump to 22% by 2050. The total number of people aged 60 years and over is expected to increase from 605 million to 2 billion over the same period. This will have a significant impact on areas such as public health and economic prosperity.

DOI: 10.4018/978-1-4666-9992-2.ch013

Highly significant changes are expected to occur in the age structure of the EU population. While in 2015 the most numerous male and female cohorts are around 45 years old, in 2060 the number of elderly people is expected to account for a rising share of the population (European Commission, 2015). This is due to the combined effect of the numerous cohorts born in the 1950s and 1960s – the baby boomers- and the continual increase in life expectancy. At the same time, the base of the age pyramid is decreasing on account of reduced replacement fertility rates.

This rapid change in the structure of the population has already placed significant pressure on social security systems. Dependency ratios (people aged 65 or above in relation to those aged 15-64) have rapidly increased in all developed countries and the rising costs of retirement and health care have produced an increasingly heavy burden. In the EU as a whole, the demographic old age dependency ratio is predicted to increase from the 2013 27.8% figure to 50.1% in 2060. This would mean that instead of having approximately four working-age technician for every person aged over 65 years, there would be only two working-age people (European Commission, 2015). Ageing also puts the supply and quality of social and health care services (including occupational health services) at risk (Reday-Mulvey, 2005).

These predictions have made European governments increasingly aware of the economic importance of older workers, since their participation in the labor market could help to secure economic productivity and sustain social welfare and pension systems. To this end, the Lisbon European Council (2000) and the Stockholm European Council (2001) developed policies containing joint strategic aims for strengthening employment, economic reform and social cohesion in a knowledge-based economy. Their main aim was to increase the average employment rate of older people aged 55–64 years to 50% by 2010 (Winkelmann-Gleed, 2008). All EU states have introduced pension reforms, and we can already see the first effects of these provisions. In Europe, there are now many more workers aged ≥50 than those aged ≤25 years and this situation is expected to last for decades. This may pose a problem for companies and their health and safety services as many new jobs are designed for young workers. This means that there is a real risk that some older workers will be unable to reach the minimum performance standard required for their work. Moreover, the reduction in retirement ratios will lead to an increase in the number of workers with health problems. This will pose new problems for health and safety services in the workplace. Production requirements will force companies to face a new problem – presenteeism - specifically connected with the presence in the workplace of workers with chronic diseases.

This momentous challenge requires a dramatic change in the methods and aims of occupational health and general health services. This effort, as regards the workplace, is still at the beginning. In this chapter we will explore the necessary change in the methods and aims of occupational health, and will give some insights into the ways in which these changes are actually happening.

BACKGROUND: THE TRADITION OF OCCUPATIONAL MEDICINE

A longer working life means a rise in the number of workers affected by chronic diseases. Healthcare organizations will have to face long-term management of active, chronically ill persons.

This new situation calls for a radical change in the traditional mindset of occupational medicine, a discipline that originated 300 years ago to combat diseases caused by work. For centuries occupational physicians have helped to identify and control physical, chemical, biological and psychosocial environmental hazards. Because this prevention in the workplace has been successful, there are currently fewer workers who fall ill due to environmental causes than workers whose sickness depends on other, non-occupational causes. These sick workers want to work, and are entitled to do so under conditions of safety for themselves and for other people.

Ageing of the workforce is accompanied by a concomitant increase in chronic diseases: e.g. cardiovascular disease, obesity, dyslipidemia, hypertension, diabetes, and cancer. Because chronic diseases are increasing, employees are becoming, on average, less healthy and less productive. This is causing employers great concern as they are faced with growing demands for increased productivity in the global marketplace but have to rely on an ageing and seemingly unhealthier workforce and inadequate occupational health schemes. Sick leave has become a huge problem as the European Agency for Safety and Health at Work has calculated that, in Europe, 600 million working days are lost due to work-related illness. Indeed, Europe and USA are facing a paradox: despite better health, more automation and less manual work, an increasing proportion of the working-age population is economically inactive and in receipt of disability benefits (Ferrie, Virtanen, & Kivimaki, 2014). One of the proposed explanations of the conundrum is that employees are under tremendous pressure at the workplace as the current unfavorable economic environment and working conditions have led to higher demands and workloads accompanied by a reduction in rewards and control.

The traditional aims of occupational medicine, that is to say, the identification of toxic substances in the workplace or an assessment of symptoms and early signs of intoxication in workers, have little to do with this problem. The Second Industrial Revolution has demonstrated the importance of human factors, work organization and the work climate for workers' health. Assessing work-related stress has become a common practice and is a mandatory requirement for all companies. However, in most cases, risk assessment is not followed by a significant improvement in working life. One of the reasons for this is that the action of the occupational physician is confined to occupational hazards and cannot include lifestyles and habits outside work, unless there is a specific health promotion program funded by the company and developed with the agreement of the workers. The traditional, labor approach to occupational health and safety, and the legislation that derives from this model (still the most common in developed countries), thought that the surveillance would apply only to aspects related to the work environment. Consequently, despite the high prevalence of diseases among the general population and therefore in adults at work, these non-occupational diseases are still not considered pertaining to work. Fortunately, a new holistic approach to occupational health is raising awareness that a number of stakeholders (employers, physicians, sickness insurance, health and environment authorities, and the workers themselves) must work together to control all risk factors, both occupational and non-occupational.

BACKGROUND: ENGAGEMENT IN THE WORKPLACE

Health and safety management in the workplace is quite different than clinical medicine. The latter deals with (presumably ill) patient, the former focuses on (presumably healthy) worker. Consequently, clinical medicine promotes patient engagement and his/her participation in healthcare (Graffigna, Barello, & Triberti, 2015), while occupational health focuses on engagement in work and participatory ergonomics.

Engagement in professional activities and positive attitudes towards work are of significant importance to functioning and health of employees. Employee engagement, conceptualized as a positive, work-related mindset including feelings of vigor, dedication and absorption in one's work, has demonstrated an association with a number of important worker outcomes, including safety attitudes and workers' behavior (Daugherty Biddison et al., 2015).

The concept of engagement should not be confused with that of workaholism. The latter has negative consequences, related to an increase of psychological distress, physical complaints, work-to-family conflict and to a decrease in life satisfaction, whereas work engagement has positive consequences in terms of well-being, life satisfaction and work performance (Shimazu & Schaufeli, 2009; Shimazu, Schaufeli, Kubota, & Kawakami, 2012; Hakanen & Peeters, 2015; Shimazu, Schaufeli, Kamiyama, & Kawakami 2015). Hence, workaholism should be prevented and work engagement should be stimulated.

Employee engagement, health behavior, and physical health indices are simultaneously associated with job performance and also, negatively, with absenteeism (Merrill et al., 2013; Airila, Hakanen, Punakallio, Lusa, & Luukkonen, 2012; Rongen, RobroekJ, Schaufeli, & Burdorf, 2014) and presenteeism (Admasachew & Dawson, 2011). Efforts to improve worker productivity should take a holistic approach encompassing employee health improvement and engagement strategies.

As well as engagement, other key factors influence work ability: frequent exercise, good sleep, non-smoking, low job demands, low physical workload, and high task resources (Airila et al., 2012). Being actively engaged in one's work is associated with lower occupational sitting times for men (vigor and dedication) and to a limited extent for women (vigor only). This suggests that interventions such as introducing sit-stand workstations to reduce sitting times, might also be beneficial for work engagement (Munir et al., 2015). Studies also indicated that individuals who are frequently engaged in poor sleep hygiene behaviors had lower self-regulatory capacity, experience higher subjective depletion and are less engaged at work. Specifically, poor sleep hygiene results in the loss of self-regulatory resources needed to be engaged in work tasks by impairing the after-work recovery process (Barber, Grawitch, & Munz, 2013).

There is also a strong relationship between work engagement and work-related stress. A meta-analysis showed that job resources (such as knowledge, autonomy, and a supportive environment) motivate employees and are positively related to engagement (Nahrgang, Morgeson, & Hofmann 2011). A cross-sectional survey using the UK Health & Safety Executive's Management Standards Indicator Tool, a multi-scale indicator (Magnavita, 2012), showed that Role appears to play a major part in determining employee engagement (Ravalier, Dandil, & Limehouse, 2015). Work-related procedural justice and interactional justice are also significantly and positively associated with work engagement (Inoue et al., 2010). In longitudinal studies, higher psychological demands and decision latitude at baseline were positively and significantly associated with greater work engagement at follow-up (Inoue et al., 2013), while higher work engagement at baseline was related to better physical and especially better mental health during the follow-up (Leijten et al., 2015). More in general, workplace relationships (perceived organizational support, supervisor-employee relationships and teamwork) have direct relationships with the engagement, well-being, organizational commitment and turnover intentions of workers (Brunetto et al., 2013). In a three-way Leadership × Demands × Resources interaction, empowering leadership also had the effect of optimizing working conditions for engagement by strengthening the positive effect of a work context in which both cognitive demands and cognitive resources were high (Tuckey, Bakker, & Dollard 2012). Demands that employees tend to appraise as hindrances are negatively associated with engagement, and demands that employees tend to appraise as challenges are positively associated with engagement (Crawford, Lepine, & Rich, 2010).

The relationships between organizational factors, stress and work engagement are very complex and deserve to be studied. Results show empirical support for the predicting role that professional self-efficacy plays in the perception of challenge (i.e., mental overload) and hindrance demands (i.e., role conflict, lack of control, and lack of social support), which are in turn related to burnout (i.e., erosion process) and engagement (i.e., motivational process). Specifically, employees with more professional self-efficacy will perceive more challenge demands and fewer hindrance demands, and this will in turn relate to more engagement and less burnout (Ventura, Salanova, & Llorens, 2015).

Numerous studies have shown the positive consequences of work engagement for both companies and employees experiencing it. For instance, research has demonstrated that work-engaged employees have lower levels of turnover intentions than non-engaged employees (Tullar et al., 2015).

Anticipating the challenges of the next decade, companies are trying to achieve a higher degree of employee engagement, aiming at enhancing organizational performance and profitability.

Workplace-based health and wellness programs may be an useful strategy for promoting positive health-related behaviors among older workers and for increasing their ability to continue to work. Participation in these programs may improve the health status of older workers and reduce health care costs. Low work ability of workers, indeed, generally precedes the use of some company policies aiming to support sustainable employability of older workers (van der Meer et al., 2015). Companies have therefore begun to promote these programs, even if the first results are not always as positive as expected (Oude Hengel, Blatter, Joling, van der Beek, & Bongers, 2012). A pioneering combined social and physical environmental intervention in office workers showed promising results on engagement, absenteeism and presenteeism, even if the implementation of this kind of interventions is not yet recommended (Coffeng et al., 2015). More studies and efforts need to be done to effectively improve employee engagement with promotion programs.

THE CHALLENGE OF WORKFORCE AGEING

The Mature Aged Worker

Occupational health (OH) services have an important role in promoting the health of workers throughout their working life. OH initiatives are needed to address the challenges of an ageing workforce. These include the prevention of work-related diseases, a reduction in work performance due to chronic diseases and the promotion of health and work ability. OH services have a key role to play in 'healthy ageing management'.

Older workers represent a new challenge for occupational health services. All aspects of human resources change with age and the most tangible ones are those related to health (Seitsamo & Klockars, 1997). A survey in EU-15 countries found that work-related health problems are common among men and women >45 years of age (Paoli & Merllie, 2000). Because of reduced physical ability and greater susceptibility to acute and chronic diseases among older employees, worksite health promotion initiatives may be particularly beneficial in terms of improving the health of mature aged workers.

The prevention of work-related symptoms and diseases is a high priority in all age groups, but ageing workers are faced with new challenges: how can they manage at work when they have chronic symptoms and diseases? What can occupational health experts do to prevent the early retirement of those suffering from chronic health problems? Clearly it is not enough to simply treat the diseases. The new challenge is to discover what kind of work adjustments are needed to manage the deterioration of workers' health. If about half of the musculoskeletal and psychosocial health problems are work-related, 'treatment' must be given not only to the worker, but also to the work itself. The knowledge and experience of occupational health physicians can play an important role in making working lives longer and healthier.

The Vulnerable Worker

Nowadays the worker is expected to keep active and competitive to a very advanced age. Despite the rapid ageing of the workforce, most productive sectors lack a policy that reduces risks for the individual and the community.

Ageing is not only a physical process (the frailty of the elderly is a well-known concept in geriatrics), but also a psychosocial issue. In many cases, older workers are more isolated than younger workers, less prepared to adapt to changes and less experienced in new technologies. Older workers may have greater difficulty in acquiring new skills and new habits, in accepting transfers or competing in a rapidly changing globalized market. This puts them in a vulnerable position, often prompting them to retire early or causing them to become unemployed.

The frailty of the elderly makes them more subject to traditional occupational risk factors. The rate of injuries and work-related disorders may be higher in older workers than in younger employees. The damage caused by being exposed to occupational hazards 20 or 30 years previously may become apparent in old age. Furthermore, the majority of chronic diseases occur more frequently in the elderly.

An issue of particular importance is age-related cognitive decline. The risk of developing cognitive impairment is 1% in the over-sixties. This then doubles every 5 years, reaching 5% by the age of 70 years. In the 60 – 70 year range, the risk of having a worker with cognitive impairment is 2%, and this figure rises to 4% if we also consider mild cognitive impairment (MCI). Under the current pension scheme, one in every 20 workers over the age of 60 is unlikely to be cognitively normal. The growing increase in the elderly population may enhance the MCI rate all over the world. Although there is no complete cure for MCI and dementia, preventive measures and appropriate treatment can improve cognitive performance and retard or prevent progressive deficits.

On the other hand, older workers possess a wealth of experience that should not be wasted. Keeping mature-aged workers healthy and productive will be crucial to remaining competitive in the global economy.

In the absence of proper prevention, the growing mass of older workers may increase the number of employees who go to work despite being ill. This situation, which goes under the name of presenteeism, presents a risk not only for productivity and therefore for the employer, but also for health, and thus for the employee.

Presenteeism

Only recently has there been full recognition of the importance of employee health in improving productivity. The term 'presenteeism' is a relatively new concept in workplace health, and has come to indicate the practice of being at work despite poor health and sub-standard performance. Presenteeism – or working while ill – is sometimes seen as just an economic indicator of disease burden; however, its significance for the worker's health is more far-reaching. Emerging evidence suggests that presenteeism may best be defined as a behavior that has implications for the individual and his/her employer, and is a phenomenon that can be managed clinically.

Presenteeism, which is potentially vital for employers, has been associated with a range of psychosocial outcomes such as poor mental health and impaired employee well-being. Working when sick is a consequence of ill health but can itself be a risk for adverse health events. These include cardiovascular disease (Kivimaki et al., 2005) and depression where lost productive time due to presenteeism accounts for 80% of total lost productive time costs (Collins et al., 2005). For many chronic diseases, the 'hidden' cost of presenteeism exceeds the visible costs of absenteeism.

Presenteeism has been found to be more frequent among older workers because of the increase in chronic diseases occurring with age e.g. depression and mental disorders (Cocker et al., 2011; Stewart, Ricci, Chee, Hahn, & Morganstein, 2003; Rost, Meng, & Xu, 2014), chronic obstructive pulmonary disease (DiBonaventura et al., 2012), musculoskeletal disorders (DiBonaventura, Gupta, McDonald, & Sadosky, 2011), obesity and metabolic disorders (Kirkham et al., 2015).

Presenteeism is associated with health, personal, work and occupational factors. Since it can be a precursor to work disability, it is important to understand its clinical significance and how early warning signs can be detected in general practice.

Being present at work despite ill-health results in work outputs that are poorer quality than would be achieved at optimal health (Gifford & Jinnett, 2014), which may contribute to job dissatisfaction. Although engagement is a positive affective and motivational state, feeling a need to be physically present coupled with being psychologically absent has been linked with growing disengagement from work. Indeed, presenteeism may be linked with poorer engagement at work (Admasachew & Dawson, 2011). Preliminary studies indicate that sickness presenteeism is negatively associated with job satisfaction, and work engagement mediates the relationship between presenteeism and job satisfaction (Karanika-Murray, Pontes, Griffiths, & Biron, 2015).

The Hazardous Worker

One of the most recent advances in occupational prevention is the discovery that workers themselves may be the cause of risk in the workplace.

The prevention of work-related injury and disease has traditionally been based on the identification, measurement and control of chemical, physical, and biological environmental risk factors. However, workers themselves may represent a hazard for colleagues and clients.

An employee might endanger the health and safety of others through illness or his/her behavior. At some point in their lives, because of physical or mental illness (due to deterioration caused by ageing or loss of motor skills), workers may be unable to perform activities involving third parties with a reasonable degree of competence and safety. Diseases which impair work may include psychiatric illness, psychosexual illness, neurological/cognitive impairment and physical illness, including communicable diseases. Inappropriate behavior may be a consequence of sleepiness and fatigue at work, alcohol and drugs, stress, burnout, violence, bullying, mobbing, and many other factors.

The hazardous worker can formally jeopardize occupational health and safety systems. Security measures, in fact, are designed and implemented to protect against external hazards or those deriving directly from substances used in the working process or processing phases. These safety systems take into account the activities and transactions carried out by the workers, but only in order to assess the likelihood of a random and preventable error. The HAZOP (hazard and operability) method, FMEA (failure of mode analysis), task analysis and other theoretical frameworks do not therefore envisage the possibility that a hazardous worker may be responsible for the deliberate alteration of processes and procedures (Magnavita, 2004b).

The scientific literature, not to mention the media, are full of famous examples of safety measure failures caused by hazardous workers.

In Florida in the early 1990s, a cluster of six cases in which HIV was transmitted from a dentist to his patients (CDC, 1993) aroused alarm among patients and a general debate that led to changes in federal and state policy. In subsequent years, all countries developed measures to control health workers who are carriers of infectious diseases (Magnavita, 2006).

On 24 March 2015, the Germanwings Flight 9525 crash was deliberately caused by the co-pilot. Although previously treated for suicidal tendencies and declared "unfit to work" by a doctor, the co-pilot kept this information from his employer and reported for duty. During the flight, he locked the captain out of the cockpit before initiating a descent that caused the plane to crash into a mountain. This recent tragedy confirms once again the importance of promptly detecting hazardous workers and encouraging them to adhere to the treatment of their diseases. Dealing with this non-conventional type of risk raises a number of difficult issues.

Probably the most important of these problems is the need to solve an ethical dilemma. It is not easy to guarantee the right to work safety not only for sick workers but also for all the people (colleagues, clients, visitors, outsiders) who may directly or indirectly suffer the consequences of a worker's illness. All parties have rights that must be respected. The sick worker's interests include furthering a career, his/her role in work organization, the right to privacy and to freedom from discrimination. The client's interests include protection from harm, the right to autonomy and to informed choice. The society's interests include maintaining effective and affordable public services, as well as the benefits and burdens of any policies. What is needed is a policy that balances the rights of the sick worker, the rights of other workers, patients and clients, and also safeguards the general society's interests.

Traditional ethics, oriented toward individual relationships, have failed to find a non-controversial solution to these complex issues. Recent research has focused on trying to resolve the ethical dilemma at an organizational level (Magnavita, 2007).

SOLUTIONS AND RECOMMENDATIONS

All the aforementioned problems can be solved by collective commitment. Management, medical staff, safety technicians and workers must collaborate in addressing and solving the problems.

The aging workforce requires an increased engagement in work, to be productive and to work safely for a longer time. A high engagement is needed to reduce job stress and the appearance of symptoms. Clinical engagement is also necessary for a better clinical outcome in chronically ill workers. Occupational health physicians, psychologists, employers and employees must work together in workplace health promotion programs aiming at enhancing engagement, improving lifestyles, and diffusing best safety practices.

Presenteeism may need to be the subject of direct inquiry on the part of the physician and some suggestions have been put forward for managing this phenomenon in day-to-day practice (Sanderson & Cocker, 2013).

The issue of hazardous workers can be solved in a participatory way. While the protection of clients is undoubtedly the top ethical priority, compromising workers' rights could deter them from reporting diseases, undergoing medical testing, and/or seeking treatment. Each organization must develop a balanced, science-based analysis of the impaired worker issue and propose preventive measures in a written policy document. Policies concerning informed consent, non-compliance, confidentiality, the responsibility of workers, the disclosure of transmission risk to third parties, non-discrimination and counselling of infected or impaired workers need to be clarified. Costs and targets need to be stated, as do ways of recovering costs in order to ensure feasibility (Magnavita, 2004a).

The physician responsible for the medical surveillance of workers should judge on a case-by-case basis the employee's ability to safely carry out his/her work, in relation not only to that individual, but also to other employees and third parties (Magnavita et al., 2006; Magnavita et al., 2008; Magnavita et al., 2014; Riboldi, Carrer, Magnavita, & Porru, 2010).

The identification of hazardous workers is a critical issue. The doctor or the company cannot actively seek to identify them without violating privacy. However, waiting for a potential danger to manifest itself is not a viable prospect, as clearly shown by the countless tragedies caused by hazardous workers (see the last, but not least, Airbus A320 tragedy). Self-identification of hazardous workers is always the best choice. Workers must be given assurance that the right thing to do is to confidentially report their problem to those who can help them. Organizations must establish treatment options for hazardous workers. Work colleagues are those best placed to identify occupationally risky behavior or sub-standard performance. They are also the ones who can best provide help.

It is important to avoid putting blame on hazardous workers. It must be clear that the intention is not to find a culprit, but to improve health and safety at work. Anyone who identifies a hazardous condition has a duty to confront the colleague involved, face-to-face. The employee should be encouraged to seek help. If an employee who is sick or manifesting behavior problems does not intend to ask for help, the problem should be reported to a superior.

Illness must be treated. The worker is entitled to strict confidentiality about his/her condition. Organizations could temporarily modify their work programs to enable the employee to undergo a course of treatment. Bringing about changes in behavior requires a joint effort on the part of both the organization and the employee.

Occupational health methods, particularly the ASIA method © (Magnavita, 2004a), have proven to be effective in reducing the incidence of workplace violence in high-risk settings (Magnavita, 2009b; Magnavita, 2011).

Successful Ageing

Adequate health provision is needed to sustain work ability in an increasingly ageing population. Furthermore, an ageing working population would undoubtedly benefit from measures that could extend work ability, performance, and job satisfaction. Engagement has proven to increase all these dimensions.

Findings have revealed that older workers use a number of strategies to adapt to a change in resources, and that these strategies help them cope and maintain their activity in the workplace (Ng & Law, 2014). A recent study on older workers indicated that workplace job design (opportunities for decision-making, skill variety, coworker support, supervisor support) contributed to aspects of successful ageing (social network, emotional support, personal control, generativity). Skill variety and coworker support were the most important job design variables for successful ageing outcomes (Sanders & McCready, 2010).

A whole set of strategies must be implemented in the workplace for the successful ageing of workers. Rehabilitation experts should help workers with disabilities to overcome barriers to workplace participation and should work with clients to enhance employment outcomes (Johnson, Brown, & Knaster, 2010). Special equipment or workplace adjustments can be useful in assisting mature age workers with declining sensory ability (Crawford, Graveling, Cowie, & Dixon, 2010). Policies and human resource practices can counteract age discrimination. However, the most important issue concerns the task of educating people to accept longevity (Walker, 1999). Organizations must counteract age discrimination by using an integrated age management strategy that focuses on the prevention of workforce ageing, and also by adopting policies and human resource practices (the demand side of the labor market) that do not attempt merely to enhance the ability of older workers.

From Occupational Medicine to Occupational Health

Existing occupational health service strategies are unable to address current challenges in an adequate way. Traditional occupational medicine deals exclusively with environmental risk factors. Some countries, such as Italy, do not allow the doctor engaged by the employer to investigate the working capacity of employees.

The traditional task of occupational medicine i.e. diagnosing and treating occupational diseases, can be performed by a single person, acting alone. Nowadays the occupational physician often works alone. He/she examines workers, carries out laboratory tests and concludes his/her activity as if it were merely a question of dispensing healthcare services. However, it is clear that, without an epidemiological analysis of data obtained from medical examinations and, above all, without intervention in the workplace, there can be no prevention. We must remember that as early as 1700, Bernardino Ramazzini, the founder of occupational medicine, claimed that in order to change the work environment and control risk, physicians and workers (employers and employees) had to co-operate (Carnevale, Mendini, & Moriani, 2009).

This statement is even more valid if we consider that today most of the diseases that workers have do not originate from the work environment. In order to investigate the lifestyles and habits that increase risk, the occupational physician needs a broader mandate than that offered by traditional occupational medicine. Instead of looking for illness, he/she must seek health in its broadest sense. This means practicing occupational health rather than occupational medicine.

The old maxim that 'work affects health' must now be integrated by adding that 'health affects work'.

In occupational health, energy, vitality and well-being are considered to be essential elements of working life. These factors belong to the "salutogenesis" concept that focuses on the resources that help a person cope and are effective in avoiding or combating a range of psychosocial stressors (Antonovsky, 1979).

The different approaches of occupational medicine and occupational health, i.e. a biomedical risk-based approach focused on the individual versus a psychosocial approach focused on the working environment, are given varying degrees of importance by different countries or regions. The United States has a long tradition based both on workplace health promotion programs that focus on reducing individual health risks, and on extensive research into health and cost benefits (Aldana, 2001). Most European countries, especially those belonging to the Scandinavian area, have concentrated on analyzing the psychosocial factors of work (e.g. work organization, employee relations and work climate) and how these affect employee health.

Improved employee health can only be achieved in a sustainable manner by integrating all health-related services within an enterprise and by addressing psychosocial and organizational factors as well as individual health issues (Kirsten, 2010).

Of course the individual worker cannot be expected to succeed in adopting a healthier lifestyle without professional assistance. Advice from the occupational physician could be a first step, but it is not enough (Garbarino & Magnavita, 2014). The employee needs to take responsibility for his or her own health and should be repeatedly stimulated by the employer. Besides a good working environment, the employer, and society at large, should provide information, resources, and policies to enable the worker to change his/her behavior. Workers will usually welcome assistance and guidance for improving their lifestyles as they obtain direct benefit from this, also in their personal life (Magnavita, 2009a).

Extending the scope of work-related health activities and investigating non-occupational aspects of life can obviously create a number of problems. Personal employee data must be handled in a very sensitive way, otherwise it will be very difficult to engage employees and their representatives on such a personal issue. Employees are concerned about "giving away" personal health data if data privacy is not fully guaranteed and data properly communicated. This will remain a crucial challenge for workplace health professionals in the near future.

Another important issue is the need for highly coordinated activities. Health management involves data collection and delivery of services in a number of different company departments. The occupational health service, the prevention and safety service, human resources, auditing and control, and worker and manager training departments must all work together in a coordinated framework. The so-called "A.S.I.A. method" ©, i.e. a systematic sequence of assessment, surveillance, information, and auditing (Bevilacqua, Sacco, & Magnavita, 2003; Magnavita, 2004a) can present a considerable challenge for employers, especially in company corporations where many different offices and professionals are dealing with health-related issues.

The challenge for occupational health services dealing with an ageing workforce calls for innovation in (i) health promotion, (ii) the prevention of work-related and occupational diseases, (iii) a reduction in work impairment due to illness, (iv) better support for disabled workers and (v) the promotion of work ability.

New schemes are needed for health promotion: sustainable lifestyle changes are still the main goal but the workforce is increasingly polarized. Many workers do more physical activity, have stopped smoking and eat more healthily than before, but at the same time many still fail to adopt a healthier lifestyle. Musculoskeletal and psychosocial disorders (especially the latter) are the most prevalent cause of work disability among older workers, and the incidence of occupational diseases tends to become linear with age. Chronic symptoms and diseases often impair ability to work and a worker returning to his/her job after a prolonged absence is often confronted with work tasks and working conditions that have remained unchanged. Frequently the sick person is treated, but the reasons underlying the inability to work are ignored and go unaddressed.

A comprehensive solution for the ageing challenge at enterprise level is the promotion of work ability among the ageing workforce (Ilmarinen & Rantanen, 1999). This concept focuses on both human resources and working conditions. The essential components of human resources include health, physical and mental capacity and social functioning, competencies, attitudes and values. Principal work elements cover the contents and demands of work, the physical, ergonomic and psychosocial work environment, as well as management and leadership issues. Work ability is also linked to the microenvironment outside the workplace (family, relatives, friends, etc.) as well as to the macro-environment (infrastructure, services and other societal aspects) (Tuomi, Huuhtanen, Nykyri, & Ilmarinen, 2001). Currently, the fundamental concept underlying work ability is a balance between human resources and work. Because the employee is mainly responsible for his resources and the employer for work, good work ability can be achieved only by better cooperation between the supervisor and the employee. Integrating a series of actions that focus simultaneously on human resources and work, increasing occupational engagement, brings about an improvement in worker wellbeing and the quality of life as well as productivity and the quality of work: a win/win result for the employee and employer. The effects of engagement and work ability promotion can also be seen subsequently, in the third age: the health and life quality of retired persons are better than those who have not participated in work ability promotion.

Today's challenge arises from the fact that human resources are changing on account of ageing, while, at the same time, globalization and new technology are changing work. To achieve a balance that leads to good work ability, there must be a dynamic process of continual change during the course of a working career, continuously maintaining a high engagement. Occupational health and safety experts and other intermediary organizations also have an important role to play. Clearly, better coordination and cooperation between the different players who influence work ability and the balance within it, are urgently needed.

Health Promotion in the Workplace

Employers around the world are currently implementing and evaluating strategic wellness and health promotion initiatives in order to improve employee health and morale, control costs, and enhance workforce productivity and performance.

However, what is still lacking in general terms are successful health promotion programs and studies indicating how productivity can be increased through comprehensive and sustainable intervention. Innovative programs that aim at achieving good health for employees alongside increased productivity include two main features:

1. An integrated health management approach that breaks down existing barriers;
2. A holistic approach that addresses psychosocial factors as well as individual health issues (Kirsten, 2010).

The concept of presenteeism, linking employee health to productivity, demonstrates the need to improve the health of employees and provide good working conditions so that these enhancements can increase morale, motivation and performance. This can only be achieved on a sustainable basis by means of an integrated participatory health management approach. There is preliminary evidence that some WHP programs can have a positive effect on presenteeism (Cancelliere, Cassidy, Ammendolia, & Côté, 2011). Knowledge translation, i.e. the exchange, synthesis, and ethically-sound application of knowledge, through a dynamic and interactive system of interactions among researchers and users, has been effective in rapidly capturing the benefits of research, through improved health, more effective services and products, and a strengthened health care system in health care settings (Westergren, 2012).

A potential strategy for reducing presenteeism and improving the mental health of employees is physical activity. Some findings have demonstrated a positive association between physical activity and the psychosocial health of employees, particularly with regard to the quality of life and emotional wellbeing. However, findings are inconclusive as to the role of physical activity in promoting workplace wellbeing (Brown, Gilson, Burton, & Brown, 2011).

One of the most important principles in workplace health management is that of addressing the health of all employees, and not just the wellbeing of the sick and disabled ones. Unfortunately, most employers still focus only on the employees who are on sick leave or have short- or long-term disability so as to re-integrate them into the work process or fire them and substitute them with another, healthy subject. This attitude overlooks the fact that low-risk employees might move into the medium- or high-risk categories, so that eventually there are more high-risk workers than subjects with reduced risk. This logic stems from the prevailing belief that health means the absence of disease.

The aim of health management is to measurably improve total health (including productivity and performance) and reduce health-related costs. In fact modern OH services began to implement health promotion systems in the workplace many years ago (Magnavita, 1993; Magnavita, Sacco, & De Lorenzo 1993). This approach seems to be the mission of occupational health in the 21st century (Magnavita, De Lorenzo, & Sacco, 2014).

Participatory Ergonomics

Participatory ergonomics can be defined as "the involvement of people in planning and controlling a significant amount of their own activities, with sufficient knowledge and power to influence both process and outcomes to achieve desirable goals" (Wilson, 1995). Emerging research has shown that co-workers have a significant influence on the return-to-work outcomes of partially fit ill or injured employees. To achieve optimal outcomes, co-workers need to perceive the arrangements as fair. Perceptions of fairness might be supported by co-workers' collaborative engagement in the planning, monitoring and review of work reintegration activities (Dunstan & Maceachen, 2014). Participatory ergonomics can also indicate solutions to problems that endanger worker's health and safety. Participatory ergonomic techniques (the so-called "Gruppi di ergonomia partecipativa, GEP ©" have been used in the workplace in Italy since the early '90s and are yielding encouraging results (Bevilacqua & Magnavita, 2008, Bevilacqua et al., 2007a; Bevilacqua et al., 2007b; Magnavita et al., 2007).

Participatory improvement methods, like all actions in which human resources are the key factor, require the continual strengthening of worker motivation. Emphasis must be given to the positive results obtained and these must be made known to other workers who did not take part in the process so that they are encouraged to subscribe to the idea underlying this method: i.e. work can be improved, and it is the task of the worker to do it. On the basis of this concept, a review of the results obtained during participatory ergonomics should be the subject of seminars in a context of on-going occupational training. As stated previously, training is crucial in participatory ergonomics: "The essence of a participatory ergonomic process is learning" (Kuorinka, 1997). Workers must learn to communicate their occupational experiences to others and put forward suggestions for improvements, regardless of their varying occupational roles. Improvements in the workplace stem from indications provided by workers, and validated by the same.

The participatory process does not always follow a linear course; setbacks may often be encountered due to a lack of economic resources, but mainly because of inadequate managerial and political skills that are always essential in forwarding new projects. However, in the long term, participatory management has so many advantages compared to traditional top-down approaches that it becomes part of a process of natural selection. Time is an essential aspect of ergonomics and health promotion activity. Timely interventions achieve the best results at a lower cost.

One of the fields in which participatory ergonomics achieves the best results, especially with older workers, is management of musculoskeletal disorders. Musculoskeletal disorders (MSDs) are the principal cause of sick leave and the most frequent cause of impaired work capacity (Buckle, 2005). More and more efforts have been made in recent years to investigate the causes of MSDs and take steps to prevent them. MSDs are considered to be multifactorial: the findings of scientific research have identified physical (Winkel, & Mathiassen, 1994), psychosocial/ organizational (Theorell, Harms-Ringdahl,

Ahlberg-Hultén, & Westin, 1991), and individual (Armstrong et al., 1993) occupational risk factors for the development of work-related MSDs.

MSDs are strongly related to occupational organizational factors, such as worker dispatch system, job insecurity, use of irregular workers, and work intensification (Kang et al., 2014).

The literature shows that the traditional approach to MSD management in the workplace is inadequate. No clear evidence has emerged to demonstrate the efficacy of any type of intervention aimed at preventing MSDs among employees (Dawson et al., 2007). This includes training in manual handling (the commonest form of intervention proposed), which has not been effective in healthcare workers (Hignett, 2003) or in other categories of workers (Tveito, Hysing, & Eriksen, 2004), since it fails to reduce sick leave, the frequency of bouts of pain, the level of pain or the costs. Furthermore, controversy remains over the efficacy of programs in which training is accompanied by the use of handling devices, and there is conflicting evidence regarding the efficacy of exercise intervention (Dawson et al., 2007). Although numerous research studies have confirmed the importance of psychosocial factors, there is insufficient evidence of a positive association between stress at work and MSDs (Hartvigsen, Lings, Leboeuf-Yde, & Bakketeig, 2004), and stress control programs have not been effective in reducing the incidence rate of MSDs (Dawson et al., 2007). Recent reviews provide limited evidence that only multidimensional intervention (Dawson et al., 2007) and programs that include treatment of workers affected by MSDs (Tveito et al. 2004) have a positive effect. However, positive results have often been obtained both in industry (Laing et al. 2007; Udo & Yoshinaga, 2001; Werner, Laerum, Wormgoor, Lindh, & Indahl, 2007; Kogi, 2006) and in health care (Udo, Kobayashi, Udo, & Branlund, 2006; Hignett, 2001; Pojonen, Punakallio, & Louhevaara, 1998) by multidisciplinary programs that adopt a participatory approach. A systematic review of the literature has found partial evidence that participatory ergonomic intervention has a positive impact on MSDs since it reduces musculoskeletal symptoms, injuries, lost workdays and compensation claims (Rivilis et al., 2008).

It has been shown that a significant effect on absence from work due to MSDs is linked to a mistaken or negative conception of the etiologic role of work, often promoted by physicians themselves (Werner, Ihlebaek, Skouen, & Laerum, 2005). The idea that MSD is a medical condition similar to an injury is counterproductive as the worker becomes a patient engaged in finding a body lesion that does not exist, is not connected with his symptoms, or that does not need treatment. Participatory groups can effectively and pervasively combat this attitude by spreading the message that active intervention at work or greater control over ergonomic factors on the part of the worker can aid recovery. Furthermore, the work climate and interaction between employers and employees ("industrial relations") have a significant impact on the length of sick leave. Perceived inequalities and poor social support (inefficient communications, unsatisfactory relations, and a non-supportive work environment) are significant risk factors in the onset of MSD (Woods, 2005). Satisfaction resulting from the way the employer responds to a worker's needs becomes a significant return-to-work factor after an acute bout of MSD (Butler, Johnson, & Coté, 2007). This is another reason for encouraging the development of participatory intervention.

Since it has been demonstrated that misconceptions and negative beliefs about musculoskeletal pain precede sickness behavior (Woby, Watson, Roach, & Urmston, 2004) and hinder recovery, the prime objective should be to create a positive and active attitude to the problem and increase peer support. There is strong evidence that traditional biomechanical training based on the industrial accident model fails to diminish the incidence rate of backache or absence from work, and that, on the contrary, it is advantageous to carry on normal activities in spite of back pain (Waddel & Burton, 2001). However, it is not easy to bring about an immediate change of direction in workers whose negative attitudes are deep-rooted and often supported by physicians ill-informed on contemporary evidence-based guidelines. Prime importance should be given to training a small group of highly experienced workers and workers' representatives to become "health promoters" with the task of reassuring colleagues with MSDs and helping them find ergonomic solutions and temporary improvements in their occupational activity. These workers must receive on-going training, be given leaflets with appropriate information and instructions and must keep in touch with the physician responsible for the medical surveillance of workers so that they can provide him/her with constant feedback on the workplace.

Workers must take part in meetings where they can be informed about the principal causes of occupational MSDs, how to prevent them and possible ergonomic intervention. These meetings must put a definite emphasis on concrete problems and practical solutions, so that workers are trained to put forward autonomous proposals for work improvements.

Participatory ergonomic interventions of this kind have been implemented in Italy and have yielded successful results (Magnavita, 2009b). Whenever the onset of MSDs seemed to indicate the presence of ergonomic problems, small participatory groups were set up to study the problem and try to find a solution. These groups were not always formed in the same way; in fact their size varied according to the number of workers involved in the problem and the complexity of the question itself. The common feature was that the workers who regularly performed the task in question were involved in the process of change together with all the stakeholders who could have potentially been affected by the ergonomic intervention. In each homogeneous workplace, the group was usually formed of workers trained as health promoters and the worker or workers who manifested signs of MSD. In a small team set up to deal with ergonomic problems, the physician is always the central figure. The physician has a facilitating role, and is a leader rather than an actor. He supervises the group activity without interfering in the decision-making process and without choosing the subjects to be discussed.

The first step in participatory group work usually consists in identifying the problem. This is achieved through self-confrontation, i.e. by encouraging the worker to give a detailed description of his job. By describing his job, the worker makes a transition from concrete to abstract, thus gaining a deeper knowledge of his work. This technique is preferable to more complex ergonomic analyses that might prove difficult to apply in a participatory group. Describing work and comparing it with other workers who share the same occupational tasks also offers an opportunity for developing group dynamics. Teamwork encourages workers to subsequently suggest ways of correcting tools or work organization that may result in the reduction or solution of ergonomic problems.

Finding solutions based on the everyday experience of members of the participatory group and, to a lesser extent, the judgment of the physician, is a crucial step. The small participatory groups usually concentrate on finding practical, simple and economic solutions. In a system with limited and diminishing resources, preference should be given to low-cost solutions that can often be implemented immediately.

Solutions to ergonomic problems must be practical and viable, but also applicable in other situations and therefore generalizable. The group cannot impose these solutions, but it can suggest them to the management who will examine their feasibility and costs and decide on whether to implement them.

A randomized controlled trial intervention, aiming at maximizing work engagement and reducing work limitation, is currently in progress in USA. Volunteer employees are attending facilitated group workshop sessions to explore methods for improving comfort, adjusting work habits, communicating needs effectively, applying systematic problem solving, and dealing with negative thoughts and emotions about work (Shaw et al, 2014). Another intervention project to develop an organization-wide approach to employee workplace health through enhanced engagement has been proposed in Canada (Seymour & Dupré, 2008).

Changing the Mindset of Medicine

Change is also needed in the mindset of general medicine as the mere diagnosis and treatment of diseases is no longer sufficient. The patient must remain active for as long as possible, and this means connecting medical intervention that takes place in the health care unit with medical surveillance in the workplace. The occupational physician, the management and the person in charge of preventive services in the workplace must receive guidance on reorganizing the workplace so that it can accommodate the sick worker. This means that the traditional "letter" dispatched from the hospital to the general practitioner must become a letter to the company with all the advice needed for a full recovery. An experiment of this kind is in place at the A. Gemelli General Hospital of the Università Cattolica del Sacro Cuore, Rome. The occupational physician and a hospital department specialist collaborate to prepare a letter for the physician who is in charge of the sick worker in the company. This letter contains recommendations on the measures to be adopted in the workplace in order to promote the gradual reintegration of the sick worker in productive activities and an early recovery of working capacity.

FUTURE RESEARCH DIRECTIONS

Research in workplaces should support activities that provide workers with effective assistance for improving their work life and keeping healthy and fit. Studies should take into consideration selective longitudinal health profiling, employment prerequisites, and socio-economic and psychological scales that could indicate health measures significantly associated with work sustainability. Probably only the combination of individual, environmental and work organization interventions will ensure the success of programs to increase employee engagement. Best health practices could be used by workers at an early stage in their working life so as to sustain and improve work ability at a mature age (Vatsalya & Karch, 2013).

In order to transform an occupational environment and organize work in a way that facilitates recovery of the sick worker, or increase the productivity and satisfaction of the healthy one, all the stakeholders (management, health and safety staff, workers) must participate. Employees usually have a profound understanding of the ways in which work can be organized and adapted to accommodate the worker. The occupational physician can stimulate this process by creating groups of participatory ergonomics.

CONCLUSION

Transformations in society call for a change in both occupational and general medicine methods. These two disciplines must cooperate in their approach to health in the workplace and in general life. Patient and worker engagement, participatory medicine and participatory ergonomics, are the milestones of future health and safety. All members of society are entitled to attain high levels of wellbeing. In order to achieve this aim, all social partners (employers and employees) must engage fully in health promotion.

REFERENCES

Admasachew, L., & Dawson, J. (2011). The association between presenteeism and engagement of National Health Service staff. *Journal of Health Services Research & Policy*, *16*(Suppl. 1), 29–33. doi:10.1258/jhsrp.2010.010085 PMID:21460347

Airila, A., Hakanen, J., Punakallio, A., Lusa, S., & Luukkonen, R. (2012). Is work engagement related to work ability beyond working conditions and lifestyle factors? *International Archives of Occupational and Environmental Health*, *85*(8), 915–925. doi:10.1007/s00420-012-0732-1 PMID:22270385

Aldana, S. (2001). Financial impact of health promotion programs: A comprehensive review of the literature. *American Journal of Health Promotion*, *15*(5), 296–320. doi:10.4278/0890-1171-15.5.296 PMID:11502012

Antonovsky, A. (1979). *Health, Stress and Coping*. San Francisco: Jossey-Bass Publishers.

Armstrong, T. J., Buckle, P., Fine, L. J., Hagberg, M., Jonsson, B., & Kilbom, A. et al. (1993). A conceptual model for work-related neck and upper-limb musculoskeletal disorders. *Scandinavian Journal of Work, Environment & Health*, *19*(2), 73–84. doi:10.5271/sjweh.1494 PMID:8316782

Barber, L., Grawitch, M. J., & Munz, D. C. (2013). Are better sleepers more engaged workers? A self-regulatory approach to sleep hygiene and work engagement. *Stress and Health*, *29*(4), 307–316. doi:10.1002/smi.2468 PMID:23086901

Bevilacqua, L., Del Piano, A., De Matteis, B., Luciani, E., Magnavita, L., & Mammi, F. et al. (2007a). The participatory approach to injury prevention appeared to be an useful tool of safety education and ergonomic improvement. *Giornale Italiano di Medicina del Lavoro Ed Ergonomia*, *29*(3), 560–561. PMID:18409831

Bevilacqua, L., & Magnavita, N. (2008). Quality improvement of risk assessment procedures in maritime work. *Giornale Italiano di Medicina del Lavoro Ed Ergonomia*, *30*(Suppl. 2), 447–449.

Bevilacqua, L., Magnavita, N., Becchetti, G., Mammi, F., Roccia, K., & Pupp, N. (2007b). Participatory risk evaluation. The role of the surveillance. *Giornale Italiano di Medicina del Lavoro Ed Ergonomia*, *29*(3), 657–658. PMID:18409891

Bevilacqua, L., Sacco, A., & Magnavita, N. (2003). Health surveillance audit of wood dust exposure. *La Medicina del Lavoro*, *94*, 224–230. PMID:12852205

Biddison, E. L. D., Paine, L., Murakami, P., Herzke, C., & Weaver, S. J. (2015). Associations between safety culture and employee engagement over time: a retrospective analysis. *BMJ quality & safety*. doi:10.1136/bmjqs-2014-003910

Brown, H. E., Gilson, N. D., Burton, N. W., & Brown, W. J. (2011). Does physical activity impact on presenteeism and other indicators of workplace well-being? *Sports Medicine (Auckland, N.Z.)*, *41*(3), 249–262. doi:10.2165/11539180-000000000-00000 PMID:21395366

Brunetto, Y., Xerri, M., Shriberg, A., Farr-Wharton, R., Shacklock, K., Newman, S., & Dienger, J. (2013). The impact of workplace relationships on engagement, well-being, commitment and turnover for nurses in Australia and the USA. *Journal of Advanced Nursing*, *69*(12), 278627–278699. doi:10.1111/jan.12165 PMID:23651183

Buckle, P. (2005). Ergonomics and musculoskeletal disorders: An overview. *Occupational Medicine*, *55*(3), 164–167. doi:10.1093/occmed/kqi081 PMID:15857895

Butler, R. J., Johnson, W. G., & Coté, P. (2007). It pays to be nice: Employer-worker relationships and the management of back pain claims. *Journal of Occupational and Environmental Medicine*, *49*, 214–225. doi:10.1097/jom.0b013e318032211d PMID:17293761

Cancelliere, C., Cassidy, J. D., Ammendolia, C., & Côté, P. (2011). Are workplace health promotion programs effective at improving presenteeism in workers? A systematic review and best evidence synthesis of the literature. *BMC Public Health*, *11*, 395. doi:10.1186/1471-2458-11-395 PMID:21615940

Carnevale, F., Mendini, M., & Moriani, G. (Eds.). (2009). Bernardino Ramazzini. Works. Verona: Cierre Edizioni. CDC- Centers for Disease Control and Prevention. (1993). Investigations of persons treated by HIV-infected-health care workers. Morbility Mortality Weekly Report, 42, 329–331.

Cocker, F., Martin, A., Scott, J., Venn, A., Otahal, P., & Sanderson, K. (2011). Factors associated with presenteeism among employed Australian adults reporting lifetime major depression with 12-month symptoms. *Journal of Affective Disorders*, *135*(1-3), 231–240. doi:10.1016/j.jad.2011.07.028 PMID:21880374

Coffeng, J. K., Hendriksen, I. J., Duijts, S. F., Twisk, J. W., van Mechelen, W., & Boot, C. R. (2014). Effectiveness of a combined social and physical environmental intervention on presenteeism, absenteeism, work performance, and work engagement in office employees. *Journal of Occupational and Environmental Medicine*, *56*(3), 258–265. doi:10.1097/JOM.0000000000000116 PMID:24603201

Collins, J., Baase, C., Shardra, C., Ozminkowski, R. J., Nicholson, S., & Billotti, G. M. et al. (2005). The assessment of chronic health conditions of work performance, absence, and total economic impact for employers. *Journal of Occupational and Environmental Medicine*, *47*(6), 547–557. doi:10.1097/01.jom.0000166864.58664.29 PMID:15951714

Crawford, E. R., Lepine, J. A., & Rich, B. L. (2010). Linking job demands and resources to employee engagement and burnout: A theoretical extension and meta-analytic test. *The Journal of Applied Psychology*, *95*(5), 834–848. doi:10.1037/a0019364 PMID:20836586

Crawford, J. O., Graveling, R. A., Cowie, H. A., & Dixon, K. (2010). The health safety and health promotion needs of older workers. *Occupational Medicine*, *60*(3), 184–192. doi:10.1093/occmed/kqq028 PMID:20423949

Dawson, A. P., McLennan, S. N., Schiller, S. D., Jull, G. A., Hodges, P. W., & Stewart, S. (2007). Interventions to prevent back pain and back injury in nurses: A systematic review. *Occupational and Environmental Medicine*, *64*(10), 642–650. doi:10.1136/oem.2006.030643 PMID:17522134

DiBonaventura, M., Paulose-Ram, R., Su, J., McDonald, M., Zou, K. H., Wagner, J. S., & Shah, H. (2012). The impact of COPD on quality of life, productivity loss, and resource use among the elderly United States workforce. *Chronic Obstructive Pulmonary Disease.*, *9*(1), 46–57. doi:10.3109/15412555.2011.634863 PMID:22292597

DiBonaventura, M. C., Gupta, S., McDonald, M., & Sadosky, A. (2011). Evaluating the health and economic impact of osteoarthritis pain in the workforce: Results from the National Health and Wellness Survey. *BMC Musculoskeletal Disorders*, *12*(1), 83. doi:10.1186/1471-2474-12-83 PMID:21527024

Dunstan, D. A., & Maceachen, E. (2014). A theoretical model of co-worker responses to work reintegration processes. *Journal of Occupational Rehabilitation*, *24*(2), 189–198. doi:10.1007/s10926-013-9461-x PMID:23912179

European Commission. (2014). *The 2015 Ageing Report. Underlying Assumptions and Projection Methodologies*. Retrieved from http://ec.europa.eu/economy_finance/publications/european_economy/2014/pdf/ee8_en.pdf

Ferrie, J. E., Virtanen, M., & Kivimaki, M. (2014). The healthy population-high disability paradox. *Occupational and Environmental Medicine*, *71*(4), 232–233. doi:10.1136/oemed-2013-101945 PMID:24492070

Garbarino, S., & Magnavita, N. (2014). Obstructive sleep apnea syndrome (OSAS), metabolic syndrome and mental health in small enterprise workers. Feasibility of an action for health. *PLoS ONE*, *9*(5), e97188. doi:10.1371/journal.pone.0097188 PMID:24810290

Gifford, B., & Jinnett, K. (2014). Employees' work responses to episodes of illness: Evidence from the American time use survey. *Journal of Occupational and Environmental Medicine*, *56*(2), 224–229. doi:10.1097/JOM.0000000000000090 PMID:24504249

Graffigna, G., Barello, S., & Triberti, S. (Eds.). (2015). *Patient Engagement. A Consumer-Centered Model to Innovate Healthcare*. Warsaw, Berlin: De Gruyter Open Ltd. doi:10.1515/9783110452440

Hakanen, J., & Peeters, M. (2015). How Do Work Engagement, Workaholism, and the Work-to-Family Interface Affect Each Other? A 7-Year Follow-Up Study. *Journal of Occupational and Environmental Medicine*, *57*(6), 601–609. doi:10.1097/JOM.0000000000000457 PMID:26053362

Hartvigsen, J., Lings, S., Leboeuf-Yde, C., & Bakketeig, L. (2004). Psychosocial factors at work in relation to low back pain and consequences of low back pain; a systematic, critical review of prospective cohort studies. *Occupational and Environmental Medicine*, *61*(1), e2. PMID:14691283

Hignett, S. (2001). Embedding ergonomics in hospital culture: Top-down and bottom-up strategies. *Applied Ergonomics*, *32*(1), 61–69. doi:10.1016/S0003-6870(00)00029-6 PMID:11209833

Hignett, S. (2003). Intervention strategies to reduce musculoskeletal injuries associated with handling patients: A systematic review. *Occupational and Environmental Medicine*, *60*(9), e6. doi:10.1136/oem.60.9.e6 PMID:12937202

Ilmarinen, J., & Rantanen, J. (1999). Promotion of work ability during ageing. *American Journal of Industrial Medicine*, *36*(Suppl. 1), 21–23. doi:10.1002/(SICI)1097-0274(199909)36:1+<21::AID-AJIM8>3.0.CO;2-S PMID:10519773

Inoue, A., Kawakami, N., Ishizaki, M., Shimazu, A., Tsuchiya, M., & Tabata, M. et al. (2010). Organizational justice, psychological distress, and work engagement in Japanese workers. *International Archives of Occupational and Environmental Health, 83*(1), 29–38. doi:10.1007/s00420-009-0485-7 PMID:19904552

Inoue, A., Kawakami, N., Tsuno, K., Shimazu, A., Tomioka, K., & Nakanishi, M. (2013). Job demands, job resources, and work engagement of Japanese employees: A prospective cohort study. *International Archives of Occupational and Environmental Health, 86*(4), 441–449. doi:10.1007/s00420-012-0777-1 PMID:22562520

Johnson, K. L., Brown, P. A., & Knaster, E. S. (2010). Aging with disability in the workplace. *Physical Medicine and Rehabilitation Clinics of North America, 21*(2), 267–279. doi:10.1016/j.pmr.2009.12.004 PMID:20494276

Kang, D., Kim, Y., Lee, Y. I., Koh, S., Kim, I., & Lee, H. (2014). Work-related Musculoskeletal Disorders in Korea Provoked by Workers' Collective Compensation Claims against Work Intensification. *Annals of Occupational and Environmental Medicine, 26*(1), 19. doi:10.1186/2052-4374-26-19 PMID:25089205

Karanika-Murray, M., Pontes, H. M., Griffiths, M. D., & Biron, C. (2015). Sickness presenteeism determines job satisfaction via affective-motivational states. *Social Science & Medicine, 139*, 100–106. doi:10.1016/j.socscimed.2015.06.035 PMID:26183017

Kirkham, H. S., Clark, B. L., Bolas, C. A., Lewis, G. H., Jackson, A. S., Fisher, D., & Duncan, I. (2015). Which modifiable health risks are associated with changes in productivity costs? *Population Health Management, 18*(1), 30–38. doi:10.1089/pop.2014.0033 PMID:25375893

Kirsten, W. (2010). Making the link between health and productivity at the workplace--a global perspective. *Industrial Health, 48*(3), 251–255. doi:10.2486/indhealth.48.251 PMID:20562499

Kivimaki, M., Head, J., Ferrie, J. E., Hemingway, H., Shipley, M. J., Vahtera, J., & Marmot, M. G. (2005). Working while ill as a risk factor for serious coronary events: The Whitehall II Study. *American Journal of Public Health, 95*(1), 98–100. doi:10.2105/AJPH.2003.035873 PMID:15623867

Kogi, K. (2006). Participatory methods effective for ergonomic workplace improvement. *Applied Ergonomics, 37*(4), 547–554. doi:10.1016/j.apergo.2006.04.013 PMID:16756940

Kuorinka, I. (1997). Tools and means of implementing participatory ergonomics. *International Journal of Industrial Ergonomics, 19*(4), 267–270. doi:10.1016/S0169-8141(96)00035-2

Laing, A. C., Cole, D. C., Theberge, N., Wells, R. P., Kerr, M. S., & Frazer, M. B. (2007). Effectiveness of a participatory ergonomics intervention in improving communication and psychosocial exposures. *Ergonomics, 50*(7), 1092–1109. doi:10.1080/00140130701308708 PMID:17510824

Leijten, F. R., van den Heuvel, S. G., van der Beek, A. J., Ybema, J. F., Robroek, S. J., & Burdorf, A. (2015). Associations of work-related factors and work engagement with mental and physical health: A 1-year follow-up study among older workers. *Journal of Occupational Rehabilitation, 25*(1), 86–95. doi:10.1007/s10926-014-9525-6 PMID:24928413

Lisbon Special European Council. (2000, March). Towards a Europe of Innovation and Knowledge. Retrieved from: http://eur-lex.europa.eu/legal-content/EN/TXT/?uri=uriserv:c10241

Magnavita, N. (1993). Workplace action for health. Prevention of obesity and hyperlipaemia in a small company. *Paper presented at the International Conference "Work & Health"*, Copenhagen, Denmark.

Magnavita, N. (2004a). Applicazione di modelli organizzativi originali per la prevenzione del rischio chimico in aziende di diverse dimensioni. Metodo A.S.I.A. Roma: IIMS Istituto Italiano di Medicina Sociale. Retrieved from http://www.puntosicuro.info/documenti/documenti/111201_sirsrer_rischio_chimico.pdf

Magnavita, N. (2004b). *Tutela del lavoratore rischioso per gli altri*. Milano: ISU Università Cattolica del Sacro Cuore.

Magnavita, N. (2006). Management of impaired physicians in Europe. *La Medicina del Lavoro*, *97*(6), 762–773. PMID:17219765

Magnavita, N. (2007). The unhealthy physician. *Journal of Medical Ethics*, *33*(4), 210–214. doi:10.1136/jme.2006.017533 PMID:17400618

Magnavita, N. (2009a). *Lavoro umano. Il benessere nei luoghi di lavoro*. Milano: EDUCatt.

Magnavita, N. (2009b). Experience of prevention activities in local health units. Assaults and musculoskeletal disorders. *La Medicina del Lavoro*, *100*(Suppl. 1), 24–28. PMID:19848097

Magnavita, N. (2011). Violence prevention in a small-scale psychiatric unit: Program planning and evaluation. *International Journal of Occupational and Environmental Health*, *17*(4), 336–344. doi:10.1179/oeh.2011.17.4.336 PMID:22069932

Magnavita, N. (2012). Validation of the Italian version of the HSE Indicator Tool. *Occupational Medicine*, *62*(4), 288–294. doi:10.1093/occmed/kqs025 PMID:22661665

Magnavita, N., Bergamaschi, A., Chiarotti, M., Colombi, A., Deidda, B., & De Lorenzo, G. et al. (2008). Workers with alcohol and drug addiction problems. Consensus Document of the Study Group on Hazardous Workers. *La Medicina del Lavoro*, *99*(Suppl. 2), 3–58. PMID:19248471

Magnavita, N., Castorina, S., Ciavarella, M., Mammi, F., Roccia, K., & Saffioti, C. (2007). Participative approach to the in hospital management of muscoloskeletal disorders. *Giornale Italiano di Medicina del Lavoro Ed Ergonomia*, *29*(3), 561–563. PMID:18409832

Magnavita, N., Cicerone, M., Cirese, V., De Lorenzo, G., Di Giannantonio, M., & Fileni, A. et al. (2006). Critical aspects of the management of "hazardous" health care workers. Consensus Document. *La Medicina del Lavoro*, *97*(5), 715–725. PMID:17171984

Magnavita, N., De Lorenzo, G., Gallo, M., Garbarino, S., Goggiamani, A., & Janiri, L. et al. (2014). Alcohol and work. Consensus Document of the La. R.A. group. *La Medicina del Lavoro*, *105*(Suppl. 1), 3–68. PMID:25488525

Magnavita, N., De Lorenzo, G., & Sacco, A. (2014). Health promotion in the workplace. *La Medicina del Lavoro*, *105*(6), 473–474. PMID:25431984

Magnavita, N., Sacco, A., & De Lorenzo, G. (1993). Hypertension and hypercholesterolemia prevention in lead-exposed workers. *Paper presented at the International Conference "Work & Health"*, Copenhagen, Denmark.

Merrill, R. M., Aldana, S. G., Pope, J. E., Anderson, D. R., Coberley, C. R., Grossmeier, J. J., ... & HERO, R. S. S. (2013). Self-rated job performance and absenteeism according to employee engagement, health behaviors, and physical health. *Journal of occupational and environmental medicine/American College of Occupational and Environmental Medicine, 55*(1), 10-8. doi:10.1097/JOM.0b013e31827b73af

Munir, F., Houdmont, J., Clemes, S., Wilson, K., Kerr, R., & Addley, K. (2015). Work engagement and its association with occupational sitting time: Results from the Stormont study. *BMC Public Health, 15*(1), 30. doi:10.1186/s12889-015-1427-9 PMID:25631579

Nahrgang, J. D., Morgeson, F. P., & Hofmann, D. A. (2011). Safety at work: A meta-analytic investigation of the link between job demands, job resources, burnout, engagement, and safety outcomes. *The Journal of Applied Psychology, 96*(1), 71–94. doi:10.1037/a0021484 PMID:21171732

Ng, E. S., & Law, A. (2014). Keeping up! Older workers' adaptation in the workplace after age 55. *Canadian Journal on Aging, 33*(1), 1–14. doi:10.1017/S0714980813000639 PMID:24345532

Oude Hengel, K. M., Blatter, B. M., Joling, C. I., van der Beek, A. J., & Bongers, P. M. (2012). Effectiveness of an intervention at construction worksites on work engagement, social support, physical workload, and need for recovery: Results from a cluster randomized controlled trial. *BMC Public Health, 12*, 1008. doi:10.1186/1471-2458-12-1008 PMID:23171354

Paoli, P., & Merllie, D. (2001). *Third European Working Conditions Survey 2000*. European foundation for the improvement of Living and Working Conditions, Office for official publications of the European Communities, Luxemburg. Retrieved from http://www.eurofound.eu.int/publications/EF0121.htm

Pohjonen, T., Punakallio, A., & Louhevaara, V. (1998). Participatory ergonomics for reducing load and strain in home care work. *International Journal of Industrial Ergonomics, 21*(5), 345–352. doi:10.1016/S0169-8141(96)00083-2

Ravalier, J. M., Dandil, Y., & Limehouse, H. (2015). Employee engagement and management standards: A concurrent evaluation. *Occupational Medicine, 65*(6), 496–498. doi:10.1093/occmed/kqv071 PMID:26078417

Reday-Mulvey, G. (2005). *Working Beyond 60. Key Policies and Practices in Europe*. Great Britain: Palgrave Macmillan. doi:10.1057/9780230504981

Riboldi, L., Carrer, P., Magnavita, N., & Porru, S. (2010). Biological risk. Relevant problems: Risk to third parties. *Giornale Italiano di Medicina del Lavoro Ed Ergonomia, 32*(3), 304–311. PMID:21061714

Rivilis, I., Van Eerd, D., Cullen, K., Cole, D. C., Irvin, E., Tyson, J., & Mahood, Q. (2008). Effectiveness of participatory ergonomic interventions on health outcomes: A systematic review. *Applied Ergonomics, 39*(3), 342–358. doi:10.1016/j.apergo.2007.08.006 PMID:17988646

Rongen, A., Robroek, S. J., Schaufeli, W., & Burdorf, A. (2014). The contribution of work engagement to self-perceived health, work ability, and sickness absence beyond health behaviors and work-related factors. *Journal of Occupational and Environmental Medicine, 56*(8), 892–897. doi:10.1097/JOM.0000000000000196 PMID:25099418

Rost, K. M., Meng, H., & Xu, S. (2014). Work productivity loss from depression: Evidence from an employer survey. *BMC Health Services Research*, *14*(1), 597. doi:10.1186/s12913-014-0597-y PMID:25519705

Sanders, M. J., & McCready, J. W. (2010). Does work contribute to successful aging outcomes in older workers? *International Journal of Aging & Human Development*, *71*(3), 209–229. doi:10.2190/AG.71.3.c PMID:21166334

Sanderson, K., & Cocker, F. (2013). Presenteeism--implications and health risks. *Australian Family Physician*, *42*(4), 172–175. PMID:23550237

Seitsamo, J., & Klockars, M. (1997). Aging and changes in health. *Scandinavian Journal of Work, Environment & Health*, *23*(Suppl. 1), 27–35. PMID:9247993

Seymour, A., & Dupré, K. (2008). Advancing employee engagement through a healthy workplace strategy. *Journal of Health Services Research & Policy*, *13*(Suppl. 1), 35–40. doi:10.1258/jhsrp.2007.007031 PMID:18325167

Shaw, W. S., Besen, E., Pransky, G., Boot, C. R., Nicholas, M. K., McLellan, R. K., & Tveito, T. H. (2014). Manage at work: A randomized, controlled trial of a self-management group intervention to overcome workplace challenges associated with chronic physical health conditions. *BMC Public Health*, *14*(1), 515. doi:10.1186/1471-2458-14-515 PMID:24885844

Shimazu, A., & Schaufeli, W. B. (2009). Is workaholism good or bad for employee well-being? The distinctiveness of workaholism and work engagement among Japanese employees. *Industrial Health*, *47*(5), 495–502. doi:10.2486/indhealth.47.495 PMID:19834258

Shimazu, A., Schaufeli, W. B., Kamiyama, K., & Kawakami, N. (2015). Workaholism vs. work engagement: The two different predictors of future well-being and performance. *International Journal of Behavioral Medicine*, *22*(1), 18–23. doi:10.1007/s12529-014-9410-x PMID:24696043

Shimazu, A., Schaufeli, W. B., Kubota, K., & Kawakami, N. (2012). Do workaholism and work engagement predict employee well-being and performance in opposite directions? *Industrial Health*, *50*(4), 316–321. doi:10.2486/indhealth.MS1355 PMID:22673364

Stewart, W. F., Ricci, J. A., Chee, E., Hahn, S. R., & Morganstein, D. (2003). Cost of lost productive work time among US workers with Depression. *Journal of the American Medical Association*, *289*(23), 3135–3144. doi:10.1001/jama.289.23.3135 PMID:12813119

Stockholm European Council. (2001, March 23-24). Presidency conclusions and annexes. Retrieved from http://aei.pitt.edu/43341/

Theorell, T., Harms-Ringdahl, K., Ahlberg-Hultén, G., & Westin, B. (1991). Psychosocial job factors and symptoms from the locomotor system-a multicausal analysis. *Scandinavian Journal of Rehabilitative Medicine*, *23*(3), 165–173. PMID:1962160

Tuckey, M. R., Bakker, A. B., & Dollard, M. F. (2012). Empowering leaders optimize working conditions for engagement: A multilevel study. *Journal of Occupational Health Psychology*, *17*(1), 15–27. doi:10.1037/a0025942 PMID:22409390

Tullar, J. M., Amick, B. C. III, Brewer, S., Diamond, P. M., Kelder, S. H., & Mikhail, O. (2015). Improve employee engagement to retain your workforce. *Health Care Management Review*. doi:10.1097/HMR.0000000000000079 PMID:26207655

Tuomi, K., Huuhtanen, P., Nykyri, E., & Ilmarinen, J. (2001). Promotion of work ability, the quality of work and retirement. *Occupational Medicine (Oxford, England)*, *51*(5), 318–324. doi:10.1093/occmed/51.5.318 PMID:11473138

Tveito, T. H., Hysing, M., & Eriksen, H. R. (2004). Low back pain interventions at the workplace: A systematic literature review. *Occupational Medicine*, *54*(1), 3–13. doi:10.1093/occmed/kqg109 PMID:14963248

Udo, H., Kobayashi, M., Udo, A., & Branlund, B. (2006). Participatory ergonomic improvement in nursing home. *Industrial Health*, *44*(1), 128–134. doi:10.2486/indhealth.44.128 PMID:16610548

Udo, H., & Yoshinaga, F. (2001). The role of the industrial medical doctor in planning and implementing ergonomic measures at the workplaces. *International Journal of Industrial Ergonomics*, *28*(3-4), 237–246. doi:10.1016/S0169-8141(01)00037-3

van der Meer, L., Leijten, F. R., Heuvel, S. G., Ybema, J. F., de Wind, A., Burdorf, A., & Geuskens, G. A. (2015). Company Policies on Working Hours and Night Work in Relation to Older Workers' Work Ability and Work Engagement: Results From a Dutch Longitudinal Study with 2 Year Follow-Up. *Journal of Occupational Rehabilitation*, 2015, 1–9. PMID:26250870

Vatsalya, V., & Karch, R. (2013). Evaluation of health determinants for sustaining workability in aging US workforce. *Advanced Aging Research*, *2*(3), 106–108. doi:10.4236/aar.2013.23015 PMID:25285260

Ventura, M., Salanova, M., & Llorens, S. (2015). Professional self-efficacy as a predictor of burnout and engagement: The role of challenge and hindrance demands. *The Journal of Psychology*, *149*(3), 277–302. doi:10.1080/00223980.2013.876380 PMID:25590343

Waddell, G., & Burton, A. K. (2001). Occupational health guidelines for the management of low back pain at work: Evidence review. *Occupational Medicine*, *51*(2), 124–135. doi:10.1093/occmed/51.2.124 PMID:11307688

Walker, A. (1999). Combating age discrimination at the workplace. *Experimental Aging Research*, *25*(4), 367–377. doi:10.1080/036107399243823 PMID:10553519

Werner, E. L., Ihlebaek, C., Skouen, J. S., & Laerum, E. (2005). Beliefs about low back pain in the Norwegian general population: Are they related to pain experiences and health professionals? *Spine*, *30*(15), 1770–1776. doi:10.1097/01.brs.0000171909.81632.fe PMID:16094280

Werner, E. L., Laerum, E., Wormgoor, M. E. A., Lindh, E., & Indahl, A. (2007). Peer support in an occupational setting preventing LBP-related sick leave. *Occupational Medicine*, *57*(8), 590–595. doi:10.1093/occmed/kqm094 PMID:17916863

Westergren, A. (2012). Action-oriented study circles facilitate efforts in nursing homes to "go from feeding to serving": Conceptual perspectives on knowledge translation and workplace learning. *Journal of Aging Research*, *2012*, 627371. doi:10.1155/2012/627371 PMID:22991666

Wilson, J. R. (1995). Ergonomic and participation. In J. R. Wilson & E. N. Corlett (Eds.), *Evaluation of Human Work: A Practical Ergonomics Methodology* (pp. 1071–1096). London: Taylor and Francis.

Winkel, J., & Mathiassen, S. E. (1994). Assessment of physical work load in epidemiologic studies: Concepts, issues and operational considerations. *Ergonomics*, *37*(6), 979–988. doi:10.1080/00140139408963711 PMID:8026455

Winkelmann-Gleed, A. (2008). *Demographic change and implications for workforce ageing in Europe: raising awareness and improving practice*. London: Working Lives Research Institute.

Woby, S. R., Watson, P. J., Roach, N. K., & Urmston, M. (2004). Adjustment to chronic low back pain--the relative influence of fear-avoidance beliefs, catastrophizing, and appraisals of control. *Behaviour Research and Therapy*, *42*(7), 761–774. doi:10.1016/S0005-7967(03)00195-5 PMID:15149897

Woods, V. (2005). Work-related musculoskeletal health and social support. *Occupational Medicine*, *55*(3), 177–189. doi:10.1093/occmed/kqi085 PMID:15857897

KEY TERMS AND DEFINITIONS

Active Ageing: The process of optimizing opportunities for health, participation and safety in order to enhance the quality of life as people age.

Ergonomics: Ergonomics is the scientific discipline concerned with understanding interactions among humans and other elements of a system, and the profession that applies theory, principles, data and methods to design in order to optimize human wellbeing and overall system performance.

Hazardous Worker: A worker who may put the health or safety of other workers or third parties at risk because of his/her health condition or behavior.

Occupational Health: A scientific discipline aimed at promoting workers' health and working capacity; at improving the working environment and work culture, and at protecting third parties and the environment outside the workplace.

Participatory Ergonomics: Programs seeking to maximize the involvement of the workers in implementing ergonomic knowledge, procedures and changes with the intention of improving working conditions, safety, productivity, quality, morale and/or comfort.

Presenteeism: Reduced productivity at work due to health problems.

Successful Ageing: Physical, mental and social wellbeing in old age.

Worksite Health Promotion: The combined efforts of employers, employees and society to improve the health and wellbeing of people at work.

Afterword

This edited book hosts contributions by scholars belonging to many different disciplinary domains and Athenaeums from across the world, all attempting a conceptual foundation of what the promotion of patients' participation and engagement is and how this may be achieved.

On the one hand, the variety of theoretical and research glances assumed by authors in the different chapters testifies to the richness (and the ferment) of this ongoing literature debate. Furthermore, these research efforts testify the multifaceted nature and the novelty of the patient engagement phenomenon, which is not reducible to only some of its phenomenological manifestations, neither assumable for granted or on the basis of traditional (and developed "there and then") perspectives and paradigms.

On the other hand, the contributions to this book also cast light on the still fragmented approach of academic research in this area: while important insights already exist, often they are circumscribed to only some aspects of the phenomenon. Wider approaches and theorizations able to cast light on the whole complexity of the phenomenon are missed.

These premises confirm the importance of promoting occasions of dialogue and sharing among scholars in order to better joint research efforts towards the common goal of a theoretical foundation of the patient engagement phenomenon. From our perspective, this edited book can be rightly considered as a first concrete step in this direction: In these last pages we shall summarize the main insights which have emerged from this joint endeavor and offer some "food for future thoughts" in this field.

PROMOTING PATIENTS ENGAGEMENT AND PARTICIPATION: STATE OF THE ART

The chapters of this book discuss what patient engagement and participation are and what may promote it from the micro analysis of the individual characteristics of the patients (at the psychological, medical, sociological and cultural level) that play a role in determining their attitude to being engaged in health management; to the analysis of dyadic relational dynamics (occurring mainly between a patient and his/her formal or informal caregivers) which may sustain or not sustain patient engagement; to the analysis of networks and peer group exchanges of their roles in this process; finally to the analysis of the organizational, structural and systemic elements that may influence patients' engagement and participation. This book well explained how many elements are play when patient engagement concerned (see Figure 1 for a conceptual summary). This should sensitize the readers against an iper-simplified approach to the analysis of patient engagement and make them aware of the multiple elements that should be taken into consideration when approaching the problem.

Figure 1. Conceptual map of the elements that may favor or hinder patient engagement and participation

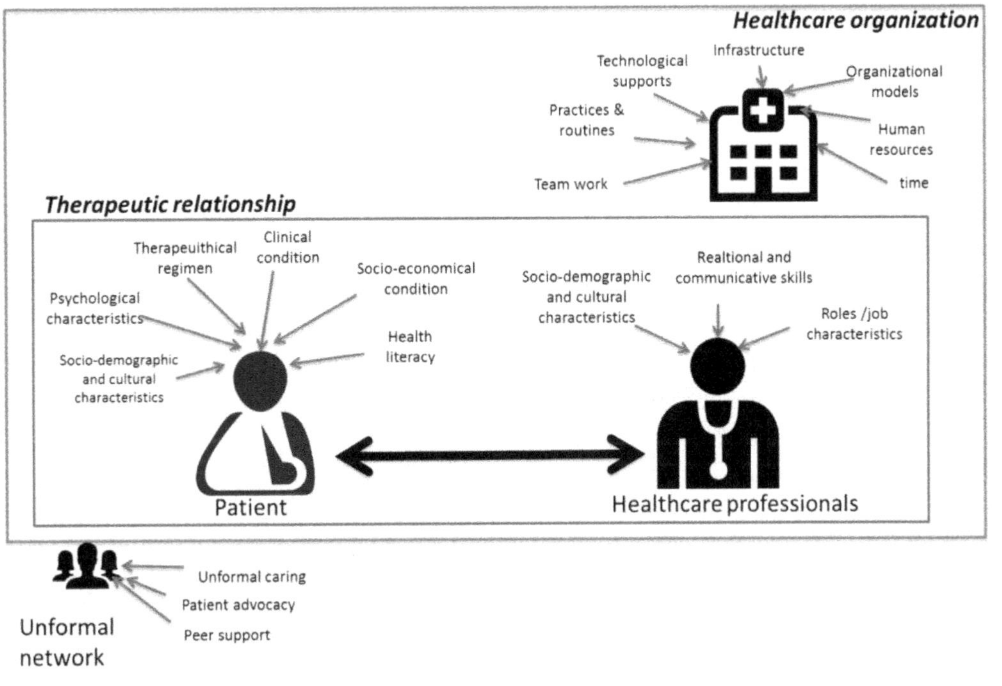

PATIENT ENGAGEMENT: TOWARDS A SHARED DEFINITION

Definitions of patients' engagement and participation vary in the literature. Although not always moving forward from the same definition of patient engagement, the chapters of this book all share the same logic when considering this phenomenon: patient engagement and participation are conceived an umbrella concept which overcomes and structures other similar ones such as "adherence," "compliance," "self-management" or "shared decision making." According to evidence which has emerged from these book chapters, patient engagement is not solely referable to the dyadic interaction between patients and healthcare professionals; neither it is describable as simply a psychological state or attitude that the patients may or may not assume during their care management. Patient engagement should rather be conceived as the kind of healthcare fruition that the patient may experience along his/her care journey. A fruition experience which characterized by the deliberate decision of playing an active and negotiating role: opting for an engaged approach to healthcare management, from the perspective of a patient, thus, means to take the decision of being an actor (and of being perceived and treated as such by the others actors on the scene) able to co-authoring the plot of his/her care journey. However, becoming an actor of one owns healthcare doesn't mean to opt for an "anarchic" or uncontrolled position towards care, rather to become aware of the potentiality of one-own role and deliberately choosing when being active, when passive, when partners, when not…of the healthcare systems. Finally, being able to became engaged patients means to better understand one owns healthcare rights, duties, needs and expectations.

PATIENT ENGAGEMENT: PERSPECTIVES FOR THE FUTURE

A lot has been done, but still much needs to be done in order to finally locate the concepts of patients' engagement and participation and to effectively orient practices. The main consideration is that this book has offered some encouraging first contributions in this direction. The auspice is to move steps forward in a better joint and orchestrated way, and by promoting the dialogue among the different research groups involved in this field.

Foremost one shared consideration which appears key to us to the continuation in this shared endeavor: the importance of opting for a process-like approach to patient engagement and, thus, to its implications for the practice. Patient engagement should not simplistically conceived such as an "on-off" of patients' status, but it should be recognized as a dynamic trajectory which is mutable, framed and influenced by several psychological, relational, contextual and organizational factors. Patient engagement is a dynamic, volatile, mutable, complex and implies different levels of manifestation and analysis. Furthermore, patient engagement is not "one" and defined "once and for all," but may change according to the different trajectories of disease and of life; depending on the different socio-demographic characteristics of actors involved and on their possible encounters and exchanges, since patient engagement concerns persons and their human subjectivities. Patient engagement thus must advocate for a humanistic and multidisciplinary approach in order to be further studied and promoted. A long path-way is still ahead: this book intends to be coinceived as a first (important) step in this direction.

Guendalina Graffigna
Catholic University of the Sacred Heart, Milan, Italy

A. Claudio Bosio
Catholic University of the Sacred Heart, Milan, Italy

Compilation of References

Acitelli, L. K., & Bard, H. (2005). My illness or our illness? Attending to the relationship when one partner is ill. In T. A. Revenson, K. Kayser, & G. Bodenmann (Eds.), *Emerging perspectives on couples' coping with stress* (pp. 121–136). Washington, DC: American Psychological Association. doi:10.1037/11031-006

Admasachew, L., & Dawson, J. (2011). The association between presenteeism and engagement of National Health Service staff. *Journal of Health Services Research & Policy*, *16*(Suppl. 1), 29–33. doi:10.1258/jhsrp.2010.010085 PMID:21460347

Agren, S., Evangelista, L. S., Davidson, T., & Stromberg, A. (2013). Cost-effectiveness of a nurse-led education and psychosocial programme for patients with chronic heart failure and their partners. *Journal of Clinical Nursing*, *22*(15-16), 2347–2353. doi:10.1111/j.1365-2702.2012.04246.x PMID:23829407

Airila, A., Hakanen, J., Punakallio, A., Lusa, S., & Luukkonen, R. (2012). Is work engagement related to work ability beyond working conditions and lifestyle factors? *International Archives of Occupational and Environmental Health*, *85*(8), 915–925. doi:10.1007/s00420-012-0732-1 PMID:22270385

Alberici, A. I., & Milesi, P. (2015, July 7-10). "The right thing to do": discussing online and the moral pathway to collective mobilization. *Paper presented atThe 14th European Congress of Psychology*, Milan (Italy).

Alberici, A. I., & Milesi, P. (2013). The influence of the internet on the psychosocial predictors of collective action. *Journal of Community & Applied Social Psychology*, *23*(5), 373–388. doi:10.1002/casp.2131

Alberici, A. I., & Milesi, P. (in press). Online discussion, politicized identity, and collective action. *Group Processes & Intergroup Relations*. doi:10.1177/1368430215581430

Aldana, S. (2001). Financial impact of health promotion programs: A comprehensive review of the literature. *American Journal of Health Promotion*, *15*(5), 296–320. doi:10.4278/0890-1171-15.5.296 PMID:11502012

Aldosary, A. S., & Garba, S. B. (1999). An analysis of factors contributing to college student dropout in a medium sized technical university: The case of the King Fahd University of Petroleum and Minerals Dhahran, Saudi Arabia. *Higher Education Policy*, *12*(4), 313–328. doi:10.1016/S0952-8733(99)00021-5

Alegría, M., Sribney, W., Perez, D., Laderman, M., & Keefe, K. (2009). The role of patient activation on patient–provider communication and quality of care for US and foreign born Latino patients. *Journal of General Internal Medicine*, *24*(3), 534–541. doi:10.1007/s11606-009-1074-x PMID:19842003

Allsop, J., Jones, K., & Baggott, R. (2004). Health consumer groups in the UK: A new social movement? *Sociology of Health & Illness*, *26*(6), 737–756. doi:10.1111/j.0141-9889.2004.00416.x PMID:15383039

Als, H., Duffy, F. H., McAnulty, G. B., Rivkin, M. J., Vajapeyam, S., Mulkern, R. V., & Eichenwald, E. C. et al. (2004). Early Experience Alters Brain Function and Structure. *Pediatrics*, *113*(4), 846–857. doi:10.1542/peds.113.4.846 PMID:15060237

Altimier, L., Kenner, C., & Damus, K. (2015). The Wee Care Neuroprotective NICU Program (Wee Care): The Effect of a Comprehensive Developmental Care Training Program on Seven Neuroprotective Core Measures for Family-Centered Developmental Care of Premature Neonates. *Newborn and Infant Nursing Reviews; NAINR*, *15*(1), 6–16. doi:10.1053/j.nainr.2015.01.006

Altuncu, E., Akman, I., Kulekci, S., Akdas, F., Bilgen, H., & Ozek, E. (2009). Noise levels in neonatal intensive care unit and use of sound absorbing panel in the isolette. *International Journal of Pediatric Otorhinolaryngology*, *73*(7), 951–953. doi:10.1016/j.ijporl.2009.03.013 PMID:19406484

American College of Physicians. (2010). *Healthcare Transparency-Focus on Price and Clinical Performance Information*. Philadelphia.

American Heart Association. (1994). Cardiac rehabilitation programs: A statement for healthcare professionals from the American Heart Association. *Circulation*, *90*(3), 1602–1610http://circ.ahajournals.org/content/90/3/1602.full.pdf+html?ijkey=c95f4e77ee2deea285d9361fb53c32d71957c126&keytype2=tf_ipsecsha. doi:10.1161/01.CIR.90.3.1602 PMID:8087975

American Hospital Association Board of Trustees. (1999). *Accountability – the pathway to restoring public trust and confidence for hospitals and other health care organizations*.

American Psychiatric Association. (2013). *Diagnostic and statistical manual of mental disorders* (5th ed.). Arlington, VA: American Psychiatric Publishing.

Andrews, G. J. (2002). Towards a more place-sensitive nursing research: An invitation to medical and health geography. *Nursing Inquiry*, *9*(4), 221–238. doi:10.1046/j.1440-1800.2002.00157.x PMID:12460418

Andrews, G. J., & Shaw, D. (2008). Clinical geography: Nursing practice and the (re) making of institutional space. *Journal of Nursing Management*, *16*(4), 463–473. doi:10.1111/j.1365-2834.2008.00866.x PMID:18405263

Andrews, M. H., & Matthews, S. G. (2004). Programming of the hypothalamo-pituitary-adrenal axis: Serotonergic involvement. *Stress (Amsterdam, Netherlands)*, *7*(1), 15–27. doi:10.1080/10253890310001650277 PMID:15204029

Antonovsky, A. (1979). *Health, Stress and Coping*. San Francisco: Jossey-Bass Publishers.

Aristotle. (2009). The Nicomachean ethics (trans. by L. Brown, ed. by W. D. Ross). Oxford: Oxford University Press.

Armstrong, T. J., Buckle, P., Fine, L. J., Hagberg, M., Jonsson, B., & Kilbom, A. et al. (1993). A conceptual model for work-related neck and upper-limb musculoskeletal disorders. *Scandinavian Journal of Work, Environment & Health*, *19*(2), 73–84. doi:10.5271/sjweh.1494 PMID:8316782

Arneil, A. B., & Devlin, A. S. (2002). Perceived quality of care: The influence of the waiting room environment. *Journal of Environmental Psychology*, *22*(4), 345–360. doi:10.1006/jevp.2002.0274

Arnetz, J. E., Winblad, U., Höglund, A. T., Lindahl, B., Spångberg, K., Wallentin, L., & Arnetz, B. B. et al. (2010). Is patient involvement during hospitalization for acute myocardial infarction associated with post-discharge treatment outcome? An exploratory study. *Health Expectations*, *13*, 298–311. PMID:20579120

Arnold, M. (2008). Polypharmacy and older adults: A role for psychology and psychologists. *Professional Psychology, Research and Practice*, *39*(3), 283–289. doi:10.1037/0735-7028.39.3.283

Arnstein, S. (1969). A ladder of citizen participation. *Journal of the American Institute of Planners*, *26*(4), 216–233. doi:10.1080/01944366908977225

Arora, N. K. (2003). Interacting with cancer patients: The significance of physicians' communication behavior. *Social Science & Medicine*, *57*(5), 791–806. doi:10.1016/S0277-9536(02)00449-5 PMID:12850107

Ashbaugh, J. B., Leick-Rude, M. K., & Kilbride, H. W. (1999). Developmental care teams in the neonatal intensive care unit: Survey on current status. *Journal of Perinatology*, *19*(1), 48–52. doi:10.1038/sj.jp.7200101 PMID:10685202

Atwal, A., & Caldwell, K. (2002). Do multidisciplinary integrated care pathways improve interprofessional collaboration? *Scandinavian Journal of Caring Sciences*, *16*(4), 360–367. doi:10.1046/j.1471-6712.2002.00101.x PMID:12445105

Babakus, E., & Mangold, W. G. (1992). Adapting the SERVQUAL scale to hospital services: An empirical investigation. *Health Services Research*, *26*(6), 767–786. PMID:1737708

Back, L. (2002). Aryans reading Adorno: Cyber-culture and twenty-first century racism. *Ethnic and Racial Studies*, *25*(4), 628–651. doi:10.1080/01419870220136664

Backman, G., Hunt, P., Khosla, R., Jaramillo-Strouss, C., Fikre, B. M., & Rumble, C. et al. (2008). Health systems and the right to health: An assessment of 194 countries. *Lancet*, *372*(9655), 2047–2085. doi:10.1016/S0140-6736(08)61781-X PMID:19097280

Bader, L. (2015). Brain-oriented care in the NICU: A case study. *Neonatal Network*, *33*(5), 263–267. doi:10.1891/0730-0832.33.5.263 PMID:25161134

Badr, H., Acitelli, L. K., & Carmack Taylor, C. L. (2007). Does couple identity mediate the stress experienced by caregiving spouses. *Psychology & Health*, *22*(2), 211–229. doi:10.1080/14768320600843077

Badr, H., Acitelli, L. K., & Carmack Taylor, C. L. (2008). Does talking about their relationship affect couples' marital and psychological adjustment to lung cancer? *Journal of Cancer Survivorship: Research and Practice*, *2*(1), 53–64. doi:10.1007/s11764-008-0044-3 PMID:18648987

Badr, H., & Carmack Taylor, C. L. (2008). Effects of relationship maintenance on psychological distress and dyadic adjustment among couples coping with lung cancer. *Health Psychology*, *27*(5), 616–627. doi:10.1037/0278-6133.27.5.616 PMID:18823188

Badr, H., Carmack Taylor, C. L., Kashy, D. A., Cristofanilli, M., & Revenson, T. A. (2010). Dyadic coping in metastatic breast cancer. *Health Psychology*, *29*(2), 169–180. doi:10.1037/a0018165 PMID:20230090

Badri, M. (2014). Medical malpractice litigation. *Journal of the American College of Cardiology*, *64*(4), 418–419. doi:10.1016/j.jacc.2014.06.013 PMID:25060379

Bainton, D., van der Steeg, H., & Weeda, L. (1995). Restructuring. Building blocks. *The Health Service Journal*, *105*(5445), 26–27. PMID:10141857

Balint, E. (1969). The possibilities of patient-centred medicine. *The British Journal of General Practice*, *17*(82), 269–276. PMID:5770926

Balint, M. (1957). *The doctor, his patient and the illness*. London: Tavistock Publications.

Barber, L., Grawitch, M. J., & Munz, D. C. (2013). Are better sleepers more engaged workers? A self-regulatory approach to sleep hygiene and work engagement. *Stress and Health*, *29*(4), 307–316. doi:10.1002/smi.2468 PMID:23086901

Bardes, C. L. (2012). Defining "patient-centered medicine". *The New England Journal of Medicine*, *366*(9), 782–783. doi:10.1056/NEJMp1200070 PMID:22375968

Barello, S. & Graffigna, G. (2015b). Patient engagement in healthcare: pathways for effective medical decision making. *Neuropsychogical Trends,* 2015, 53.

Barello, S., Graffigna, G., Savarese, M., Donato, S., & Bertoni, A. (2014). Patient engagement in chronic disease management: The pivotal role of partners. *Paper presented at the EACH - International conference on communication in healthcare*, Amsterdam, NL.

Barello, S., Graffigna, G., Vegni, E., & Bosio, A. C. (2014). The challenges of conceptualizing patient engagement in health care: A lexicographic literature review. *Journal of Participatory Medicine, 6*.

Barello, S., & Graffigna, G. (2014b). Engaging patients to recover life projectuality: An Italian cross-disease framework. *Quality of Life Research: An International Journal of Quality of Life Aspects of Treatment, Care and Rehabilitation, 24*(5), 1087–1096. doi:10.1007/s11136-014-0846-x PMID:25373927

Barello, S., & Graffigna, G. (2015). Patient engagement in healthcare: Pathways for effective medical decision making. *Neuropsychological Trends, 17*(1), 53–65. doi:10.7358/neur-2015-017-bare

Barello, S., Graffigna, G., Savarese, M., & Bosio, A. C. (2014a). Engaging patients in health management: Towards a preliminary theoretical conceptualization. *Psicologia della Salute, 3*(3), 11–33. doi:10.3280/PDS2014-003002

Barello, S., Graffigna, G., & Vegni, E. (2012). Patient engagement as an emerging challenge for healthcare services: Mapping the literature. *Nursing Research and Practice, 1*, 1–7. doi:10.1155/2012/905934 PMID:23213497

Barello, S., Graffigna, G., Vegni, E., Savarese, M., Lombardi, F., & Bosio, A. C. (2015). 'Engage me in taking care of my heart': A grounded theory study on patient–cardiologist relationship in the hospital management of heart failure. *BMJ Open, 5*(3), e005582. doi:10.1136/bmjopen-2014-005582 PMID:25776041

Barello, S., Savarese, M., & Graffigna, G. (2015). The role of caregivers in the elderly healthcare journey: insights for sustaining elderly patient engagement. In G. Graffigna, S. Barello, & S. Triberti (Eds.), *Patient engagement: A consumer-centered model to innovate healthcare* (pp. 108–119). Warsaw: De Gruyter Open. doi:10.1515/9783110452440-010

Barfod, T. S., Hecht, F. M., Rubow, C., & Gerstoft, J. (2006). Physicians' communication with patients about adherence to HIV medication in San Francisco and Copenhagen: A qualitative study using grounded theory. *BMC Health Services Research, 6*(1), 154. doi:10.1186/1472-6963-6-154 PMID:17144910

Barnes, M., & Bennet, G. (1998). Frail bodies, courageous voices: Older people influencing community care. *Health & Social Care in the Community, 6*(2), 102–111. doi:10.1046/j.1365-2524.1998.00105.x PMID:11560582

Barnett, J., Fife-Schaw, C., Shepherd, R., Timotijevic, L., Fletcher, J., & Fletcher, D. (2008). *Online deliberative engagement: A pilot study. A report for the Wellcome Trust*. Surrey, U.K.: University of Surrey/Brook Lyndhurst/White October.

Barnett, K., Mercer, S. W., Norbury, M., Watt, G., Wyke, S., & Guthrie, B. (2012). Epidemiology of multimorbidity and implications for health care, research, and medical education: A cross-sectional study. *Lancet, 380*(9836), 37–43. doi:10.1016/S0140-6736(12)60240-2 PMID:22579043

Barnoy, S., Bar-tal, Y., & Zisser, B. (2006). Correspondence in informational coping styles: How important is it for cancer patients and their spouses? *Personality and Individual Differences, 41*(1), 105–115. doi:10.1016/j.paid.2005.12.013

Barry, M. J., & Edgman-Levitan, S. (2012). Shared decision making – The pinnacle of patient-centered care. *The New England Journal of Medicine, 366*(9), 780–781. doi:10.1056/NEJMp1109283 PMID:22375967

Batalden, P., & Davidoff, F. (2007). What is quality improvement and how it can transform healthcare. *Quality & Safety in Health Care, 16*(1), 2–3. doi:10.1136/qshc.2006.022046 PMID:17301192

Battersby, M. W., Ask, A., Reece, M. M., Markwick, M. J., & Collins, J. P. (2003). The Partners in Health scale: The development and psychometric properties of a generic assessment scale for chronic condition self-management. *Australian Journal of Primary Health, 9*(3), 41–52. doi:10.1071/PY03022

Bauer, U. E., Briss, P. A., Goodman, R. A., & Bowman, B. A. (2014). Prevention of chronic disease in the 21st century: Elimination of the leading preventable causes of premature death and disability in the USA. *Lancet*, *384*(9937), 45–52. doi:10.1016/S0140-6736(14)60648-6 PMID:24996589

Bauman, Z. (2007). *Consuming life*. Cambridge: Polity Press.

Beaglehole, R., Epping-Jordan, J., Patel, V., Chopra, M., Ebrahim, S., Kidd, M., & Haines, A. (2008). Improving the prevention and management of chronic disease in low-income and middle-income countries: A priority for primary health care. *Lancet*, *372*(9642), 940–949. doi:10.1016/S0140-6736(08)61404-X PMID:18790317

Beauchamp, T. L., & Childress, J. F. (2012). *Principles of biomedical ethics* (7th ed.). New York: Oxford University Press.

Becker, E. R., & Roblin, D. W. (2008). Translating primary care practice climate into patient activation: The role of patient trust in physician. *Medical Care*, *46*(8), 795–805. doi:10.1097/MLR.0b013e31817919c0 PMID:18665059

Becker, F., & Douglass, S. (2008). The Ecology of the Patient Visit. Physical Attractiveness, Waiting Times, and Perceived Quality of Care. *The Journal of Ambulatory Care Management*, *31*(2), 128–141. doi:10.1097/01.JAC.0000314703.34795.44 PMID:18360174

Becker, L. C. (1992). Good Lives: Prolegomena. *Social Philosophy & Policy*, *9*(02), 5–37. doi:10.1017/S0265052500001382

Becker, L. C. (2000). The Good of Agency. In L. P. Francis & A. Silvers (Eds.), *Americans with disabilities: Exploring implications of the law for individuals and institutions* (pp. 54–63). New York: Routledge.

Becker, L. C. (2003). Human Health and Stoic Moral Norms. *The Journal of Medicine and Philosophy*, *28*(2), 221–238. doi:10.1076/jmep.28.2.221.14206 PMID:12943215

Becker, L. C. (2012). *Habilitation, health, and agency: A framework for basic justice*. New York: Oxford University Press. doi:10.1093/acprof:oso/9780199917549.001.0001

Becker, L. C., & Becker, C. B. (2001). *Encyclopedia of ethics* (2nd ed.). New York: Routledge.

Becker, L. C., & Becker, C. B. (2003). *A history of western ethics* (2nd ed.). New York: Routledge. doi:10.4324/9780203426937

Beckman, H. B., Markakis, K. M., Suchman, A. L., & Frankel, R. M. (1994). The doctor-patient relationship and malpractice: Lessons from plaintiff depositions. *Archives of Internal Medicine*, *154*(12), 1365–1370. doi:10.1001/archinte.1994.00420120093010 PMID:8002688

Beech, N. (2011). Liminality and the practices of identity reconstruction. *Human Relations*, *64*(2), 285–302. doi:10.1177/0018726710371235

Belcher, A. J., Laurenceau, J. P., Graber, E. C., Cohen, L. H., Dash, K. B., & Siegel, S. D. (2011). Daily support in couples coping with early stage breast cancer: Maintaining intimacy during adversity. *Health Psychology*, *30*(6), 665–673. doi:10.1037/a0024705 PMID:21823795

Bensing, J. (2000). Bridging the gap.: The separate worlds of evidence-based medicine and patient-centered medicine. *Patient Education and Counseling*, *39*(1), 17–25. doi:10.1016/S0738-3991(99)00087-7 PMID:11013544

Beresford, P., & Branfield, F. (2006). Developing inclusive partnerships: User-defined outcomes, networking and knowledge – a case study. *Health & Social Care in the Community*, *14*(5), 436–444. doi:10.1111/j.1365-2524.2006.00654.x PMID:16918836

Berg, C. A., Meegan, S. P., & Deviney, F. P. (1998). A social contextual model of coping with everyday problems across the life span. *International Journal of Behavioral Development*, *22*, 239–261. doi:10.1080/016502598384360

Berg, C. A., Wiebe, D. J., Butner, J., Bloor, L., Bradstreet, C., Upchurch, R., & Patton, G. et al. (2008). Collaborative coping and daily mood in couples dealing with prostate cancer. *Psychology and Aging*, *23*(3), 505–516. doi:10.1037/a0012687 PMID:18808241

Bergeson, S. C., & Dean, J. D. (2006). A systems approach to patient-centered care. *Journal of the American Medical Association*, *296*(23), 2848–2851. doi:10.1001/jama.296.23.2848 PMID:17179462

Berghuis, J. P., & Stanton, A. L. (2002). Adjustment to a dyadic stressor: A longitudinal study of coping and depressive symptoms in infertile couples over an insemination attempt. *Journal of Consulting and Clinical Psychology*, *70*(2), 433–438. doi:10.1037/0022-006X.70.2.433 PMID:11952202

Bertoni, A., Barni, D., Bodenmann, G., Charvoz, L., Gagliardi, S., Iafrate, R., & Rosnati, R. (2007). Comunicazione dello stress, coping diadico e benessere della coppia: Uno studio cross-sectional e cross-nazionale. *Età Evolutiva*, *86*, 58–66.

Bertoni, A., & Bodenmann, G. (2010). Satisfied and dissatisfied couples: Positive and negative dimensions, conflict styles, and relationships with family of origin. *European Psychologist*, *15*(3), 175–184. doi:10.1027/1016-9040/a000015

Bertoni, A., Donato, S., Graffigna, G., Barello, S., & Parise, M. (2015). Engaged patients, engaged partnerships: Singles and partners dealing with an acute cardiac event. *Psychology Health and Medicine*, *20*(5), 505–517. doi:10.1080/13548506.2014.969746 PMID:25506636

Bertoni, A., Donato, S., Morgano, A., Iafrate, R., & Rosnati, R. (in press). A Qualitative Evaluation of a Preventive Intervention for Parents: The Groups for Family Enrichment_Parent Version (GFE_P). *Themed Issue of Journal of Prevention & Intervention in the Community*.

Bertoni, A., Parise, M., & Iafrate, R. (2012). Beyond Satisfaction: Generativity as a New Outcome of Couple Functioning. In P. E. Esposito & C. I. Lombardi (Eds.), *Marriage: Psychological Implications, Social Expectations, and Role of Sexuality* (pp. 115–131). New York, US: Nova Science Publishers.

Berwick, D. M. (2009). What a "Patient-Centered" should mean: Confession of an extremist. *Health Affairs*, *28*(4), 555–565. doi:10.1377/hlthaff.28.4.w555 PMID:19454528

Berwick, D. M., James, B., & Coye, M. J. (2003). Connections between quality measurement and improvement. *Medical Care*, *41*(Suppl. 1), I30–I38. doi:10.1097/00005650-200301001-00004 PMID:12544814

Berwick, D. M., Nolan, T. W., & Whittington, J. (2008). The triple aim: Care, health, and cost. *Health Affairs*, *27*(3), 759–769. doi:10.1377/hlthaff.27.3.759 PMID:18474969

Betsch, C., Renkewitz, F., Betsch, T., & Ulshöfer, C. (2010). The influence of vaccine-critical websites on perceiving vaccination risks. *Journal of Health Psychology*, *15*(3), 446–455. doi:10.1177/1359105309353647 PMID:20348365

Bevilacqua, L., Del Piano, A., De Matteis, B., Luciani, E., Magnavita, L., & Mammi, F. et al. (2007a). The participatory approach to injury prevention appeared to be an useful tool of safety education and ergonomic improvement. *Giornale Italiano di Medicina del Lavoro Ed Ergonomia*, *29*(3), 560–561. PMID:18409831

Bevilacqua, L., & Magnavita, N. (2008). Quality improvement of risk assessment procedures in maritime work. *Giornale Italiano di Medicina del Lavoro Ed Ergonomia*, *30*(Suppl. 2), 447–449.

Bevilacqua, L., Magnavita, N., Becchetti, G., Mammi, F., Roccia, K., & Pupp, N. (2007b). Participatory risk evaluation. The role of the surveillance. *Giornale Italiano di Medicina del Lavoro Ed Ergonomia*, *29*(3), 657–658. PMID:18409891

Bevilacqua, L., Sacco, A., & Magnavita, N. (2003). Health surveillance audit of wood dust exposure. *La Medicina del Lavoro*, *94*, 224–230. PMID:12852205

Beyes, T., & Steyaert, C. (2012). Spacing organization: Non-representational theory and performing organizational space. *Organization*, *19*(1), 45–61. doi:10.1177/1350508411401946

Biddison, E. L. D., Paine, L., Murakami, P., Herzke, C., & Weaver, S. J. (2015). Associations between safety culture and employee engagement over time: a retrospective analysis. *BMJ quality & safety*. doi:10.1136/bmjqs-2014-003910

Biggs, S. (2001). Toward critical narrativity: Stories of aging in contemporary social policy. *Journal of Aging Studies*, *15*(4), 303–316. doi:10.1016/S0890-4065(01)00025-1

Bismark, M., Dauer, E., Paterson, R., & Studdert, D. (2006). Accountability sought by patients following adverse events from medical care: The New Zealand experience. *Canadian Medical Association Journal*, *175*(8), 889–894. doi:10.1503/cmaj.060429 PMID:17030939

Blackwood, L. M., & Louis, W. R. (2012). If it matters for the group then it matters to me: Collective action outcomes for seasoned activists. *The British Journal of Social Psychology*, *51*(1), 72–92. doi:10.1111/j.2044-8309.2010.02001.x PMID:21294752

Boaden, R., Harvey, G., Moxham, C., & Proudlove, N. (2008). *Quality improvement: theory and practice in healthcare*. National Health Service Institute for Innovation and Improvement/ University of Manchester Business School.

Bock, J., Rether, K., Gröger, N., Xie, L., & Braun, K. (2014). Perinatal programming of emotional brain circuits: An integrative view from systems to molecules. *Frontiers in Neuroscience*, *8*(8), 1–16. PMID:24550772

Bodenmann, G. (1997). Dyadic coping - a systemic-transactional view of stress and coping among couples: Theory and empirical findings. *European Review of Applied Psychology*, *47*, 137–140.

Bodenmann, G. (2000). *Stress und Coping bei Paaren*. Göttingen: Hogrefe.

Bodenmann, G. (2005). Dyadic coping and its significance for marital functioning. In T. Revenson, K. Kayser, & G. Bodenmann (Eds.), *Couples coping with stress: Emerging perspectives on dyadic coping* (pp. 33–50). Washington: American Psychological Association. doi:10.1037/11031-002

Bodenmann, G., & Bertoni, A. (2004). *Promuovere le competenze della coppia. Il Couple Coping Enhancement Training*. Roma: Carocci.

Bok, S. (2008). Rethinking the WHO Definition of Health. In K. Heggenhougen & S. Quah (Eds.), *International encyclopedia of public health* (Vol. 6, pp. 590–597). San Diego, CA: Academic Press. doi:10.1016/B978-012373960-5.00550-5

Bolger, N., DeLongis, A., Kessler, R. C., & Wethington, E. (1989). The contagion of stress across multiple roles. *Journal of Marriage and the Family*, *51*(1), 175–183. doi:10.2307/352378

Bonner, M., & Mynatt, E. D. (2014). Gauging the patient-centered potential of online health seeking. *Proceedings of the 8th International Conference on Pervasive Computing Technologies for Healthcare PervasiveHealth '14*. Retrieved from https://research.cc.gatech.edu/ecl/sites/edu.ecl/files/PH-paper-v5-cameraReady.pdf

Boorse, C. (1975). On the Distinction between Disease and Illness. *Philosophy & Public Affairs*, *5*(1), 49–68.

Boorse, C. (1976). What a Theory of Mental Health Should Be. *Journal for the Theory of Social Behaviour*, *6*(1), 61–84. doi:10.1111/j.1468-5914.1976.tb00359.x

Boorse, C. (1977). Health as a Theoretical Concept. *Philosophy of Science*, *44*(4), 542–573. doi:10.1086/288768

Boorse, C. (1997). A Rebuttal on Health. In J. Humber & R. Almeder (Eds.), *What is disease?* (pp. 1–134). Totowa, NJ: Humana Press. doi:10.1007/978-1-59259-451-1_1

Braithwaite, D. O., Waldron, V. R., & Finn, J. (1999). Communication of social supportin computer-mediated groups for people with disabilities. *Health Communication, 11*(2), 123–151. doi:10.1207/s15327027hc1102_2 PMID:16370973

Braithwaite, J., Runciman, W. B., & Merry, F. (2009). Towards safer, better healthcare: Harnessing the natural properties of complex sociotechnical systems. *Quality & Safety in Health Care, 18*(1), 37–41. doi:10.1136/qshc.2007.023317 PMID:19204130

Branin, J. J. (2001). The role of memory strategies in medication adherence among the elderly. *Home Health Care Services Quarterly, 20*(2), 1–16. doi:10.1300/J027v20n02_01 PMID:11987652

Brashers, D. E., Goldsmith, D. J., & Hsieh, E. (2002). Information seeking and avoiding in health contexts. *Human Communication Research, 28*(2), 258–271. doi:10.1111/j.1468-2958.2002.tb00807.x

Brashers, E., Haas, M., Klingle, S., & Neidig, L. (2000). Collective AIDS activism and individuals' perceived self-advocacy in physician-patient communication. *Human Communication Research, 26*(3), 372–402. doi:10.1111/j.1468-2958.2000.tb00762.x

Brinkerhoff, D. (2003). *Accountability and Health Systems: Overview, Framework, and Strategies*. Bethesda, MD: The Partners for Health Reformplus Project, Abt Associates Inc.

Broadbent, E., Petrie, K. J., Main, J., & Weinman, J. (2006). The brief illness perception questionnaire. *Journal of Psychosomatic Research, 60*(6), 631–637. doi:10.1016/j.jpsychores.2005.10.020 PMID:16731240

Brodersen, J., & Thorwid, J. (1997). Enabling sustainable change for healthcare in Stockholm. *British Journal of Healthcare Computing and Information Management, 14*, 22–25.

Bromley, E. (2012). Building patient-centeredness: Hospital design as an interpretive act. *Social Science & Medicine, 75*(6), 1057–1066. doi:10.1016/j.socscimed.2012.04.037 PMID:22703887

Brown, B. B. (1987). Territoriality. In D. Stokols & I. Altman (Eds.), *Handbook of environmental psychology* (pp. 505–531). New York: Wiley.

Brown, G. (2009). NICU noise and the preterm infant. *Neonatal Network, 28*(3), 165–173. doi:10.1891/0730-0832.28.3.165 PMID:19451078

Brown, G., Lawrence, T. B., & Robinson, S. (2005). Territoriality in organizations. *Academy of Management Review, 30*(3), 577–594. doi:10.5465/AMR.2005.17293710

Brown, H. E., Gilson, N. D., Burton, N. W., & Brown, W. J. (2011). Does physical activity impact on presenteeism and other indicators of workplace well-being? *Sports Medicine (Auckland, N.Z.), 41*(3), 249–262. doi:10.2165/11539180-000000000-00000 PMID:21395366

Brown, P., Zavestoski, S., McCormick, S., Mayer, B., Morello-Frosch, R., & Gasior Altman, R. (2004). Embodied health movements: New approaches tosocial movements in health. *Sociology of Health & Illness, 26*(1), 50–80. doi:10.1111/j.1467-9566.2004.00378.x PMID:15027990

Brummelte, S., Grunau, R. E., Zaidman-Zait, A., Weinberg, J., Nordstokke, D., & Cepeda, I. L. (2011). Cortisol levels in relation to maternal interaction and child internalizing behavior in preterm and full-term children at 18 months corrected age. *Developmental Psychobiology, 53*(2), 184–195. doi:10.1002/dev.20511 PMID:21298633

Brunetto, Y., Xerri, M., Shriberg, A., Farr-Wharton, R., Shacklock, K., Newman, S., & Dienger, J. (2013). The impact of workplace relationships on engagement, well-being, commitment and turnover for nurses in Australia and the USA. *Journal of Advanced Nursing, 69*(12), 278627–278699. doi:10.1111/jan.12165 PMID:23651183

Brunsting, S., & Postmes, T. (2002). Social movement participation in the digital age: Predicting offline and online collective action. *Small Group Research, 33*(5), 525–554. doi:10.1177/104649602237169

Bruscaglioni, L. (2013). Rapporto sulle evidenze emerse durante la fase di ricerca sul campo - flusso ambulatoriale. In A. Simoncini, M. C. Torricelli, L. Chiesi, & S. Surrenti (Eds.), Lo Spazio dei Diritti. L'effettività del diritto alla salute nelle strutture ospedaliere (pp. 116–144). Firenze: Edi Toscana.

Bruscaglioni, L. (2015). Theorizing in Grounded Theory and creative abduction. *Quality & Quantity*, 2015, 1–16. DOI 10.1007/s11135-015-0248-3

Buck, H. G., Harkness, K., Wion, R., Carroll, S. L., Cosman, T., Kaasalainen, S., & Arthur, H. M. et al. (2015). Caregivers' contributions to heart failure self-care: A systematic review. *European Journal of Cardiovascular Nursing, 14*(1), 79–89. doi:10.1177/1474515113518434 PMID:24399843

Buckle, P. (2005). Ergonomics and musculoskeletal disorders: An overview. *Occupational Medicine, 55*(3), 164–167. doi:10.1093/occmed/kqi081 PMID:15857895

Butler, R. J., Johnson, W. G., & Coté, P. (2007). It pays to be nice: Employer-worker relationships and the management of back pain claims. *Journal of Occupational and Environmental Medicine, 49*, 214–225. doi:10.1097/jom.0b013e318032211d PMID:17293761

Buunk, B. P., Berkhuysen, M. A., Sanderman, R., Nieuwland, W., & Ranchon, A. V. (1996). The role of partner in heart disease: Active engagement, protective buffering, and overprotection. *Gedrag en Gezondheid, 24*, 304–313.

Cacace, M., Ettelt, S., Brereton, L., Pedersen, J., & Nolte, E. (2011). *How health systems make available information on service providers. Experience in seven countries.* United Kingdom: RAND and London School of Hygiene and Tropical Medicine.

Calciolari, G., & Montirosso, R. (2011). The sleep protection in the preterm infants. *The Journal of Maternal-Fetal & Neonatal Medicine, 24*(Suppl.1), 12–14. doi:10.3109/14767058.2011.607563 PMID:21942583

Campbell, S. M., Roland, M. O., & Buetow, S. A. (2000). Defining quality of care. *Social Science & Medicine, 51*(11), 1611–1625. doi:10.1016/S0277-9536(00)00057-5 PMID:11072882

Cancelliere, C., Cassidy, J. D., Ammendolia, C., & Côté, P. (2011). Are workplace health promotion programs effective at improving presenteeism in workers? A systematic review and best evidence synthesis of the literature. *BMC Public Health, 11*, 395. doi:10.1186/1471-2458-11-395 PMID:21615940

Cantù, C., & Tzannis, A. (2011). *From health service quality to health system quality. A network innovation adoption and diffusion* (Working paper). Retrieved from http://www.impgroup.org/uploads/papers/7696.pdf

Carey, R. G. (2003). *Improving healthcare with control charts: basic and advanced SPC methods and case studies.* Milwaukee: ASQ Quality Press.

Carman, K. L., Dardess, P., Maurer, M., Sofaer, S., Adams, K., Bechtel, C., & Sweeney, J. (2013). Patient and family engagement: A framework for understanding the elements and developing interventions and policies. *Health Affairs, 32*(2), 223–231. doi:10.1377/hlthaff.2012.1133 PMID:23381514

Carmichael, B. D. (1994). Business process reengineering: A remedy for health care. *Healthcare Management Forum, 7*(4), 44–50. doi:10.1016/S0840-4704(10)61077-0 PMID:10140167

Carnevale, F., Mendini, M., & Moriani, G. (Eds.). (2009). Bernardino Ramazzini. Works. Verona: Cierre Edizioni. CDC- Centers for Disease Control and Prevention. (1993). Investigations of persons treated by HIV-infected-health care workers. Morbility Mortality Weekly Report, 42, 329–331.

Carpenter, D. M., Elstad, E. A., Sage, A. J., Geryk, L. L., DeVellis, R. F., & Blalock, S. J. (2015). The relationship between partner information-seeking, information-sharing, and patient medication adherence. *Patient Education and Counseling*, *98*(1), 120–124. doi:10.1016/j.pec.2014.10.001 PMID:25455797

Carter, T., & Beresford, P. (2000). *Age and change: Models of involvement for older people*. New York, NY: Joseph Rowntree Foundation.

Cellini, E. (2008). *L'osservazione nelle scienze umane*. Milano: Franco Angeli.

Center for Advancing Health. (2010). *A New Definition of Patient Engagement: What is Engagement and Why is it Important?* Retrieved from http://www.cfah.org/pdfs/CFAH_Engagement_Behavior_Framework_current.pdf

Champagne, F. A., & Curley, J. P. (2009). Epigenetic mechanisms mediating the long-term effects of maternal care on development. *Neuroscience and Biobehavioral Reviews*, *33*(4), 593–600. doi:10.1016/j.neubiorev.2007.10.009 PMID:18430469

Chanlat, J. F. (2006). Space, organization and management thinking: a socio-historical perspective. In S. Clegg & M. Kornberger (Eds.), *Space, Organization and Management Theory* (pp. 17–43). Copenhagen: Copenhagen Business School Press.

Charles, C., Gafni, A., & Whelan, T. (1997). Shared decision-making in the medical encounter: What does it mean? (Or it takes, at least two to tango). *Social Science & Medicine*, *44*(5), 681–692. doi:10.1016/S0277-9536(96)00221-3 PMID:9032835

Charmaz, K. (1991). *Good days, bad days: The self in chronic illness and time*. New Brunswick, NJ: Rutgers University Press.

Charmaz, K. (2006). *Constructing Grounded A Practical Guide through Qualitative Analysis*. Rohnert Park: Sonoma State University.

Chassin, M. R., Loeb, J. M., Schmaltz, S. P., & Wachter, R. M. (2010). Accountability Measures - Using Measurement to Promote Quality Improvement. *The New England Journal of Medicine*, *363*(7), 683–688. doi:10.1056/NEJMsb1002320 PMID:20573915

Chau, C. M. Y., Ranger, M., Sulistyoningrum, D., Devlin, A. M., Oberlander, T. F., & Grunau, R. E. (2014). Neonatal pain and COMT Val158Met genotype in relation to serotonin transporter (SLC6A4) promoter methylation in very preterm children at school age. *Frontiers in Behavioral Neuroscience*, *8*, 1–12. doi:10.3389/fnbeh.2014.00409 PMID:25520635

Chiu, Y. C. (2010). What drives patients to sue doctors? The role of cultural factors in the pursuit of malpractice claims in Taiwan. *Social Science & Medicine*, *71*(4), 702–707. doi:10.1016/j.socscimed.2010.04.040 PMID:20646806

Choi, S. (2014). Flow, diversity, form, and influence of political talk in social-media-based public forums. *Human Communication Research*, *40*(2), 209–237. doi:10.1111/hcre.12023

Chretien, K., & Kind, T. (2013). Social media as a tool in medicine. *Circulation*, *127*, 1351–1443. doi:10.1161/CIRCULATIONAHA.112.128017

Chung, M. L., Moser, D. K., Lennie, T. A., & Rayers, M. K. (2009). The effect of depressive symptoms and anxiety on quality of life in patients with heart failure and their spouses: Testing dyadic using Actor-Partner Interdependence Model. *Journal of Psychosomatic Research*, *67*(1), 29–35. doi:10.1016/j.jpsychores.2009.01.009 PMID:19539816

Cigoli, V., & Scabini, E. (2006). *Family identity: Ties, symbols, and transitions*. New York: Lawrence Erlbaum Associates Publishers.

Clancy, C. M. (2011). Patient Engagement in Health Care. *Health Services Research*, *46*(2), 389–393. doi:10.1111/j.1475-6773.2011.01254.x PMID:21371026

Clegg, S. R., & Kornberger, M. (2006). *Space, Organizations and Management Theory*. Frederiksberg: CBS Press.

Cocker, F., Martin, A., Scott, J., Venn, A., Otahal, P., & Sanderson, K. (2011). Factors associated with presenteeism among employed Australian adults reporting lifetime major depression with 12-month symptoms. *Journal of Affective Disorders*, *135*(1-3), 231–240. doi:10.1016/j.jad.2011.07.028 PMID:21880374

Codman, E. A. (1975). *A Study of Hospital Efficiency: As Demonstrated by the Case Report of the First Five Years of a Private Hospital*. Joint Commission.

Coffeng, J. K., Hendriksen, I. J., Duijts, S. F., Twisk, J. W., van Mechelen, W., & Boot, C. R. (2014). Effectiveness of a combined social and physical environmental intervention on presenteeism, absenteeism, work performance, and work engagement in office employees. *Journal of Occupational and Environmental Medicine*, *56*(3), 258–265. doi:10.1097/JOM.0000000000000116 PMID:24603201

Cohen, G. A. (1989). On the Currency of Egalitarian Justice. *Ethics*, *99*(4), 906–944. doi:10.1086/293126

Cohen, G. A. (2008). *Rescuing justice and equality*. Cambridge, MA: Harvard University Press. doi:10.4159/9780674029651

Cohen, J. W. (1988). *Statistical power analysis for the behavioral sciences* (2nd ed.). Hillsdale, NJ: Lawrence Erlbaum Associates.

Collins, K., & Ison, R. (2006). Dare we jump off Arnstein's ladder? Social learning as a new policy paradigm. *Proceedings of the PATH Conference*, Scotland. Retrieved from http://www.macaulay.ac.uk/PATHconference/outputs/PATH_abstract_3.1.2.pdf

Collins, J., Baase, C., Shardra, C., Ozminkowski, R. J., Nicholson, S., & Billotti, G. M. et al. (2005). The assessment of chronic health conditions of work performance, absence, and total economic impact for employers. *Journal of Occupational and Environmental Medicine*, *47*(6), 547–557. doi:10.1097/01.jom.0000166864.58664.29 PMID:15951714

Collins, S. R., & Davis, K. (2006). *Transparency in Health Care: The Time Has Come*. The Commonwealth Fund.

Colmers, J. M. (2007). *Public Reporting and Transparency*. The Commonwealth Fund.

Cong, X., Ludington-Hoe, S. M., & Walsh, S. (2011). Randomized crossover trial of kangaroo care to reduce biobehavioral pain responses in preterm infants: A pilot study. *Biological Research for Nursing*, *13*(2), 204–216. doi:10.1177/1099800410385839 PMID:21196428

Conry, M. C., Humphries, N., Morgan, K., McGowan, Y., Montgomery, A., Vedhara, K., & Mc Gee, H. A. et al. (2012). A 10 year (2000-2010) systematic review of interventions to improve quality of care in hospitals. *Health Services Research*, *12*(1), 275. doi:10.1186/1472-6963-12-275 PMID:22925835

Cook, G., & Klein, B. (2005). Involvement of older people in care, service and policy planning. *International Journal of Older People Nursing in association with Journal of Clinical Nursing, 14*(S1), 43-47.

Cooper, C., Carpenter, I., Katona, C., Schroll, M., Wagner, C., Fialova, D., & Livingstone, G. (2005). The AdHOC study of older adults' adherence to medication in 11 countries. *The American Journal of Geriatric Psychiatry*, *13*(12), 1067–1076. doi:10.1097/00019442-200512000-00006 PMID:16319299

Corrigan, P. W., & Penn, D. L. (1999). Lessons from social psychology on discrediting psychiatric stigma. *The American Psychologist*, *54*(9), 765–776. doi:10.1037/0003-066X.54.9.765 PMID:10510666

Costand, M. K., MacDermid, J. C., Dal Bello-Hass, V., & Law, M. (2014). Scoping review of patient-centered care approaches in healthcare. *BMC Health Services Research*, *14*(1), 271. doi:10.1186/1472-6963-14-271 PMID:24947822

Coulson-Thomas, C. (1996). Re-engineering hospitals and health care processes. *British Journal of Health Care Management*, *2*(6), 338–342.

Coulter, A. (1997). Partnerships with patients: The pros and cons of shared clinical decision-making. *Journal of Health Services Research & Policy*, *2*, 112–121. PMID:10180362

Coulter, A. (2012). Patient engagement—what works? *The Journal of Ambulatory Care Management*, *35*(2), 80–89. doi:10.1097/JAC.0b013e318249e0fd PMID:22415281

Coulter, A., & Dunn, N. (2002). After Bristol: putting patients at the centre. Commentary: Patient centered care: timely, but is it practical? *British Medical Journal*, *324*(7338), 648–651. doi:10.1136/bmj.324.7338.648 PMID:11895824

Coulter, A., & Ellins, J. (2007). Effectiveness of strategies for informing, educating, and involving patients. *BMJ: British Medical Journal*, *335*(7609), 24–27. doi:10.1136/bmj.39246.581169.80 PMID:17615222

Cox, M., & Klinger, E. (2004). Systematic motivational counseling: The motivational structure questionnaire in action. In W. M. Cox & E. Klinger (Eds.), *Handbook of motivational counselling: Concepts, approaches, and assessment* (pp. 3–28). Chichester: John Willey & Sons.

Coyne, J. C., & DeLongis, A. (1986). Going beyond social support: The role of social relationships in adaptation. *Journal of Consulting and Clinical Psychology*, *54*(4), 454–460. doi:10.1037/0022-006X.54.4.454 PMID:3745597

Coyne, J. C., Ellard, J. H., & Smith, D. A. (1990). Unsupportive relationships, interdependence, and unhelpful exchanges. In I. G. Sarason, B. R. Sarason, & G. Pierce (Eds.), *Social support: An interactional view* (pp. 129–149). New York: Wiley.

Coyne, J. C., & Smith, D. A. F. (1991). Couples coping with a myocardial infarction: A contextual perspective on wives' distress. *Journal of Personality and Social Psychology*, *61*(3), 404–412. doi:10.1037/0022-3514.61.3.404 PMID:1941511

Crawford, E. R., Lepine, J. A., & Rich, B. L. (2010). Linking job demands and resources to employee engagement and burnout: A theoretical extension and meta-analytic test. *The Journal of Applied Psychology*, *95*(5), 834–848. doi:10.1037/a0019364 PMID:20836586

Crawford, J. O., Graveling, R. A., Cowie, H. A., & Dixon, K. (2010). The health safety and health promotion needs of older workers. *Occupational Medicine*, *60*(3), 184–192. doi:10.1093/occmed/kqq028 PMID:20423949

Crisp, R. (2013). *The Oxford handbook of the history of ethics*. Oxford: Oxford University Press. doi:10.1093/oxfordhb/9780199545971.001.0001

Crosby, P. B. (1979). *Quality is free: The art of making quality certain*. New York: McGraw Hill.

Cumming, E., & Henry, W. E. (1961). *Growing old: The process of disengagement*. New York, NY: Basic Books.

Cunliffe, A. L. (2003). Reflexive inquiry in organizational research: Questions and possibilities. *Human Relations*, *56*(8), 983–1003. doi:10.1177/00187267030568004

Cutrona, C. E. (1996). *Social support in couples: Marriage as a resource in times of stress*. Thousand Oaks: Sage. doi:10.4135/9781483327563

Dale, K., & Burrell, G. (2008). *The Spaces of Organization and the Organization of Space: Power Identity and Materiality at Work*. Basingstoke: Palgrave Macmillan.

Daley, D., Deane, K., Gray, R., Hill, R., & Myint, P. (2015). Qualitative evaluation of adherence therapy in Parkinson's disease: A multidirectional model. *Patient Preference and Adherence*, *9*, 989–998. doi:10.2147/PPA.S80158 PMID:26203231

Dall, T. M., Gallo, P. D., Chakrabarti, R., West, T., Semilla, A. P., & Storm, M. V. (2013). An aging population and growing disease burden will require a large and specialized health care workforce by 2025. *Health Affairs*, *32*(11), 2013–2020. doi:10.1377/hlthaff.2013.0714 PMID:24191094

Daly, J., Sindone, A. P., Thompson, D. R., Hancock, K., Chang, E., & Davidson, P. (2007). Barriers to participation in and adherence to cardiac rehabilitation programs: A critical literature review. *Progress in Cardiovascular Nursing*, *17*(1), 8–17. doi:10.1111/j.0889-7204.2002.00614.x PMID:11872976

Daniel, J. (2012). *Sampling essentials: Practical guidelines for making sampling choices*. Thousand Oaks, CA: Sage Publications Inc.

Daniels, N. (1985). *Just health care*. New York: Cambridge University Press. doi:10.1017/CBO9780511624971

Daniels, N. (2000). Accountability for reasonableness. *BMJ (Clinical Research Ed.)*, *321*(7272), 1300–1301. doi:10.1136/bmj.321.7272.1300 PMID:11090498

Daniels, N. (2007). *Just health: Meeting health needs fairly*. New York: Cambridge University Press. doi:10.1017/CBO9780511809514

Daskalki, M., Butler, G. L., & Petrovic, J. (2015). Somewhere In-Between: Narratives of Place, Identity, and Translocal Work. *Journal of Management Inquiry*, *7*(3).

Davies, T. (2009). The blossoming field of online deliberation. In *Online deliberation: Design, research, and practice* (pp. 1-19).

Davies, P., Taylor, F., Beswick, A., Wise, F., Moxham, T., Rees, K., & Ebrahim, S. (2010). Promoting patient uptake and adherence in cardiac rehabilitation. *Cochrane Database of Systematic Reviews*. doi:10.1002/14651858.CD007131.pub2 PMID:20614453

Davis, M. S. (1968). Variations in patients' compliance with doctors' advice: An empirical analysis of patterns of communication. *American Journal of Public Health*, *58*(2), 274–288. doi:10.2105/AJPH.58.2.274 PMID:5688773

Davis, M. S., & von der Lippe, R. P. (1968). Discharge from Hospital Against Medical Advice: A Study of Reciprocity in the Doctor-Patient Relationship. *Social Science & Medicine*, *1*, 336–342.

Davis, R. E., Jacklin, R., Sevdalis, N., & Vincent, C. A. (2007). Patient involvement in patient safety: What factors influence patient participation and engagement. *Health Expectations*, *10*(3), 259–267. doi:10.1111/j.1369-7625.2007.00450.x PMID:17678514

Davis, R. E., Koutantji, M., & Vincent, C. A. (2008). How willing are patients to question healthcare staff on issues related to the quality and safety of their healthcare? An exploratory study. *Quality & Safety in Health Care*, *17*(2), 90–96. doi:10.1136/qshc.2007.023754 PMID:18385400

Dawson, A. P., McLennan, S. N., Schiller, S. D., Jull, G. A., Hodges, P. W., & Stewart, S. (2007). Interventions to prevent back pain and back injury in nurses: A systematic review. *Occupational and Environmental Medicine*, *64*(10), 642–650. doi:10.1136/oem.2006.030643 PMID:17522134

De Certeau, M. (1990). *L'invention du quotidien. 1. Arts de faire*. Paris: Gallimard.

De Cindio, F., Macintosh, A., & Peraboni, C. (2010). From e-Participation to Online Deliberation.*Proceedings of the Fourth International Conference on Online Deliberation OD2010*, Leeds, UK.

De Haes, H. (2006). Dilemmas in patient centerdness and shared decision making: A case for vulnerability. *Patient Education and Counseling*, *62*(3), 291–298. doi:10.1016/j.pec.2006.06.012 PMID:16859860

Dearing, R. L., Barrick, C., Dermen, K. H., & Walitzer, K. S. (2005). Indicators of client engagement: Influences on alcohol treatment satisfaction and outcomes. *Psychology of Addictive Behaviors*, *19*(1), 71–78. doi:10.1037/0893-164X.19.1.71 PMID:15783280

Dekel, R., Vilchinsky, N., Liberman, G., Leibowitz, M., Khaskia, A., & Mosseri, M. (2014). Marital satisfaction and depression among couples following men's acute coronary syndrome: Testing dyadic dynamics in a longitudinal design. *British Journal of Health Psychology*, *19*(2), 347–362. doi:10.1111/bjhp.12042 PMID:23552169

DeLongis, A., & O'Brien, T. (1990). An interpersonal framework for stress and coping: An application to the families of alzheimer's patients. In M. A. P. Stephens, J. H. Crowther, S. E. Hobfoll, & D. L. Tennenbaum (Eds.), *Stress and coping in later-life families* (pp. 221–240). New York: Hemisphere Publishing Corporation.

Deming, W. E. (1986). *Out of the crisis*. Cambridge, MA: Centre of Advanced Engineering Study, MIT.

Department of Health. (1998). *A first class service: quality in the new NHS*. London: HMSO.

Devlin, A. M., Brain, U., Austin, J., & Oberlander, T. F. (2010). Prenatal exposure to maternal depressed mood and the MTHFR C677T variant affect SLC6A4 methylation in infants at birth. *PLoS ONE*, *5*(8), e12201. doi:10.1371/journal.pone.0012201 PMID:20808944

Di Nunno, N., Vimercati, L., Viola, L., & Vimercati, F. (2005). Epidemiological case survey of medical malpractice in some medical and surgical specialties. *Forensic Science International*, *149*(2-3), 139–142. doi:10.1016/j.forsciint.2004.06.029 PMID:15749354

Diamond, J. (2005). *Collapse: How societies choose to fail or succeed*. New York: Viking.

DiBonaventura, M. C., Gupta, S., McDonald, M., & Sadosky, A. (2011). Evaluating the health and economic impact of osteoarthritis pain in the workforce: Results from the National Health and Wellness Survey. *BMC Musculoskeletal Disorders*, *12*(1), 83. doi:10.1186/1471-2474-12-83 PMID:21527024

DiBonaventura, M., Paulose-Ram, R., Su, J., McDonald, M., Zou, K. H., Wagner, J. S., & Shah, H. (2012). The impact of COPD on quality of life, productivity loss, and resource use among the elderly United States workforce. *Chronic Obstructive Pulmonary Disease.*, *9*(1), 46–57. doi:10.3109/15412555.2011.634863 PMID:22292597

Dickerson, S. S., Posluszny, M., & Kennedy, M. C. (2000). Help seeking in a support group for recipients of implantable cardioverter defibrillators and their support persons. *Heart & Lung*, *29*(2), 87–96. doi:10.1067/mhl.2000.104138 PMID:10739484

Dickson, A., Allan, D., & O'Carroll, R. (2008). Biographical disruption and the experience of loss following a spinal cord injury: An interpretative phenomenological analysis. *Psychology & Health*, *23*(4), 407–425. doi:10.1080/14768320701219136 PMID:25160576

Dijkers, M. P., Yavuzer, G., Ergin, S., Weitzenkamp, D., & Whiteneck, G. G. (2002). A tale of two countries: Environmental impacts on social participation after spinal cord injury. *Spinal Cord*, *40*(7), 351–362. doi:10.1038/sj.sc.3101310 PMID:12080463

DiMatteo, M. R. (2004). Variations in patients' adherence to medical recommendations: A quantitative review of 50 years of research. *Medical Care*, *42*(3), 200–209. doi:10.1097/01.mlr.0000114908.90348.f9 PMID:15076819

DiMatteo, M. R., Reiter, R. C., & Gambone, J. C. (1994). Enhancing medication adherence through communication and informed collaborative choice. *Health Communication*, *6*(4), 253–265. doi:10.1207/s15327027hc0604_2

Diniz, A. M., & Amado, N. (2014). Procedures for successful data collection through psychological tests in the elderly. *Psychology/Psicologia. Reflexão e Crítica, 27*(3), 491–497. doi:10.1590/1678-7153.201427309

Dixon-Woods, M. (2010). Why is patient safety so hard? A selective review of ethnographic studies. *Journal of Health Services Research & Policy, 15*(Suppl. 1), 11–16. doi:10.1258/jhsrp.2009.009041 PMID:20075122

Domingos, S. (2014). *Alimentação com conta, peso e medida: Um estudo exploratório da representação mental e da quantificação subjetiva do consumo de carne vermelha, numa amostra de idosos.* [Estimating, weighing and measuring food consumption: An exploratory study of the mental representation and subjective quantification of meat consumption, in an elderly sample] [Master thesis]. University of Évora, Évora, Portugal.

Donabedian, A. (1966). Evaluating the quality of medical care. *The Milbank Memorial Fund Quarterly, 44*(3), 166–206. doi:10.2307/3348969 PMID:5338568

Donabedian, A. (1980). The Definition of Quality and Approaches to Its Assessment (Vol. 1). *Explorations in Quality Assessment and Monitoring.* Ann Arbor, MI: Health Administration Press.

Donabedian, A. (1988). The Quality of Care How Can It Be Assessed? *Journal of the American Medical Association, 260*(12), 1743–1748. doi:10.1001/jama.1988.03410120089033 PMID:3045356

Donabedian, A. (1990). The seven pillars of quality. *Archives of Pathology & Laboratory Medicine, 114*, 1115–1118. PMID:2241519

Donabedian, A. (2005). Evaluating the quality of medical care. *The Milbank Quarterly, 83*(4), 691–729. doi:10.1111/j.1468-0009.2005.00397.x PMID:16279964

Donato, S. (2014). Il coping diadico, ovvero far fronte allo stress insieme: Una rassegna della letteratura. *Giornale Italiano di Psicologia, 36*, 471–499. doi:10.1421/78499

Donato, S., Canzi, E., Parise, M., & Ferrari, L. (2014). Partnership Questionnaire: Factorial structure, gender invariance, and concurrent validity. *TPM - Testing, Psychometrics. Methodology in Applied Psychology, 21*, 161–180. doi:10.4473/TPM21.2.4

Donato, S., Iafrate, R., Barni, D., Bertoni, A., Bodenmann, G., & Gagliardi, S. (2009). Measuring dyadic coping: The factorial structure of Bodenmann's "Dyadic Coping Questionnaire" in an Italian sample. *TPM - Testing, Psychometrics. Methodology in Applied Psychology, 16*, 25–47.

Donato, S., Iafrate, R., Bradbury, T. N., & Scabini, E. (2012). Acquiring dyadic coping: Partners and parents as models. *Personal Relationships, 19*(2), 386–400. doi:10.1111/j.1475-6811.2011.01368.x

Donato, S., & Parise, M. (2012). The role of enacted and perceived dyadic coping for young couples' satisfaction. In B. Molinelli & V. Grimaldo (Eds.), *Handbook of the Psychology of Coping: New research* (pp. 261–278). Hauppauge, NY: Nova Science Publisher.

Donato, S., Parise, M., Iafrate, R., Bertoni, A., Finkenauer, C., & Bodenmann, G. (2015). Dyadic coping responses and partners' perceptions for relationship satisfaction: An actor-partner longitudinal analysis. *Journal of Social and Personal Relationships, 32*, 580–600. doi:10.1177/0265407514541071

Donato, S., Parise, M., Pagani, A. F., Bertoni, A., & Iafrate, R. (2014). Demand-withdraw, couple satisfaction and relationship duration. *Procedia: Social and Behavioral Sciences, 140*, 200–206. doi:10.1016/j.sbspro.2014.04.410

Donnini, M., & Lumini, E. (2008). Non aprite quella porta. Le percezioni e i bisogni dei familiari in sala di attesa. *Paper presented at 27' Aniarti Conference/3rd EfCCNa Congress: Influencing Critical Care Nursing in Europe*, Florence.

Douglas, K. M. (2007). Psychology, discrimination and hate groups online. In A. N. Joinson, K. Y. A. McKenna, T. Postmes, & U. D. Reips (Eds.), *The Oxford handbook of Internet psychology* (pp. 155–163). Oxford: Oxford University Press.

Douglas, K. M., & McGarty, C. (2002). Internet identifiability and beyond: A model of the effects of identifiability on communicative behavior. *Group Dynamics*, *6*(1), 17–26. doi:10.1037/1089-2699.6.1.17

Duke, C. C., Lynch, W. D., Smith, B., & Winstanley, J. (2015). Validity of a New Patient Engagement Measure: The Altarum Consumer Engagement (ACE) Measure™. *The Patient-Patient-Centered Outcomes Research*, *8*(6), 559–568. doi:10.1007/s40271-015-0131-2 PMID:26097010

Dunstan, D. A., & Maceachen, E. (2014). A theoretical model of co-worker responses to work reintegration processes. *Journal of Occupational Rehabilitation*, *24*(2), 189–198. doi:10.1007/s10926-013-9461-x PMID:23912179

Dunston, R., Lee, A., Boud, D., Brodie, P., & Chiarella, M. (2009). Co-Production and Health System Reform–From Re-Imagining To Re-Making. *Australian Journal of Public Administration*, *68*(1), 39–52. doi:10.1111/j.1467-8500.2008.00608.x

Durand, M. A., Moulton, B., Cockle, E., Mann, M., & Elwyn, G. (2015). Can shared decision-making reduce medical malpractice litigation? A systematic review. *BMC Health Services Research*, *15*(1), 167. doi:10.1186/s12913-015-0823-2 PMID:25927953

Eagle, C. J., & Davies, J. M. (1993). Current models of "quality" – an introduction for anaesthetists. *Canadian Journal of Anaesthesia*, *40*(9), 851–862. doi:10.1007/BF03009257 PMID:8403179

Eaton, S., Roberts, S., & Turner, B. (2015). Delivering person centred care in long term conditions. *British Medical Journal*, *350*(feb10 14), 181. doi:10.1136/bmj.h181 PMID:25670186

Edwards, W. (1962). Dynamic decision theory and probabilistic information processings. *Human Factors: The Journal of the Human Factors and Ergonomics Society*, *4*(2), 59–74.

Ekman, I., Wolf, A., Olsson, L. E., Taft, C., Dudas, K., Schaufelberger, M., & Swedberg, K. (2012). Effects of person-centred care in patients with chronic heart failure: The PCC-HF study. *European Heart Journal*, *33*(9), 1112–1119. doi:10.1093/eurheartj/ehr306 PMID:21926072

Ekman, J., & Amnå, E. (2012). Political participation and civic engagement: Towards a new typology. *Human Affairs*, *22*(3), 283–300. doi:10.2478/s13374-012-0024-1

el-Kebbi, I. M., Ziemer, D. C., Gallina, D. L., Dunbar, V., & Phillips, L. S. (1999). Diabetes in urban African-Americans. XV: Identification of barriers to provider adherence to management protocols. *Diabetes Care*, *22*(10), 1617–1620. doi:10.2337/diacare.22.10.1617 PMID:10526724

Ellemers, N. (2002). Social identity and relative deprivation. In I. Walker & H. Smith (Eds.), *Relative deprivation: Specification, development and integration* (pp. 239–264). Cambridge, UK: Cambridge University Press.

Ellis, R., & Whittington, R. (1993). *Quality assurance in health care: A handbook*. London: Arnold.

Emanuel, E. J., & Emanuel, L. L. (1996). What Is Accountability in Health Care? *Annals of Internal Medicine*, *124*(2), 229–239. doi:10.7326/0003-4819-124-2-199601150-00007 PMID:8533999

Endler, N. S., & Parker, J. D. A. (1990). Multidimensional assessment of coping: A critical evaluation. *Journal of Personality and Social Psychology*, *58*(5), 844–854. doi:10.1037/0022-3514.58.5.844 PMID:2348372

Engel, G. L. (1977). The need for a new medical model: A challenge for biomedicine. *Science*, *196*(4286), 129–136. doi:10.1126/science.847460 PMID:847460

Engel, G. L. (1981). The clinical application of the biopsychosocial model. *The Journal of Medicine and Philosophy*, *6*(2), 101–124. doi:10.1093/jmp/6.2.101 PMID:7264472

Essex, M. J., Boyce, W. T., Hertzman, C., Lam, L. L., Armstrong, J. M., Neumann, S. M., & Kobor, M. S. (2013). Epigenetic vestiges of early developmental adversity: Childhood stress exposure and DNA methylation in adolescence. *Child Development*, *84*(1), 58–75. doi:10.1111/j.1467-8624.2011.01641.x PMID:21883162

European Commission. (2012). The 2012 Ageing Report: Economic and budgetary projections for the EU27 Member States (2010-2060), European Economy 2/2012.

European Commission. (2014). *The 2015 Ageing Report. Underlying Assumptions and Projection Methodologies*. Retrieved from http://ec.europa.eu/economy_finance/publications/european_economy/2014/pdf/ee8_en.pdf

Evans, S., & Vallely, S. (2007). *Social well-being in extra care housing*. New York, NY: Joseph Rowntree Foundation.

Evenson, K. R., & Fleury, J. (2000). Barriers to outpatient cardiac rehabilitation participation and *adherence. Journal of Cardiopulmonary Rehabilitation*, *20*(4), 241–246. doi:10.1097/00008483-200007000-00005 PMID:10955265

Faber, M., Bosch, M., Wollersheim, H., Leatherman, S., & Grol, R. (2009). Public reporting in health care: How do consumers use quality-of-care information? A systematic review. *Medical Care*, *47*(1), 1–8. doi:10.1097/MLR.0b013e3181808bb5 PMID:19106724

Fagiolini, M., Jensen, C. L., & Champagne, F. A. (2009). Epigenetic influences on brain development and plasticity. *Current Opinion in Neurobiology*, *19*(2), 207–212. doi:10.1016/j.conb.2009.05.009 PMID:19545993

Falanga, R. (2013). Participation and Public Sector: A Democratic Challenge. *Universitas Humanas*, *10*, 11–20.

Falanga, R. (2014). Changes need change. A psychosociological perspective on participation and social inclusion. *Rivista di Psicologia Clinica*, *2*, 24–38.

Farrington, J., Bebbington, A., Wellard, K., & Lewis, D. J. (1993). *Reluctant Partners: Non-governmental Organisations, the State and Sustainable Agricultural Development*. London: Routledge.

Feldman, R., Eidelman, A. I., Sirota, L., & Weller, A. (2002). Comparison of skin-to-skin (kangaroo) and traditional care: Parenting outcomes and preterm infant development. *Pediatrics*, *110*(1), 16–26. doi:10.1542/peds.110.1.16 PMID:12093942

Ferlie, E., Fitzgerald, L., Wood, M., & Hawkins, C. (2013). The Nonspread of Innovations: The Mediating Role of Professionals. *Academy of Management Journal*, *48*(1), 117–134. doi:10.5465/AMJ.2005.15993150

Ferrie, J. E., Virtanen, M., & Kivimaki, M. (2014). The healthy population-high disability paradox. *Occupational and Environmental Medicine*, *71*(4), 232–233. doi:10.1136/oemed-2013-101945 PMID:24492070

Ficarra, B. J. (1976). A history of legal medicine. In C. Wecht (Ed.), *Legal medicine annual*. New York: Appleton Century Crofts.

Field, D., Draper, E. S., Fenton, A., Papiernik, E., Zeitlin, J., Blondel, B., & Van Reempts, P. et al. (2009). Rates of very preterm birth in Europe and neonatal mortality rates. *Archives of Disease in Childhood. Fetal and Neonatal Edition*, *94*(4), F253–F256. doi:10.1136/adc.2008.150433 PMID:19066186

Fileni, A., & Magnavita, N. (1995). Malpractice lawsuits in Radiology - Comparison of the Italian and American situations. *Radiology*, *197*(2), 548–549. doi:10.1148/radiology.197.2.548-b PMID:7480715

Finucane, M. L., & Lees, N. B. (2005). Decision-making competence of older adults: Models and methods. Retrieved from http://citeseerx.ist.psu.edu/viewdoc/download?doi=10.1.1.116.7585&rep=rep1&type=pdf

Fischer, F. (2003). *Reframing Public Policy. Discursive Politics and Deliberative Practices*. New York, NY: Oxford University Press. doi:10.1093/019924264X.001.0001

Fiske, V., Coyne, J. C., & Smith, D. A. (1991). Couples coping with myocardial infarction: An empirical reconsideration of the role of overprotectiveness. *Journal of Family Psychology*, *5*(1), 4–20. doi:10.1037/0893-3200.5.1.4

Flacking, R., Ewald, U., Nyqvist, K. H., & Starrin, B. (2006). Trustful bonds: A key to "becoming a mother" and to reciprocal breastfeeding. Stories of mothers of very preterm infants at a neonatal unit. *Social Science & Medicine*, *62*(1), 70–80http://www.scopus.com/inward/record.url?eid=2-s2.0-28444467433&partnerID=40&md5=3132a5f7c93c56a18 7af23f82e6cc43c. doi:10.1016/j.socscimed.2005.05.026 PMID:15992983

Fleischacker, S. (2004). *A short history of distributive justice*. Cambridge, MA: Harvard University Press.

Folger, R. (1986). A referent cognitions theory of relative deprivation. In J. M. Olson, C. P. Herman, & M. P. Zanna (Eds.), *Relative deprivationand social comparison: The Ontario symposium* (Vol. 4, pp. 217–242). Hillsdale, NJ: Erlbaum.

Folger, R. (1987). Reformulating the conditions of resentment: A referent cognition model. In J. C. Masters & W. P. Smith (Eds.), *Social comparison, social justice, and relative deprivation* (pp. 183–215). London: Erlbaum.

Fortin, A. H., Dwamena, F. C., Frankel, R. M., & Smith, R. C. (2012). *Smith's Patient Centered Interviewing: An Evidence-Based Method: An Evidence-Based Method*. McGraw Hill Professional.

Foster, M. D. (2015). Tweeting about sexism: The well-being benefits of a social media collective action. *The British Journal of Social Psychology*, *54*(4), 629–647. doi:10.1111/bjso.12101 PMID:25639601

Francis, D., Diorio, J., Liu, D., & Meaney, M. J. (1999). Nongenomic transmission across generations of maternal behavior and stress responses in the rat. *Science*, *286*(5442), 1155–1158. doi:10.1126/science.286.5442.1155 PMID:10550053

Frank, A. W. (1997). Enacting illness stories: When, what, and why. In H. L. Nelson (Ed.), *Stories and their limits: Narrative approach to bioethics* (pp. 31–49). New York: Routledge.

Freidson, E. (1988). *Profession of Medicine. A Study of sociology of applied knowledge*. Chicago: The University of Chicago Press.

French, D. P., Cooper, A., & Weinman, J. (2006, December). Illness perceptions predict attendance at cardiac rehabilitation following acute myocardial infarction: A systematic review with meta-analysis. *Journal of Psychosomatic Research*, *61*(6), 757–767. doi:10.1016/j.jpsychores.2006.07.029 PMID:17141663

Freund, P., & McGuire, M. (1999). *Health, illness, andthe social body: A critical sociology*. Upper Saddle River, NJ: Prentice Hall.

Frohlich, D. O., & Zmyslinski-Seelig, A. N. (in press). How Uncover Ostomy challenges ostomy stigma, and encourages others to do the same. *New Media & Society*. doi:1461444814541943

Fung, A. (2006). Varieties of Participation in Complex Governance. *Public Administration Review*, *66*(s1), 66–75. doi:10.1111/j.1540-6210.2006.00667.x

Gagliardi, S., Bodenmann, G., Heinrichs, N., Bertoni, A., Iafrate, R., & Donato, S. (2013). Unterschiede in der Partnerschaftsqualität und imdyadischen Coping beiverschiedenenbindungsbezogenenPaartypen[Differences in relationship quality and dyadic coping for attachment-related couple types]. *Psychotherapie, Psychosomatik, Medizinische Psychologie*, *63*, 185–192. doi:10.1055/s-0032-1333291

Gambetti, R. C., & Graffigna, G. (2010). The concept of engagement: A systematic analysis of the ongoing marketing debate. *International Journal of Market Research*, *52*(6), 7. doi:10.2501/S147078531020166

Gamson, W. A. (1992). The social psychology of collective action. In A. D. Morris & C. M. Mueller (Eds.), *Frontiers in social movement theory* (pp. 53–76). New Haven, CT: Yale University Press.

Garbarino, S., & Magnavita, N. (2014). Obstructive sleep apnea syndrome (OSAS), metabolic syndrome and mental health in small enterprise workers. Feasibility of an action for health. *PLoS ONE*, *9*(5), e97188. doi:10.1371/journal.pone.0097188 PMID:24810290

Gasbarrini, M. F., Snyder, D. K., Iafrate, R., Bertoni, A., Donato, S., & Margola, D. (in press). Investigating the Relation Between Shared Stressors and Marital Satisfaction: The Moderating Effects of Dyadic Coping and Communication. *Special Section of Family Science*. doi:10.1080/19424620.2015.1082044

Gaspar, R., Carvalho, J., Luís, S., & Lima, M. L. (2014). Food risk communication: Empirical studies and practical resources. *Transcultural*, *4*, 25–37.

Gaspar, R., Luís, S., Seibt, B., Lima, M. L., Marcu, A., Rutsaert, P., & Barnett, J. et al. (2015). Consumers' avoidance of information on red meat risks: Information exposure effects on attitudes and perceived knowledge. *Journal of Risk Research*, 1–17. doi:10.1080/13669877.2014.1003318

Gaventa, J. (2006). Finding the spaces for change: A power analysis. *Ids Bulletin-Institute of Development Studies*, *37*(6), 23–33. doi:10.1111/j.1759-5436.2006.tb00320.x

Gee, A., Khalaf, A., & McGarty, C. (2007). Using group-based interaction to change stereotypes about people with mental disorders. *Australian Psychologist*, *42*(2), 98–105. doi:10.1080/00050060701280581

Gerteis, M., Edgman-Levitan, S., Daley, J., & Delbanco, T. (1993). *Through the patient's eyes: Understanding and Promoting Patient-Centered Care Paperback*. San Francisco: Jossey-Bass.

Gesler, W. M. (1992). Therapeutic landscapes: Medical issues in light of the new cultural geography. *Social Science & Medicine*, *34*(7), 735–746. doi:10.1016/0277-9536(92)90360-3 PMID:1376497

Gifford, B., & Jinnett, K. (2014). Employees' work responses to episodes of illness: Evidence from the American time use survey. *Journal of Occupational and Environmental Medicine*, *56*(2), 224–229. doi:10.1097/JOM.0000000000000090 PMID:24504249

Gilardi, S., Guglielmetti, C., Casati, S., & Monti, P. (2014). Promuovere l'engagement dei pazienti con malattie croniche: un percorso di ricerca collaborativa. *Psicologia della salute, 3*(3), 58-79.

Gilleard, C., & Higgs, P. (1998). Old people as users and consumers of healthcare: A third age rhetoric for a fourth age reality? *Ageing and Society*, *18*(2), 233–248. doi:10.1017/S0144686X98006904

Gilmour, J. A. (2006). Hybrid space: Constituting the hospital as a home space for patients. *Nursing Inquiry*, *13*(1), 16–22. doi:10.1111/j.1440-1800.2006.00276.x PMID:16494663

Glaser, B. G. (2004). Remodeling Grounded Theory. *Forum Qualitative Social Research*, 5(2). Retrieved from http://nbn-resolving.de/urn:nbn:de:0114-fqs040245

Glaser, B. G., & Strauss, A. L. (1965). *Awareness of Dying*. Chicago, IL: Aldine Pub. Co.

Glaser, B. G., & Strauss, A. L. (1967). *The Discovery of Grounded Theory: strategies for qualitative research*. Chicago: Aldine de Gruyter.

Glendinning, C. (2008). Increasing Choice and Control for Older and Disabled People: A Critical review of New Developments in England. *Social Policy and Administration*, *42*(5), 451–469. doi:10.1111/j.1467-9515.2008.00617.x

Gobo, G. (2001). *Descrivere il mondo. Teoria e pratica del metodo etnografico in sociologia*. Roma: Carocci.

Godinho, C., Alvarez, M. J., & Lima, M. L. (2013). Formative research on HAPA model determinants for fruit and vegetable intake: Target beliefs for audiences at different stages of change. *Health Education Research*, *28*(6), 1014–1028. doi:10.1093/her/cyt076 PMID:23856178

Goffman, E. (1961). *Asylums: Essays on the Social Situation of Mental Patients and Other Inmates*. New York: Doubleday Anchor.

Goodin, R. E. (1992). *Motivating political morality*. Oxford: Wiley–Blackwell.

Gorli, M., Galuppo, L., & Liberati, E. G. (2015a). Hospital innovations in the light of patient engagement. Insights from the organizational field. In G. Graffigna, S. Barello, & S. Triberti (Eds.), *Patient engagement: a consumer-centered model to innovate healthcare* (pp. 120–137). Warsaw, Poland: Gruyter Open. doi:10.1515/9783110452440-011

Gorli, M., Nicolini, D., & Scaratti, G. (2015b). Reflexivity in practice. Tools and conditions for developing organizational authorship. *Human Relations*, *68*(8), 1347–1375. doi:10.1177/0018726714556156

Graffigna, G., Barello, S., Bonanomi, A., Menichetti, J. (in press). The Motivating Function of Healthcare Professional in eHealth and mHealth Interventions for Type 2 Diabetes Patients and the Mediating Role of Patient Engagement, *Journal of Diabetes Research.*

Graffigna, G., Barello, S., Riva, G., & Bosio, A. C. (2014a). Patient Engagement: The Key to Redesign the Exchange Between the Demand and Supply for Healthcare in the Era of Active Ageing. *Active Ageing and Healthy Living: A Human Centered Approach in Research and Innovation as Source of Quality of Life, 203*, 85

Graffigna, G., & Barello, S. (2015). Modelling Patient Engagement in Healthcare: Insight for Research and Practice. In G. Graffigna, S. Barello, & S. Triberti (Eds.), *Patient Engagement: a consumer-centered model to innovate healthcare* (pp. 27–43). Warsaw, Poland: De Gruyter Open. doi:10.1515/9783110452440-004

Graffigna, G., Barello, S., Bonanomi, A., & Lozza, E. (2015a). Measuring patient engagement: Development and psychometric properties of the patient health engagement (PHE) scale. *Frontiers in Psychology*, 2015, 6. PMID:25870566

Graffigna, G., Barello, S., Bonanomi, A., & Lozza, E. (2015a). Measuring patient engagement: Development and psychometric properties of the Patient Health Engagement (PHE) scale. *Frontiers in Psychology*, 2015, 6. PMID:25870566

Graffigna, G., Barello, S., Bonanomi, A., Lozza, E., & Hibbard, J. (2015b). Measuring patient activation in Italy: Translation, adaptation and validation of the Italian version of the patient activation measure 13 (PAM13-I). *BMC Medical Informatics and Decision Making*, *15*(1), 1. doi:10.1186/s12911-015-0232-9 PMID:26699852

Graffigna, G., Barello, S., Libreri, C., & Bosio, C. A. (2014b). How to engage type-2 diabetic patients in their own health management: Implications for clinical practice. *BMC Public Health*, *14*(1), 648. doi:10.1186/1471-2458-14-648 PMID:24966036

Graffigna, G., Barello, S., & Riva, G. (2013). Technologies for patient engagement. *Health Affairs*, *32*(6), 1172. doi:10.1377/hlthaff.2013.0279 PMID:23733998

Graffigna, G., Barello, S., Riva, G., & Bosio, A. C. (2014). Patient engagement: The key to redesign the exchange between the demand and supply for healthcare in the era of active ageing. *Active Ageing and Healthy Living*, *203*, 85–95. doi:10.3233/978-1-61499-425-1-85 PMID:26630515

Graffigna, G., Barello, S., Riva, G., & Bosio, A. C. (2014). Patient Engagement: The Key to Redesign the Exchange Between the Demand and Supply for Healthcare in the Era of Active Ageing. *Studies in Health Technology and Informatics*, *203*, 85–95. PMID:26630515

Graffigna, G., Barello, S., Riva, G., & Bosio, A. C. (2014). Patient engagement: the key to redesign the exchange in between the demand and supply for healthcare in the era of active ageing. In G. Riva, P. Ajmone Marsan, & C. Grassi (Eds.), *Active Ageing and Healthy Living: A Human Centered Approach in Research and Innovation as Source of Quality of Life* (pp. 85–95). Amsterdam: IOS Press.

Graffigna, G., Barello, S., Riva, G., & Bosio, C. (2014). Patient Engagement: The Key to Redesign the Exchange Between the Demand and Supply for Healthcare in the Era of Active Ageing. In *G. Riva, P. Ajmone Marsan & C. Grasso, Active Ageing and Healthy Living* (pp. 85–95). Amsterdam: IOS Press.

Graffigna, G., Barello, S., & Triberti, S. (2015b). *Patient engagement: a consumer-centered model to innovate healthcare*. Warsaw, Poland: DeGruyter Open. doi:10.1515/9783110452440

Graffigna, G., Barello, S., Wiederhold, B. K., Bosio, A. C., & Riva, G. (2013). Positive technology as a driver for health engagement. *Studies in Health Technology and Informatics*, *191*, 9–17. PMID:23792833

Grant, J. S., Glandon, G. L., Elliot, T. R., Giger, J. N., & Weaver, M. (2004). Caregiving problems and feelings experienced by family caregivers of stroke survivors the first month after discharge. *International Journal of Rehabilitation Research. Internationale Zeitschrift fur Rehabilitationsforschung. Revue Internationale de Recherches de Readaptation*, *27*(2), 105–111. doi:10.1097/01.mrr.0000127639.47494.e3 PMID:15167107

Graven, S. N. (2004). Early neurosensory visual development of the fetus and newborn. *Clinics in Perinatology*, *31*(2), 199–216. doi:10.1016/j.clp.2004.04.010 PMID:15289028

Greeneich, D. (1993). The link between new and return business and quality of care: Patient satisfaction. *ANS. Advances in Nursing Science*, *16*(1), 62–72. doi:10.1097/00012272-199309000-00008 PMID:8311426

Greene, J., & Hibbard, J. H. (2012). Why does patient activation matter? An examination of the relationships between patient activation and health-related outcomes. *Journal of General Internal Medicine*, *27*(5), 520–526. doi:10.1007/s11606-011-1931-2 PMID:22127797

Greene, S. M., Tuzzio, L., & Cherkin, D. (2012). A framework for making patient-centered care front and center. *The Permanente Journal*, *16*(3), 49–53. PMID:23012599

Greisen, G., Mirante, N., Haumont, D., Pierrat, V., Pallás-Alonso, C. R., & Warren, I. et al. (2009). Parents, siblings and grandparents in the Neonatal Intensive Care Unit A survey of policies in eight European countries. *Acta Paediatrica: International Journal of Pediatrics*, *98*(11), 1744–1750.

Griffin, K. W., Friend, R., Kaell, A. T., & Bennet, R. S. (2001). Distress and disease status among patients with rheumatoid arthritis: Roles of coping styles and perceived responses from support providers. *Annals of Behavioral Medicine*, *23*(2), 133–138. doi:10.1207/S15324796ABM2302_8 PMID:11394555

Griffiths, B. B., & Hunter, R. G. (2014). Neuroepigenetics of stress. *Neuroscience*, *275*, 420–435. doi:10.1016/j.neuroscience.2014.06.041 PMID:24976514

Groene, O., Kringos, D., Sunol, R. (2014). *Seven ways to improve quality and safety in hospitals. An evidence-based guide*. DUQuE Collaboration.

Gruman, J., Rovner, M. H., French, M. E., Jeffress, D., Sofaer, S., Shaller, D., & Prager, D. J. (2010). From patient education to patient engagement: Implications for the field of patient education. *Patient Education and Counseling*, *78*(3), 350–356. doi:10.1016/j.pec.2010.02.002 PMID:20202780

Grunau, R. E. (2013). Neonatal pain in very preterm infants: Long-term effects on brain, neurodevelopment and pain reactivity. *Rambam Maimonides Medical Journal*, *4*(4), e0025. PMID:24228168

Grunau, R. E., Holsti, L., Haley, D. W., Oberlander, T., Weinberg, J., Solimano, A., & Yu, W. et al. (2005). Neonatal procedural pain exposure predicts lower cortisol and behavioral reactivity in preterm infants in the NICU. *Pain*, *113*(3), 293–300. doi:10.1016/j.pain.2004.10.020 PMID:15661436

Grunau, R. E., Whitfield, M. F., Petrie-Thomas, J., Synnes, A. R., Cepeda, I. L., Keidar, A., & Johannesen, D. et al. (2009). Neonatal pain, parenting stress and interaction, in relation to cognitive and motor development at 8 and 18 months in preterm infants. *Pain*, *143*(1-2), 138–146. doi:10.1016/j.pain.2009.02.014 PMID:19307058

Grüninger, U. J. (1995). Patient education: An example of one-to-one communication. *Journal of Human Hypertension*, *9*(1), 15–25. PMID:7730996

Guyatt, G. H., Mulla, S. M., Scott, I. A., Jackevicius, C. A., & You, J. J. (2014). Patient engagement and shared decision-making. *Journal of General Internal Medicine*, *29*(4), 562. doi:10.1007/s11606-013-2727-3 PMID:24464283

Hagedoorn, M., Dagan, M., Puterman, E., Hoff, C., Meijerink, W. J., Delongis, A., & Sanderman, R. (2011). Relationship satisfaction in couples confronted with colorectal cancer: The interplay of past and current spousal support. *Journal of Behavioral Medicine*, *34*(4), 288–297. doi:10.1007/s10865-010-9311-7 PMID:21222025

Hagedoorn, M., Kuijer, R. G., Buunk, B. P., DeJong, G. M., Wobbes, T., & Sanderman, R. (2000). Marital satisfaction in patients with cancer: Does support from intimate partners benefit those who need it most? *Health Psychology*, *19*(3), 274–282. doi:10.1037/0278-6133.19.3.274 PMID:10868772

Hagedoorn, M., Sanderman, R., Bolks, H., Tuinstra, J., & Coyne, J. C. (2008). Distress in couples coping with cancer: A meta-analysis and critical review of role and gender effects. *Psychological Bulletin*, *134*(1), 1–30. doi:10.1037/0033-2909.134.1.1 PMID:18193993

Hajjar, E. R., Cafiero, A. C., & Hanlon, J. T. (2007). Polypharmacy in elderly patients. *The American Journal of Geriatric Pharmacotherapy*, *5*(4), 345–351. doi:10.1016/j.amjopharm.2007.12.002 PMID:18179993

Hakanen, J., & Peeters, M. (2015). How Do Work Engagement, Workaholism, and the Work-to-Family Interface Affect Each Other? A 7-Year Follow-Up Study. *Journal of Occupational and Environmental Medicine*, *57*(6), 601–609. doi:10.1097/JOM.0000000000000457 PMID:26053362

Haley, D. W., Weinberg, J., & Grunau, R. E. (2006). Cortisol, contingency learning, and memory in preterm and full-term infants. *Psychoneuroendocrinology*, *31*(1), 108–117. doi:10.1016/j.psyneuen.2005.06.007 PMID:16122876

Halford, S., & Leonard, P. (2003). Space and place in the construction and performance of gendered nursing identities. *Journal of Advanced Nursing*, *42*(2), 201–208. doi:10.1046/j.1365-2648.2003.02601.x PMID:12670387

Hall, J., Peat, M., Birks, Y., Golder, S., Entwistle, V., Gilbody, S., & Wright, J. et al. (2010). Effectiveness of interventions designed to promote patient involvement to enhance safety: A systematic review. *Quality & Safety in Health Care*, *19*, 1–7. PMID:20427301

Hall, M. A., Camacho, F., Dugan, E., & Balkrishnan, R. (2002). Trust in the medical profession: Conceptual and measurement issues. *Health Services Research*, *37*(5), 1419–1439. doi:10.1111/1475-6773.01070 PMID:12479504

Halpern, D., & Gibbs, J. (2013). Social media as a catalyst for online deliberation? Exploring the affordances of Facebook and YouTube for political expression. *Computers in Human Behavior*, *29*(3), 1159–1168. doi:10.1016/j.chb.2012.10.008

Hardin, R. (1971). Collective action as an agreeable "n"-Prisoners' dilemma. *Behavioral Science*, *16*(5), 472–481. doi:10.1002/bs.3830160507

Hartvigsen, J., Lings, S., Leboeuf-Yde, C., & Bakketeig, L. (2004). Psychosocial factors at work in relation to low back pain and consequences of low back pain; a systematic, critical review of prospective cohort studies. *Occupational and Environmental Medicine*, *61*(1), e2. PMID:14691283

Haug, M., & Lavin, B. (1981). Practitioner or patient – who's in charge? *Journal of Health and Social Behavior*, *22*(3), 212–229. doi:10.2307/2136517 PMID:7288129

Hayden, C., & Boaz, A. (2000) *Making a Difference: Better Government for Older People Programme Evaluation Report.* The University of Warwick, Local Government Centre.

Haynes, R. B., Ackloo, E., Sahota, N., McDonald, H. P., & Yao, X. (2008). Interventions for enhancing medication adherence. *Cochrane Database of Systematic Reviews*. doi:10.1002/14651858.CD000011.pub3 PMID:18425859

Health Services Research Group. (1992). Quality of care. *Canadian Medical Association Journal*, *146*, 2153–2158. PMID:1611571

Heart and Stroke Foundation of Barbados. (n. d.). *Cardiac disease prevention and rehabilitation programme.* Retrieved from http://www.hsfbarbados.org/GymCDPR.aspx

Henbest, R. J., & Stewart, M. A. (1989). Patient-centredness in the consultation. 1: A method for measurement. *Family Practice*, *6*(4), 249–253. doi:10.1093/fampra/6.4.249 PMID:2632300

Henke, N., Kelsey, T., & Whately, H. (2011). Transparency the most powerful driver of healthcare improvement? *Health International*, *11*, 65–73.

Hernandez, S. E., Conrad, D. A., Marcus-Smith, M. S., Reed, P., & Watts, C. (2013). Patient centered innovation in healthcare organizations: A conceptual framework and case study application. *Health Care Management Review*, *38*(2), 166–175. doi:10.1097/HMR.0b013e31825e718a PMID:22669050

Hernes, T. (2004). *The Spatial Construction of Organization.* Amsterdam: John Benjamin. doi:10.1075/aios.12

Hibbard, J. H., Stockard, J., Mahoney, E. R., & Tusler, M. (2004). Development of the Patient Activation Measure (PAM): conceptualizing and measuring activation in patients and consumers. *Health services research,* 39(4 Part 1), 1005-1026.

Hibbard, J. H. (2009). Using systematic measurement to target consumer activation strategies. *Medical Care Research and Review*, *66*(1Suppl.), 9S–27S. doi:10.1177/1077558708326969 PMID:19052169

Hibbard, J. H., & Greene, J. (2013). What the evidence shows about patient activation: Better health outcomes and care experiences; fewer data on costs. *Health Affairs*, *32*(2), 207–214. doi:10.1377/hlthaff.2012.1061 PMID:23381511

Hibbard, J. H., Greene, J., & Overton, V. (2013). Patients with lower activation associated with higher costs; delivery systems should know their patients' scores. *Health Affairs*, *32*(2), 216–222. doi:10.1377/hlthaff.2012.1064 PMID:23381513

Hibbard, J. H., & Mahoney, E. (2010). Toward a theory of patient and consumer activation. *Patient Education and Counseling*, *78*(3), 377–381. doi:10.1016/j.pec.2009.12.015 PMID:20188505

Hibbard, J. H., Mahoney, E. R., Stock, R., & Tusler, M. (2007). Do Increases in Patient Activation Result in Improved Self-Management Behaviors? *Health Services Research*, *42*(4), 1443–1463. doi:10.1111/j.1475-6773.2006.00669.x PMID:17610432

Hibbard, J. H., Stockard, J., Mahoney, E. R., & Tusler, M. (2004). Development of the Patient Activation Measure (PAM): Conceptualizing and measuring activation in patients and consumers. *Health Services Research*, *39*(4p14 Part 1), 1005–1026. doi:10.1111/j.1475-6773.2004.00269.x PMID:15230939

Hickson, G. B., Clayton, E. W., Entman, S. S., Miller, C. S., Githens, P. B., Whetten-Goldstein, K., & Sloan, F. A. (1994). Obstetricians' prior malpractice experience and patients' satisfaction with care. *Journal of the American Medical Association, 272*(20), 1583–1587. doi:10.1001/jama.1994.03520200039032 PMID:7966867

Hickson, G. B., Clayton, E. W., Githens, P. B., & Sloan, F. A. (1992). Factors that prompted families to file medical malpractice claims following prenatal injuries. *Journal of the American Medical Association, 267*(10), 1359–1363. doi:10.1001/jama.1992.03480100065032 PMID:1740858

Hignett, S. (2001). Embedding ergonomics in hospital culture: Top-down and bottom-up strategies. *Applied Ergonomics, 32*(1), 61–69. doi:10.1016/S0003-6870(00)00029-6 PMID:11209833

Hignett, S. (2003). Intervention strategies to reduce musculoskeletal injuries associated with handling patients: A systematic review. *Occupational and Environmental Medicine, 60*(9), e6. doi:10.1136/oem.60.9.e6 PMID:12937202

Hinshaw, A. (1992). *Welcome Patient outcomes research conference, In Patient Outcomes Research Examining the Effectiveness of Nursing Practice Proceedings of the state of the science conference sponsored by the National Center for Nursing Research*. Rockville, MD: National Institutes of Health Publication.

Holtzman, S., & DeLongis, A. (2007). One day at time: The impact of daily spouse support on pain, negative affect and catastrophizing among individuals with rheumatoid arthritis. *Pain, 131*, 1633–1655. doi:10.1016/j.pain.2007.04.005

Howie, J. G., Heaney, D. J., Maxwell, M., & Walker, J. J. (1998). A comparison of a Patient Enablement Instrument (PEI) against two established satisfaction scales as an outcome measure of primary care consultations. *Family Practice, 15*(2), 165–171. doi:10.1093/fampra/15.2.165 PMID:9613486

Høybye, M. T., Dalton, S. O., Deltour, I., Bidstrup, P. E., Frederiksen, K., & Johansen, C. (2010). Effect of Internet peer-support groups on psychosocial adjustment to cancer: A randomised study. *British Journal of Cancer, 102*(9), 1348–1354. doi:10.1038/sj.bjc.6605646 PMID:20424614

Hsieh, E. (2004). Stories in action and the dialogic management of identities: Storytelling in transplant support group meetings. *Research on Language and Social Interaction, 37*(1), 39–70. doi:10.1207/s15327973rlsi3701_2

Huizinga, M. M., Bleich, S. N., Beach, M. C., Clark, J. M., & Cooper, L. A. (2010). Disparity in physician perception of patients' adherence to medications by obesity status. *Obesity (Silver Spring, Md.), 18*(10), 1932–1937. doi:10.1038/oby.2010.35 PMID:20186132

Humber, J., & Almeder, R. (1997). *What is disease?* Totowa, NJ: Humana Press. doi:10.1007/978-1-59259-451-1

Hume, D. (1993). Enquiry concerning the principles of morals (2nd Ed., E. Steinberg). Indianapolis: Hackett Publishing Company.

Hume, D. (1978). *Treatise of human nature* (L. A. Selby-Bigge, Ed.). Oxford: Oxford University Press.

Hurst, K. (1995). *Progress with Patient Focused Care in the United Kingdom*. United Kingdom: NHS Executive.

Hyman, S. E. (2009). How adversity gets under the skin. *Nature Neuroscience, 12*(3), 241–243. doi:10.1038/nn0309-241 PMID:19238182

Iafrate, R., Bertoni, A., Barni, D., & Donato, S. (2009). Congruenza percettiva nella coppia e stili di coping diadico. *Psicologia Sociale, 1*, 95–114.

Iafrate, R., Bertoni, A., Donato, S., & Finkenauer, C. (2012). Perceived similarity and understanding in dyadic coping among young and mature couples. *Personal Relationships, 19*(3), 401–419. doi:10.1111/j.1475-6811.2011.01369.x

Iafrate, R., Bertoni, A., Margola, D., Cigoli, V., & Acitelli, L. K. (2012). The link between perceptual congruence and couple relationship satisfaction in dyadic coping. *European Psychologist*, *17*(1), 73–82. doi:10.1027/1016-9040/a000069

Iafrate, R., & Donato, S. (2012). Coping in a relational context: The case of dyadic coping. In B. Molinelli & V. Grimaldo (Eds.), *Handbook of the Psychology of Coping: New research* (pp. 111–132). Hauppauge, NY: Nova Science Publisher.

Iedema, R., Long, D., & Carroll, K. (2012). Corridor communication, spatial design and patient safety: enacting and managing complexities. In A. Van Marrewijk & D. Yanow (Eds.), *Organizational Spaces. Rematerializing the Workaday World* (pp. 41–57). Northampton, Massachusetts, USA: Edward Elgar Publishing.

Ilmarinen, J., & Rantanen, J. (1999). Promotion of work ability during ageing. *American Journal of Industrial Medicine*, *36*(Suppl. 1), 21–23. doi:10.1002/(SICI)1097-0274(199909)36:1+<21::AID-AJIM8>3.0.CO;2-S PMID:10519773

Inoue, A., Kawakami, N., Ishizaki, M., Shimazu, A., Tsuchiya, M., & Tabata, M. et al. (2010). Organizational justice, psychological distress, and work engagement in Japanese workers. *International Archives of Occupational and Environmental Health*, *83*(1), 29–38. doi:10.1007/s00420-009-0485-7 PMID:19904552

Inoue, A., Kawakami, N., Tsuno, K., Shimazu, A., Tomioka, K., & Nakanishi, M. (2013). Job demands, job resources, and work engagement of Japanese employees: A prospective cohort study. *International Archives of Occupational and Environmental Health*, *86*(4), 441–449. doi:10.1007/s00420-012-0777-1 PMID:22562520

Institute of Medicine (US) Roundtable on Evidence-Based Medicine. (2010). The Healthcare Imperative: Lowering Costs and Improving Outcomes. In P. L. Yong, R. S. Saunders, & L. Olsen (Eds.), *Washington (DC)*. US: National Academies Press.

Institute of Medicine. (1990). *Medicare: a strategy for quality assurance*. Washington, D.C.: National Academy Press.

Institute of Medicine. (2001). Crossing the quality chasm: a new health system for the 21st century. In *Committee on Quality of Health Care in America*. Washington: National Academies Press.

Institute of Medicine. (2001). *Crossing the Quality Chasm: A New Health System for the Twenty-First Century*. Washington, D.C.: National Academies Press.

International Alliance of Patients Organizations. (2007). *What is patient-centered healthcare? A review of definition and principles*. Retrieved from http://iapo.org.uk/sites/default/files/files/IAPO%20Patient-Centred%20Healthcare%20Review%202nd%20edition.pdf

Jaarsma, T., & Stromberg, A. (2014). Heart failure clinics are still useful (more than ever?). *The Canadian Journal of Cardiology*, *30*(3), 272–275. doi:10.1016/j.cjca.2013.09.022 PMID:24468418

Jackson, J. L., Kroenke, K., & Chamberlin, J. (1999). Effects of physician awareness of symptom-related expectations and mental disorders: A controlled trial. *Archives of Family Medicine*, *8*(2), 135–142. doi:10.1001/archfami.8.2.135 PMID:10101984

Jahoda, M. (1958). *Current concepts of positive mental health*. New York: Basic Books. doi:10.1037/11258-000

James, J. (2012). Health Policy Brief: Public Reporting on Quality and Costs. *Health Affairs*.

Jamieson, D. (2013). Constructing Practical Ethics. In R. Crisp (Ed.), *The Oxford handbook of the history of ethics* (pp. 843–866). Oxford University Press.

Jansen, J., Beijers, R., Riksen-Walraven, M., & de Weerth, C. (2010). Cortisol reactivity in young infants. *Psychoneuroendocrinology*, *35*(3), 329–338. doi:10.1016/j.psyneuen.2009.07.008 PMID:19651476

Jena, A. B., Seabury, S., Lakdawalla, D., & Chandra, A. (2011). Malpractice risk according to physician specialty. *The New England Journal of Medicine*, *365*(7), 629–636. doi:10.1056/NEJMsa1012370 PMID:21848463

Jennings, M. K. (1999). Political responses to pain and loss. *The American Political Science Review*, *93*(1), 1–15. doi:10.2307/2585757

Jetten, J., Haslam, C., & Haslam, S. A. (2012). *The social cure: Identity, health, and well-being*. London, UK: Psychology Press.

Joekes, K., Van Elderen, T., & Schreurs, K. (2007). Self-efficacy and overprotection are related to quality of life, psychological well-being and self-management in cardiac patients. *Journal of Health Psychology*, *12*(1), 4–16. doi:10.1177/1359105306069096 PMID:17158836

Johnson, K. L., Brown, P. A., & Knaster, E. S. (2010). Aging with disability in the workplace. *Physical Medicine and Rehabilitation Clinics of North America*, *21*(2), 267–279. doi:10.1016/j.pmr.2009.12.004 PMID:20494276

Joosten, T., Bongers, I., & Janssen, R. (2009). Application of lean thinking to health care: Issues and observations. *International Journal for Quality in Health Care*, *21*(5), 341–347. doi:10.1093/intqhc/mzp036 PMID:19696048

Jost, J. T., & Major, B. (2001). *The psychology of legitimacy: Emerging perspectives on ideology, justice, and inter-group relations*. New York: Cambridge University Press.

Juran, J. M. (1988). *Juran on planning for quality*. New York: McGraw-Hill.

Jutapakdeegul, N., Casalotti, S. O., Govitrapong, P., & Kotchabhakdi, N. (2003). Postnatal touch stimulation acutely alters corticosterone levels and glucocorticoid receptor gene expression in the neonatal rat. *Developmental Neuroscience*, *25*(1), 26–33. doi:10.1159/000071465 PMID:12876428

Kaluzny, A. D., McLaughlin, C. P., & Simpson, K. (1992). Applying total quality management concepts to public health organizations. *Public Health Reports*, *107*(3), 257–264. PMID:1594734

Kang, D., Kim, Y., Lee, Y. I., Koh, S., Kim, I., & Lee, H. (2014). Work-related Musculoskeletal Disorders in Korea Provoked by Workers' Collective Compensation Claims against Work Intensification. *Annals of Occupational and Environmental Medicine*, *26*(1), 19. doi:10.1186/2052-4374-26-19 PMID:25089205

Kantake, M., Yoshitake, H., Ishikawa, H., Araki, Y., & Shimizu, T. (2014). Postnatal epigenetic modification of glucocorticoid receptor gene in preterm infants: A prospective cohort study. *BMJ Open*, *4*(7), e005318. doi:10.1136/bmjopen-2014-005318 PMID:25023132

Kapiriri, L., Norheim, O. F., & Martin, D. K. (2007). Priority setting at the micro-, mesoandmacro-levels in Canada, Norway and Uganda. *Health Policy (Amsterdam)*, *82*(1), 78–94. doi:10.1016/j.healthpol.2006.09.001 PMID:17034898

Kaplan, S. H., Greenfield, S., & Ware, J. E. Jr. (1989). Assessing the effects of physician-patient interactions on the outcomes of chronic disease. *Medical Care*, *27*(3Suppl.), S110–S127. doi:10.1097/00005650-198903001-00010 PMID:2646486

Karanika-Murray, M., Pontes, H. M., Griffiths, M. D., & Biron, C. (2015). Sickness presenteeism determines job satisfaction via affective-motivational states. *Social Science & Medicine*, *139*, 100–106. doi:10.1016/j.socscimed.2015.06.035 PMID:26183017

Karatsoreos, I. N., & McEwen, B. S. (2013). Resilience and vulnerability: A neurobiological perspective. *F1000prime Reports*, *5*, 13. PMID:23710327

Kayser, K., Feldman, B. N., Borstelmann, N. A., & Daniels, A. A. (2010). Effects of a randomized couple-based intervention on quality of life of breast cancer patients and their partners. *Social Work Research*, *34*(1), 20–32. doi:10.1093/swr/34.1.20

Kayser, K., Watson, L. E., & Andrade, J. T. (2007). Cancer as a "we-disease": Examining the process of coping from a relational perspective. *Families, Systems & Health*, *25*(4), 404–418. doi:10.1037/1091-7527.25.4.404

Kearns, R. A., & Joseph, A. E. (1993). Space in its place: Developing the link in medical geography. *Social Science & Medicine*, *37*(6), 711–717. doi:10.1016/0277-9536(93)90364-A PMID:8211286

Kember, R. L., Dempster, E. L., Lee, T. H., Schalkwyk, L. C., Mill, J., & Fernandes, C. (2012). Maternal separation is associated with strain-specific responses to stress and epigenetic alterations to Nr3c1, Avp, and Nr4a1 in mouse. *Brain and Behavior*, *2*(4), 455–467. doi:10.1002/brb3.69 PMID:22950049

Keren, M., Feldman, R., Eidelman, A. I., Sirota, L., & Lester, B. (2003). Clinical interview for high-risk parents of premature infants (CLIP) as a predictor of early disruptions in the mother-infant relationship at the nursery. *Infant Mental Health Journal*, *24*(2), 93–110. doi:10.1002/imhj.10049

Keyes, C. L. (2009). Toward a Science of Mental Health. In C. R. Snyder & S. J. Lopez (Eds.), *Oxford handbook of positive psychology* (2nd ed., pp. 89–96). New York: Oxford University Press.

Keyes, C. L., & Annas, J. (2009). Feeling Good and Functioning Well: Distinctive Concepts in Ancient Philosophy and Contemporary Science. *The Journal of Positive Psychology*, *4*(3), 197–201. doi:10.1080/17439760902844228

Khan, S. S., Hopkins, N., Reicher, S., Tewari, S., Srinivasan, N., & Stevenson, C. (2014). Shared identity predicts enhanced health at a mass gathering. *Group Processes & Intergroup Relations*, *18*(4), 504–522. doi:10.1177/1368430214556703

Kiechl-Kohlendorfer, U., Merkle, U., Deufert, D., Neubauer, V., Peglow, U. P., & Griesmaier, E. (2015). Effect of developmental care for very premature infants on neurodevelopmental outcome at 2 years of age. *Infant Behavior and Development*, *39*, 166–172. doi:10.1016/j.infbeh.2015.02.006 PMID:25867251

King, K. B., & Reis, H. T. (2012). Marriage and long-term survival coronary artery bypass grafting. *Health Psychology*, *31*(1), 55–62. doi:10.1037/a0025061 PMID:21859213

Kinmonth, A. L., Woodcock, A., Griffin, S., Spiegal, N., & Campbell, M. J. (1998). Randomised controlled trial of patient centred care of diabetes in general practice: Impact on current wellbeing and future disease risk. *British Medical Journal*, *317*(7167), 1202–1208. doi:10.1136/bmj.317.7167.1202 PMID:9794859

Kinnersley, P., Stott, N., Peters, T. J., & Harvey, I. (1999). The patient-centredness of consultations and outcome in primary care. *The British Journal of General Practice*, *49*(446), 711–716. PMID:10756612

Kirkham, H. S., Clark, B. L., Bolas, C. A., Lewis, G. H., Jackson, A. S., Fisher, D., & Duncan, I. (2015). Which modifiable health risks are associated with changes in productivity costs? *Population Health Management*, *18*(1), 30–38. doi:10.1089/pop.2014.0033 PMID:25375893

Kirsten, W. (2010). Making the link between health and productivity at the workplace--a global perspective. *Industrial Health*, *48*(3), 251–255. doi:10.2486/indhealth.48.251 PMID:20562499

Kittay, E. (1998). *Love's labor: Essays on women, equality, and dependency*. New York: Routledge.

Kivimaki, M., Head, J., Ferrie, J. E., Hemingway, H., Shipley, M. J., Vahtera, J., & Marmot, M. G. (2005). Working while ill as a risk factor for serious coronary events: The Whitehall II Study. *American Journal of Public Health*, *95*(1), 98–100. doi:10.2105/AJPH.2003.035873 PMID:15623867

Kjeldmand, D., Holmstrom, I., & Rosenqvist, U. (2006). How patient-centered am I? A new method to measure physicians' patient-centredness. *Patient Education and Counseling*, *62*, 31–37. doi:10.1016/j.pec.2005.05.017 PMID:16024208

Klandermans, B. (1984). Mobilization and participation: Social-psychological expansions of resource mobilization theory. *American Sociological Review*, *49*(5), 583–600. doi:10.2307/2095417

Klandermans, B. (1997). *The social psychology of protest*. Oxford: Basic Blackwell.

Klandermans, B. (2004). The demand and supply of participation: Social-psychological correlates of participation in social movements. In D. A. Snow, S. A. Soule, & H. Kriesi (Eds.), *The Blackwell Companion to Social Movements* (pp. 360–379). Blackwell Publishing; doi:10.1002/9780470999103.ch16

Klandermans, B., & Oegema, D. (1987). Potentials, networks, motivations, and barriers: Steps toward participationin social movements. *American Sociological Review*, *52*(4), 519–531. doi:10.2307/2095297

Klandermans, B., & Van Stekelenburg, J. (2013). Social movements and participation in collective Action. In D. O. Sears, L. Huddy, & R. Jervis (Eds.), *Oxford handbook of Political psychology* (pp. 774–812). Oxford: University Press; doi:10.1093/oxfordhb/9780199760107.013.0024

Klawiter, M. (1999). Racing for the cure, walking women, andtoxic touring. Mapping cultures of action within the BayArea terrain of breast cancer: Programs and organizationalprocesses. *Social Problems*, *46*(1), 104–126. doi:10.2307/3097164

Kleinman, A. (1988). *The illness narrative: Suffering, healing, and the human condition*. New York: Basic Books.

Kleinman, A. (1989). *The illness narratives: suffering, healing, and the human condition*. New York: Basic Books.

Klinger, E., & Cox, M. (2004). Motivation and the Theory of Current Concerns. In W. M. Cox & E. Klinger (Eds.), *Handbook of motivational counselling: Concepts, approaches, and assessment* (pp. 3–28). Chichester: John Willey & Sons.

Kodner, D. L., & Spreeuwenberg, C. (2002). Integrated care: Meaning, logic, applications, and implications–a discussion paper. *International Journal of Integrated Care*, 2002, 2. PMID:16896389

Kogi, K. (2006). Participatory methods effective for ergonomic workplace improvement. *Applied Ergonomics*, *37*(4), 547–554. doi:10.1016/j.apergo.2006.04.013 PMID:16756940

Kohn, L. T., Corrigan, J. M., & Donaldson, M. S. (2000). *To err is human: building a safer health system*. Washington: National Academic Press.

Korraa, A. A., El Nagger, A. A., Mohamed, R. A. E. S., & Helmy, N. M. (2014). Impact of kangaroo mother care on cerebral blood flow of preterm infants. *Italian Journal of Pediatrics*, *40*(1), 1–6. doi:10.1186/s13052-014-0083-5 PMID:25391600

Korsgaard, C. M. (2008). *The constitution of agency: Essays on practical reason and moral psychology*. New York: Oxford University Press. doi:10.1093/acprof:oso/9780199552733.001.0001

Kostova, Z., Caiata-Zufferey, M., & Schulz, P. J. (2014). The process of acceptance among rheumatoid arthritis patients in Switzerland: A qualitative study. *Pain Research & Management*, *19*(2), 61–68. doi:10.1155/2014/168472 PMID:24527466

Kravitz, R. L., Callahan, E. J., Azari, R., Antonius, D., & Lewis, C. E. (1997). Assessing patients' expectations in ambulatory medical practice. *Journal of General Internal Medicine*, *12*(1), 67–72. doi:10.1007/s11606-006-0010-6 PMID:9034949

Kreckler, S., Catchpole, K., McCulloch, P., & Handa, A. (2009). Factors influencing incident reporting in surgical care. *Quality & Safety in Health Care*, *18*(2), 116–120. doi:10.1136/qshc.2008.026534 PMID:19342525

Krueger, K. P., Berger, B. A., & Felkey, B. (2005). Medication adherence and persistence: A comprehensive review. *Advances in Therapy*, *22*(4), 313–356. doi:10.1007/BF02850081 PMID:16418141

Kumpunen, S., Trigg, L., & Rodrigues, R. (2014). *Public reporting in health and long-term care to facilitate provider choice*. Denmark: WHO Regional Office for Europe and European Observatory on Health Systems and Policies.

Kuorinka, I. (1997). Tools and means of implementing participatory ergonomics. *International Journal of Industrial Ergonomics*, *19*(4), 267–270. doi:10.1016/S0169-8141(96)00035-2

Lafollette, H. (2013). *International encyclopedia of ethics*. Hoboken, NJ: Wiley-Blackwell.

Laing, A. C., Cole, D. C., Theberge, N., Wells, R. P., Kerr, M. S., & Frazer, M. B. (2007). Effectiveness of a participatory ergonomics intervention in improving communication and psychosocial exposures. *Ergonomics*, *50*(7), 1092–1109. doi:10.1080/00140130701308708 PMID:17510824

Lakshminarayana, R., Wang, D., Burn, D., Chaudhuri, K. R., Cummins, G., Galtrey, C., & Williams, A. et al.SMART-PD Investigators. (2014). Smartphone- and internet-assisted self-management and adherence tools to manage Parkinson's disease (SMART-PD): Study protocol for a randomised controlled trial. *Trials*, *15*(1), 374. doi:10.1186/1745-6215-15-374 PMID:25257518

Lamiell, J. T. (1995). Rethinking the role of quantitative methods in psychology. In J. A. Smith, R. Harré, & L. Van Langenhove (Eds.), *Rethinking methods in psychology* (pp. 143–162). London: Sage. doi:10.4135/9781446221792.n10

Langer, E. J. (1989). *Mindfulness*. Boston: Perseus Books.

Langer, E. J. (2009). *Counterclockwise: Mindful health and the power of possibility*. New York: Ballantine Books.

Laplante, P., Diorio, J., & Meaney, M. J. (2002). Serotonin regulates hippocampal glucocorticoid receptor expression via a 5-HT7 receptor. *Brain Research. Developmental Brain Research*, *139*(2), 199–203. doi:10.1016/S0165-3806(02)00550-3 PMID:12480134

Latva, R., Lehtonen, L., Salmelin, R. K., & Tamminen, T. (2004). Visiting less than every day: A marker for later behavioral problems in Finnish preterm infants. *Archives of Pediatrics & Adolescent Medicine*, *158*(12), 1153–1157. doi:10.1001/archpedi.158.12.1153 PMID:15583100

Latva, R., Lehtonen, L., Salmelin, R. K., & Tamminen, T. (2007). Visits by the family to the neonatal intensive care unit. *Acta Paediatrica (Oslo, Norway)*, *96*(2), 215–220. doi:10.1111/j.1651-2227.2007.00053.x PMID:17429908

Laubie, R., & Elie-Dit-Cosaque, C. (2012, December 16-19). Exploring and predicting online collective action on patients' virtual communities: a multi-method investigation in France. *Research Paper presented at ICIS12*, Orlando, Florida, USA.

Lazarus, R. S., & Folkman, S. (1984). *Stress, appraisal, and coping*. New York: Springer Publishing Company.

Leatherman, S., & McCarthy, D. (1999). Counterpoint. Public disclosure of health care performance reports: Experience, evidence and issues for policy. *International Journal for Quality in Health Care*, *11*(2), 93–98. doi:10.1093/intqhc/11.2.93 PMID:10442837

Lee, C. S., Vellone, E., Lyons, K. S., Cocchieri, A., Bidwell, J. T., & D'Agostino, F. et al. (2015). Pattern and predictors of patient and caregiver engagement in heart failure care: A multi-level dyadic study. *International Journal of Nursing Studies*, *52*(2), 588–597. doi:10.1016/j.ijnurstu.2014.11.005 PMID:25468283

Lee, E. J. (2007). Deindividuation effects on group polarization in computer-mediated communication: The role of group identification, public-self-awareness, and perceived argument quality. *Journal of Communication*, *57*(2), 385–403. doi:10.1111/j.1460-2466.2007.00348.x

Lee, Y.-H., Malakooti, N., & Lotas, M. (2005). A comparison of the light-reduction capacity of commonly used incubator covers. *Neonatal Network*, *24*(2), 37–44. doi:10.1891/0730-0832.24.2.37 PMID:15835478

Lefebvre, H. (1991). *The Production of Space*. Oxford: Blackwell.

Lega, F., & DePietro, C. (2005). Converging patterns in hospital organization: Beyond the professional bureaucracy. *Health Policy (Amsterdam, Netherlands)*, *74*(3), 261–281. doi:10.1016/j.healthpol.2005.01.010 PMID:16226138

Légaré, F., & Witteman, H. O. (2013). Shared decision making: Examining key elements and barriers to adoption into routine clinical practice. *Health Affairs*, *32*(2), 276–284. doi:10.1377/hlthaff.2012.1078 PMID:23381520

Leijten, F. R., van den Heuvel, S. G., van der Beek, A. J., Ybema, J. F., Robroek, S. J., & Burdorf, A. (2015). Associations of work-related factors and work engagement with mental and physical health: A 1-year follow-up study among older workers. *Journal of Occupational Rehabilitation*, *25*(1), 86–95. doi:10.1007/s10926-014-9525-6 PMID:24928413

Leon, A. S., Franklin, B. A., Costa, F., Balady, G. J., Berra, K. A., & Stewart, K. J. et al.. (2005). Cardiac rehabilitation and secondary prevention of coronary heart disease. *Circulation*, *111*(3), 369–376. doi:10.1161/01.CIR.0000151788.08740.5C PMID:15668354

Lesch, K. P. (2011). When the serotonin transporter gene meets adversity: The contribution of animal models to understanding epigenetic mechanisms in affective disorders and resilience. *Current Topics in Behavioral Neurosciences*, *7*, 251–280. doi:10.1007/7854_2010_109 PMID:21225411

Lester, B. M., Hawes, K., Abar, B., Sullivan, M., Miller, R., Bigsby, R., & Padbury, J. F. et al. (2014). Single-Family Room Care and Neurobehavioral and Medical Outcomes in Preterm Infants. *Pediatrics*, *134*(4), 754–760. doi:10.1542/peds.2013-4252 PMID:25246623

Lester, B. M., Tronick, E., Nestler, E., Abel, T., Kosofsky, B., Kuzawa, C. W., & Wood, M. A. et al. (2011). Behavioral epigenetics. *Annals of the New York Academy of Sciences*, *1226*(1), 14–33. doi:10.1111/j.1749-6632.2011.06037.x PMID:21615751

Levasseur, M., Richard, L., Gauvin, L., & Raymond, É. (2010). Inventory and analysis of definitions of social participation found in the aging literature: Proposed taxonomy of social activities. *Social Science & Medicine*, *71*(12), 2141–2149. doi:10.1016/j.socscimed.2010.09.041 PMID:21044812

Levenstein, J. H., Mccracken, E. C., Mcwhinney, I. R., Stewart, M. A., & Brown, J. B. (1986). The patient-centered clinical method. A model for the doctor-patient interaction in family medicine. *Family Practice*, *3*(1), 24–30. doi:10.1093/fampra/3.1.24 PMID:3956899

Leventhal, H., Benyamini, Y., Brownlee, S., Diefenbach, M., Leventhal, E. A., Patrick-Miller, L., & Robitaille, C. (1997). Illness representations: theoretical foundations. In *Perceptions of health and illness* (Vol. 2, pp. 19-46).

Leventhal, G. S. (1980). What should be done with equity theory? Newapproaches to the study of fairness in social relationships. In K. Gergen, M. Greenberg, & R. Willis (Eds.), *Social exchanges: Advances in theoryand research* (pp. 27–55). New York: Plenum. doi:10.1007/978-1-4613-3087-5_2

Levin, J. B., Sher, T. G., & Theodos, V. (1997). The effect of intracouple coping concordance on psychological and marital distress in infertility patients. *Journal of Clinical Psychology in Medical Settings*, *4*(4), 361–372. doi:10.1023/A:1026249317635

Levinson, W., Kao, A., Kuby, A., & Thisted, R. A. (2005). Not all patients want to participate in decision making: A national study of public preferences. *Journal of General Internal Medicine*, *20*(6), 531–535. doi:10.1111/j.1525-1497.2005.04101.x PMID:15987329

Levinson, W., Roter, D. L., Mullooly, J. P., Dull, V. T., & Frankel, R. M. (1997). Physician-patient communication: The relationship with malpractice claims among primary care physicians and surgeons. *Journal of the American Medical Association*, *277*(7), 553–559. doi:10.1001/jama.1997.03540310051034 PMID:9032162

Liang, J., Krause, N. M., & Bennett, J. M. (2001). Social exchange and well-being: Is giving better than receiving? *Psychology and Aging*, *16*(3), 511–523. doi:10.1037/0882-7974.16.3.511 PMID:11554527

Liberati, E. G., Gorli, M., Moja, L., Galuppo, L., Ripamonti, S., & Scaratti, G. (2015). Exploring the practice of patient centered care: The role of ethnography and reflexivity. *Social Science & Medicine*, *133*, 45–52. doi:10.1016/j.socscimed.2015.03.050 PMID:25841094

Liberati, E. G., Gorli, M., & Scaratti, G. (in press). Reorganising hospitals to implement a patient-centered model of care: The effects on clinical practice and professional relationships in the Italian NHS. *Journal of Health Organization and Management*. PMID:26556155

Lincoln, Y. S., & Guba, E. G. (1985). *Naturalistic inquiry* (Vol. 75). Sage.

Lind, E. A., & Tyler, T. R. (1988). *The social psychology of proceduraljustice*. New York: Plenum.

Linderman, K., Schroeder, R. G., Zaheer, S., & Choo, A. S. (2003). Six Sigma: A goal-theoretic perspective. *Journal of Operations Management*, *21*(2), 193–203. doi:10.1016/S0272-6963(02)00087-6

Li, Q., & Loke, A. Y. (2014). A systematic review of spousal couple-based intervention studies for couples coping with cancer: Direction for the development of interventions. *Psycho-Oncology*, *23*(7), 731–739. doi:10.1002/pon.3535 PMID:24723336

Lisbon Special European Council. (2000, March). Towards a Europe of Innovation and Knowledge. Retrieved from: http://eur-lex.europa.eu/legal-content/EN/TXT/?uri=uriserv:c10241

Little, P., Everitt, H., Williamson, I., Warner, G., Moore, M., Gould, C., & Payne, S. et al. (2001). Preferences of patients for patient centered approach to consultation in primary care: Observational study. *British Medical Journal*, *322*(7284), 468–472. doi:10.1136/bmj.322.7284.468 PMID:11222423

Long, A. A. (1986). *Hellenistic Philosophy: Stoics, Epicureans, Sceptics* (2nd ed.). Berkeley: University of California Press.

Longtin, Y., Sax, H., Leape, L. L., Sheridan, S. E., Donaldson, L., & Pittet, D. (2010). Patient participation: Current knowledge and applicability to patient safety. *Mayo Clinic Protocol*, *85*(1), 53–62. doi:10.4065/mcp.2009.0248 PMID:20042562

Luxford, K., Safran, D. G., & Delbanco, T. (2011). Promoting patient-centered care: A qualitative study of facilitators and barriers in healthcare organizations with a reputation for improving the patient experience. *International Journal for Quality in Health Care*, *23*(5), 510–515. doi:10.1093/intqhc/mzr024 PMID:21586433

Lyons, K. S., Bennett, J. A., Nail, L. M., Fromme, E. K., Dieckmann, N., & Sayer, A. G. (2014). The role of patient pain and physical function on depressive symptoms in couples with lung cancer: A longitudinal dyadic analysis. *Journal of Family Psychology*, *28*(5), 692–700. doi:10.1037/fam0000017 PMID:25090253

Lyons, R., Mickelson, K. D., Sullivan, M. J. L., & Coyne, J. C. (1998). Coping as a communal process. *Journal of Social and Personal Relationships*, *15*(5), 579–605. doi:10.1177/0265407598155001

Mackintosh, N., & Sandall, J. (2010). Overcoming gendered and professional hierarchies in order to facilitate escalation of care in emergency situations: The role of standardised communication protocols. *Social Science & Medicine*, *71*(9), 1683–1686. doi:10.1016/j.socscimed.2010.07.037 PMID:20850919

Maddalena, P. (2013). Long term outcomes of preterm birth: The role of epigenetics. *Newborn and Infant Nursing Reviews; NAINR*, *13*(3), 137–139. doi:10.1053/j.nainr.2013.06.010

Magnavita, N. (1993). Workplace action for health. Prevention of obesity and hyperlipaemia in a small company. *Paper presented at the International Conference "Work & Health"*, Copenhagen, Denmark.

Magnavita, N. (2004a). Applicazione di modelli organizzativi originali per la prevenzione del rischio chimico in aziende di diverse dimensioni. Metodo A.S.I.A. Roma: IIMS Istituto Italiano di Medicina Sociale. Retrieved from http://www.puntosicuro.info/documenti/documenti/111201_sirsrer_rischio_chimico.pdf

Magnavita, N. (2009a). *Lavoro umano. Il benessere nei luoghi di lavoro*. Milano: EDUCatt.

Magnavita, N., Sacco, A., & De Lorenzo, G. (1993). Hypertension and hypercholesterolemia prevention in lead-exposed workers. *Paper presented at the International Conference "Work & Health"*, Copenhagen, Denmark.

Magnavita, N. (2004b). *Tutela del lavoratore rischioso per gli altri*. Milano: ISU Università Cattolica del Sacro Cuore.

Magnavita, N. (2006). Management of impaired physicians in Europe. *La Medicina del Lavoro*, *97*(6), 762–773. PMID:17219765

Magnavita, N. (2007). The unhealthy physician. *Journal of Medical Ethics*, *33*(4), 210–214. doi:10.1136/jme.2006.017533 PMID:17400618

Magnavita, N. (2009b). Experience of prevention activities in local health units. Assaults and musculoskeletal disorders. *La Medicina del Lavoro*, *100*(Suppl. 1), 24–28. PMID:19848097

Magnavita, N. (2011). Violence prevention in a small-scale psychiatric unit: Program planning and evaluation. *International Journal of Occupational and Environmental Health*, *17*(4), 336–344. doi:10.1179/oeh.2011.17.4.336 PMID:22069932

Magnavita, N. (2012). Validation of the Italian version of the HSE Indicator Tool. *Occupational Medicine*, *62*(4), 288–294. doi:10.1093/occmed/kqs025 PMID:22661665

Magnavita, N., Bergamaschi, A., Chiarotti, M., Colombi, A., Deidda, B., & De Lorenzo, G. et al. (2008). Workers with alcohol and drug addiction problems. Consensus Document of the Study Group on Hazardous Workers. *La Medicina del Lavoro*, *99*(Suppl. 2), 3–58. PMID:19248471

Magnavita, N., Castorina, S., Ciavarella, M., Mammi, F., Roccia, K., & Saffioti, C. (2007). Participative approach to the in hospital management of muscoloskeletal disorders. *Giornale Italiano di Medicina del Lavoro Ed Ergonomia*, *29*(3), 561–563. PMID:18409832

Magnavita, N., Cicerone, M., Cirese, V., De Lorenzo, G., Di Giannantonio, M., & Fileni, A. et al. (2006). Critical aspects of the management of "hazardous" health care workers. Consensus Document. *La Medicina del Lavoro*, *97*(5), 715–725. PMID:17171984

Magnavita, N., De Lorenzo, G., Gallo, M., Garbarino, S., Goggiamani, A., & Janiri, L. et al. (2014). Alcohol and work. Consensus Document of the La. R.A. group. *La Medicina del Lavoro*, *105*(Suppl. 1), 3–68. PMID:25488525

Magnavita, N., De Lorenzo, G., & Sacco, A. (2014). Health promotion in the workplace. *La Medicina del Lavoro*, *105*(6), 473–474. PMID:25431984

Magnavita, N., Fileni, A., Mirk, P., Magnavita, G., Ricci, S., & Cotroneo, A. R. (2013). Malpractice Claims in interventional radiology: Frequency, characteristics and protective measure. *Radiological Medicine*, *118*(3), 504–517. doi:10.1007/s11547-012-0878-7 PMID:22986698

Mahmud, S. (2004). Citizen participation in the health sector in rural Bangladesh: Perceptions and reality. *IDS Bulletin, 35*(2), 11–18. doi:10.1111/j.1759-5436.2004.tb00116.x

Maisiak, R., Austin, J., West, S., & Heck, L. (1996). The effect of person-centered counseling on the psychological status of persons with systemic lupus erythematosus or rheumatoid arthritis. A randomized, controlled trial. *Arthritis and Rheumatism, 9*(1), 60–66. doi:10.1002/art.1790090111 PMID:8945114

Major, B. (1994). In M. P. Zanna (Ed.), *From social inequality to personal entitlement: The role of social comparisons, legitimacy appraisals, and group membership* (Vol. 26, pp. 293–355). Advances in experimental social psychologySan Diego, CA: Academic Press.

Makai, P., Perry, M., Robben, S. H., Schers, H. J., Heinen, M. M., Olde Rikkert, M. G., & Melis, R. R. (2014). Evaluation of an eHealth intervention in chronic care for frail older people: Why adherence is the first target. *Journal of Medical Internet Research, 16*(6), e156. doi:10.2196/jmir.3057 PMID:24966146

Manne, S. L. (1998). Cancer in the marital context: A review of the literature. *Cancer Investigation, 16*(3), 188–202. doi:10.3109/07357909809050036 PMID:9541634

Manne, S. L., & Badr, H. (2008). Intimacy and relationship processes in couples' psychosocial adaptation to cancer. *Cancer, 112*(S11), 2541–2555. doi:10.1002/cncr.23450 PMID:18428202

Manne, S. L., Badr, H., & Kashy, D. A. (2012). A longitudinal analysis of intimacy processes and psychological distress among couples coping with head and neck or lung cancers. *Journal of Behavioral Medicine, 35*(3), 334–346. doi:10.1007/s10865-011-9349-1 PMID:21556790

Manne, S. L., Ostroff, J. S., Norton, T. R., Fox, K., Goldstein, L., & Grana, G. (2006). Cancer-related relationship communication in couples coping with early stage breast cancer. *Psycho-Oncology, 15*(3), 234–247. doi:10.1002/pon.941 PMID:15926198

Manne, S. L., Ostroff, J., Rini, C., Fox, K., Goldstein, L., & Grana, G. (2004). The interpersonal process model of intimacy: The role of self-disclosure, partner disclosure, and partner responsiveness in interactions between breast cancer patients and their partners. *Journal of Family Psychology, 18*(4), 589–599. doi:10.1037/0893-3200.18.4.589 PMID:15598164

Manne, S. L., & Zautra, A. J. (1989). Spouse criticism and support: Their association with coping and psychological adjustment among women with rheumatoid arthritis. *Journal of Personality and Social Psychology, 56*(4), 608–617. doi:10.1037/0022-3514.56.4.608 PMID:2709309

Manne, S. L., & Zautra, A. J. (1990). Couples coping with chronic illness: Women with rheumatoid arthritis and their healthy husband. *Journal of Behavioral Medicine, 13*(4), 327–342. doi:10.1007/BF00844882 PMID:2246781

Manne, S., & Badr, H. (2010). Intimacy processes and psychological distress among couples coping with head and neck or lung cancers. *Psycho-Oncology, 19*(9), 941–954. doi:10.1002/pon.1645 PMID:19885852

Manne, S., Badr, H., Zaider, T., Nelson, C., & Kissane, D. (2010). Cancer-related communication, relationship intimacy, and psychological distress among couples coping with localized prostate cancer. *Journal of Cancer Survivorship: Research and Practice, 4*(1), 74–85. doi:10.1007/s11764-009-0109-y PMID:19967408

Marcu, A., Gaspar, R., Rutsaert, P., Seibt, B., Fletcher, D., Verbeke, W., & Barnett, J. (2014). Analogies, metaphors, and wondering about the future: Lay sense-making around synthetic meat. *Public Understanding of Science (Bristol, England), 24*(5), 547–562. doi:10.1177/0963662514521106 PMID:24553438

Marcum, Z. A., Sevick, M. A., & Handler, S. M. (2013). Medication non-adherence: A diagnosable and treatable medical condition. *Journal of the American Medical Association, 309*, 2105–2106. doi:10.1001/jama.2013.4638 PMID:23695479

Marengoni, A., Angleman, S., Melis, R., Mangialasche, F., Karp, A., Garmen, A., & Fratiglioni, L. et al. (2011). Aging with multimorbidity: A systematic review of the literature. *Ageing Research Reviews*, *10*(4), 430–439. doi:10.1016/j.arr.2011.03.003 PMID:21402176

Marin, T., Holtzman, S., DeLongis, A., & Robinson, L. (2007). Coping and the response of others. *Journal of Social and Personal Relationships*, *24*(6), 951–969. doi:10.1177/0265407507084192

Markus, T. A., & Cameron, D. (2002). *The Words Between the Spaces: Buildings and Language*. Psychology Press.

Marriot, C., & Thompson, A. R. (2008). Managing Threat to femininity: Personal and interpersonal experience of living with vulval pain. *Psychology & Health*, *23*(2), 243–258. doi:10.1080/14768320601168185 PMID:25160053

Marshall, M. N., Shekelle, P. G., Davies, H. T., & Smith, P. C. (2003). Public reporting on quality in the United States and the United Kingdom. *Health Affairs*, *22*(3), 134–148. doi:10.1377/hlthaff.22.3.134 PMID:12757278

Martire, L. M., Lustig, A. P., Schulz, R., Miller, G. E., & Helgeson, V. S. (2004). Is it beneficial to involve a family member? A meta-analysis of psychosocial interventions for chronic illness. *Health Psychology*, *23*(6), 599–611. doi:10.1037/0278-6133.23.6.599 PMID:15546228

Marwell, G., & Oliver, P. (1993). *The critical mass in collective action: A micro-social theory*. Cambridge: Cambridge University Press. doi:10.1017/CBO9780511663765

Marzano, M. (2002). La medicina, la morte e la modernità: Un'analisi sociologica. *Rassegna Italiana di Sociologia*, *43*(2), 267–294.

Marzolini, S., Brooks, D., & Oh, I. P. (2008, December). Sex differences in completion of a 12-month cardiac rehabilitation programme: An analysis of 5922 women and men. *European Journal of Cardiovascular Prevention and Rehabilitation*, *15*(6), 698–703. doi:10.1097/HJR.0b013e32830c1ce3 PMID:18981927

Matricardi, S., Agostino, R., Fedeli, C., & Montirosso, R. (2013). Mothers are not fathers: differences between parents in the reduction of stress levels after a parental intervention in a NICU. *Acta Paediatrica, 102*(1), 8–14.

Matsui, D. (2013). Medication adherence issues on patients: Focus on cost. *Clinical Audit*, *5*, 33–42. doi:10.2147/CA.S30125

Maxwell, R. J. (1992). Dimensions of quality revisited: From thought to action. *Quality in Health Care*, *1*(3), 171–177. doi:10.1136/qshc.1.3.171 PMID:10136859

Mayr, E. (2011). *Understanding human agency*. New York: Oxford University Press. doi:10.1093/acprof:oso/9780199606214.001.0001

Mazanderani, F., O'Neill, B., & Powell, J. (2013). "People power" or "pester power"? YouTube as a forum for the generation of evidence and patient advocacy. *Patient Education and Counseling*, *93*(3), 420–425. doi:10.1016/j.pec.2013.06.006 PMID:23830239

Mazzoni, D., & Cicognani, E. (2014). Sharing experiences and social support requests in an Internet forum for patients with Systemic Lupus Erythematosus (SLE). *Journal of Health Psychology*, *19*(5), 689–696. doi:10.1177/1359105313477674 PMID:23479300

Mazzoni, D., Van Zomeren, M., & Cicognani, E. (2015). The motivating role of perceived right violation and efficacy beliefs in identification with the Italian Water Movement. *The Journal of Positive Psychology*, *36*(3), 315–330. doi:10.1111/pops.12101

McBride, T., & Korczak, V. (2007). Community consultation and engagement in healthcare reform. *Australian Health Review*, *31*(5), 13–15. doi:10.1071/AH070S13 PMID:17402899

McCarthy, J. D., & Zald, M. N. (1977). Resource mobilization and social movements: A partial theory. *American Journal of Sociology*, *82*(6), 1212–1241. doi:10.1086/226464

McIntyre, A. (2006). *A short history of ethics* (2nd ed.). New York: Routledge.

McIntyre, A. (2007). *After virtue* (3rd ed.). South Bend, IN: Notre Dame Press.

McKee, M., & Healy, J. (2002). *Hospital in a changing Europe*. Buckingham: Open University Press.

McMahon, M. E., Gremore, T. M., Cella, D., & Sher, T. G. (2014). Partners empowered: A couple-based intervention for newly diagnosed cancer. *Psycho-Oncology*, *23*(7), 832–834. doi:10.1002/pon.3490 PMID:24497302

McMillan, S. S., Kendall, E., Sav, A., King, M. A., Whitty, J. A., Kelly, F., & Wheeler, A. J. (2013). Patient-centered approaches to health care: A systematic review of randomized controlled trials. *Medical Care Research and Review*, *70*(6), 567–596. doi:10.1177/1077558713496318 PMID:23894060

McWhinney, I. (1989). The need for a transformed clinical method. In M. Stewart & D. Roter (Eds.), *Communicating with medical patients*. London: Sage.

McWhinney, I. (1993). Why we need a new clinical method. *Scandinavian Journal of Primary Health Care*, *11*(1), 3–7. doi:10.3109/02813439308994894 PMID:8484077

Mead, N., & Bower, P. (2000). Patient-centredness: A conceptual framework and review of the empirical literature. *Social Science & Medicine*, *51*(7), 1087–1110. doi:10.1016/S0277-9536(00)00098-8 PMID:11005395

Mead, N., & Bower, P. (2002). Patient-centred consultations and outcomes in primary care: A review of the literature. *Patient Education and Counseling*, *48*(1), 51–61. doi:10.1016/S0738-3991(02)00099-X PMID:12220750

Meaney, M. J., & Szyf, M. (2005). Maternal care as a model for experience-dependent chromatin plasticity? *Trends in Neurosciences*, *28*(9), 456–463. doi:10.1016/j.tins.2005.07.006 PMID:16054244

Meegan, S. P., & Berg, C. A. (2002). Contexts, functions, forms, and processes of collaborative everyday problem solving in older adulthood. *International Journal of Behavioral Development*, *26*(1), 6–15. doi:10.1080/01650250143000283

Meglic, M., Furlan, M., Kuzmanic, M., Kozel, D., Baraga, D., Kuhar, I., & Brodnik, A. et al. (2010). Feasibility of an ehealth service to support collaborative depression care: Results of a pilot study. *Journal of Medical Internet Research*, *12*(5), e63. doi:10.2196/jmir.1510 PMID:21172765

Mehta, D., Klengel, T., Conneely, K. N., Smith, A. K., Altmann, A., Pace, T. W., & Binder, E. B. et al. (2013). Childhood maltreatment is associated with distinct genomic and epigenetic profiles in posttraumatic stress disorder. *Proceedings of the National Academy of Sciences of the United States of America*, *110*(20), 8302–8307. doi:10.1073/pnas.1217750110 PMID:23630272

Meij, L., W., , Stroebe, M., Schut, H., Stroebe, W., van den Bout, J., & Dijkstra, I. et al. (2008). Parents grieving the loss of their child: Interdependence in coping. *The British Journal of Clinical Psychology*, *47*(1), 31–42. doi:10.1348/014466507X216152 PMID:17588295

Merrill, R. M., Aldana, S. G., Pope, J. E., Anderson, D. R., Coberley, C. R., Grossmeier, J. J., ... & HERO, R. S. S. (2013). Self-rated job performance and absenteeism according to employee engagement, health behaviors, and physical health. *Journal of occupational and environmental medicine/American College of Occupational and Environmental Medicine*, *55*(1), 10-8. doi:10.1097/JOM.0b013e31827b73af

Metcalfe, J., & Terrace, H. S. (2013). *Agency and joint attention*. New York: Oxford University Press. doi:10.1093/acprof:oso/9780199988341.001.0001

Mickelson, K. D., Lyons, R. F., Sullivan, M. J. L., & Coyne, J. C. (2001). Yours, mine, ours: The relational context of communal coping. In B. R. Sarason & S. Duck (Eds.), *Personal relationships: Implications for clinical and community psychology* (pp. 181–200). New York: Wiley.

Mikesell, L., & Bromley, E. (2012). Patient centered, nurse averse? Nurses' care experiences in a 21st-century hospital. *Qualitative Health Research*, *22*(12), 1659–1671. doi:10.1177/1049732312458180 PMID:22923388

Miles, M. S., Holditch-Davis, D., Schwartz, T. A., & Scher, M. (2007). Depressive symptoms in mothers of prematurely born infants. *Journal of Developmental and Behavioral Pediatrics*, *28*(1), 36–44. doi:10.1097/01.DBP.0000257517.52459.7a PMID:17353730

Miles, S., & Frewer, L. J. (2003). Public perception of scientific uncertainty in relation to food hazards. *Journal of Risk Research*, *6*(3), 267–283. doi:10.1080/1366987032000088883

Miller, D. T. (2001). Disrespect and the experience of injustice. *Annual Review of Psychology*, *52*(1), 527–553. doi:10.1146/annurev.psych.52.1.527 PMID:11148316

Moja, E. A., & Vegni, E. (2000). *La visita medica centrata sul paziente*. Milano: Cortina Editore.

Molloy, G. J., Johnston, D. W., & Witham, M. D. (2005). Family caregiving and congestive heart failure. Review and analysis. *European Journal of Heart Failure, 7*, 592-603. doi:10.10167j.ejheart.2004.07.008

Montirosso, R., Del Prete, A., Bellu, R., Tronick, E., & Borgatti, R.NEO-ACquA Study Group. (2012a). Level of NICU quality of developmental care and neurobehavioral performance in very preterm infants. *Pediatrics*, *129*(5), e1129–e1137. doi:10.1542/peds.2011-0813 PMID:22492762

Montirosso, R., Fedeli, C., Del Prete, A., Calciolari, G., Borgatti, R., & Mosca, F. et al.. (2014). Maternal stress and depressive symptoms associated with quality of developmental care in 25 Italian Neonatal Intensive Care Units: A cross sectional observational study. *International Journal of Nursing Studies*, *51*(7), 994–1002. doi:10.1016/j.ijnurstu.2013.11.001 PMID:24315196

Montirosso, R., & Provenzi, L. (2015). Implications of Epigenetics and Stress Regulation on Research and Developmental Care of Preterm Infants. *Journal of Obstetric, Gynecologic, and Neonatal Nursing*, *44*(2), 174–182. doi:10.1111/1552-6909.12559 PMID:25712710

Montirosso, R., Provenzi, L., Calciolari, G., & Borgatti, R.NEO-ACQUA Study Group. (2012b). Measuring maternal stress and perceived support in 25 Italian NICUs. *Acta Paediatrica (Oslo, Norway)*, *101*(2), 136–142. doi:10.1111/j.1651-2227.2011.02440.x PMID:21827551

Montirosso, R., Provenzi, L., Fumagalli, M., Sirgiovanni, I., Giorda, R., & Pozzoli, U. et al. (2016). Serotonin transporter gene (*SLC6A4*) methylation associates with Neonatal Intensive Care Unit stay and 3-month-old temperament in preterm infants. *Child Development*, 87(1), 38-48. doi:10.1111/cdev.12492

Moore, P. J., Adler, N. E., & Robertson, P. A. (2000). Medical malpractice: The effects of doctor-patient relationships on medical patient perceptions and malpractice intentions. *The Western Journal of Medicine*, *173*(4), 244–250. doi:10.1136/ewjm.173.4.244 PMID:11017984

Mörelius, E., Nelson, N., & Gustafsson, P. A. (2007). Salivary cortisol response in mother-infant dyads at high psychosocial risk. *Child: Care, Health and Development*, *33*(2), 128–136. doi:10.1111/j.1365-2214.2006.00637.x PMID:17291316

Mörelius, E., Örtenstrand, A., Theodorsson, E., & Frostell, A. (2015). A randomised trial of continuous skin-to-skin contact after preterm birth and the effects on salivary cortisol, parental stress, depression, and breastfeeding. *Early Human Development*, *91*(1), 63–70. doi:10.1016/j.earlhumdev.2014.12.005 PMID:25545453

Morgan, M. G., Fischhoff, B., Bostrom, A., & Altman, C. J. (2002). *Risk communication.* Boston, MA, USA: Cambridge University Press.

Mueller, A., Brocke, B., Fries, E., Lesch, K. P., & Kirschbaum, C. (2010). The role of the serotonin transporter polymorphism for the endocrine stress response in newborns. *Psychoneuroendocrinology, 35*(2), 289–296. doi:10.1016/j.psyneuen.2009.07.002 PMID:19647944

Mueller, C. (1994). Conflict networks and the origins of women's liberation. In H. Johnston, E. Larana, & J. R. Gusfield (Eds.), *New Social movements. From ideology toidentity* (pp. 234–263). Philadelphia: Temple University Press.

Munir, F., Houdmont, J., Clemes, S., Wilson, K., Kerr, R., & Addley, K. (2015). Work engagement and its association with occupational sitting time: Results from the Stormont study. *BMC Public Health, 15*(1), 30. doi:10.1186/s12889-015-1427-9 PMID:25631579

Murdoch, J. (1998). The Spaces of Actor-Network Theory. *Geoforum, 29*(4), 357–374. doi:10.1016/S0016-7185(98)00011-6

Nahrgang, J. D., Morgeson, F. P., & Hofmann, D. A. (2011). Safety at work: A meta-analytic investigation of the link between job demands, job resources, burnout, engagement, and safety outcomes. *The Journal of Applied Psychology, 96*(1), 71–94. doi:10.1037/a0021484 PMID:21171732

National Association of Insurance Companies. (2014). *Malpractice, the hastle. Dossier Ania about medical malpractice* [Malpractice, il grande caos. Dossier ANIA sul tema della malasanità]. Retrieved from http://www.ania.it

National Health Performance Committee. (2001). *National Health Performance Framework report.* Canberra: AIHW.

Naylor, C., Parsonage, M., McDaid, D., Knapp, M., Fossey, M., & Galea, A. (2012). *Long-term conditions and mental health: the cost of co-morbidities.* London: The King's Fund and Centre for Mental Health.

Ng, E. S., & Law, A. (2014). Keeping up! Older workers' adaptation in the workplace after age 55. *Canadian Journal on Aging, 33*(1), 1–14. doi:10.1017/S0714980813000639 PMID:24345532

Nie, N., & Verba, S. (1975). Political participation. In F. I. Greenstein & N. W. Polsby (Eds.), *Handbook of political science* (pp. 1–74). Reading, MA: Addison-Wesley.

Norelli, G. A., De Luca, F., Focardi, M., Giardiello, R., & Pinchi, V. (2015). The claims management committees trial: Experience of an Italian hospital of the National Health System. *Journal of Forensic and Legal Medicine, 29*, 6–12. doi:10.1016/j.jflm.2014.10.004 PMID:25572077

Northhouse, L. L., Katapodi, M. C., Song, L., Zhang, L., & Mood, D. W. (2010). Interventions with family caregivers of cancer patients meta-analysis of randomized trials. *CA: a Cancer Journal for Clinicians, 60*, 317–339. doi:10.3322/caac.20081 PMID:20709946

Nugus, P., Greenfield, D., Travaglia, J., Westbrook, J., & Braithwaite, J. (2010). How and where clinicians exercise power: Interprofessional relations in health care. *Social Science & Medicine, 71*(5), 898–909. doi:10.1016/j.socscimed.2010.05.029 PMID:20609507

Nussbaum, M. C. (2000). *Women and human development: The capabilities approach.* New York: Cambridge University Press. doi:10.1017/CBO9780511841286

Nussbaum, M. C. (2007). *Frontiers of justice.* Cambridge, MA: The Belknap Press of Harvard University Press.

Nussbaum, M. C. (2011). *Creating capabilities: The human development approach.* Cambridge, MA: The Belknap Press of Harvard University Press. doi:10.4159/harvard.9780674061200

O'Brien, M. A., Ellis, P. M., Whelan, T. J., Charles, C., Gafni, A., Lovrics, P., & Hodgson, N. et al. (2013). Physician-related facilitators and barriers to patient involvement in treatment decision making in early breast cancer: Perspectives of physicians and patients. *Health Expectations*, *16*(4), 373–384. doi:10.1111/j.1369-7625.2011.00712.x PMID:21923813

O'Brien, T. B., & DeLongis, A. (1997). Coping with chronic stress: An interpersonal perspective. In B. H. Gottlieb (Ed.), *Coping with chronic stress* (pp. 161–190). New York: Plenum Press. doi:10.1007/978-1-4757-9862-3_6

Oberlander, T. F., Weinberg, J., Papsdorf, M., Grunau, R., Misri, S., & Devlin, A. M. (2008). Prenatal exposure to maternal depression, neonatal methylation of human glucocorticoid receptor gene (NR3C1) and infant cortisol stress responses. *Epigenetics: Official Journal of the DNA Methylation Society*, *3*(2), 97–106. doi:10.4161/epi.3.2.6034 PMID:18536531

Oborn, E., & Dawson, S. (2010). Knowledge and practice in multidisciplinary teams: Struggle, accommodation and privilege. *Human Relations*, *63*(12), 1835–1857. doi:10.1177/0018726710371237

Okhuysen, G. A., & Bechky, B. A. (2009). Coordination in organizations: An integrative perspective. *The Academy of Management Annals*, *3*(1), 463–502. doi:10.1080/19416520903047533

Okin, S. M. (1989). *Gender, justice, and the family*. New York: Basic Books.

O'Leary, D. S., & O'Leary, M. R. (1992). From quality assurance to quality improvement. The Joint Commission on Accreditation of Healthcare Organizations and Emergency Care. *Emergency Medicine Clinics of North America*, *10*, 477–492. PMID:1628555

Olson, M. (1965). *The logic of collective action: public goods and the theory of groups*. Cambridge, MA: Harvard University Press.

Opp, K. D. (1986). Soft incentives and collective action. Participation in the Anti-Nuclear Movement. *British Journal of Political Science*, *16*(01), 87–112. doi:10.1017/S0007123400003811

Orizio, G., Schulz, P., Gasparotti, C., Caimi, L., & Gelatti, U. (2010). The world of e-patients: A content analysis of online social networks focusing on diseases. *Telemedicine Journal and e-Health*, *16*(10), 1060–1066. doi:10.1089/tmj.2010.0085 PMID:21070131

Osmond, H. (1957). Function as Basic Psychiatric Ward Design. *Psychiatric Services (Washington, D.C.)*, *8*(4), 23–27. doi:10.1176/ps.8.4.23

Osterberg, L., & Blaschke, T. (2005). Adherence to medication. *The New England Journal of Medicine*, *353*(5), 487–497. doi:10.1056/NEJMra050100 PMID:16079372

Oude Hengel, K. M., Blatter, B. M., Joling, C. I., van der Beek, A. J., & Bongers, P. M. (2012). Effectiveness of an intervention at construction worksites on work engagement, social support, physical workload, and need for recovery: Results from a cluster randomized controlled trial. *BMC Public Health*, *12*, 1008. doi:10.1186/1471-2458-12-1008 PMID:23171354

Øvretveit, J. (2009). *Does improving quality save money? A review of the evidence of which improvements to quality reduce costs to health service providers*. London: the Health Foundation.

Øvretveit, J. (2011). Understanding the conditions for improvement: Research to discover which context influences affect improvement success. *BMJ Quality & Safety*, *20*(Suppl. 1), 18–23. doi:10.1136/bmjqs.2010.045955 PMID:21450764

Owen-Smith, A., Coast, J., & Donovan, J. (2009). "I can see where they're coming from, but when you're on the end of it ... you just want to get the money and the drug.": Explaining reactions to explicit healthcare rationing. *Social Science & Medicine*, *68*(11), 1935–1942. doi:10.1016/j.socscimed.2009.03.024 PMID:19375210

Own, L. S., Iqbal, R., & Patel, P. D. (2013). Maternal separation alters serotonergic and HPA axis gene expression independent of separation duration in c57bl/6 mice. *Brain Research*, *1515*, 29–38. doi:10.1016/j.brainres.2013.03.032 PMID:23548594

Ozawa, M., Sasaki, M., & Kanda, K. (2010). Effect of procedure light on the physiological responses of preterm infants. *Japan Journal of Nursing Science*, *7*(1), 76–83. doi:10.1111/j.1742-7924.2010.00142.x PMID:20618679

Pack, Q. R., Johnson, L. L., Barr, L. M., Daniels, S. R., Wolter, A. D., Squires, R. W., & Thomas, R. J. et al. (2013). Improving cardiac rehabilitation attendance and completion through quality improvement activities and a motivational program. *Journal of Cardiopulmonary Rehabilitation and Prevention*, *33*(3), 153–159. doi:10.1097/HCR.0b013e31828db386 PMID:23595006

Pagani, A. F., Donato, S., Parise, M., Iafrate, R., Bertoni, A., & Schoebi, D. (2015). When Good Things Happen: The Effects of Implicit and Explicit Capitalization Attempts on Intimate Partners' Well-being. *Family Science*, *6*, 119–128. doi:10.1080/19424620.2015.1082013

Pallant, J. (2007). *SPSS survival manual: A step by step guide to data analysis using SPSS for windows* (3rd ed.). Berkshire, England: Open University Press.

Paoli, P., & Merllie, D. (2001). *Third European Working Conditions Survey 2000*. European foundation for the improvement of Living and Working Conditions, Office for official publications of the European Communities, Luxemburg. Retrieved from http://www.eurofound.eu.int/publications/EF0121.htm

Pascoe, G. C. (1983). Patient satisfaction in primary health care: A literature review and analysis. *Evaluation and Program Planning*, *6*(3), 185–210. doi:10.1016/0149-7189(83)90002-2 PMID:10299618

Paxton, P. (2002). Social capital and democracy: An interdependentrelationship. *American Sociological Review*, *67*(2), 254–277. doi:10.2307/3088895

Peng, N., Bachman, J., Jenkins, R., Chen, C.-H., Chang, Y.-C., Chang, Y.-S., & Wang, T.-M. (2009). Stressors and Stress Biobehavioral Responses of Preterm Infants in NICU. *The Journal of Perinatal & Neonatal Nursing*, *23*(4), 363–371. doi:10.1097/JPN.0b013e3181bdd3fd PMID:19915421

Peters, E., Hess, T. H., Västfjäll, D., & Auman, C. (2007). Implications for the role of affective and deliberative processes in older adults' decision making. *Perspectives on Psychological Science*, *2*(1), 1–23. doi:10.1111/j.1745-6916.2007.00025.x PMID:26151915

Peterson, C., & Seligman, M. (2004). *Character strengths and virtues: A handbook and classification*. New York: Oxford University Press.

Pettigrew, T. F. (1967). Social evaluation theory. In D. Levine (Ed.), *Nebraska symposium on motivation* (pp. 241–315). Lincoln: Nebraska University Press.

Philibert, R. A., Sandhu, H., Hollenbeck, N., Gunter, T., Adams, W., & Madan, A. (2008). The relationship of 5HTT (SLC6A4) methylation and genotype on mRNA expression and liability to major depression and alcohol dependence in subjects from the Iowa Adoption Studies. *American Journal of Medical Genetics*, *147B*(5), 543–549. doi:10.1002/ajmg.b.30657 PMID:17987668

Piette, J. D., Beard, A., Rosland, A. M., & McHorney, C. A. (2011). Beliefs that influence cost-related medication nonadherence among the "haves" and "have nots" with chronic disease. *Patient Preference and Adherence*, *5*, 389–396. doi:10.2147/PPA.S23111 PMID:21949602

Pillai Ridell, R., Racine, N., Turcotte, K., Uman, L. S., Horton, R., & Osmun, L. D. et al.. (2011). Nonpharmacological management of procedural pain in infants and young children. *Pain Research & Management: The Journal of the Canadian Pain Society*, *16*(5), 321–330. doi:10.1155/2011/489286 PMID:22059204

Plato. (2002). Five dialogues (trans. by J. M. Cooper, ed. by G. M. Grube). Indianapolis, IN: Hackett Publishing Company.

Plato, . (2004). *Republic* (C.D. Reeve, Trans.). Indianapolis, IN: Hackett Publishing Company.

Platt, F. W., Gaspar, D. L., Coulehan, J. L., Fox, L., Adler, A. J., & Weston, W. W. et al.. (2001). "Tell me about yourself": The patient-centered interview. *Annals of Internal Medicine*, *134*(11), 1079–1085. doi:10.7326/0003-4819-134-11-200106050-00020 PMID:11388827

Pohjonen, T., Punakallio, A., & Louhevaara, V. (1998). Participatory ergonomics for reducing load and strain in home care work. *International Journal of Industrial Ergonomics*, *21*(5), 345–352. doi:10.1016/S0169-8141(96)00083-2

Pollack, M. M., Holubkov, R., Funai, T., Clark, A., Berger, J. T., Meert, K., & Jenkins, T. L. et al. (2014). Pediatric Intensive Care Outcomes: Development of New Morbidities During Pediatric Critical Care. *Pediatric Critical Care Medicine*, *15*(9), 821–827. doi:10.1097/PCC.0000000000000250 PMID:25226501

Postmes, T. (2007). The psychological dimensions of collective action, online. In A. N. Joinson, K. Y. McKenna, T. Postmes, & U. D. Reips (Eds.), *The Oxford handbook of Internet psychology* (pp. 165–184). Oxford: Oxford University Press.

Postmes, T., Haslam, S. A., & Swaab, R. I. (2005). Social identity and social influence in small groups: Communication, consensualization and socially shared cognition. *European Review of Social Psychology*, *16*, 1–42. doi:10.1080/10463280440000062

Postmes, T., Spears, R., Lee, A. T., & Novak, R. J. (2005). Individuality and social influence in groups: Inductive and deductive routes to group identity. *Journal of Personality and Social Psychology*, *89*(5), 747–763. doi:10.1037/0022-3514.89.5.747 PMID:16351366

Pretty, J. N. (1995). Participatory learning for sustainable agriculture. *World Development*, *23*(8), 1247–1263. doi:10.1016/0305-750X(95)00046-F

Prochaska, J. O., & Di Clemente, C. C. (1982). Transtheoretical therapy: Toward a more integrative model of change. *Psychotherapy (Chicago, Ill.)*, *19*(3), 276–288. doi:10.1037/h0088437

Provenzi, L., Barello, S., & Graffigna, G. (2016). Caregiver engagement in the Neonatal Intensive Care Unit: Parental needs, engagement milestones, and action priorities for neonatal health care of preterm infants. In G. Graffigna, S. Barello, S. Triberti (Eds.), Caregiver Engagement in the Neonatal Intensive Care Unit: Parental Needs, Engagement Milestones, and Action Priorities for Neonatal Healthcare of Preterm Infants (pp. 94-107). Berlin, Germany: De Gruyter.

Provenzi, L., & Barello, S. (2015). Behavioral Epigenetics of Family-Centered Care in the Neonatal Intensive Care Unit. *JAMA Pediatrics*, *169*(7), 697–698. doi:10.1001/jamapediatrics.2015.0367 PMID:26147053

Provenzi, L., Fumagalli, M., Sirgiovanni, I., Giorda, R., Pozzoli, U., Morandi, F., & Montirosso, R. et al. (2015b). Pain-related stress during the Neonatal Intensive Care Unit stay and SLC6A4 methylation in very preterm infants. *Frontiers in Behavioral Neuroscience*, *9*, 1–9. doi:10.3389/fnbeh.2015.00099 PMID:25941480

Provenzi, L., Menichetti, J., Coin, R., & Aschieri, F. (2016). (in press). Psychological assessment as an intervention with couples: Single case application of collaborative techniques in clinical practice. *Professional Psychology*.

Provenzi, L., & Montirosso, R. (2015). Epigenethics" in the Neonatal Intensive Care Unit Conveying Complexity in Health Care for Preterm Children. *JAMA Pediatrics*, *169*(7), 617–618. doi:10.1001/jamapediatrics.2015.43 PMID:25938864

Provenzi, L., & Santoro, E. (2015). The lived experience of fathers of preterm infants in the Neonatal Intensive Care Unit: A systematic review of qualitative studies. *Journal of Clinical Nursing*, *24*(13-14), 1784–1794. doi:10.1111/jocn.12828 PMID:25850518

Putnam, R. (2000). *Bowling Alone: The Collapse and Revival of American Community*. New York: Simon and Schuster. doi:10.1145/358916.361990

Rabeharisoa, V. (2006). From representation to mediation: The shaping of collective mobilization on muscular dystrophy in France. *Social Science & Medicine*, *62*(3), 564–576. doi:10.1016/j.socscimed.2005.06.036 PMID:16051407

Rabinow, P. (2002). Artificiality and enlightnment: From sociobiology to biosociality. In M. Biagioli (Ed.), The Science Studies Reader. New York: Routledge.

Radin, P. (2006). "To me, it's my life": Medical communication, trust, and activism in cyberspace. *Social Science & Medicine*, *62*(3), 591–601. doi:10.1016/j.socscimed.2005.06.022 PMID:16039031

Randall, A. K., & Bodenmann, G. (2009). The role of stress on close relationships and marital satisfaction. *Clinical Psychology Review*, *29*(2), 105–115. doi:10.1016/j.cpr.2008.10.004 PMID:19167139

Ranger, M., Synnes, A. R., Vinall, J., & Grunau, R. E. (2014). Internalizing behaviours in school-age children born very preterm are predicted by neonatal pain and morphine exposure. *European Journal of Pain (London, England)*, *18*(6), 844–852. doi:10.1002/j.1532-2149.2013.00431.x PMID:24318537

Rankin-Esquer, L. A., Deeter, A. K., & Barr Taylor, C. (2000). Coronary heart disease and couples. In K. B. Schmaling & T. Goldman Sher (Eds.), *The psychology of couples and illness: Theory, research and practice* (pp. 43–70). Washington: American Psychological Association. doi:10.1037/10360-002

Rao, J. K., Weinberger, M., & Kroenke, K. (2000). Visit-specific expectations and patient-centered outcomes: A literature review. *Archives of Family Medicine*, *9*(10), 1148–1155. doi:10.1001/archfami.9.10.1148 PMID:11115222

Rask, K. J., Ziemer, D. C., Kohler, S. A., Hawley, J. N., Arinde, F. J., & Barnes, C. S. (2009). Patient activation is associated with healthy behaviors and ease in managing diabetes in an indigent population. *The Diabetes Educator*, *35*(4), 622–630. doi:10.1177/0145721709335004 PMID:19419972

Rathert, C., Wyrwich, M. D., & Boren, S. A. (2013). Patient-Centered Care and Outcomes A Systematic Review of the Literature. *Medical Care Research and Review*, *70*(4), 351–379. doi:10.1177/1077558712465774 PMID:23169897

Ravalier, J. M., Dandil, Y., & Limehouse, H. (2015). Employee engagement and management standards: A concurrent evaluation. *Occupational Medicine*, *65*(6), 496–498. doi:10.1093/occmed/kqv071 PMID:26078417

Rawls, J. (1971). *A theory of justice*. Cambridge, MA: The Belknap Press of Harvard University Press.

Reday-Mulvey, G. (2005). *Working Beyond 60. Key Policies and Practices in Europe*. Great Britain: Palgrave Macmillan. doi:10.1057/9780230504981

Regan, Á., McConnon, Á., Kuttschreuter, M., Rutsaert, P., Shan, L., Pieniak, Z., & Wall, P. et al. (2014). The impact of communicating conflicting risk and benefit messages: An experimental study on red meat information. *Food Quality and Preference*, *38*, 107–114. doi:10.1016/j.foodqual.2014.05.019

Regan, T. M., Lambert, S. D., Kelly, B., Falconier, M., Kissane, D., & Levesque, J. V. (2015). Couples coping with cancer: Exploration of theoretical frameworks from dyadic studies. *Psycho-Oncology*, *24*(12), 1605–1617. doi:10.1002/pon.3854 PMID:26059915

Reicher, S. (1984). The St Paul's riot: An explanation ofthe limits of crowd action in terms of a socialidentity model. *European Journal of Social Psychology*, *14*(1), 1–21. doi:10.1002/ejsp.2420140102

Reicher, S., Spears, R., & Postmes, T. (1995). A social identity model of deindividuation phenomena. *European Review of Social Psychology*, *6*(1), 161–198. doi:10.1080/14792779443000049

Reinhardt, J. (2001). Effects of positive and negative support received and provided on adaptation to chronic visual impairment. *Applied Developmental Science*, *5*(2), 76–85. doi:10.1207/S1532480XADS0502_3

Reis, H. T., & Collins, N. (2000). Measuring relationship properties and interactions relevant to social support. In S. Cohen, L. G. Underwood, & B. J. Gottlieb (Eds.), *Social support measurement and intervention* (pp. 136–192). New York: Oxford University Press. doi:10.1093/med:psych/9780195126709.003.0005

Reis, H. T., & Shaver, P. (1988). Intimacy as an interpersonal process. In S. Duck (Ed.), *Handbook of personal relationships* (pp. 367–389). Chichester, England: Wiley.

Renkema, E., Broekhius, M., & Ahaus, K. (2014). Conditions that influence the impact of malpractice litigation risk on physicians' behavior regarding patient safety. *BMC Health Services Research*, *14*(1), 38. doi:10.1186/1472-6963-14-38 PMID:24460754

Renn, O. (2008). *Risk governance: coping with uncertainty in a complex world.* Earthscan.

Repetti, R. L. (1989). Effects of daily workload on subsequent behavior during marital interaction: The roles of social withdrawal and spouse support. *Journal of Personality and Social Psychology*, *57*(4), 651–659. doi:10.1037/0022-3514.57.4.651 PMID:2795436

Revenson, T. A. (1994). Social support and marital coping with chronic illness. *Annals of Behavioral Medicine*, *16*, 122–130.

Revenson, T. A. (2003). Scenes from a marriage: Examining support, coping, and gender within the context of chronic illness. In J. Suls & K. Wallston (Eds.), *Social psychological foundation of health and illness* (pp. 530–559). Oxford: Blackwell Publishers. doi:10.1002/9780470753552.ch19

Revenson, T. A., Abraido-Lanza, A. F., Majerovitz, S. D., & Jordan, C. (2005). Couples coping with chronic illness: What's gender got to do with it? In T. A. Revenson, K. Kayser, & G. Bodenmann (Eds.), *Couples coping with stress: Emerging perspectives on dyadic coping* (pp. 121–136). Washington, DC: American Psychological Association. doi:10.1037/11031-007

Revenson, T. A., & DeLongis, A. (2011). Couples coping with chronic illness. In S. Folkman (Ed.), *The Oxford Handbook of Stress, Health, and Coping* (pp. 101–123). New York: Oxford University Press.

Revenson, T. A., Kayser, K., & Bodenmann, G. (2005). *Couples coping with stress: Emerging perspectives on dyadic coping*. Washington, DC: American Psychological Association. doi:10.1037/11031-000

Riboldi, L., Carrer, P., Magnavita, N., & Porru, S. (2010). Biological risk. Relevant problems: Risk to third parties. *Giornale Italiano di Medicina del Lavoro Ed Ergonomia*, *32*(3), 304–311. PMID:21061714

Rice, T. (2001). Should consumer choice be encouraged in health care? In J. B. Davis (Ed.), *The social economics of health care* (pp. 9–39). London: Routledge. doi:10.4324/9780203459898.pt1

Richardson, S. S., Daniels, C. R., Gillman, M. W., Golden, J. L., Kukla, R., Kuzawa, C., & Rich-Edwards, J. (2014). Don't blame the mothers. *Nature*, *512*(7513), 131–132. doi:10.1038/512131a PMID:25119222

Ried, L. D. (2010). Cost sharing and adherence, medication burden and adherence, and beta receptor selectivity. *Journal of the American Pharmacists Association*, *50*(3), 440. doi:10.1331/JAPhA.2010.10521 PMID:20452925

Riegel, B., Lee, C. S., & Dickson, V. V. (2011). Self-care in patients with chronic heart failure. *Nature Reviews. Cardiology*, *8*(11), 644–654. doi:10.1038/nrcardio.2011.95 PMID:21769111

Ripamonti, S., Galuppo, L., Gorli, M., Scaratti, G., & Cunliffe, A. L. (2015). Pushing action-research towards reflexive practice. *Journal of Management Inquiry*. doi:10.1177/1056492615584972

Rivilis, I., Van Eerd, D., Cullen, K., Cole, D. C., Irvin, E., Tyson, J., & Mahood, Q. (2008). Effectiveness of participatory ergonomic interventions on health outcomes: A systematic review. *Applied Ergonomics*, *39*(3), 342–358. doi:10.1016/j.apergo.2007.08.006 PMID:17988646

Robben, S. H., Huisjes, M., van Achterberg, T., Zuidema, S. U., Olde Rikkert, M. G., Schers, H. J., ... & Zowel N.N. Study Group. (2012a). Filling the gaps in a fragmented health care system: Development of the Health and Welfare Information Portal (ZWIP). *JMIR Research Protocols, 1,* e10. doi:10.2196/resprot.1945

Robben, S. H., Perry, M., Huisjes, M., van Nieuwenhuijzen, L., Schers, H. J., van Weel, C., & Melis, R. J. F. et al. (2012b). Implementation of an innovative web-based conference table for community-dwelling frail older people, their informal caregivers and professionals: A process evaluation. *BMC Health Services Research*, *12*(1), 251. doi:10.1186/1472-6963-12-251 PMID:22894654

Roberts, K. J., & Volberding, P. (1999). Adherence communication: A qualitative analysis of physician-patient dialogue. *AIDS (London, England)*, *13*(13), 1771–1778. doi:10.1097/00002030-199909100-00022 PMID:10509580

Roberts, S., Lester, K. J., Hudson, J. L., Rapee, R. M., Creswell, C., Cooper, P. J., & Eley, T. C. et al. (2014). Serotonin transporter methylation and response to cognitive behaviour therapy in children with anxiety disorders. *Translational Psychiatry*, *4*(9), e444–e445. doi:10.1038/tp.2014.83 PMID:25226553

Robinson, J. H., Callister, L. C., Berry, J. A., & Dearing, K. A. (2008). Patient-centered care and adherence: Definitions and applications to improve outcomes. *Journal of the American Academy of Nurse Practitioners*, *20*(12), 600–607. doi:10.1111/j.1745-7599.2008.00360.x PMID:19120591

Rohrbaugh, M. J., Shoham, V., & Coyne, J. C. (2006). Effect of marital quality on eight-year survival of patients with heart failure. *The American Journal of Cardiology*, *98*(8), 1069–1072. doi:10.1016/j.amjcard.2006.05.034 PMID:17027573

Rongen, A., Robroek, S. J., Schaufeli, W., & Burdorf, A. (2014). The contribution of work engagement to self-perceived health, work ability, and sickness absence beyond health behaviors and work-related factors. *Journal of Occupational and Environmental Medicine*, *56*(8), 892–897. doi:10.1097/JOM.0000000000000196 PMID:25099418

Rosenberg, E. E., Lussier, M. T., & Beaudoin, C. (1997). Lessons for clinicians from physician-patient communication literature. *Archives of Family Medicine*, *6*(3), 279–283. doi:10.1001/archfami.6.3.279 PMID:9161356

Rost, K. M., Meng, H., & Xu, S. (2014). Work productivity loss from depression: Evidence from an employer survey. *BMC Health Services Research*, *14*(1), 597. doi:10.1186/s12913-014-0597-y PMID:25519705

Roter, D. (2006). The patient-physician relationship and its implications for malpractice litigation. *Journal of Health Care Law & Policy*, *9*, 304–314.

Roter, D. L. (1991). *Roter Interaction Analysis System: Coding Manual*. Baltimore, USA: Johns Hopkins University.

Roter, D., & Larson, S. (2002). The Roter interaction analysis system (RIAS): Utility and flexibility for analysis of medical interactions. *Patient Education and Counseling*, *46*(4), 243–251. doi:10.1016/S0738-3991(02)00012-5 PMID:11932123

Runciman, B., Merry, A., & Walton, M. (2007). *Safety and Ethics in Healthcare: A Guide to Getting it Right*. Burlington, VT: Ashgate.

Runciman, W. G. (1966). *Relative deprivation and social justice: A study of attitudes to social inequality in twentieth-century England*. Berkeley: University of California Press.

Russell, C. L., Conn, V. S., & Jantarakupt, P. (2006). Older adult medication compliance: Integrated review of randomized controlled trials. *American Journal of Health Behavior*, *6*(6), 636–650. doi:10.5993/AJHB.30.6.10 PMID:17096621

Rutsaert, P., Barnett, J., Gaspar, R., Marcu, A., Pieniak, Z., Seibt, B., & Verbeke, W. et al. (2015). Beyond information seeking: Consumers' online deliberation about the risks and benefits of red meat. *Food Quality and Preference*, *39*, 191–201. doi:10.1016/j.foodqual.2014.07.011

Sabate, E. (2003). Adherence to long-term therapies: Evidence for action. Geneva: World Health Organization; Retrieved from http://www.who.int/chronic_conditions/en/adherence_report.pdf

Safran, D. G., Neuman, P., Schoen, C., Kitchman, M. S., Wilson, I. B., Cooper, B., et al. (2005). *Prescription drug coverage and seniors: Findings from a 2003 national survey*. Retrieved from http://content.healthaffairs.org/content/early/2005/04/19/hlthaff.w5.152

Safran, D. G., Taira, D. A., Rogers, W. H., Kosinski, M., Ware, J. E., & Tarlov, A. R. (1998). Linking primary care performance to outcomes of care. *The Journal of Family Practice*, *47*(3), 213–220. PMID:9752374

Samra, H., McGrath, J. M., Fischer, S., Schumacher, B., Dutcher, J., & Hansen, J. (2015). The NICU Parent Risk Evaluation and Engagement Model and Instrument (PREEMI) for Neonates in Intensive Care Units. *Journal of Obstetric, Gynecologic, and Neonatal Nursing*, *44*(1), 114–126. doi:10.1111/1552-6909.12535 PMID:25580952

Samuel, O., Grant, J., & Irvine, D. (1994). *Quality and audit in general practice: Meanings and definitions*. London: Royal College of General Practitioners.

Sanders, M. J., & McCready, J. W. (2010). Does work contribute to successful aging outcomes in older workers? *International Journal of Aging & Human Development*, *71*(3), 209–229. doi:10.2190/AG.71.3.c PMID:21166334

Sanderson, K., & Cocker, F. (2013). Presenteeism--implications and health risks. *Australian Family Physician*, *42*(4), 172–175. PMID:23550237

Santos, V. (2014). *Determinantes da resposta de adesão ao medicamento em idosos: Uma abordagem experimental* [Determinants of response to drug adherence in the elderly: An experimental approach] [Master thesis]. University of Évora, Évora, Portugal.

Saunders, M., Lewis, P., & Thornhill, A. (2009). *Research methods for business students* (5th ed.). Essex, England: Pearson Education Limited.

Scally, G., & Donaldson, L. J. (1998). Clinical governance and the drive for quality improvement in the new NHS in England. *British Medical Journal*, *317*(7150), 61–65. doi:10.1136/bmj.317.7150.61 PMID:9651278

Scaratti, G., Gorli, M., & Ripamonti, S. (2009). The power of professionally situated practice analysis in redesigning organisations: A psychosociological approach. *Journal of Workplace Learning*, *21*(7), 538–554. doi:10.1108/13665620910985531

Schauer, F. (2011). Transparency in Three Dimensions. *University of Illinois Law Review*, *4*, 1339–1342.

Scher, M. S., Ludington-Hoe, S., Kaffashi, F., Johnson, M. W., Holditch-Davis, D., & Loparo, K. (2009). Neurophysiologic assessment of brain maturation after an 8-week trial of skin-to-skin contact on preterm infants. *Clinical Neurophysiology*, *120*(10), 1812–1818. doi:10.1016/j.clinph.2009.08.004 PMID:19766056

Schinka, J., Busch, R. M., & Robichaux-Keene, N. (2004). A meta-analysis of the association between the serotonin transporter gene polymorphism (5-HTTLPR) and trait anxiety. *Molecular Psychiatry*, *9*(2), 197–202. doi:10.1038/sj.mp.4001405 PMID:14966478

Schneider, E. C., & Epstein, A. M. (1998). Use of public performance reports: A survey of patients undergoing cardiac surgery. *Journal of the American Medical Association*, *279*(20), 1638–1642. doi:10.1001/jama.279.20.1638 PMID:9613914

Schoebi, D. (2008). The coregulation of daily affect in marital relationships. *Journal of Family Psychology*, *22*(4), 595–604. doi:10.1037/0893-3200.22.3.595 PMID:18729673

Schur, L., Shields, T., & Schriner, K. (2003). Can I make a difference? Efficacy, employment, and disability. *Political Psychology*, *24*(1), 119–149. doi:10.1111/0162-895X.00319

Schüz, B., Marx, C., Wurm, S., Warner, L. M., Ziegelmann, J. P., Schwarzer, R., & Tesch-Römer, C. (2011). Medication beliefs predict medication adherence in older adults with multiple illnesses. *Journal of Psychosomatic Research*, *70*(2), 179–187. doi:10.1016/j.jpsychores.2010.07.014 PMID:21262421

Schüz, B., Wolff, J. K., Warner, L. M., Ziegelmann, J. P., & Wurm, S. (2014). Multiple illness perceptions in older adults: Effects on physical functioning and medication adherence. *Psychology & Health*, *29*(4), 442–457. doi:10.1080/08870446.2013.863884 PMID:24224651

Schüz, B., Wurm, S., Warner, L. M., Wolff, J. K., & Schwarzer, R. (2013). Health motives and health behaviour self-regulation in older adults. *Journal of Behavioral Medicine*, *37*(3), 491–500. doi:10.1007/s10865-013-9504-y PMID:23512197

Schwarzer, R. (1992). Self-efficacy in the adoption and maintenance of health behaviours: Theoretical approaches and a new model. In R. Schwarzer (Ed.), *Self-efficacy: Thought control of action* (pp. 217–242). Washington, DC: Hemisphere.

Schwarzer, R. (2008). Modeling health behaviour change: How to predict and modify the adoption and maintenance of health behaviours. *Applied Psychology*, *57*, 1–29. doi:10.1111/j.1464-0597.2007.00325.x

Scotch, R. K. (1988). Disability as the basis of a social movement: Advocacy and the politics of definition. *The Journal of Social Issues*, *44*(1), 159–172. doi:10.1111/j.1540-4560.1988.tb02055.x

Scott, J. L., & Kayser, K. (2009). A review of couple-based interventions for enhancing women's sexual adjustment and body image after cancer. *Cancer Journal (Sudbury, Mass.)*, *15*(1), 48–56. doi:10.1097/PPO.0b013e31819585df PMID:19197174

Scourfield, P., & Burch, S. (2010). Ethical Considerations when involving older people in public service participation processes. *Ethics and Social Welfare*, *4*(3), 236–253. doi:10.1080/17496535.2010.516120

Sebern, M. D. (1996). Explication of the construct of shared care and the prevention of pressure ulcers in home health care. *Research in Nursing & Health*, *19*(3), 183–192. doi:10.1002/(SICI)1098-240X(199606)19:3<183::AID-NUR2>3.0.CO;2-G PMID:8628907

Sebern, M. D. (2005). Psychometric evaluation of the Shared Care Instrument in a sample of home health care family dyads. *Journal of Nursing Measurement*, *13*(3), 175–191. doi:10.1891/jnum.13.3.175 PMID:16605041

Sebern, M. D., & Woda, A. (2012). Shared care dyadic intervention: Outcome patterns for heart failure care partners. *Western Journal of Nursing Research*, *34*(3), 289–316. doi:10.1177/0193945911399088 PMID:21383082

Segall, S. (2010). *Health, luck, and justice*. Princeton, NJ: Princeton University Press.

Seitsamo, J., & Klockars, M. (1997). Aging and changes in health. *Scandinavian Journal of Work, Environment & Health*, *23*(Suppl. 1), 27–35. PMID:9247993

Sen, A. (2009). *The idea of justice*. Cambridge, MA: The Belknap Press of Harvard University Press.

Seymour, A., & Dupré, K. (2008). Advancing employee engagement through a healthy workplace strategy. *Journal of Health Services Research & Policy*, *13*(Suppl. 1), 35–40. doi:10.1258/jhsrp.2007.007031 PMID:18325167

Shah, D. V., Cho, J., Eveland, W. P., & Kwak, N. (2005). Information and expression in a digital age: Modeling Internet effects on civic participation. *Communication Research*, *32*(5), 531–565. doi:10.1177/0093650205279209

Shahian, D. M., Edwards, F. H., Jacobs, J. P., Prager, R. L., Normand, S. L., Shewan, C. M., & Grover, F. L. et al. (2011). Public reporting of cardiac surgery performance: Part 1--history, rationale, consequences. *The Annals of Thoracic Surgery*, *92*(Suppl. 3), S2–S11. doi:10.1016/j.athoracsur.2011.06.100 PMID:21867789

Shaller, D. (2007). Patient-centered care: What does it take?. *The Commonwealth Fund* N. 1067.

Shaw, B. R., McTavish, F., Hawkins, R., Gustafson, D. H., & Pingree, S. (2000). Experienceso f women with breast cancer; Exchanging social support over the CHESS computer network. *Journal of Health Communication*, *5*(2), 135–159. doi:10.1080/108107300406866 PMID:11010346

Shaw, W. S., Besen, E., Pransky, G., Boot, C. R., Nicholas, M. K., McLellan, R. K., & Tveito, T. H. (2014). Manage at work: A randomized, controlled trial of a self-management group intervention to overcome workplace challenges associated with chronic physical health conditions. *BMC Public Health*, *14*(1), 515. doi:10.1186/1471-2458-14-515 PMID:24885844

Shepherd, S., & Kay, A. C. (2012). On the perpetuation of ignorance: System dependence, system justification, and the motivated avoidance of sociopolitical information. *Journal of Personality and Social Psychology*, *102*(2), 264–280. doi:10.1037/a0026272 PMID:22059846

Shimazu, A., & Schaufeli, W. B. (2009). Is workaholism good or bad for employee well-being? The distinctiveness of workaholism and work engagement among Japanese employees. *Industrial Health*, *47*(5), 495–502. doi:10.2486/indhealth.47.495 PMID:19834258

Shimazu, A., Schaufeli, W. B., Kamiyama, K., & Kawakami, N. (2015). Workaholism vs. work engagement: The two different predictors of future well-being and performance. *International Journal of Behavioral Medicine*, *22*(1), 18–23. doi:10.1007/s12529-014-9410-x PMID:24696043

Shimazu, A., Schaufeli, W. B., Kubota, K., & Kawakami, N. (2012). Do workaholism and work engagement predict employee well-being and performance in opposite directions? *Industrial Health*, *50*(4), 316–321. doi:10.2486/indhealth.MS1355 PMID:22673364

Shortt, H. (2014). Liminality, space and the importance of 'transitory dwelling places' at work. *Human Relations*, 2014, 1–26.

Sidgwick, H. (1902). *Outlines of the history of ethics* (4th ed.). London: Macmillan.

Silenzi, A., Falvo, R., Lazzari, A., Marino, M., Pelone, F., Basso, D., & Ricciardi, W. (2013). Health systems reviews and policy. Quality in public reporting: where do we go? An overview of systematic reviews. *The European Journal of Public Health,* 23(Suppl. 1).

Silverman, D. (2010). *Doing Qualitative Research: A Practical Handbook* (4th ed.). SAGE.

Simmons, L. A., Wolever, R. Q., Bechard, E. M., & Snyderman, R. (2014). Patient engagement as a risk factor in personalized health care: A systematic review of the literature on chronic disease. *Genome Medicine*, *6*(2), 1–21. doi:10.1186/gm533 PMID:24571651

Simon, B., & Grabow, O. (2010). The politicization of migrants: Further evidence that politicized collective identity is a dual identity. *Political Psychology*, *31*(5), 717–738. doi:10.1111/j.1467-9221.2010.00782.x

Simon, B., & Klandermans, B. (2001). Politicized collective identity: A social psychological analysis. *The American Psychologist*, *56*(4), 319–331. doi:10.1037/0003-066X.56.4.319 PMID:11330229

Simon, B., Loewy, M., Stürmer, S., Weber, U., Freytag, P., & Habig, C. et al. (1998). Collective identification and social movement participation. *Journal of Personality and Social Psychology*, *74*(3), 646–658. doi:10.1037/0022-3514.74.3.646

Simoni, S. (2001). Salute e Cultura organizzative. In M. Bucchi & F. Neresini (Eds.), *Sociologia della salute* (pp. 122–138). Roma: Carocci.

Singer, P. (2011). *Practical Ethics* (3rd ed.). New York: Cambridge University Press. doi:10.1017/CBO9780511975950

Sintomer, Y. (2007). *Le pouvoir au people: Jurys citoyens, tirage au sort et démocratie partecipative*. Paris: La Découverte.

Sjöberg, L. (2002). Factors in risk perception. *Risk Analysis*, *20*(1), 1–12. doi:10.1111/0272-4332.00001 PMID:12017352

Skitka, L. J., Bauman, C. W., & Sargis, E. G. (2005). Moral conviction: Another contributor to attitude strength or something more? *Journal of Personality and Social Psychology*, *88*(6), 895–917. doi:10.1037/0022-3514.88.6.895 PMID:15982112

Skolasky, R. L., Mackenzie, E. J., Wegener, S. T., & Riley, L. H. III. (2008). Patient activation and adherence to physical therapy in persons undergoing spine surgery. *Spine*, *33*(21), E784–E791. doi:10.1097/BRS.0b013e31818027f1 PMID:18827683

Slovic, P., Finucane, M., Peters, E., & MacGregor, D. G. (2002). The affective heuristic. In T. Gilovich, D. Griffin, & D. Kahneman (Eds.), *Heuristics and biases: The psychology of intuitive judgment* (pp. 397–420). New York, NY: Cambridge University Press. doi:10.1017/CBO9780511808098.025

Slovic, P., Peters, E., Finucane, M., & MacGregor, D. G. (2005). Affect, risk and decision making. *Health Psychology*, *24*(4Suppl. 4), S35–S40. doi:10.1037/0278-6133.24.4.S35 PMID:16045417

Smith, P., Mossialos, E., &, Papanicolas, I. (2008). *Performance measurement for health system improvement: experiences, challenges and prospects*. Copenhagen: World Health Organization on behalf of the European Observatory on Health Systems and Policies.

Smith, G. C., Gutovich, J., Smyser, C., Pineda, R., Newnham, C., Tjoeng, T. H., & Inder, T. et al. (2011). Neonatal intensive care unit stress is associated with brain development in preterm infants. *Annals of Neurology*, *70*(4), 541–549. doi:10.1002/ana.22545 PMID:21976396

Smith, J. A. (1995). Semi-structured interviewing and qualitative analysis. In J. A. Smith, R. Hark, & L. Van Langenhove (Eds.), *Rethinking Methods in Psychology*. London: Sage. doi:10.4135/9781446221792.n2

Smith, J. A. (1996). Beyond the divide between cognition and discourse: Using interpretative phenomenological analysis in health psychology. *Psychology & Health*, *11*(2), 261–217. doi:10.1080/08870449608400256

Smith, J. A., Flowers, P., & Osborn, M. (1997). Interpretative phenomenological analysis and the psychology of health and illness. In L. Yardley (Ed.), *Material discourses of health and illness*. London: Routledge.

Snyder, L., & Leffler, C. (2005). Ethics and Human Rights Committee, American College of Physicians, Ethics manual: fifth edition. Annals of Internal Medicine, 142(7), 560-82.

Snyder, C. R., & Lopez, S. J. (2009). *Oxford handbook of positive psychology* (2nd ed.). New York: Oxford University Press.

Sorrentino, M., Guglielmetti, C., Gilardi, S., & Marsilio, M. (2015). Health Care Services and the Coproduction Puzzle: Filling in the Blanks. *Administration & Society*. doi:10.1177/0095399715593317

Spears, R., & Lea, M. (1994). Panacea or panopticon? The hidden power of computer-mediated communication. *Communication Research, 21*(4), 427–459. doi:10.1177/009365094021004001

Spears, R., Lea, M., Corneliussen, R. A., Postmes, T., & Ter Haar, W. (2002). Computer mediated communication as a channel for social resistance - The strategic side of SIDE. *Small Group Research, 33*(5), 555–574. doi:10.1177/104649602237170

Specchia, M. L., Poscia, A., Volpe, M., Parente, P., Capizzi, S., Cambieri, A., & De Belvis, A. G. et al. (2015, December). Does clinical governance influence the appropriateness of hospital stay? *Health Services Research, 15*(1), 142. doi:10.1186/s12913-015-0795-2 PMID:25889675

Spiegel, A. D., & Kavaler, F. (1997). America's first medical malpractice crisis, 1835-1865. *Journal of Community Health, 22*(4), 283–308. doi:10.1023/A:1025104520383 PMID:9247851

Stanton, A. L. (1991). Cognitive appraisals, coping processes, and adjustment to infertility. In A. L. Stanton & C. Dunkel-Schetter (Eds.), *Infertility: Perspectives from stress and coping research* (pp. 87–108). New York: Plenum Press. doi:10.1007/978-1-4899-0753-0_5

Stanton, A. L., Tennen, H., Affleck, G., & Mendola, R. (1992). Coping and adjustment to infertility. *Journal of Social and Clinical Psychology, 11*(1), 1–13. doi:10.1521/jscp.1992.11.1.1

Steffen, G. E. (1988). Quality medical care: A definition. *Journal of the American Medical Association, 260*(1), 56–61. doi:10.1001/jama.1988.03410010064036 PMID:3379723

Stein, M. (2007). Toxicity and the unconscious experience of the body at the employee-customer interface. *Organization Studies, 28*(8), 1223–1241. doi:10.1177/0170840607079527

Steverink, N., Lindenberg, S., & Slaets, J. P. J. (2005). How to understand and improve older people's self-management of wellbeing. *European Journal of Ageing, 2*(4), 235–244. doi:10.1007/s10433-005-0012-y

Stewart, M., Brown, J. B., & Weston, W. W., NcWhinney, I. R., McWilliam, C.L., & Freeman, T.R. (2003). Patient-centered medicine-Transforming the clinical method. Bristol, UK: Radcliffe medical Press.

Stewart, M. (2001). Towards a global definition of patient centered care: The patient should be the judge of patient centred care. *British Medical Journal, 322*(7284), 444. doi:10.1136/bmj.322.7284.444 PMID:11222407

Stewart, M., Brown, J. B., Donner, A., McWhinney, I. R., Oates, J., Weston, W. W., & Jordan, J. (2000). The impact of patient-centered care on outcomes. *The Journal of Family Practice, 49*(9), 796–804. PMID:11032203

Stewart, W. F., Ricci, J. A., Chee, E., Hahn, S. R., & Morganstein, D. (2003). Cost of lost productive work time among US workers with Depression. *Journal of the American Medical Association, 289*(23), 3135–3144. doi:10.1001/jama.289.23.3135 PMID:12813119

Stockholm European Council. (2001, March 23-24). Presidency conclusions and annexes. Retrieved from http://aei.pitt.edu/43341/

Stoll, B. J., Hansen, N. I., Bell, E. F., Shankaran, S., Laptook, A. R., Walsh, M. C., & Higgins, R. D. et al. (2010). Neonatal outcomes of extremely preterm infants from the NICHD Neonatal Research Network. *Pediatrics, 126*(3), 443–456. doi:10.1542/peds.2009-2959 PMID:20732945

Stouffer, S. A., Suchman, E. A., DeVinney, L. C., Star, S. A., & Williams Jr, R. M. (1949). Adjustment during army Me. In *Studies in social psychology in World War II* (Vol. 1, pp. 379-387).

Strauss, A. L., & Corbin, J. (1990). *Basics of qualitative research.* Thousand Oaks: Sage.

Strauss, A. L., & Corbin, J. (1994). Grounded theory methodology: an overview. In N. K. Denzin & Y. S. Lincoln (Eds.), *Handbook of qualitative research.* London: Sage.

Street, R. L. Jr, & De Haes, H. (2013). Designing a curriculum for communication skills training from a theory and evidence-based perspective. *Patient Education and Counseling*, *93*(1), 27–33. doi:10.1016/j.pec.2013.06.012 PMID:23890580

Street, R. L. Jr, Gordon, H. S., Ward, M. M., Krupat, E., & Kravitz, R. L. (2005). Patient participation in medical consultations: Why some patients are more involved than others. *Medical Care*, *43*(10), 960–969. doi:10.1097/01.mlr.0000178172.40344.70 PMID:16166865

Street, R. L. Jr, Makoul, G., Arora, N. K., & Epstein, R. M. (2009). How does communication heal? Pathways linking clinician–patient communication to health outcomes. *Patient Education and Counseling*, *74*(3), 295–301. doi:10.1016/j.pec.2008.11.015 PMID:19150199

Streiner, D. L., & Norman, G. R. (2008). *Health Measurement Scales: A Practical Guide to Their Development and Use* (4th ed.). Oxford, UK: Oxford University Press. doi:10.1093/acprof:oso/9780199231881.001.0001

Stroebe, M., Finkenauer, C., Wijngaards-de Meij, L., Schut, H., Van den Bout, J., & Stroebe, W. (2013). Partner-oriented self-regulation among bereaved parents: The cost of holding in grief for the partner sake. *Psychological Science*, *24*(4), 1–8. doi:10.1177/0956797612457383 PMID:23406609

Stromer-Galley, J., & Wichowski, A. (2010). Political discussion online. In R. M. Burnett, M. Consalvo, & C. Ess (Eds.), *The handbook of Internet studies* (pp. 168–187). Chichester, UK: John Wiley & Sons.

Stryker, S., Owens, T. J., & White, R. W. (2000). *Self, identity, and social movements* (Vol. 13). Minneapolis: University of Minnesota Press.

Stuart, A., Thomas, E. F., Donaghue, N., & Russell, A. (2013). "We may be pirates, but we are not protesters": Identity in the Sea Shepherd Conservation Society. *Political Psychology*, *34*, 753–777. doi:10.1111/pops.12016

Sturdy, A. (2006). *Knowledge Evolution in Action: Consultancy-Client Relationships.* Economic & Social Research Council.

Stürmer, S., & Simon, B. (2004). The role of collective identification in social movement participation: A panel study in the context of the German gay movement. *Personality and Social Psychology Bulletin*, *30*(3), 263–277. doi:10.1177/0146167203256690 PMID:15030619

Sullivan, C. F. (2003). Gendered cybersupport: A thematic analysis of two online cancersupport groups. *Journal of Health Psychology*, *8*(1), 83–104. doi:10.1177/1359105303008001446 PMID:22113903

Symington, A., & Pinelli, J. (2006). Developmental care for promoting development and preventing morbidity in preterm infants. *Cochrane Database of Systematic Reviews*, *2*, CD001814. PMID:16625548

Szasz, T. S., & Hollender, M. H. (1956). A contribution to the philosophy of medicine: The basic models of the doctor-patient relationship. *A.M.A. Archives of Internal Medicine*, *97*(5), 585–592. doi:10.1001/archinte.1956.00250230079008 PMID:13312700

Tajfel, H., & Turner, J. (1986). The social identity theory of intergroup behaviour. In S. Worchel & W. G. Austin (Eds.), *Psychology of intergroup relations* (pp. 33–47). Chicago: Nelson.

Taylor, S., & Spicer, A. (2007). Time for space: A narrative review of research on organizational spaces. *International Journal of Management Reviews*, *9*(4), 325–346. doi:10.1111/j.1468-2370.2007.00214.x

Tetlock, P. E. (2002). Social functionalist frameworks for judgment and choice: Intuitive politicians, theologians, and prosecutors. *Psychological Review*, *109*(3), 451–471. doi:10.1037/0033-295X.109.3.451 PMID:12088240

Theorell, T., Harms-Ringdahl, K., Ahlberg-Hultén, G., & Westin, B. (1991). Psychosocial job factors and symptoms from the locomotor system-a multicausal analysis. *Scandinavian Journal of Rehabilitative Medicine*, *23*(3), 165–173. PMID:1962160

Thomas, E. F., Mavor, K. I., & McGarty, C. (2012). Social identities facilitate and encapsulate action-relevant constructs: A test of the social identity model of collective action. *Group Processes & Intergroup Relations*, *15*(1), 75–88. doi:10.1177/1368430211413619

Thomas, E. F., & McGarty, C. (2009). The role of efficacy and moral outrage norms in creating the potential for international development activism through group-based interaction. *The British Journal of Social Psychology*, *48*(1), 115–134. doi:10.1348/014466608X313774 PMID:18534045

Thomas, E. F., Smith, L. G. E., McGarty, C., & Postmes, T. (2010). Nice and nasty: The formation of prosocial and hostile social movements. *Revue Internationale de Psychologie Sociale*, *23*(2), 5–43.

Thompson, A., & Bolger, N. (1999). Emotional transmission in couples under stress. *Journal of Marriage and the Family*, *61*(1), 38–48. doi:10.2307/353881

Thórarinsdóttir, K., & Kristjánsson, K. (2014). Patients' perspectives on person-centred participation in healthcare: A framework analysis. *Nursing Ethics*, *21*(2), 129–147. doi:10.1177/0969733013490593 PMID:23812560

Timonen, V. (2008). *Ageing societies: A comparative introduction*. London: McGraw Hill Open University Press.

Totten, A. M., Wagner, J., Tiwari, A., O'Haire, C., Griffin, J., & Walker, M. (2012). *Public Reporting as a Quality Improvement Strategy. Closing the Quality Gap: Revisiting the State of the Science*, Evidence Report No. 208. AHRQ Publication No. 12-E011-EF, Rockville, MD, Agency for Healthcare Research and Quality. Retrieved from http://www.effectivehealthcare.ahrq.gov/ehc/products/343/1199/EvidReport208_CQGPublicReporting_FinalReport_20120724.pdf

Traina, F. (2009). Medical Malpractice. The experience in Italy. *Clinical Orthopaedics and Related Research*, *467*(2), 434–442. doi:10.1007/s11999-008-0582-z PMID:18985423

Trigg, L. (2011). Patients' opinions of health care providers for supporting choice and quality improvement. *Journal of Health Services Research & Policy*, *16*(2), 102–107. doi:10.1258/jhsrp.2010.010010 PMID:20870690

Tsigos, C., & Chrousos, G. P. (2002). Hypothalamic-pituitary-adrenal axis, neuroendocrine factors and stress. *Journal of Psychosomatic Research*, *53*(4), 865–871. doi:10.1016/S0022-3999(02)00429-4 PMID:12377295

Tuckey, M. R., Bakker, A. B., & Dollard, M. F. (2012). Empowering leaders optimize working conditions for engagement: A multilevel study. *Journal of Occupational Health Psychology*, *17*(1), 15–27. doi:10.1037/a0025942 PMID:22409390

Tullar, J. M., Amick, B. C. III, Brewer, S., Diamond, P. M., Kelder, S. H., & Mikhail, O. (2015). Improve employee engagement to retain your workforce. *Health Care Management Review*. doi:10.1097/HMR.0000000000000079 PMID:26207655

Tuomi, K., Huuhtanen, P., Nykyri, E., & Ilmarinen, J. (2001). Promotion of work ability, the quality of work and retirement. *Occupational Medicine (Oxford, England)*, *51*(5), 318–324. doi:10.1093/occmed/51.5.318 PMID:11473138

Turner, J. C. (1982). Towards a cognitive redefinition of the social group. In H. Tajfel (Ed.), *Social identity and intergroup relations* (pp. 15–40). Cambridge: Cambridge University Press.

Turner, J. C., Hogg, M. A., Oakes, P. J., Reicher, S. D., & Wetherell, M. S. (1987). *Rediscovering the social group: A self-categorization perspective*. Oxford: Basil Blackwell.

Turner, J. W., Grube, J. A., & Meyers, J. (2001). Developing an optimal match withinonline communities: An exploration of CMC support community and traditional support. *Journal of Communication, 51*(2), 231–251. doi:10.1111/j.1460-2466.2001.tb02879.x

Turner, V. W. (1969). *The Ritual Process: Structure and Anti-structure*. Chicago: Aldine.

Turner, V. W. (1974). *Dramas, Fields, and Metaphors: Symbolic Action in Human Society*. London: Cornell University Press.

Tveito, T. H., Hysing, M., & Eriksen, H. R. (2004). Low back pain interventions at the workplace: A systematic literature review. *Occupational Medicine, 54*(1), 3–13. doi:10.1093/occmed/kqg109 PMID:14963248

Tyler, T. R., Boeckmann, R. J., Smith, H. J., & Huo, Y. J. (1997). *Social justice in a diverse society*. Oxford, England: Westview Press.

Tzannis, A., & Nadin, G. (2011, September 1-3). Elderly and health care services: the elements characterizing the patient satisfaction. *Proceedings of the 14th Toulon-Verona Conference "Organizational Excellence in services"*, University of Alicante & University of Oviedo (pp. 1201-1017).

Uchino, B. N. (2006). Social support and health: A review of physiological processes potentially underlying links to disease outcomes. *Journal of Behavioral Medicine, 29*(4), 377–387. doi:10.1007/s10865-006-9056-5 PMID:16758315

Udo, H., Kobayashi, M., Udo, A., & Branlund, B. (2006). Participatory ergonomic improvement in nursing home. *Industrial Health, 44*(1), 128–134. doi:10.2486/indhealth.44.128 PMID:16610548

Udo, H., & Yoshinaga, F. (2001). The role of the industrial medical doctor in planning and implementing ergonomic measures at the workplaces. *International Journal of Industrial Ergonomics, 28*(3-4), 237–246. doi:10.1016/S0169-8141(01)00037-3

Vaillant, G. (2003). Mental health. *The American Journal of Psychiatry, 160*(8), 1373–1384. doi:10.1176/appi.ajp.160.8.1373 PMID:12900295

van den Akker, M., Buntinx, F., Metsemakers, J. M., Roos, S., & Knottnerus, A. (1998). Multimorbidity in general practice: Prevalence, incidence, and determinants of co-occurring chronic and recurrent diseases. *Journal of Clinical Epidemiology, 51*(5), 367–375. doi:10.1016/S0895-4356(97)00306-5 PMID:9619963

Van den Bos, K., & Lind, E. A. (2002). In M. P. Zanna (Ed.), *Uncertainty management by meansof fairness judgments* (Vol. 34, pp. 1–60). Advances in experimentalsocial psychologySan Diego, CA: Academic Press.

van der Meer, L., Leijten, F. R., Heuvel, S. G., Ybema, J. F., de Wind, A., Burdorf, A., & Geuskens, G. A. (2015). Company Policies on Working Hours and Night Work in Relation to Older Workers' Work Ability and Work Engagement: Results From a Dutch Longitudinal Study with 2 Year Follow-Up. *Journal of Occupational Rehabilitation*, 2015, 1–9. PMID:26250870

Van Gennep, A. (1960). *The rites of Passage*. Chicago: University of Chicago Press. (Original work published 1909)

Van Kleef, E., Frewer, L. J., Chryssochoidis, G. M., Houghton, J. R., Korzen-Bohr, S., Krystallis, T., & Rowe, G. et al. (2006). Perceptions of food risk management among key stakeholders: Results from a cross-European study. *Appetite, 47*(1), 46–63. doi:10.1016/j.appet.2006.02.002 PMID:16584811

Van Marrewijk, A., & Yanow, D. (2012). *Organizational Spaces. Rematerializing the Workaday World*. Northampton, Massachusetts, USA: Edward Elgar Publishing.

Van Stekelenburg, J., & Klandermans, B. (2009). Social movement theory: Past, present and prospect. *Movers and shakers: Social movements in Africa, 8*, 17.

Van Stekelenburg, J. (2013). The political psychology of protest: Sacrificing for a cause. *European Psychologist, 18*(4), 224–234. doi:10.1027/1016-9040/a000156

Van Stekelenburg, J., & Klandermans, B. (2013). The social psychology of protest. *Current Sociology Review, 61*(5-6), 886–905. doi:10.1177/0011392113479314

van Uden-Kraan, C. F., Drossaert, C. H., Taal, E., Shaw, B. R., Seydel, E. R., & van de Laar, M. A. (2008). Empowering processes and outcomes of participation in online support groups for patients with breast cancer, arthritis, or fibromyalgia. *Qualitative Health Research, 18*(3), 405–417. doi:10.1177/1049732307313429 PMID:18235163

Van Zomeren, M. (2011). Four core social-psychological motivations to undertake collective action. *Social and Personality Psychology Compass, 7*(6), 378–388. doi:10.1111/spc3.12031

Van Zomeren, M., & Iyer, A. (2009). Introduction to the social and psychological dynamics of collective action. *The Journal of Social Issues, 65*(4), 645–660. doi:10.1111/j.1540-4560.2009.01618.x

Van Zomeren, M., & Lodewijkx, H. F. M. (2005). Motivated responses to 'senseless' violence: Explaining emotional and behavioural responses through person and position identification. *European Journal of Social Psychology, 35*(6), 755–766. doi:10.1002/ejsp.274

Van Zomeren, M., Postmes, T., & Spears, R. (2008). Toward an integrative social identity model of collective action: A quantitative research synthesis of three socio-psychological perspectives. *Psychological Bulletin, 134*(4), 504–535. doi:10.1037/0033-2909.134.4.504 PMID:18605818

Van Zomeren, M., Postmes, T., & Spears, R. (2012). On conviction's collective consequences: Integrating moral conviction with the socialidentity model of collective action. *The British Journal of Social Psychology, 51*(1), 52–71. doi:10.1111/j.2044-8309.2010.02000.x PMID:22435846

Van Zomeren, M., Postmes, T., Spears, R., & Bettache, K. (2011). Can moral convictions motivate the advantaged to challenge social inequality? Extending the social identity model of collective action. *Group Processes & Intergroup Relations, 14*(5), 735–753. doi:10.1177/1368430210395637

Van Zomeren, M., Saguy, T., & Schellhaas, F. M. H. (2013). Believing in "making a difference" to collective efforts: Participative efficacy beliefs as a unique predictor of collective action. *Group Processes & Intergroup Relations, 16*(5), 618–634. doi:10.1177/1368430212467476

Van Zomeren, M., & Spears, A. (2009). Metaphors of protest: A classification of motivations for collective action. *The Journal of Social Issues, 65*(4), 661–680. doi:10.1111/j.1540-4560.2009.01619.x

Van Zomeren, M., Spears, R., Fischer, A. H., & Leach, C. W. (2004). Put your money where your mouth is!: Explaining collective action tendencies through group-based anger and group efficacy. *Journal of Personality and Social Psychology, 87*(5), 649–664. doi:10.1037/0022-3514.87.5.649 PMID:15535777

Vatsalya, V., & Karch, R. (2013). Evaluation of health determinants for sustaining workability in aging US workforce. *Advanced Aging Research, 2*(3), 106–108. doi:10.4236/aar.2013.23015 PMID:25285260

Vegeris, S., Barnes, H., Campbell-Barr, V., Mackinnon, K., Taylor, R., Martin, D., & Harris, J. (2007). *Beyond the tick box: Older citizen engagement in UK local government*. London: Policy Studies Institute PSI and Better Government OPAG.

Velasco, V., Miglioretti, M., Strada, M., & Vecchio, L. (2014). Patient satisfaction regarding general practitioners: A theoretical model based on patients' experience and engagement in care process. [La soddisfazione dei pazienti rispetto ai medici di medicina generale: Un modello teorico basato sull'esperienza e l'engagement dei pazienti nei processi di cura]. *Psicologia della salute, 2*, 34-57.

Vellone, E., Chung, M. L., Cocchieri, A., Rocco, G., Alvaro, R., & Riegel, B. (2014). Effects of self-care on quality of life in adults with heart failure and their spousal caregivers: Testing dyadic dynamics using the actor-partner interdependence model. *Journal of Family Nursing*, *20*(1), 120–141. doi:10.1177/1074840713510205 PMID:24189325

Ventura, M., Salanova, M., & Llorens, S. (2015). Professional self-efficacy as a predictor of burnout and engagement: The role of challenge and hindrance demands. *The Journal of Psychology*, *149*(3), 277–302. doi:10.1080/00223980.2013.876380 PMID:25590343

Vera, A., & Kuntz, L. (2007). Process-based organization design and hospital efficiency. *Health Care Management Review*, *32*(1), 55–65. doi:10.1097/00004010-200701000-00008 PMID:17245203

Vermeire, E., Hearnshaw, H., Van Royen, P., & Denekens, J. (2001). Patient adherence to treatment: Three decades of research. A comprehensive review. *Journal of Clinical Pharmacy and Therapeutics*, *26*(5), 331–342. doi:10.1046/j.1365-2710.2001.00363.x PMID:11679023

Victoor, A., Delnoij, D. M. J., Friele, R. D., & Rademakers, J. J. (2012). Determinants of patient choice of healthcare providers: A scoping review. *BMC Health Services Research*, *12*(1), 272. doi:10.1186/1472-6963-12-272 PMID:22913549

Vijayendran, M., Beach, S., Plume, J. M., Brody, G., & Philibert, R. (2012). Effects of genotype and child abuse on DNA methylation and gene expression at the serotonin transporter. *Frontiers in Psychiatry*, *3*, 55. doi:10.3389/fpsyt.2012.00055 PMID:22707942

Vilchinsky, N., Dekel, R., Leibowitz, M., Reges, O., Khaskia, A., & Mosseri, M. (2011). Dynamics of support perceptions among couples with cardiac illness: The effect on recovery outcomes. *Health Psychology*, *30*(4), 411–419. doi:10.1037/a0023453 PMID:21480711

Villa, S., Barbieri, M., & Lega, F. (2009). Restructuring patient flow logistics around patient care needs: Implications and practicalities from three critical cases. *Health Care Management Science*, *12*(2), 155–165. doi:10.1007/s10729-008-9091-6 PMID:19469455

Vincent, C., Young, M., & Phillips, A. (1994). Why do people sue doctors? A study of patients and relatives taking legal action. *Lancet*, *343*(8913), 1609–1613. doi:10.1016/S0140-6736(94)93062-7 PMID:7911925

Vlieland, V. T. P. (2002). Managing chronic disease: Evidence-based medicine or patient centred medicine? *Health Care Analysis*, *10*(3), 289–298. doi:10.1023/A:1022951808151 PMID:12769416

Vos, L., Chalmers, S. E., Dückers, M. L., Groenewegen, P. P., Wagner, C., & Van Merode, G. G. (2011). Towards an organisation-wide process-oriented organisation of care: A literature review. *Implementation Science; IS*, *6*(1), 8. doi:10.1186/1748-5908-6-8 PMID:21247491

Waddell, G., & Burton, A. K. (2001). Occupational health guidelines for the management of low back pain at work: Evidence review. *Occupational Medicine*, *51*(2), 124–135. doi:10.1093/occmed/51.2.124 PMID:11307688

Walker, A. (1999). Combating age discrimination at the workplace. *Experimental Aging Research*, *25*(4), 367–377. doi:10.1080/036107399243823 PMID:10553519

Walker, A. (2006). Aging and politics: An international perspective. In R. H. Binstock & L. K. George (Eds.), *Handbook of aging and the social sciences* (6th ed., pp. 339–359). San Diego, CA: Academic Press. doi:10.1016/B978-012088388-2/50022-5

Walker, I., & Smith, H. J. (2002). *Relative deprivation: Specification, development, and integration*. Cambridge, England: Cambridge University Press.

Walston, S. L., Lawton, R. B., & Kimberly, J. R. (2000). Does reengineering really work? An examination of the context and outcomes of hospital reengineering initiatives. *Health Services Research*, *34*(6), 1363–1388. PMID:10654836

Wang, D., Szyf, M., Benkelfat, C., Provencal, N., Turecki, G., Caramaschi, D., & Booij, L. et al. (2012). Peripheral SLC6A4 DNA methylation is associated with in vivo measures of human brain serotonin synthesis and childhood physical aggression. *PLoS ONE*, *7*(6), e39501. doi:10.1371/journal.pone.0039501 PMID:22745770

Ward, B. W. (2013). Prevalence of multiple chronic conditions among US adults: Estimates from the National Health Interview Survey, 2010. *Preventing Chronic Disease*, 2013, 10. PMID:23618545

Ward, B. W., & Schiller, J. S. (2013). Prevalence of multiple chronic conditions among US adults: Estimates from the national health interview survey, 2010. *Preventing Chronic Disease*, *10*, 1–15. doi:10.5888/pcd10.120203 PMID:23618545

Ware, J. E. Jr, Davies-Avery, A., & Stewart, A. L. (1978). The measurement and meaning of patient satisfaction. *Health & Medical Care Services Review*, *1*(1), 1–3. PMID:10297474

Ware, J. E. Jr, & Davis, A. R. (1983). Behavioral consequences of consumer dissatisfaction with medical care. *Evaluation and Program Planning*, *6*(3), 291–297. doi:10.1016/0149-7189(83)90009-5 PMID:10267257

Warf, B., & Arias, S. (2009). *The spatial turn. Interdisciplinary perspectives*. Abingdon, New York: Routledge.

Waring, J. J. (2005). Beyond blame: Cultural barriers to medical incident reporting. *Social Science & Medicine*, *60*(9), 1927–1935. doi:10.1016/j.socscimed.2004.08.055 PMID:15743644

Weaver, I. C. G., Cervoni, N., Champagne, F., D'Alessio, A. C., Sharma, S., Seckl, J. R., & Meaney, M. J. et al. (2004). Epigenetic programming by maternal behavior. *Nature Neuroscience*, *7*(8), 847–854. doi:10.1038/nn1276 PMID:15220929

Weinberg, N., Schmale, J. D., Uken, J., & Wessel, K. (1996). Online help: Cancer patients participate in a computer mediated support group. *Health & Social Work*, *21*, 24–29. doi:10.1093/hsw/21.1.24 PMID:8626154

Weisberg, H. F. (2005). *The total survey error approach: A guide to the new science of survey research*. Chicago, IL: The University of Chicago Press. doi:10.7208/chicago/9780226891293.001.0001

Welberg, L. A., & Seckl, J. R. (2001). Prenatal stress, glucocorticoids and the programming of the brain. *Journal of Neuroendocrinology*, *13*(2), 113–128. doi:10.1111/j.1365-2826.2001.00601.x PMID:11168837

Wells, K. B., Rogers, W., Burnam, A., Greenfield, S., & Ware, J. E. Jr. (1991). How the medical comorbidity of depressed patients differs across health care settings: Results from the Medical Outcomes Study. *The American Journal of Psychiatry*, *148*(12), 1688–1696. doi:10.1176/ajp.148.12.1688 PMID:1957931

Wenger, E. (1998). *Communities of Practice: Learning, Meaning and Identity*. Cambridge, UK: Cambridge University Press. doi:10.1017/CBO9780511803932

Wens, J., Vermeire, E., Van Royen, P., Sabbe, B., & Denekens, J. (2005). GPs' perspectives of type 2 diabetes patients' adherence to treatment: A qualitative analysis of barriers and solutions. *BMC Family Practice*, *6*(1), 20. doi:10.1186/1471-2296-6-20 PMID:15890071

Werner, E. L., Ihlebaek, C., Skouen, J. S., & Laerum, E. (2005). Beliefs about low back pain in the Norwegian general population: Are they related to pain experiences and health professionals? *Spine*, *30*(15), 1770–1776. doi:10.1097/01.brs.0000171909.81632.fe PMID:16094280

Werner, E. L., Laerum, E., Wormgoor, M. E. A., Lindh, E., & Indahl, A. (2007). Peer support in an occupational setting preventing LBP-related sick leave. *Occupational Medicine*, *57*(8), 590–595. doi:10.1093/occmed/kqm094 PMID:17916863

Werner, R. M., & Asch, D. A. (2005). The unintended consequences of publicly reporting quality information. *Journal of the American Medical Association*, *293*(10), 1239–1244. doi:10.1001/jama.293.10.1239 PMID:15755946

Westergren, A. (2012). Action-oriented study circles facilitate efforts in nursing homes to "go from feeding to serving": Conceptual perspectives on knowledge translation and workplace learning. *Journal of Aging Research*, *2012*, 627371. doi:10.1155/2012/627371 PMID:22991666

Westrup, B. (2007). Newborn Individualized Developmental Care and Assessment Program (NIDCAP) - family-centered developmentally supportive care. *Early Human Development*, *83*(7), 443–449. doi:10.1016/j.earlhumdev.2007.03.006 PMID:17459617

Wiederhold, B. K., Riva, G., & Graffigna, G. (2013). Ensuring the best care for our increasing aging population: Health engagement and positive technology can help patients achieve a more active role in future healthcare. *Cyberpsychology, Behavior, and Social Networking*, *16*(6), 411–412. doi:10.1089/cyber.2013.1520 PMID:23751102

Williams, S., Weinman, J., & Dale, J. (1998). Doctor-patient communication and patient satisfaction: A review. *Family Practice*, *15*(5), 480–492. doi:10.1093/fampra/15.5.480 PMID:9848436

Wilson, J. R. (1995). Ergonomic and participation. In J. R. Wilson & E. N. Corlett (Eds.), *Evaluation of Human Work: A Practical Ergonomics Methodology* (pp. 1071–1096). London: Taylor and Francis.

Wilton, R., & Cranford, C. (2002). Toward an understanding of the spatiality of social movements: Labor organizing at a private university in Los Angeles. *Social Problems*, *49*(3), 374–394. doi:10.1525/sp.2002.49.3.374

Winkel, J., & Mathiassen, S. E. (1994). Assessment of physical work load in epidemiologic studies: Concepts, issues and operational considerations. *Ergonomics*, *37*(6), 979–988. doi:10.1080/00140139408963711 PMID:8026455

Winkelmann-Gleed, A. (2008). *Demographic change and implications for workforce ageing in Europe: raising awareness and improving practice*. London: Working Lives Research Institute.

Witteman, H. O., & Zikmund-Fisher, B. J. (2012). The defining characteristics of Web 2.0 and their potential influence in the online vaccination debate. *Vaccine*, *30*(25), 3734–3740. doi:10.1016/j.vaccine.2011.12.039 PMID:22178516

Wittmer, M., Volpatti, M., Piazzalonga, S., & Hoffmann, A. (2012, October). Expectation, satisfaction, and predictors of dropout in cardiac rehabilitation. *European Journal of Preventive Cardiology*, *19*(5), 1082–1088. doi:10.1177/1741826711418163 PMID:21788251

Witzmann, S. R., Turner, J. D., Meriaux, S. B., Meijer, O. C., & Muller, C. P. (2012). Epigenetic regulation of the glucocorticoid receptor promoter 1(7) in adult rats. *Epigenetics : Official Journal of the DNA Methylation Society*, *7*(11), 1290–1301. doi:10.4161/epi.22363 PMID:23023726

Woby, S. R., Watson, P. J., Roach, N. K., & Urmston, M. (2004). Adjustment to chronic low back pain--the relative influence of fear-avoidance beliefs, catastrophizing, and appraisals of control. *Behaviour Research and Therapy*, *42*(7), 761–774. doi:10.1016/S0005-7967(03)00195-5 PMID:15149897

Wojcieszak, M. E. (2011). Computer-mediated false consensus: Radical online groups, social networks and news media. *Mass Communication & Society*, *14*(4), 527–546. doi:10.1080/15205436.2010.513795

Wong, H. S., McNamara, P., & Greenberg, W. (2004). Provider competition and health care quality: Challenges and opportunities for research. *International Journal of Health Care Finance and Economics*, *4*(2), 99–111. doi:10.1023/B:IHFE.0000032418.86010.5d PMID:15211101

Woods, V. (2005). Work-related musculoskeletal health and social support. *Occupational Medicine*, *55*(3), 177–189. doi:10.1093/occmed/kqi085 PMID:15857897

World Bank. (n. d.). *World databank.* Retrieved from http://data.worldbank.org/indicator/SP.POP.TOTL

World Health Organization. (1993). *Needs and actions priorities in cardiac rehabilitation and secondary prevention in patients with CHD.* Retrieved from http://whqlibdoc.who.int/euro/-1993/EUR_ICP_CVD_125.pdf

World Health Organization. (2001). *International Classification of Functioning, Disability and Health.* Geneva: WHO. Retrieved from http://psychiatr.ru/download/1313?view=1&name=ICF_18.pdf

World Health Organization. (2002). *Active ageing: A policy framework.* Retrieved from http://apps.who.int/iris/bitstream/10665/67215/1/WHO_NMH_NPH_02.8.pdf

World Health Organization. (2006). *Quality of care, a process for making strategic choices in health systems.* Geneva: WHO Press. Retrieved from http://www.who.int/management/quality/assurance/QualityCare_B.Def.pdf

Wright, K. (2002). Social support within an online cancer community: An assessment of emotional support, perceptions of advantages and disadvantages, and motives for usingthe community from a communication perspective. *Journal of Applied Communication*, *30*(3), 195–209. doi:10.1080/00909880216586

Wright, S. C., Taylor, D. M., & Moghaddam, F. M. (1990). Responding to membership in a disadvantaged group: From acceptance to collective protest. *Journal of Personality and Social Psychology*, *58*(6), 994–1003. doi:10.1037/0022-3514.58.6.994

Yang, H., & Schuler, T. A. (2009). Marital quality and survivorship: Slowed recovery for breast cancer patients in distressed relationships. *Cancer*, *115*(1), 217–228. doi:10.1002/cncr.23964 PMID:18951520

Ybema, J. F., Kuijer, R. G., Buunk, B. P., DeJong, G. M., & Saderman, R. (2001). Depression and perceptions of inequity among couples facing cancer. *Personality and Social Psychology Bulletin*, *27*(1), 3–13. doi:10.1177/0146167201271001

Yohannes, A. M., Yalfani, A., Doherty, P., & Bundy, C. (2007, March). Predictors of drop-out from an outpatient cardiac rehabilitation programme. *Journal of Clinical Rehabilitation*, *21*(3), 222–229. doi:10.1177/0269215506070771 PMID:17329279

Zarani, F., Besharat, A. M., Sadeghian, S., & Sarami, G. (2010, September). The effectiveness of the Information-Motivation-Behavioral skills model in promoting adherence in CABG patients. *Journal of Health Psychology*, *15*(6), 828–837. doi:10.1177/1359105309357092 PMID:20453057

Zelazo, P. D. (2013). *The oxford handbook of developmental psychology.* Oxford: Oxford University Press.

Zikmund, W. G. (2003). *Business research methods* (7th ed.). Mason, OH: South-Western.

Zoller, H. (2005). Health activism: Communication theory and action for social change. *Communication Theory*, *15*(4), 341–364. doi:10.1111/j.1468-2885.2005.tb00339.x

Zwicker, J. G., Grunau, R. E., Adams, E., Chau, V., Brant, R., Poskitt, K. J., & Miller, S. P. et al. (2013). Score for neonatal acute physiology-II and neonatal pain predict Corticospinal tract development in premature newborns. *Pediatric Neurology*, *48*(2), 123–129. doi:10.1016/j.pediatrneurol.2012.10.016 PMID:23337005

About the Contributors

Guendalina Graffigna received a PhD in Social Psychology at Catholic University of the Sacred Hearth of Milan (Italy) where she actually is Associate Professor. At the same University she teaches "Qualitative Methodology", she is Associate Director for the II level Master Degree in "Qualitative Methods applied to Social and Marketing Research" and she is member of the Scientific Committee for the PhD School in Psychology. Before her actual appointments, Guendalina has been a Post Doc fellow (A.A. 2007-2008) and visiting professor in Qualitative Methods (A.A. 2008-2009) at the International Institute for Qualitative Methodology, University of Alberta, with which she still collaborate for several research and teaching initiatives. Beside her academic achievements, Guendalina acts as Scientific Advisor of the Consortium for Patient Engagement (COPE) and she is Director the Study and Training Centre of ASSIRM (Italian Association of Marketing Research Institutes). In July 2012 Guendalina was awarded with the prize of Qualitative Health Research Leadership 2012 from the Global Congress for Qualitative Health Research Committee. Her research and scientific activities are mainly devoted to patient engagement in health and wellbeing, healthcare organization innovation and digital health. She has spent the last 10 years of activity in constructing a bridges between scientific/academic knowledge and professional practice, in the particularly sectors of consumer and health research. At present she is coordinating and intra and inter university reflection for contributing to priorities and policies discussions at the European Level on patient health engagement.

* * *

Emmanuel Adugu, Ph.D., is a research methodologist and lecturer at the Department of Government, Sociology and Social Work at the University of West Indies, Cave Hill Campus. His current area of research focuses on citizens using the marketplace to influence public policy with the goal of promoting sustainable development and global welfare.

Augusta Isabella Alberici is Assistant Professor in Social Psychology, at the Catholic University of Milan (Italy). After getting her Ph.D. in Political Psychology at the Catholic University of Milan, she taught Research Methods at the University of Urbino, and then Social Psychology and Political Psychology at the University of Pavia. Presently, she teaches Social Psychology and Psychology of Communication. She is a full member of the European Association of Social Psychology and the International Society of Political Psychology. Her research interests include: political psychology, political communication, mass media effects on citizens' attitudes, collective action. She recently focused her research interests on the role of online communication in fostering collective action.

Precious Arnan's academic training is in project management, evaluation and accounting. She has over six years working experience encompassing project management and evaluation, financial advisory, customer relations management and tax consultancy. She is a tutor at the Department of Management Studies, University of West Indies, Cave Hill campus.

Serena Barello is a health psychologist and received a PhD in Psychology at the Catholic University of the Sacred Hearth of Milan (Italy) where she actually teaches Qualitative Marketing Research. She is currently member of the "European Association for Communication in Healthcare" (EACH) and her main domain of inquiry includes the study of effective clinical/organizational models and the role of new technologies (ehealth) to make patients actively engaged in their health and healthcare.

Lawrence C. Becker received his PhD in philosophy from the University of Chicago in 1965. He is a Fellow of Hollins University, and is Kenan Professor of Philosophy Emeritus, College of William & Mary in Virginia. He is the author of books and articles in ethical theory, social, political, and legal philosophy, and the co-editor with Charlotte B. Becker of the multivolume Encyclopedia of Ethics (2001). His five monographs include Reciprocity (1986), A New Stoicism (1998), and Habilitation, Health, and Agency (2012). From 2001-2005, he served on the national advisory committee on medical rehabilitation research at the National Institutes of Health (US), and, from 2000-2011, he was on the Board of Directors at Post-Polio Health International and its affiliated International Ventilator Users Network, serving as their president from 2006-2009. Most recently, he has been working on ethical questions involving disability, agency, and aging with significant physical disabilities.

Anna Bertoni obtained her PhD in Social Psychology at Catholic University of the Sacred Hearth of Milan (Italy) where she actually is Associate Professor. At the same University she teaches "Methods and Techniques on Family and Community Interventions", "Groups and Community Psychology" and "Social Psychology". Furthermore, she is trainer and member of the scientific committee of a post-graduate course on family preventive intervention. She is member of the Internal Executive Committee of Catholic University Centre for Family Studies and Research at the UCSC-Milano. Her research focused primarily on the study of couple relationship, in particular stress and coping in couples, with specific attention to the role of dyadic coping for partners' wellbeing in both everyday life and acute/chronic illness. Her interests extend, moreover, to partners' interpersonal perceptions, divorce and childrens' wellbeing, preventive psychosocial interventions and their evaluation.

Lidia Borghi is scholarship holder of clinical psychology, Department of Health Sciences at the University of Milan. She holds a 5-yrs degree in Cognitive Neuroscience and a PhD in Clinical Psychology. She teaches occupational therapist students at the University of Milan and she serves as a consultant neuro-psychologist at the Clinic of infectious Disease of San Paolo Hospital. Her research experience has focused on clinical and health psychology, clinician-patient communication, and patients' illness experience. She has been trained by D. Roter in the use of the Roter Interaction Analysis System, one of the most frequently used system of analysis for physician–patient communication. She is author of national and international articles.

Livia Bruscaglioni, psychologist, PhD in Methodology of Social Science at the University of Florence, is involved in research projects for CIMESS (Centro interuniversitario di Metodologia delle Scienze Sociali), University of Florence. She has been Marie Curie fellow at the Maison Méditerranéenne des Sciences de l'Homme at the University of Aix-Marseille and post doc fellow at the Faculty of Political Science, University of Florence. Her research and scientific activities are mainly devoted to healthcare, organization analysis, qualitative research and research-intervention. She has explored methodological aspects of qualitative research, particularly of the Grounded Theory method, as bases for action research. Recent publications: Grounded Theory. La teoria, il metodo, le tecniche. Bonanno: Catania (2013), Theorizing in Grounded Theory and qualitative abduction, Quality and Quantity (2015).

Sabina Bucci graduated from the Università Cattolica del Sacro Cuore (Health Economics) in 2012. Since 2014 she has been Ph. D. student in Epidemiology and Public Health at the Università Cattolica del Sacro Cuore.

António M. Diniz has a License (Pre-Bologna's Process) in Clinical Psychology and a PhD in Educational Psychology, and is an assistant professor in the Department of Psychology, School of Social Sciences, University of Évora, Portugal, where he teaches, mainly, research methods. His research interests include quantitative and qualitative methods and data analysis applied to psychological assessment and psychosocial aspects of aging. His research work is currently undertaken at the Research Center in Education and Psychology (CIEP-UE), University of Évora.

Silvia Donato is a researcher in Social Psychology for the Faculty of Psychology at the UCSC-Milano, where she teaches "Methods and Techniques on Family and Community Interventions" and "Social Psychology". She is member of the Catholic University Centre for Family Studies and Research at the UCSC-Milano. Furthermore, she is trainer and member of the scientific committee of a post-graduate course on family preventive intervention. Her research focused primarily on the study of stress and coping in couples, with particular attention to the role of dyadic coping for partners' wellbeing in both everyday life and illness, as well as the intergenerational transmission of coping competences. Her interests extend, moreover, to partners' interpersonal perceptions, partners' support in response to positive events, scale psychometrics, preventive psychosocial interventions and their evaluation.

Roberta Falanga is a Psychologist and Doctor of Sociology. His main research interests concern participatory processes with civil society at different scale. Civic participation is understood as the set of principles and mechanisms aimed at including citizens in policy making. In the last few years, the focus of his studies has included participatory initiatives aimed at enhancing senior citizens' power of decision in matters that affect them. He is member of international research projects related with civic participation and active ageing. He is also expert advisor for national and local participatory policy programmes in Portugal.

Federica Galli is a Clinical Psychologist, PhD and Researcher at the Department of Health Sciences of the University of Milan. She graduated at "Sapienza" University of Rome, where, afterwards, she had a PhD in Neuroscience and a post-graduation in Clinical Psychology and Psychotherapy. She is assistant professor of Clinical Psychology at the University of Milan and Developmental Psychopathology at the University of Pavia. Her research area has been primarily focused on psychological components of chronic pain disorders (mainly headache) both in paediatric age and adulthood, and it is now shifting towards relational and communicative skills of the medical encounter. She is Author of many national and international papers on psychological and psychopathological components of headache and other pain disorders.

Laura Galuppo is Assistant Professor in Work and Organizational Psychology at the Faculty of Psychology, Catholic University of Milan. Her current research focuses on CSR and sustainability in organizations, organizational learning and change and ethnographic methods in organizational studies. Laura is author and co-author of several publications, including book chapters and papers in journals. She has published in journal such as Systemic Practice and Action Research, European Journal of Psychology of Education, Implementation Science, Social Science and Medicine, Journal of Management Inquiry, Social Sustainability Journal.

Rui Gaspar has a PhD in Social Psychology and is a research fellow at the William James Center for Research, ISPA-Instituto Universitário with a research focus on Social Psychology applied to health, environmental and consumer issues. His work comprises various aspects of health communication, crisis communication and social media analysis. The current research interests include: risk perception and communication in crisis (e.g. health epidemics) and non-crisis situations (e.g. food risks and benefits; water intake; etc.); psychosocial analysis of the new social media (Twitter, facebook, ...); personal and situational determinants of health recommendations adherence, in vulnerable population groups (e.g. elderly); barriers/constraints to sustainable consumption.

Mara Gorli, PhD in Social and Applied Psychology, is Assistant Professor of Organizational Psychology at the Faculty of Economics, Catholic University of Milan, Italy. Her main research interests are on the social consequences of change in organizations; practice-based approaches to the study of knowing, learning and change in organizations; organizational reflection. She mainly focuses on collaborative research and action research perspective, with specific attention to ethnographic and qualitative methods for researching in organizations. Mara is author and co-author of several publications, as book chapters and papers in journals like Human Relations, Implementation Science, Social Science and Medicine, Journal of Management Inquiry, Social Sustainability Journal, Qualitative Research in Organizations and Management, Systemic Practice and Action Research, Journal of Workplace Learning.

Elisa Giulia Liberati is a PhD candidate in Catholic University of Milan and a visiting researcher in Leicester University. During her master in Organizational Psychology, she trained in ethnographic methods and developed an interest for quality, safety and professional relationships in health care. Her PhD project analyses how professional relationships and roles in health care affects the impact of initiatives to improve quality of care within the Italian NHS. Her broader research interests comprise: organizational and technological innovation in healthcare, professional boundaries and sociology of profession, practice based studies. She is also interested in participatory methods to transform the knowledge emerged from the research in actionable knowledge that can sustain internal development in organizational contexts. She has published in journals such as Implementation Science, Social Science and Medicine, Journal of Health Organization and Management.

Livio Provenzi is a developmental psychologist and infant researcher, Psy.D. and PhD. He works at the 0-3 Center for the at-Risk Infant of the Scientific Institute IRCCS Eugenio Medea in Bosisio Parini, Lecco, Italy. His main research interests encompass preterm birth, socio-emotional stress regulation, psychobiological development, behavioral epigenetics.

Nicola Magnavita, Aggregate Professor (Senior researcher) in Occupational Medicine in the Università Cattolica del Sacro Cuore of Rome, M.D. in the hospital ward of Occupational Medicine in the Agostino Gemelli Hospital of Rome (Italy), he is currently working in the Public Health Department of the same hospital. He has published more than 580 scientific papers and books, has directed 23 research projects, and has so far played >209 courses of teaching in the University.

Francesca Mariani is a lawyer. In 2013 she graduated in clinical psychology at the University of Milan Bicocca in Milan, in 2014 successfully passed the qualification test for being a professional psychologist and in 2015 she received the title of family mediator. Finally enrolled at the school of specialization in psychotherapy at the Milan Centre for Family Therapy.

Davide Mazzoni obtained his PhD in Social Psychology at the University of Bologna, with a dissertation on the role of moral conviction and perceived injustice in collective action processes. In the last years, he took part in multinational research projects funded by the European Commission, like PIDOP (Processes Influencing Democratic Ownership and Participation) and CATCH-EyoU (Constructing AcTive CitizensHip with European Youth: Policies, Practices, Challenges and Solutions). He is currently researcher at the University of Bologna. His activities are mainly located in the field of social and community psychology. His research interests include the processes of civic and political engagement. He is also interested in health psychology, with a specific focus on well-being of individuals living with a chronic disease.

Massimo Miglioretti is assistant professor of work and organizational psychology at the Psychology Department of the University of Milano-Bicocca. Health psychologist. After a period spent as head of Psychological Unit of Cardiovascular Rehabilitation Clinic, in 2006 he started his academic career at the University of Milano-Bicocca, where he still works. In the recent years his main research interests have been: quality and development of health care systems, well-being at work, focusing on return to work after illness and Work-health Balance.

Rosario Montirosso is a developmental psychologist and infant researcher. He is the director of the 0-3 Center for the Study of Social-Emotional Development of the at-Risk Infant of the Scientific Institute IRCCS Eugenio Medea in Bosisio Parini, Lecco, Italy. His main research interests encompass preterm birth, socio-emotional stress regulation, psychobiological development, mirror neurons, and behavioral epigenetics.

Giuseppe Scaratti is Professor of Work and Organizational Psychology at the Faculty of Economics, Catholic University of Milan, Italy. His research interests include the study of knowing, learning and change in organizations; reflexivity in organizations; qualitative methodologies for the study of organizational life; evaluation and assessment of complex and transformative actions. He has published numerous articles and chapters, published in Management Learning, Qualitative Inquiry, Social Responsibility Journal, Journal of Workplace Learning, Qualitative Research in Organizations and Management. He is also a founding member of the Digital KBC -Knowledge Boundaries Crossing and of the Center of interdisciplinary researches for transformative actions.

Maria Tanzariello graduated from Università Cattolica del Sacro Cuore (Health Economics) in 2011. Since 2013 she has been Ph. D. student in Economics and Management in Public Health.

Luca Vecchio is Professor of work and organizational psychology at the Psychology Department of the University of Milano-Bicocca. He received his PhD in Cognitive Psychology at the University of Pavia in 1992. After a period spent at the marketing company Eurisko s.p.a (now GfK-Eurisko srl) as a researcher in the Health Department, in 2001 he started his academic career at the University of Milano-Bicocca, where he still works. In the recent years his main research interests have been: well-being at work, focusing on people working in healthcare organizations, and sustainability in organizations, with particular attention to environmental sustainability and its promotion.

Elena Vegni is Associate Professor of clinical psychology, Department of Health Sciences at the University of Milan. She holds a 4-yrs degree in Philosophy, a 5-yrs degree in Psychology and a training in Psychotherapy. She teaches medical students at the University of Milan and she also serves as a clinical psychologist at San Paolo Hospital with a special interest on group counseling for patients affected by physical illnesses. Her academic work has focused on clinician-patient communication, patient education and patients' illness experience. She is an expert of interaction analysis processes, in particular she has been trained by D. Roter in the use of the Roter Interaction Analysis System. She has experience also in qualitative research, in particular on the principles of Interpretative Phenomenological Analysis. She is author of several national and international articles and co-authored a book titled "The patient centred clinical consultation", published by Cortina, Milan, Italy.

Index

K

L

M

N

O

P

Q

R

S

T

W

www.ingramcontent.com/pod-product-compliance
Lightning Source LLC
LaVergne TN
LVHW081251011026
849162LV00006BA/1406